Imaging of

Bone Tumors

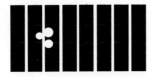

Imaging of

Bone Tumors

A Multimodality Approach

EDITOR

George B. Greenfield, M.D.
Professor of Radiology
University of South Florida
Attending Radiologist
H. Lee Moffitt Cancer Center
    and Research Institute
Consultant Radiologist
Shriner's Hospital for Crippled
    Children
Tampa, Florida

CO-EDITOR

John A. Arrington, M.D.
Associate Professor of Radiology
University of South Florida
Attending Radiologist
H. Lee Moffitt Cancer Center
    and Research Institute
Consultant Radiologist
Shriner's Hospital for Crippled
    Children
Tampa, Florida

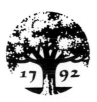

J. B. LIPPINCOTT COMPANY
Philadelphia

Acquisitions Editor: James Ryan
Sponsoring Editor: Kimberley J. Cox
Project Editor: Molly E. Dickmeyer
Indexer: Julia Figures
Designer: Doug Smock
Production Manager: Caren Erlichman
Production Coordinator: Wendell Love
                        David Yurkovich
Compositor: Compset, Inc.
Printer/Binder: Quebecor/Kingsport
Color Insert Printer: Walsworth Publishing Company

6 5 4 3 2 1

Library of Congress Cataloging-in-Publications Data

Imaging of bone tumors : a multimodality approach / editor, George B.
  Greenfield ; co-editor, John A. Arrington.
     p.   cm.
    Includes bibliographical references and index.
    ISBN 0-397-51274-0
    1. Bones—Tumors—Imaging.   I. Greenfield, George B., 1928–
II. Arrington, John A.
    [DNLM: 1. Bone Neoplasms—diagnosis. 2. Bone Neoplasms—therapy.
3. Diagnostic Imaging—methods.   WE 258 I31 1995]
RC280.B6I43 1995
616.99′2710754—dc20
DNLM/DLC
for Library of Congress   94-11143
                                           CIP

The authors and publisher have exerted every effort to ensure that drug selection
and dosage set forth in this text are in accord with current recommendations and
practice at the time of publication. However, in view of ongoing research, changes
in government regulations, and the constant flow of information relating to drug
therapy and drug reactions, the reader is urged to check the pacakage insert for
each drug for any change in indications and dosage and for added warnings and pre-
cautions. This is particularly important when the recommended agent is a new or
infrequently employed drug.

Many of the images in this book have been previously published in *Radiology
of Bone Diseases, fifth edition,* by George B. Greenfield, published by J. B.
Lippincott Company, Philadelphia, 1990.

To Our Families

CONTRIBUTORS

John A. Arrington, M.D.
Assistant Professor of Radiology
University of South Florida
Attending Radiologist
H. Lee Moffitt Cancer Center and Research Institute
Consultant Radiologist
Shriner's Hospital for Crippled Children
Tampa, Florida

Jaime Estrada, M.D.
Clinical Associate Professor of Pediatrics
University of Texas Health Science Center
    at San Antonio
San Antonio, Texas

Stephanie D. Holman Ferris, M.D.
Assistant Professor
University of South Florida
Department of Radiology
Chief of Interventional Radiology
H. Lee Moffitt Cancer Center and Research Institute
Tampa, Florida

Harvey M. Greenberg, M.D.
Associate Professor and Director
Division of Radiation Oncology
University of South Florida
Director of Radiation Oncology
H. Lee Moffitt Cancer Center and Research Institute
Tampa, Florida

George B. Greenfield, M.D.
Professor of Radiology
University of South Florida
Attending Radiologist
H. Lee Moffitt Cancer Center and Research Institute
Consultant Radiologist
Shriner's Hospital for Crippled Children
Tampa, Florida

George Douglas Letson, M.D.
Assistant Professor of Surgery
University of South Florida
Musculoskeletal Tumor Surgery
H. Lee Moffitt Cancer Center and Research Institute
Tampa, Florida

Kenneth R. Schroer, M.D.
Associate Professor of Pathology
University of South Florida
Chief, Surgical Pathology
H. Lee Moffitt Cancer Center and Research Institute
Tampa, Florida

Martin L. Silbiger, M.D., M.B.A.
Professor and Chairman
University of South Florida College of Medicine
Department of Radiology
Staff
H. Lee Moffitt Cancer Center and Research Institute
Tampa, Florida

Arthur K. Walling, M.D.
Clinical Associate Professor of Orthopaedics
University of South Florida
Program Director
Tampa Orthopaedic Program
Tampa General Hospital
Tampa, Florida

PREFACE

A new era of imaging has evolved that is yet to be fully explored. Bone tumor pathology has been sharply refined, allowing more precise definition of the various entities. Surgical techniques have greatly improved, permitting the sparing of functional limbs that previously would have been amputated. Survival rates have increased. The imaging of musculoskeletal tumors is of central importance in their diagnosis and treatment. This book addresses these issues.

The parameters of interpretation of each modality and the practical issues in magnetic resonance imaging of musculoskeletal lesions are presented. Recent concepts in pathology are given and illustrated with color plates and electron micrographs. The multimodality imaging appearances of malignant and benign tumors of bone and soft tissue, as well as metastases and entities that enter into the differential diagnosis, are discussed and illustrated. This integrated approach allows direct comparison of the utility of each of the various modalities for each major disease entity and provides a foundation for the reader to choose for himself or herself the most appropriate modality to investigate the problem at hand. It will also provide a basis for identification of an incidental focal bone or soft-tissue lesion found on MRI. Finally, a brief clinical perspective, along with the treatment options for osteosarcoma and radiotherapy of soft tissue sarcoma, is presented.

George B. Greenfield, M.D.
John A. Arrington, M.D.

ACKNOWLEDGMENT

We would like to thank Don Pillai for his excellent photography.

CONTENTS

     The color plates fall between pages 14 and 15.

Imaging of

Bone Tumors

Imaging of Bone Tumors: A Multimodality Approach,
edited by George B. Greenfield and John A. Arrington,
J. B. Lippincott Company, Philadelphia © 1995.

chapter

ONE

Methodology and Pathology of Bone Tumors

The challenges of musculoskeletal tumor imaging in this multimodality era are formidable. An organ system concept must be supplemented with a thorough knowledge of the high-tech systems available, and the nuances of conventional radiology must be appreciated. An understanding of the basic pathology and clinical picture that define each clinicopathologic entity is essential. Equal with an understanding of the clinical problem is the ability to work with the referring physician or surgeon in precise evaluation, treatment planning, and follow-up. The indications for each type of examination must be understood, and the modalities should be carefully chosen.

Effective image interpretation requires an organized approach to the analysis of the lesion, the involved bone, and the adjacent structures. The essentials of analysis hold true regardless of the imaging modality used. Table 1-1 outlines a systematic approach to evaluating the imaging parameters or lesion characteristics. The parameters can be divided into three categories, depending on whether they involve the analysis of the lesion, the involved bone, or the adjacent structures. The effectiveness of the various imaging modalities is quantified in Table 1-1.

The imaging pattern should be analyzed objectively with respect to the distinct features presented by each modality employed. On the basis of this analysis, a list of differential diagnoses can be prepared and applied to the case in question. The age and sex of the patient are important in establishing the probabilities for many tumors, as are the clinical and biochemical findings. This effectively reduces the list to a few possibilities. An optimal biopsy site, if indicated, may then be determined using the most suitable imaging modality, and adequate, representative biopsy material is delivered to the pathologist.

The conclusion of the objective analysis should be correlated with the clinical and laboratory findings. Care should be taken not to read features into the images that are not there, because they may be expected in a tentative clinical diagnosis.

A definitive diagnosis of some asymptomatic, benign entities, such as benign cortical defect, osteochondroma, or nonossifying fibroma, may be made on radiologic grounds. Malignant tumors and atypical lesions require a biopsy. Some lesions require only periodic follow-up examinations.

The bone marrow is of special interest because of the unique ability of magnetic resonance imaging (MRI) to define changes. Types of marrow include red or blood-forming marrow, yellow or fatty marrow, fibrous marrow, and mixed marrow. In the infant, all marrow spaces are filled with red marrow. In the adult, red marrow is normally found in the bones of the trunk and proximal metaphyseal segments of the long bones. Marrow ischemia can hasten the conversion of red to yellow marrow. Reconversion of yellow to red marrow occurs in certain disease states.

IMAGING FEATURES OF BONE TUMORS AND TUMOR-LIKE LESIONS

The decision-making process in establishing an imaging diagnosis should be based on the objective analysis of the features of each modality used, and it should conform to established criteria. In many instances, we may not be able to make a specific diagnosis but are able to determine the aggressiveness of the lesion. Understanding the bases of the features seen on diagnostic images elucidates their significance in determining the causal lesion. The parameters employed in evaluating a musculoskeletal tumor are described in this section.

Loss of bone density may occur as a result of the general metabolic diseases of osteoporosis, osteomalacia, and hyperparathyroidism or because of bone infiltration. Localized osteoporosis produces aggressive, painful lesions. Conventional radiographs display a qualitative picture of local osteoporosis, with a periarticular pattern generated for aggressive lesions. Computed tomography (CT) allows quantitative measurements of bone density, as does dual photon absorbtiometry. MRI is limited in this respect, although it can show cortical infiltration and permeation.

Alteration of bone texture manifested by a coarsened trabecular pattern is caused by resorption or destruction of bone trabeculae, allowing the remaining trabeculae to be more conspicuous. Apposition of the

TABLE 1-1.
Effectiveness of Imaging Modalities

Site Analyzed	Radiograph	CT	MRI	Scintigram
LESION				
Origin and location	+ + +	+ +	+ + + +	+ +
Extension	+ +	+ +	+ + + +	+
Size and shape	+ + +	+ + +	+ + +	
Margination	+ + +	+ + + +	+ +	
Bone destruction	+ +	+ + + +		
Bone production	+ + +	+ + + +	+	
Calcification	+ + +	+ + + +	+	
Vascularity		+ +	+ + + +	+ +
Tissue characterization	+ +	+ +	+ + + +	
INVOLVED BONE				
Cortex and periosteum	+ + +	+ + + +	+ +	
Size and shape of bone	+ + + +	+	+ + +	
Expansion of bone	+ + +	+ + + +	+ +	
Trabeculation	+ +	+ + + +		
Density	+ +	+ + + +		
Pathologic fracture	+ + +	+ + + +	+ +	
ADJACENT STRUCTURES				
Marrow	+	+	+ + + +	
Joint space		+	+ + + +	
Soft tissues		+ +	+ + + +	
Edema patterns		+ +	+ + + +	

Pluses indicate degree of effectiveness on a scale of + to + + + + .

remaining trabeculae causes true thickening of the bone. These changes commonly appear in infiltrative disease of the marrow cavity and in conditions having increased bone marrow activity. This finding can be the clue to underlying disease in evaluating a solitary lesion. Bone texture can best be assessed on conventional radiographs, and the bone marrow is best assessed with MRI. MRI is particularly sensitive to changes within the medullary cavity, showing generalized or focal disease. CT scans can show changes in attenuation of the medullary cavity.

The *cortex* is composed of cancellous bone. The internal architecture, the haversian system, is continuously remodeled. Cortical destruction can be caused by malignant and benign processes. Some well-developed malignant processes sweep away the entire involved segment of cortex. Some benign processes, such as osteomyelitis, destroy areas segmentally with draining sinuses, leaving intact cortex between the areas. An exception is Ewing sarcoma, which usually permeates the cortex. Permeative cortical destruction may be evident on CT scans as tiny, low-density foci within the cortex (Fig. 1-1) or as an intact cortex with

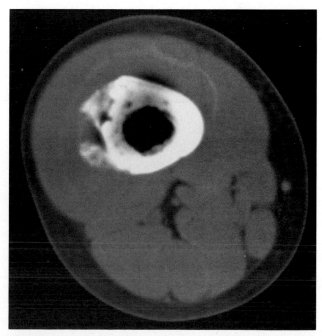

FIGURE 1-1. In the CT scan of a Ewing tumor, low-density foci of permeative destruction are seen in the cortex.

a surrounding soft-tissue mass. MRI shows the intact cortex as a signal void on all pulse sequences (Fig. 1-2). A permeated cortex may show tiny, high-signal foci within it on T2-weighted or proton density (PD) MR images (see Magnetic Resonance Imaging). Cortical thickening characterizes some processes, such as Paget disease.

The *endosteum* is the membrane that covers the trabeculae and the inner margin of the cortex. Its single layer has osteoblastic and osteoclastic properties. Endosteal scalloping of the inner margin of the cortex characterizes some disease processes. Chondrosarcoma and multiple myeloma are malignant tumors that characteristically cause foci of endosteal destruction. The

endosteum is active in expanding lesions. An interrupted endosteal line may be an indicator of a subtle lesion. This may be appreciated on conventional films, CT scans, and MR images.

The *periosteum* is the membrane surrounding bone. It comprises the outer or fibrous layer and the inner or cambium layer. The cambium layer has osteoblastic and osteoclastic properties. Edema, hemorrhage, pus, or tumor cells can lift the periosteum from the shaft, after which reactive periosteal new bone formation takes place. The basic patterns of periosteal reaction are simple or solid (Fig. 1-3), laminated (Fig. 1-4), and spiculated (Figs. 1-5 and 1-6). Long, thin, filiform spicules are seen in malignant processes, and

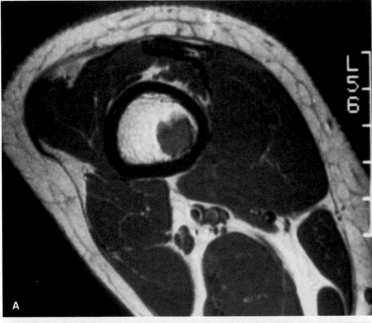

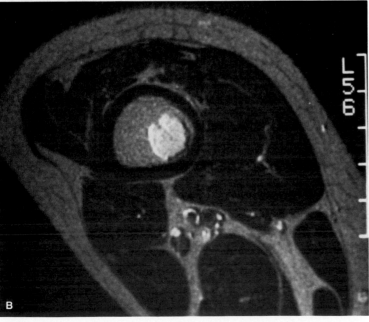

FIGURE 1-2. Intact cortex. (**A,B**) Axial MR images (for **A**, repetition time msec/echo time msec = SE 1500/25; **B**, SE 1500/75) show the cortex as a solid black ring, regardless of the pulse sequence or plane of imaging. Diagnosis: intramedullary metastasis from breast carcinoma. (From Greenfield GB, Warren DL, Clark RA: MR imaging of periosteal and cortical changes of bone. Radiographics 11(4):611–624, 1991)

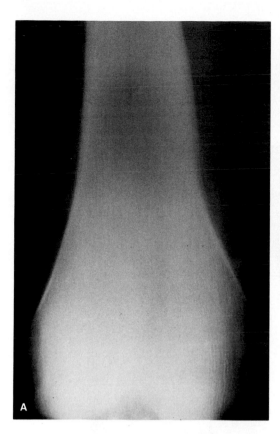

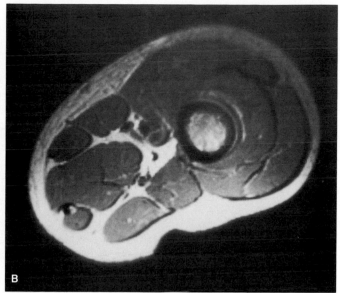

FIGURE 1-3. Simple periosteal elevation. (**A**) Plain radiograph of the distal left femur shows medial and lateral simple periosteal elevations. (**B**) Axial MR image (SE 2700/20) shows an intact cortical black ring and a thin black line representing elevated periosteum. White stripes of edema and tumor are on both sides of the periosteal black line. Diagnosis: osteosarcoma. (From Greenfield GB, Warren DL, Clark RA: MR imaging of periosteal and cortical changes of bone. Radiographics 11(4):611–624, 1991)

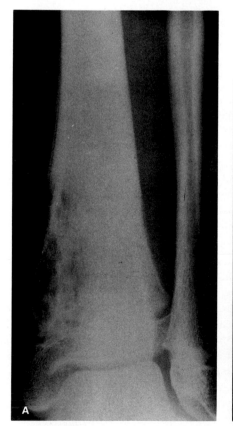

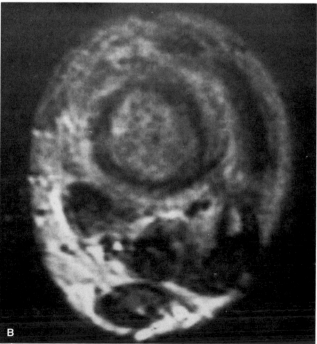

FIGURE 1-4. Laminated periosteum. (**A**) Plain radiograph of the left distal tibia shows laminated periosteum superior to the gross bone destruction by tumor. (**B**) Axial MR image (SE 2700/80) demonstrates concentric black periosteal lines representing laminated periosteum. Area of high signal intensity may represent tumor or edema. Diagnosis: Ewing sarcoma. (From Greenfield GB, Warren DL, Clark RA: MR imaging of periosteal and cortical changes of bone. Radiographics 11(4):611–624, 1991)

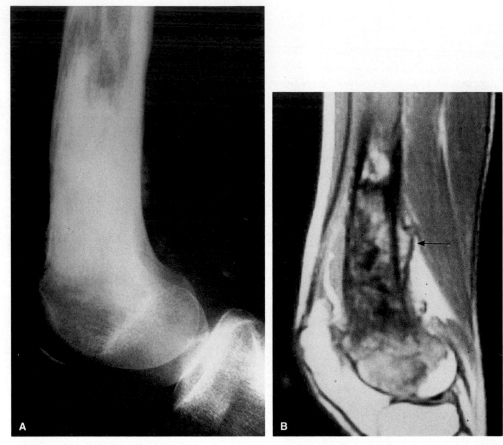

FIGURE 1-5. Spiculated periosteal reaction. (**A**) A plain film of the right femur shows a sclerotic reaction in the distal femur with anterior and posterior spiculated periosteal reactions. (**B**) A sagittal MR image (SE 800/20) demonstrates extensive marrow infiltration by a tumor, anterior disruption of the black cortical stripe, and posterior elevation of a thin, periosteal line. There are additional black periosteal lines, representing spiculated periosteum, posteriorly between and perpendicular to the cortex and elevated periosteum (*arrow*). Diagnosis: osteosarcoma.

short, thick spicules may be seen in some benign processes (Fig. 1-7). A periosteal cuff called the Codman triangle may be seen (Fig. 1-8). This can be caused by malignant or aggressive benign processes. All of these changes can be well seen on MR images.

Changes in bone size and shape can be localized or part of a generalized process. Any lesion that interferes with enchondral bone formation can result in a shortened bone. Lengthening of bone can be the result of localized causes or generalized disease, such as giantism. Vascular malformations or soft-tissue tumors such as hemangiomas, lipomas, or neurofibromas may cause lengthening of a bone during the growth period. Underconstriction or undertubulation of bone results from a failure of normal modeling processes. The normal proportion between diaphyseal and metaphyseal diameter is altered, resulting in a rectangular bone or an "Erlenmeyer flask" deformity. The latter may be caused by a local lesion that interferes with metaphyseal remodeling of bone. Changes in contour or defor-

mities of bone may be a significant diagnostic finding, as in exostoses.

Expansion of bone is caused by endosteal resorption and periosteal apposition in a localized area. The rate of enlargement of the lesion must be slower than the ability of the periosteum to form new bone, or destruction would result. This feature indicates a slow rate of growth. Certain lesions are characterized by an expansile, lightly trabeculated appearance without a periosteal reaction. These include giant cell tumor, brown tumor or cyst of hyperparathyroidism, nonossifying fibroma, unicameral bone cyst, and aneurysmal bone cyst (Fig. 1-9). If a lesion of this type is seen, determinations of serum calcium, phosphorus, and alkaline phosphatase should be done to rule out hyperparathyroidism. After tumor therapy, the lesion forms a limiting shell, which may calcify, resulting in an expansile appearance (Fig. 1-10).

Destruction of bone can be caused by osteoclastic activity stimulated by the lesion. An osteoclastic front

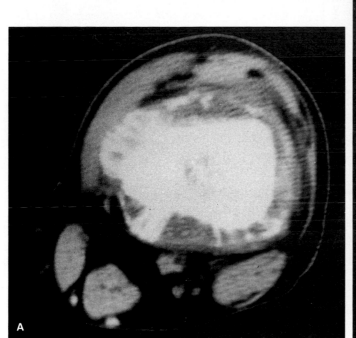
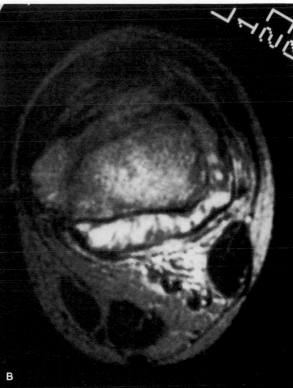

FIGURE 1-6.   Spiculated periosteal reaction. (**A**) Axial CT section through the left femur. (**B**) Axial MR image (SE 2700/80). The CT and MR images demonstrate tumor surrounding the femur. The spiculated periosteum is seen as radially oriented white lines on the CT scan and black lines on the MR image. On the MR image, the high-signal tumor surrounds the spiculated periosteum. Diagnosis: osteosarcoma.

FIGURE 1-7. Thyroid acropachy involving the hands. Spiculated periosteal new bone has formed bilaterally and symmetrically. The first and second rays show the most pronounced changes at the radial side, and the fifth ray shows most pronounced changes at the ulnar side. Soft tissue masses are associated with the periosteal new bone formation. The spicules are short and squat, characteristic of a benign spiculative process. (From Greenfield GB, Escamilla CH, Schorsch HA: The hand as an indicator of generalized disease. AJR Am J Roentgenol 99:736–745, 1967)

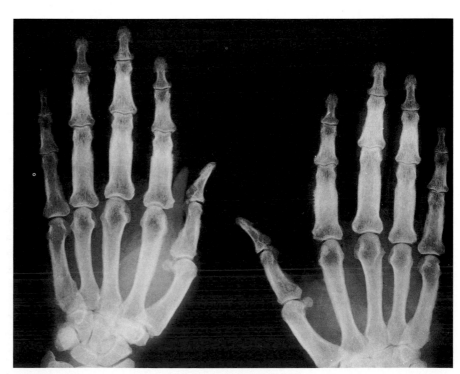

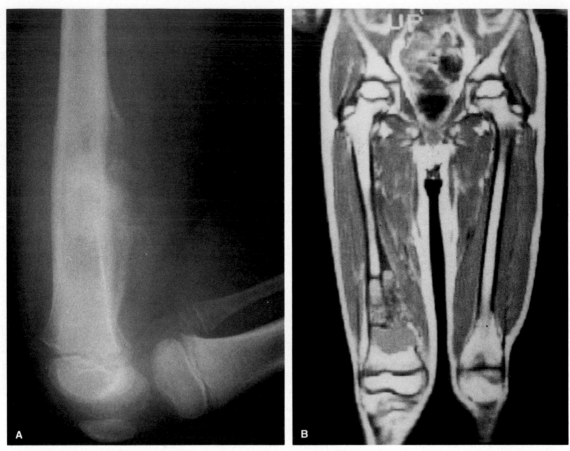

FIGURE 1-8. (A) The lateral plain film of the distal right femur demonstrates posterior Codman triangles superiorly and inferiorly, showing destruction of the elevated periosteum in the mid-portion of the lesion. (B) Coronal MR image (SE 800/20) shows a Codman triangle superior and medial to the tumor as a black triangular region. The triangle is black because of periosteal new bone formation. Diagnosis: osteosarcoma.

precedes the tumor cells, and bone lysis involves a wider area histologically than the tumor cells. This may be reflected in radionuclide scans. Tumor cells also directly cause trabecular destruction, and osteoclasts may be difficult to find in these microscopic fields. Approximately 30% to 50% of cancellous bone must be destroyed before changes are evident on conventional films, but the exact figure depends on the margination of the lesion and the radiographic technique. Scintigraphy, CT, or MR images show early bone lesions when conventional films are negative. MRI is the most sensitive modality.

Three patterns of bone destruction that result from the degree of aggressiveness of the lesion can be differentiated: geographic, moth-eaten, and permeative.[1] Geographic lesions comprise one or several well-defined holes (Fig. 1-11). Moth-eaten lesions are multiple, moderate-sized holes, which may coalesce. The permeative pattern of destruction is composed of many tiny holes in cortical bone that become fewer in num-

ber away from the center of the lesion, causing a lack of definition. On CT scans, this may be evident as a soft-tissue mass surrounding an intact cortex. On MR images, the cortex may show tiny foci of high signal intensity on T2-weighted or PD-weighted images (Fig. 1-12).

A radionuclide bone scan may not show increased uptake in some cases of myeloma or highly anaplastic tumors.

Resorption of bone is loss of bone substance at the bone ends, as in neurotrophic changes, or subperiosteally, which is the hallmark of hyperparathyroidism. The most common areas of bone resorption are the terminal tufts of the fingers and toes and the distal clavicles. Neurotrophic disease may cause a pencil- or candlestick-like resorptive deformity.

Erosion of bone is evidenced by a smooth marginal or saucer-like cortical defect. It indicates the pressure effects of a process external to the bone, such as an aneurysm (Fig. 1-13) or lymph node. It is the hallmark

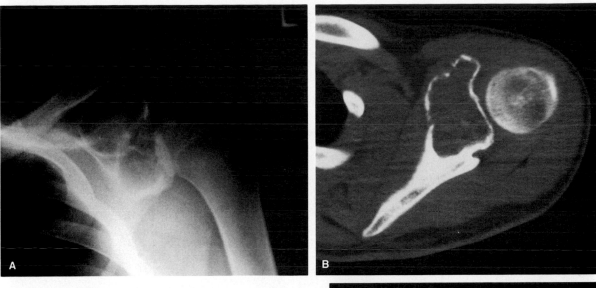

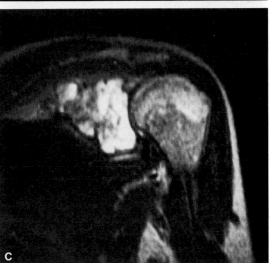

FIGURE 1-9. Expansion. (**A**) A plain film of the left shoulder shows expansion of the glenoid with thinning of the cortex and small cortical discontinuities superiorly. (**B**) An axial CT scan similarly shows expansion of the glenoid, thinning of the white cortical stripe, and small disruptions of the medial and anterior cortex. (**C**) A coronal oblique MR image (SE 500/20) demonstrates the expanded glenoid and an intact but thinned black cortical stripe with superior cortical disruptions. The image also shows blood pools within the expansile lesion (*bright signal* on T1-weighted image). Diagnosis: aneurysmal bone cyst.

of the erosive arthritides (Fig. 1-14). It must be differentiated from neoplastic invasion of bone, which has a more irregular margin. This finding may be difficult to see on MR images. If the marrow is shown to be involved, the process is invasive.

Sequestration refers to segments of the cortex that are deprived of their blood supply and become necrotic. They are detached and usually dense, and they usually occur in bacterial and tuberculous osteomyelitis. The size may range from a tiny piece to the entire cortex. The long bones are most often involved, although a sequestrum may be seen in almost any bone (Fig. 1-15). Other conditions may also be associated with sequestra, including fibrosarcoma, malignant fibrous histiocytoma, eosinophilic granuloma, desmoplastic fibroma, and lymphoma.

Bone production or sclerosis may result from malignant or benign conditions. Ossification in the tumor matrix appears as dense or patchy structureless formations. This appearance can usually be differentiated from calcifications in the cartilaginous matrix. A local lesion or a generalized process may cause osteoblasts to form new bone. This reactive bone sclerosis must be differentiated from neoplastic new bone formation, which can be caused by osteogenic tumors. Heterotopic new bone formation by metaplasia may occur in the soft tissues. Medullary bone sclerosis is reflected as a signal void in T1-weighted and T2-weighted MR images.

Calcification may be differentiated from ossification by its lack of organization. Calcification may be intraosseous or extraosseous. Calcification caused by a disturbance of calcium metabolism is called metastatic calcification. If it occurs in devitalized tissues, it is called dystrophic. Within bone, calcification is most

(*text continues on page 13*)

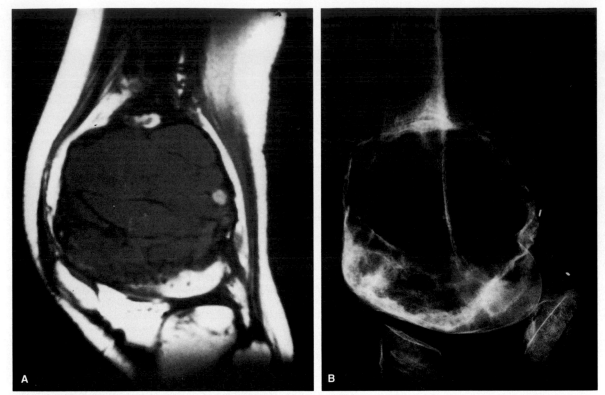

FIGURE 1-10. Expansion. (**A**) Sagittal MR image of the knee (SE 600/20) and (**B**) lateral radiograph of the amputation specimen. The MR image of the knee was performed before surgery after three courses of intraarterial chemotherapy for this osteosarcoma. The radiograph of the amputation specimen shows the expanded cortex as a thin, undulating but intact white stripe. The MR image shows the expanded cortex as a thinned, black stripe, and a small area of hemorrhagic necrosis (*focal bright signal*) is present posteriorly within the tumor mass. Diagnosis: treated osteosarcoma.

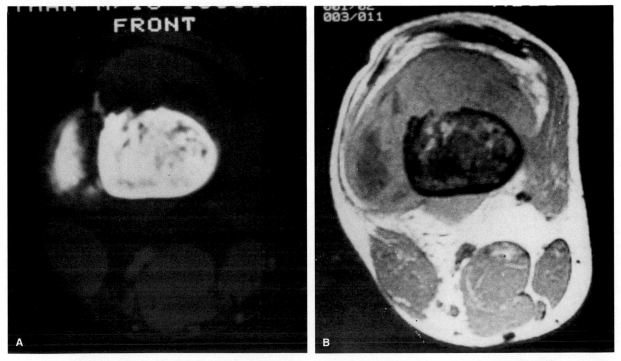

FIGURE 1-11. Geographic cortical destruction. (**A**) An axial CT cross section through the right femur shows a tumor mass, lateral tumoral bone production (*white area*), and anterior geographic cortical destruction. (**B**) An axial MR image (SE 600/20) demonstrates a tumor mass, lateral tumoral bone production (*black area*), and anterior geographic destruction of the black cortical stripe. Diagnosis: osteosarcoma.

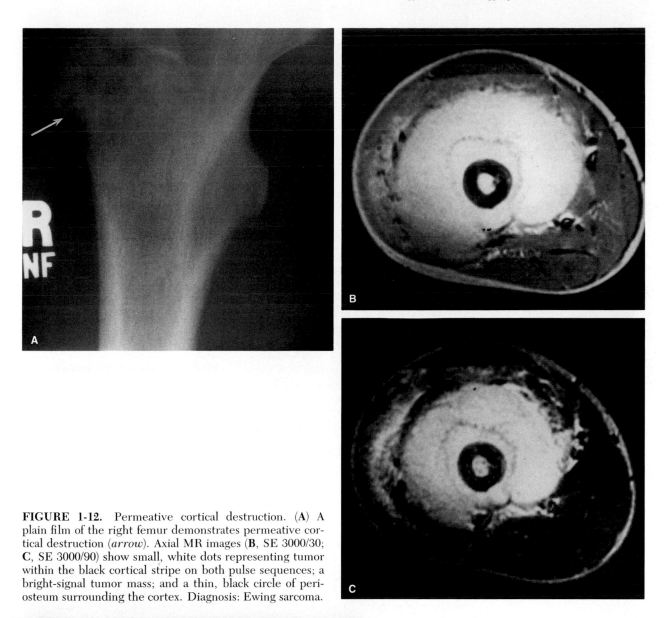

FIGURE 1-12. Permeative cortical destruction. (**A**) A plain film of the right femur demonstrates permeative cortical destruction (*arrow*). Axial MR images (**B**, SE 3000/30; **C**, SE 3000/90) show small, white dots representing tumor within the black cortical stripe on both pulse sequences; a bright-signal tumor mass; and a thin, black circle of periosteum surrounding the cortex. Diagnosis: Ewing sarcoma.

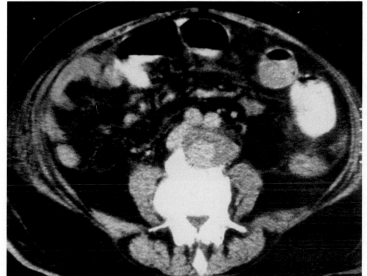

FIGURE 1-13. A leaking abdominal aortic aneurism erodes the anterior aspect of the vertebral body.

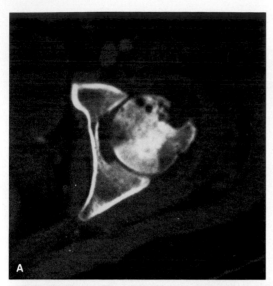

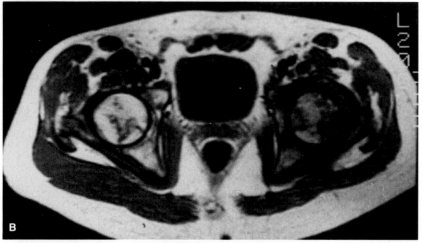

FIGURE 1-14. (**A**) An axial CT scan of the left hip demonstrates sharply marginated erosive defects in the cortex that disrupt the white cortical stripe. (**B**) An axial MR image (SE 600/20) shows erosive disruption of the black cortical stripe and better demonstrates the surrounding low-signal synovial process causing the erosions. Contralateral erosions occur in the right femoral head. Diagnosis: juvenile rheumatoid arthritis.

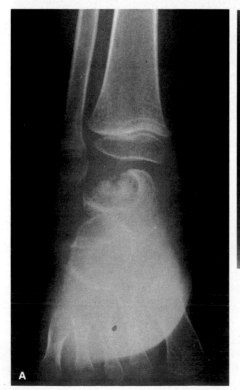

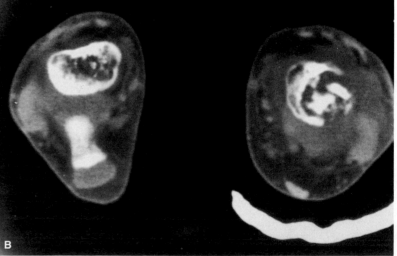

FIGURE 1-15. A 3-year-old girl with tuberculous osteomyelitis involving the talus. (**A**) An anteroposterior view of the left ankle shows a destructive area of the talar dome with a sharp sclerotic margin. Sequestered bone is seen centrally. (**B**) A CT scan shows destruction and sequestration of the talus and surrounding soft-tissue thickening.

likely to be seen in cartilaginous tumors and infarcts. Calcification in cartilage tissue appears as amorphous, stippled, linear, or ring-like. A hemangioma in soft tissues may be identified by calcified phleboliths. MR images can show dense calcification extremely well (Fig. 1-16). The greatest disadvantage of current MR techniques is that the amount and pattern of fainter calcifications cannot be accurately determined.

The *origin of the solitary lesion* is a fundamental parameter of diagnosis.[1] There are anatomic and histologic causes for the predilection for certain sites by many lesions. Bone tumors most often occur at the site and time of greatest activity of their homologous normal cells.[2] This is at the most active metaphyses, which are at the knees and proximal humeri, during the adolescent growth spurt. Tumors originating in supportive or marrow cells may occur anywhere along the bone. Hematogenous osteomyelitis has a predilection for the metaphyses because of the vascular anatomic structure.

The *location of the lesion* indicates the current disease state. For example, a giant cell tumor is thought to originate in the metaphysis, but if the cartilage plate has closed, the tumor extends to the articular surface and is located at the bone end. If the tumor occurs before epiphyseal fusion, it does not appear at the bone end but remains at its site of origin. The central or eccentric location of a lesion is also a consideration. The location with respect to epiphysis, metaphysis, or diaphysis is most important.

Invasion is another critical consideration. A bone lesion of medullary or cortical origin invading soft tissue causes cortical destruction, but one of periosteal origin may not. Soft-tissue tumors can also invade bone, with a characteristic saucerized appearance. The determination of invasion or encasement of vessels and nerves is fundamental in soft-tissue tumor staging. MRI is well suited for this evaluation.

The *size of the lesion* is important. Primary malignant bone tumors are not small when first seen, and a bone tumor size of more than 6 cm is considered by some to be a sign of malignancy. A soft-tissue tumor size of 5 cm is the dividing line between the A and B subclassifications of the American Joint Committee Task Force on Soft Tissue Sarcomas. The *shape of the lesion* is an indication of its rate of progress. A rapidly growing lesion expands uniformly and has a circular shape. A unicameral bone cyst is a good example of an elongated lesion.

Margination and the *zone of transition* between tumor and normal bone are reflections of the aggressiveness of the lesion, the rate of growth of the lesion, and the stimulation of osteoblasts. A sharply marginated lesion usually grows more slowly than a nonmarginated lesion. Faster growth results in aggressive de-

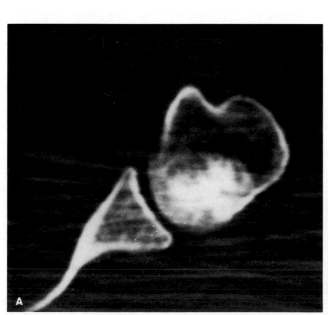
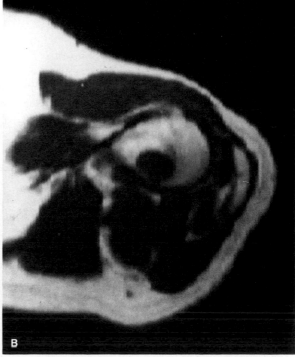

FIGURE 1-16.   Dense calcification. (**A**) An axial CT scan of the left shoulder shows dense, intraosseous calcification in the humeral head due to treated metastasis. (**B**) In the sagittal MR image (SE 500/20), the density of the calcifications is sufficient to mimic the MR appearance of cancellous bone, producing a black area of signal void in the humeral head. Diagnosis: treated prostate cancer metastasis.

structive patterns and a wide zone of transition. Some aggressive tumors, such as myeloma, show a sharp, nonsclerotic margin with an abrupt zone of transition described as a "punched-out" appearance. A thin, osteosclerotic margin is usually seen in benign tumors. Sclerosis may be seen with sharply or poorly marginated lesions. MRI can accurately depict the margin of a lesion that replaces bone marrow. Care must be taken not to mistake chemical shift artifact for a thick sclerotic marginal zone. The latter completely surrounds the tumor, but the artifact is only on one side. This is a displacement artifact between boundaries of fat and water-containing tissue that occurs in the frequency-encoding direction. It is caused by the difference in resonance frequencies between hydrogen attached to oxygen in water and hydrogen bonded to carbon in fat.

Trabeculation usually is a result of uneven cortical expansion and erosion that results in ridges in the lesion wall. The various apparent chambers usually communicate with each other. Lesions may be typically lightly trabeculated, as in a giant cell tumor. Some lesions may be truly compartmented. Bony trabeculae may be difficult to see on MR images (see Fig. 3-56), but if compartmented blood pools exist, the appearance is characteristic, as in an aneurysmal bone cyst, for example. Any tumor with focal hemorrhages or blood pools may show fluid-fluid levels.[2a] A fibrous lesion may be differentiated from a cellular or cystic lesion by T2-weighted signal intensities, which are low in the former and high in the latter.

A *fracture* may be traumatic or pathologic. If a fracture line is completely transverse, the underlying bone should be suspected of being abnormal. Callus formation, particularly in march fractures, is not to be confused with bone tumor. MRI shows subtle or trabecular fractures earlier than plain films because of marrow changes caused by edema and hemorrhage. An acute fracture of a vertebral body secondary to osteoporosis in a patient with a known primary malignancy is difficult to differentiate from metastatic collapse. On MR images, the pattern of marrow edema may be be similar in the two. A "stepladder" pattern of marrow edema with high signal intensity on T2-weighted images indicates acute vertebral body fractures.

The *soft tissues* may be the site of origin of primary benign or malignant tumors, but there can be invasion of soft tissue from bone tumors. Soft-tissue edema, calcifications, ossifications, emphysema, and atrophy may occur. MRI is particularly useful for tissue characterization and treatment planning. Determination of invasion or encasement of major vessels and nerves by soft-tissue tumors is important and best achieved by MRI.

Vascularity and vascular patterns are important for diagnosis, for localization of a suitable biopsy site, and for determination of the extent of a lesion. The vascular pattern of a bone tumor is crucial in the follow-up evaluation of the efficacy of chemotherapy. The procedures used include arteriography, arterial digital subtraction angiography, infusion CT, and MRI with or without MR angiography (MRA).

The *bone marrow* can be evaluated only with MRI. The marrow can show diffuse or focal changes on MR images, and these changes can be caused by replacement, infiltration, or conversion of the marrow. T1-weighted images show most cellular lesions as having a darker signal intensity than marrow fat, and T2-weighted images show them as having a brighter signal intensity. Marrow edema shows similar changes. Developmental and age-related marrow changes must be taken into consideration in the interpretation. The normal adult skeleton has red marrow centrally and in the proximal diametaphyseal regions of the humeri and femora. The proximal humeral epiphyses may also contain residual or reconverted red marrow normally.[3] The pattern may be a curvilinear subcortical distribution or a central patchy globular appearance. Differentiation of a recent osteoporotic compression fracture from a metastatic vertebral body collapse is difficult. Particulate contrast material that is taken up by the marrow reticuloendothelial cells has shown some promise in this respect.

The *joints* are involved in the arthritides, which can be an important clue in the diagnosis of a bone lesion. For example, if a destructive lesion of bone coincides with a joint picture of hemophilic arthropathy, hemophilic pseudotumor should be a consideration. Rheumatoid arthritis may underlie bone changes, as can neurotrophic destruction. Gout can be extremely destructive. Various malignant and benign tumors may involve the joints.

Tissue characterization is optimized with MRI. Disease processes usually have a high water content with signal characteristics that are easily differentiated from fat, marrow, hemorrhage, muscle, tendons, ligaments, flowing blood, and dense bone. Blood flow can be demonstrated and quantified. CT also provides tissue characterization, but it does not offer the superior soft-tissue contrast inherent to MRI. The types of tissue can be identified by signal intensities, as shown in Table 1-2.

IMAGING MODALITIES

The radiologist must have knowledge of the modalities and techniques available to select the most efficient imaging protocol to solve the diagnostic problem. The interpretational process has three components. The first is the detection of the lesion. If the modality chosen is not sensitive enough to show the lesion, the ra-

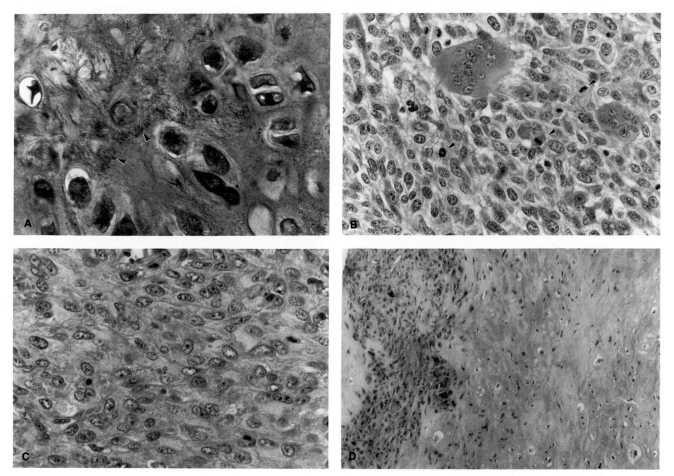

COLOR FIGURE 1-1. Osteosarcoma. (**A**) Arrows point to calcification of the osteoid matrix that is essential for the diagnosis of osteosarcoma but seen well only with limited decalcification of tumor bone. (**B**) Cellular atypical stroma with numerous mitotic figures and osteoclast-like giant cells. (**C**) Fibroblast-like spindle cell differentiation in osteosarcoma. (**D**) Mature hyaline cartilage in chondroblastic osteosarcoma.

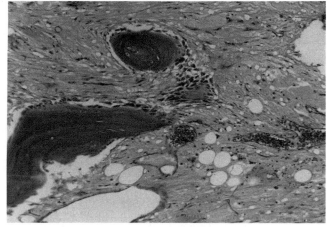

COLOR FIGURE 1-2. Bone mapping of the postchemotherapy effect in osteosarcoma requires thorough sampling of a cross section of the tumor. Shown is the intertrabecular fibrosis between areas of normal-appearing bone. The extent of tumor necrosis, although common even in untreated osteosarcoma, has been correlated with clinical outcome.

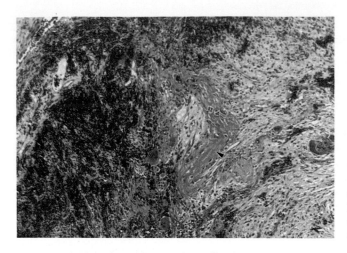

COLOR FIGURE 1-3. Aneurysmal bone cyst often simulates a malignant tumor. There is osteoid in the septae (*arrowhead*), with giant cells, hemorrhage, and hemosiderin deposition.

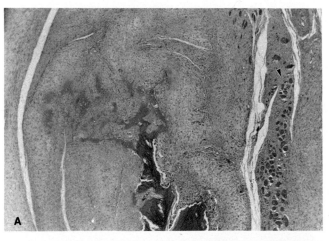

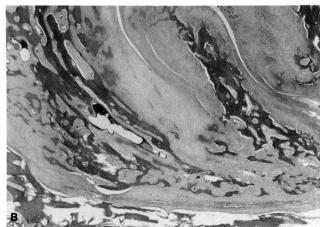

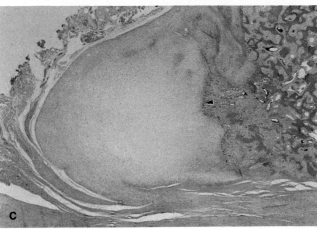

COLOR FIGURE 1-4. Parosteal osteosarcoma. (**A**) A dense but slightly hypercellular fibroblastic stroma with irregular new bone is in the extracortical component adjacent to skeletal muscle (*arrowhead*). (**B**) The mixed fibroblastic and bony tumor flares from the cortex. (**C**) Foci of normal-appearing hyaline cartilage may be present focally (*arrowhead*).

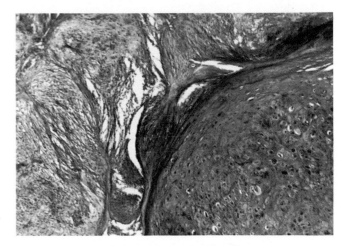

COLOR FIGURE 1-5. Lobulated mature islands of cartilage of an enchondroma.

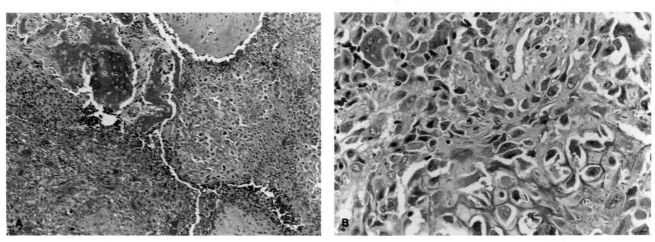

COLOR FIGURE 1-6. Chondroblastoma. (**A**) Cartilaginous differentiation is apparent with lobulated growth, fragments of nonneoplastic new bone, and hyaline cartilage. (**B**) Cytologic atypia of cells in a chicken-wire matrix, showing moderate cellularity and giant cells.

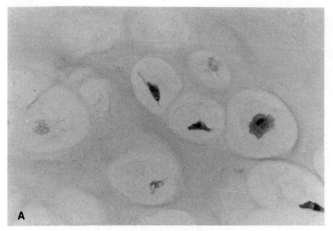

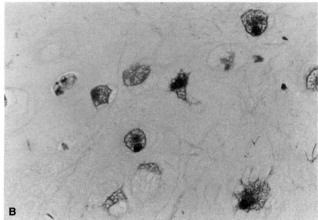

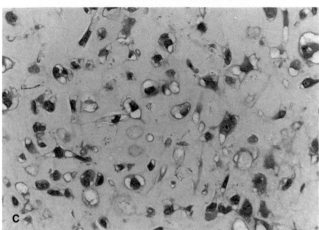

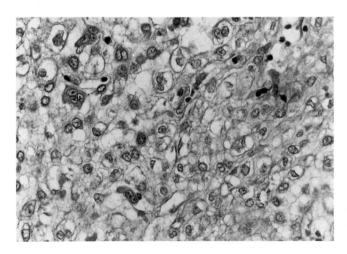

COLOR FIGURE 1-7. Chondrosarcoma grades I through III. (**A**) Grade I tumor cells show small dark nuclei, low cellularity, and no mitotic activity. (**B**) Grade II tumors have medium-sized nuclei and increased cellularity. (**C**) Grade III tumors have hyperchromatism, high cellularity, and greater than two mitoses per 10-high-power fields; mitoses are not shown.

COLOR FIGURE 1-8. Clear cell chondrosarcoma has features that may be confused with chondroblastoma, giant cell tumor, and metastatic carcinoma.

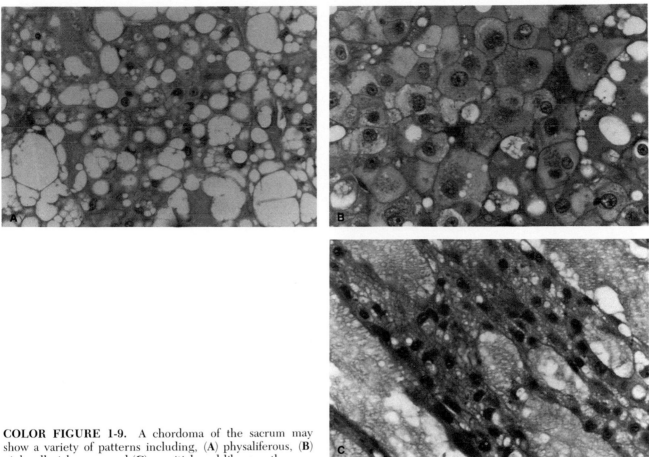

COLOR FIGURE 1-9. A chordoma of the sacrum may show a variety of patterns including, (**A**) physaliferous, (**B**) pink-cell–rich areas, and (**C**) syncitial cord-like growth.

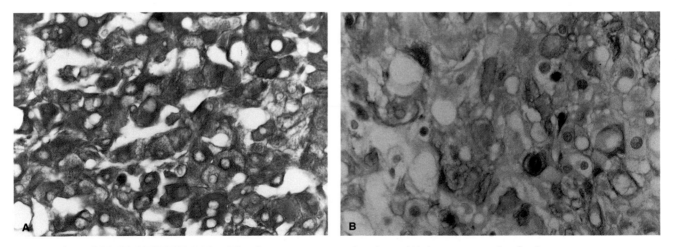

COLOR FIGURE 1-10. Chordoma immunocytochemistry. (**A**) A strong reaction for immuno-stainable cytokeratin is typical. (**B**) Tumor cells are also positive for S100 protein with nuclear and cytoplasmic staining.

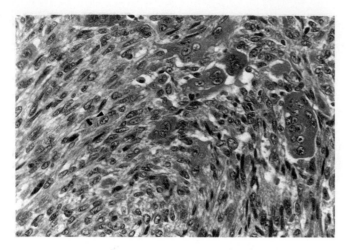

COLOR FIGURE 1-11. Giant cell tumor of bone has many regularly distributed giant cells and well-vascularized, neoplastic stromal cells that may have occasional mitotic figures (*arrowhead*).

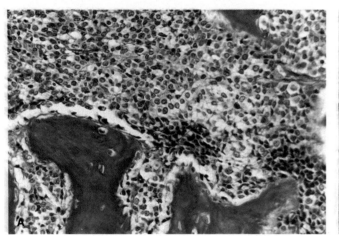
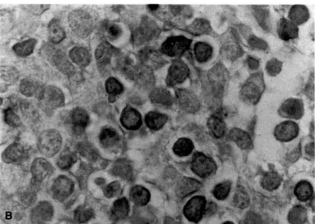

COLOR FIGURE 1-12. Peripheral neuroepithelioma, or Ewing sarcoma of bone, requires electron microscopy, cytogenetics, or immunohistochemistry for the definitive exclusion of other similar-appearing tumors. (**A**) Light microscopic appearance of a typical tumor with bland nuclei, light and dark cell populations, and no extracellular matrix. (**B**) Immunostaining of the cells of Ewing sarcoma with the p30-32^{mic} antibody HBA71 or O13. (See Figure 1-20.)

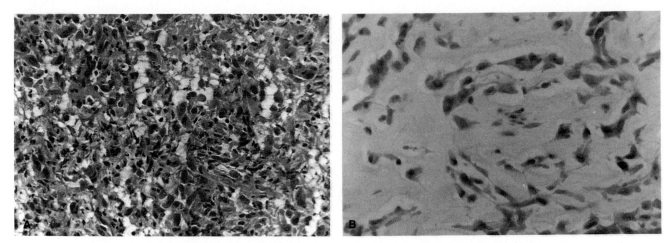

COLOR FIGURE 1-13. Epitheloid hemangioma, or histiocytoid hemangioma. (**A**) The tumor has plump cells with eosinophilic cytoplasm. (**B**) The neoplastic cells are immunohistochemically positive for factor VIII-related antigen determinants, which are markers of endothelium. (See Figure 1-21.)

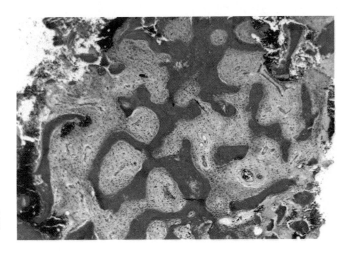

COLOR FIGURE 1-14. Fibrous dysplasia contains immature woven bone, lacking maturation or rimming by cells and composed of irregular O-, C-, and Y-shaped trabeculae.

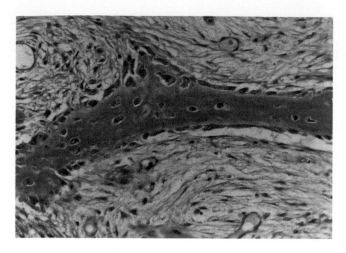

COLOR FIGURE 1-15. Osteofibrous dysplasia, or ossifying fibroma, with osteoblasts lining the narrow trabeculae.

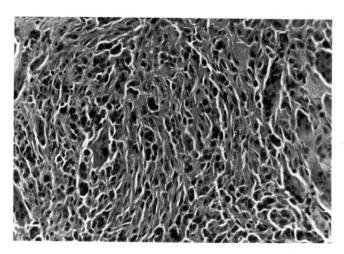

COLOR FIGURE 1-16. Nonossifying fibroma, or metaphyseal fibrous defect, shows dense storiform spindle cell proliferation with abundant hemosiderin staining but lacks the cytologically malignant features of a sarcoma.

TABLE 1-2.
Tissue Characterization by MRI Signal Intensity

Tissue	T1-Weighted Image	T2-Weighted Image
Fat, yellow marrow	High	Lower
Water-containing or highly cellular	Low	High
Subacute and chronic hemorrhage	High	High
Muscle	Intermediate	Intermediate
Fibrous tissue, scar, red marrow	Low	Low
Ligaments, tendons	very low	very low
Cortical bone, dense calcifications	Void	Void
Osteosclerosis	Void	Void

diologist can progress no further. The second problem is the actual diagnosis. In the case of a bone tumor, this would be a prediction of the histology. The third problem, particularly in the case of a bone or soft-tissue tumor, is defining the precise limits of the lesion for treatment planning. The advantages of each noninvasive modality with respect to each phase of interpretation, particularly for a solitary lesion, is presented in Table 1-3.

Conventional Radiography

Plain films are the procedure of choice for detection and diagnosis of appendicular skeletal lesions. The strengths include the characterization of peripheral lesions, skeletal mineralization, and joints. The weaknesses include detection of central skeletal lesions, early bone destruction, and soft-tissue tumors or extension.

Excellent-quality conventional radiographs can demonstrate most peripheral bone and joint lesions. Features such as sclerosis, periosteal new bone formation, cortical destruction, and the amount and patterns of calcification and osteoporosis are shown well on conventional radiographs. Attention to radiographic technique and patient positioning is critical. Additional views employing different projections, magnification,

soft-tissue technique, and conventional tomography are often helpful. Although the conventional film examination is the method of choice for the detection and diagnosis of bone tumors in the peripheral skeleton, it is extremely limited in its ability to define soft-tissue extension and soft-tissue tumors. Detection of soft-tissue extension is more critical to staging and presurgical planning than it is to diagnosis of skeletal lesions. It is not possible to show early bony destructive changes on conventional films, because 30% to 40% of bone must be destroyed before the lesion usually can be seen. CT is far superior to plain films in detecting and characterizing bone destruction.

Computed Tomography

CT is the procedure of choice for central skeletal lesions. It is based on tissue attenuation of an x-ray beam. Two features render it most useful for musculoskeletal radiology: greater tissue contrast resolution than conventional radiography and its ability to display cross-sectional anatomy.

Its strengths include detection of central skeletal lesions, display of cross-sectional anatomy, and the characterization of central skeletal lesions, cortical and trabecular bone, soft-tissue extension, and soft-tissue tumors. Its weaknesses include evaluation of the bone

TABLE 1-3.
Comparative Advantages of Imaging Modalities

Application	Radiography	Scintigraphy	CT	MRI
Detection	Limited; up to 40% destruction can be seen	Most cost effective	Better than conventional radiograph centrally	Most sensitive
Diagnosis	Superior in periphery	Limited to patterns	Superior centrally	Tissue characterization
Planning	Limited	Limited	Better	Far superior

marrow compared with that achievable with MRI, an inability to image the peripheral skeleton in the long axis except for spiral CT, and the inability to screen a large anatomic area effectively.

Tissue density is expressed in terms of the Hounsfield scale. It is calculated from the measured x-ray attenuation relations of air and water. Air has a value of -1000 Hounsfield units (HU); dense bone, between 1000 and 2000 HU; soft tissue, between 40 and 60 HU; and water, 0 HU. One Hounsfield unit corresponds to a change of 0.1% in the linear attenuation coefficient relative to water.

CT allows the evaluation of cases of trauma, neoplasms, infections, and soft-tissue masses. It is able to define soft-tissue densities, although not as well as MRI. In areas of complex anatomy, such as the shoulder, spine, pelvis, and hip, the cross-sectional view eliminates the confusing shadows of superimposed structures that are inevitable in conventional radiographs.

Three-dimensional (3D) CT reconstruction, giving a stereoscopic effect, is commonly used (Fig. 1-17), and the approach is also available for MRI. This technique is especially helpful for exophytic bony lesions and lesions around joints. Joint images can be disarticulated, which allows a lesion involving the hip to be viewed in 3D as an intact joint, with just the femur or with just the acetabulum. The 3D reconstructed image can be further manipulated by removing or cutting away portions of a structure, which allows the interior of structures to be viewed. The ability to perform cut-away views on any projection gives this technique the ability to create tomograms in any plane. The tomograms can be performed on part or all of an osseous structure.

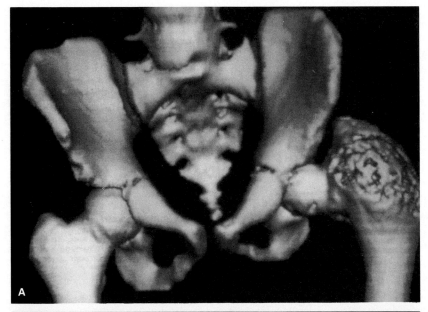

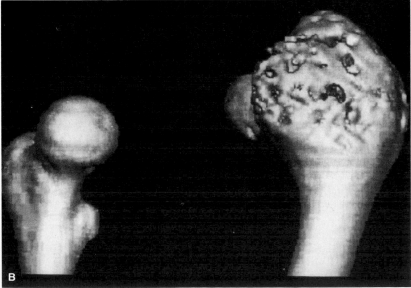

FIGURE 1-17. Three-dimensional reconstruction of a femur with fibrous dysplasia is drawn from CT scans. (**A**) The left femur shows a "shepherd's crook" deformity, with expansion and surface irregularity. (**B**) The pelvis has been electronically removed to show better detail of the left proximal femur.

Three-dimensional CT usually adds little additional diagnostic information, but it adds greatly to the surgeon's understanding of the relation between a tumor and adjacent osseous structures and joints. This information is often critical in presurgical planning.

Spiral CT shows promise of being useful for musculoskeletal imaging. It is excellent for 2D and 3D reconstruction and for data acquisition at the peak level with intravenous contrast.[4]

The diagnostic features of bone lesions in CT are the same as those in conventional radiology. The difference lies in the perspective, because the skeleton and body are seen in cross section. All of the basic parameters described for plain films apply equally well for CT scans.[5]

Radionuclide Imaging

The radionuclide bone scan is the procedure of choice to screen the entire skeleton for osseous lesions.[6] Its strengths include high sensitivity, a high cost-benefit ratio, and the ability to image the entire skeleton. Its weaknesses include low specificity, poor definition of the margin and other characteristics of the lesion, limited diagnostic capabilities, and limited usefulness in therapy planning. It displays tumors, fractures, and inflammatory processes with exquisite sensitivity but lacks specificity. Reliance must be placed on patterns of abnormality, the clinical setting, and the correlation with other examinations for a specific diagnosis. A musculoskeletal lesion is most often detected as an area of increased activity.

The radionuclide uptake in the lesion depends on the reactive or reparative osseous response to the disease process and not the disease itself. The degree of abnormal bone uptake is determined by the rate of osseous response. If there is no reparative response, there is no uptake. The lesion may, paradoxically, be seen with less than normal activity; in this case, it is called a photopenic or cold lesion. Several primary and metastatic tumors may sometimes not show increased uptake on radionuclide bone scans: myeloma, lymphoma, oat cell carcinoma, neuroblastoma, renal cell carcinoma, reticulum cell sarcoma, thyroid carcinoma, anaplastic tumors, and embryonal cell carcinoma.[7]

There are many indications for a radionuclide bone scan. It is particularly useful if multiple lesions are suspected. Tumor, trauma, and inflammatory processes can be detected. Its greatest value is in detecting early processes before sufficient change has occurred to render them visible on radiographic examination. One of its most important indications is suspected metastatic disease.

Bone scans are also used to evaluate the response of a primary sarcoma to chemotherapy. A positive response to chemotherapy is seen as decreasing uptake on serial scans. A significant reparative response to tumor necrosis is seen as increasing activity and can mimic a poor response.

The agents most commonly used in clinical practice are the technetium 99m diphosphonates (i.e., ethane-1-hydroxy-1,1-diphosphonic acid [EHDP] and ^{99m}Tc medronate methylene diphosphonate [MDP]). Gallium 67 is occasionally used. Triple-phase imaging is another technique that yields additional information. The first phase represents arterial flow. Serial images after injection provide information about vascularity and hemodynamics. The second phase represents blood pool. A static image 1 to 2 minutes after injection defines the extravascular space and soft tissues. The third phase, after 2 to 3 hours, evaluates bone uptake. Delayed images may be of further value.

Magnetic Resonance Imaging

MRI is the modality of choice for detection of central skeletal lesions and for treatment planning of central and peripheral skeletal lesions.[8,9] Its strengths include detection of skeletal lesions, evaluation of the bone marrow and soft tissues, and detection of soft-tissue tumors.[10] Its weaknesses include lack of specificity, poorer bone detail, and relative insensitivity to calcifications.

There are a multitude of MR techniques and pulse sequences to chose from, with distinct drawbacks and benefits associated with each one. A thorough understanding of the tissue contrast achieved with the various techniques and their blind spots and strengths is critical to correctly interpret the images.

Clinical MRI techniques rely on signals emitted by hydrogen nuclei after their excitation by a radio frequency (RF) pulse. Three different pulse sequences are used: spin echo (SE), gradient echo (GRE), and inversion recovery (IR). The signal strength depends on three factors: proton density (i.e., number of protons), inherent tissue relaxation times (i.e., T1 and T2 or T2*), and blood flow.[11] Depending on the pulse sequence and parameters selected, the tissue signal intensity in an MR image can primarily reflect PD, T1 relaxation time, or T2 relaxation time, and the image can be classified as PD weighted, T1 weighted, or T2 weighted. MRA is the result of sequence and parameter selection set to maximize signal from flowing blood. MRA shows blood flow, not the anatomic structure of the vessel wall.

Spin echo technique (SE) uses an initial 90-degree RF pulse followed by a 180-degree refocusing pulse and produces the most heavily T1-weighted and T2-weighted images for musculoskeletal imaging (Table 1-4). Tissue contrast in SE images is a function of the

TABLE 1-4.
Spin Echo Technique for Musculoskeletal Imaging

| Weighting | Relaxation Times | | Pulse Sequence |
	TR *(msec)*	TE *(msec)*	
T1	<700	<35	Short TR/short TE
T2	>2000	>70	Long TR/long TE
Proton density	>1000	<35	Long TR/short TE

inherent T1 and T2 relaxation times and the TR (i.e., time of repetition of the signal) and TE (i.e., time of echo) used. T1-weighted SE images offer an excellent signal-to-noise ratio (SNR) and resolution. They are extremely sensitive to marrow pathology, give excellent anatomic display with adequate detail of cortical bone, and have excellent soft-tissue contrast. T2-weighted SE images have poorer SNRs but are exquisitely sensitive to soft-tissue pathology and fluid collections or edema. PD-weighted images offer excellent anatomic display and tissue contrast with an adequate SNR. They are most helpful in detecting permeation of cortical bone and evaluating the soft tissues, but are relatively insensitive to marrow lesions. GRE pulse sequences use a partial flip angle (<90 degrees) and a gradient refocused echo to produce images with T1 and T2 contrast. Musculoskeletal imaging primarily uses T2*-weighted GRE scans. Although this technique is more sensitive to artifacts, it offers adequate T2 weighting and SNR with high resolution and decreased scan times. It is the only technique to offer 3D scanning or volume acquisition. Tissue contrast in GRE images depends on the same factors as SE images plus three additional factors: type of magnetization spoiling used, type of echo acquired, and type of RF pulse.

These pulse sequences were originally developed to obtain T2-weighted images with reduced scan times and are commonly known as the fast scan technique. At first glance, the number of GRE techniques to choose from is overwhelming. With SE pulse sequences, T1, T2, and PD weighting are determined by selecting the TR and TE. With GRE pulse sequences,

TR, TE, magnetization spoiling, echo acquired, and RF pulse determine T1, T2, and PD weighting. This is further complicated by the fact that different vendors have different names for similar sequences (Table 1-5).

STIR (short tau inversion recovery) technique is a common and important pulse sequence in musculoskeletal imaging. The signal from fat is nulled, suppressing the normal marrow signal, and the T1 and T2 contrast effects are additive. This combination provides exquisite sensitivity and conspicuity for marrow lesions.[11]

The principal advantage of MRI is its dramatic ability to define soft-tissue contrast. In addition, blood flow can be defined noninvasively. The various tissues have different inherent signal characteristics on T1- and T2-weighted images. Fat, muscle, cortical bone, red and yellow marrow, tendons, ligaments, nerves, blood vessels, tumors, hemorrhage, and fluid collections have different MRI signal characteristics. On T1-weighted images, fat, fluids with high protein content, and subacute hemorrhage have high signal intensities, but other tissues have intermediate or low signal intensities. T2-weighted images demonstrate high signal intensity for most cellular pathology and fluid collections. Fat has a high signal intensity on T1-weighted images that decreases on T2-weighted images. Cortical bone, dense calcifications, dense fibrous tissue, menisci of the knee, ligaments and tendons, rapidly flowing blood, and air are dark on both types of images.

MRI is extremely sensitive to bone marrow changes. The five types of signal intensities that can be elicited from the marrow cavity are shown in Table

TABLE 1-5.
Gradient Echo Technique for Musculoskeletal Imaging

| Weighting | Flip Angle *(degree)* | Relaxation Times | |
		TR *(msec)*	TE *(msec)*
T1	90	200–350	<15
T2	<20	200–350	20–50
Proton density	30–60	20–50	<15

TABLE 1-6.
MRI Signal Intensities for Bone Marrow

Type of Marrow	Fat (%)	T1-Weighted	T2-Weighted
Red	40	Medium low	Intermediate
Yellow	80	Bright	Darker
Replaced	Approaching 0	Dark	Bright
Postirradiation	Approaching 100	Very bright	Dark
Bony Sclerosis	Approaching 0	Dark	Dark

1-6. Hematomas have a complex pattern that depends on breakdown products.

Multiplanar imaging is a significant benefit for MRI. The coronal and sagittal planes are best for a long axis view and for determining origin, location, and extent of a lesion. The axial plane is best to define the anatomy among tumor, bone, soft-tissue, and the neurovascular structures.

MRI combines the sensitivity of radionuclide scans with the spatial resolution of CT. It is of proven value as a tool in the diagnosis of musculoskeletal diseases. Many of the basic parameters that are evaluated in conventional films and CT, particularly patterns of cortical destruction and periosteal new bone formation, are also evident on MR images.[12] Its greatest disadvantage is the inability to depict the amount and pattern of calcification.

Angiography and Arteriography

With the continued evolution and improvements of CT and MRI in the evaluation of vessels, vascularity, and flow, the role of arteriography in the evaluation of a bone or soft-tissue tumor is a supportive one. Arteriography is rarely used in the diagnostic evaluation of soft-tissue and bone neoplasms. Although arteriography best demonstrates vessel encasement, arteriovenous shunting, neovascularity, and tumor blush or hypervascularity, this vascular information adds little to the diagnosis or staging of a tumor.

Angiography is indicated when a vascular neoplasm or arteriovenous malformation is suspected and if an early or subtle recurrence of a vascular sarcoma is suspected. In patients receiving intraarterial chemotherapy, digital angiography can effectively monitor the response of sarcomas to chemotherapy by evaluating the decrease in tumor vascularity. Although arteriography gives the greatest vessel detail in diagnosing vessel displacement by large osteochondromas and vessel encasement by malignant soft-tissue and osseous neoplasms, this information is effectively obtained noninvasively with MRI, contrast-enhanced CT, or CT- or MR-guided angiography.

Several arteriographic features of malignant tumors are important.[13] *Tumor vessels* are small, deformed and tortuous, irregular in caliber, and exhibit alternate areas of narrowing and dilatation. The contrast material stays longer in the pathologic vessels than in the normal ones. An abrupt termination of a vessel may be seen, as well as a tumor stain. *Dilated capillary arteriovenous connections* with increased blood flow in the tumor region cause rapid circulation and early visualization of veins surrounding the tumor. There may be *large, abnormal draining veins* around the tumor. These veins do not demonstrate valves like those of normal veins of the extremities. *Tumor lakes* remain opacified for a considerable period of time. *Avascular areas*, usually in the center of the tumor, are related to tumor necrosis, arterial emboli, or hematoma. *Direct invasion* of large veins or arteries may occur in malignant bone or soft-tissue tumors.

Ultrasonography

Ultrasonography has a limited role in the imaging of musculoskeletal neoplasms. Its primary role is in soft-tissue imaging: determining whether a mass is cystic or solid, defining the extent of a cystic mass, evaluating the vascularity of a mass, and guiding the biopsy of a soft-tissue mass in the radiology department or in the operating room.[14] Sonography is the gold standard for differentiating a cystic mass and a simple cyst outside of bone, which is a common problem in liver and renal imaging but a rare problem in musculoskeletal imaging.[15] Real-time sonography with color flow Doppler is an effective, noninvasive, and cost-efficient way to evaluate a painful and swollen popliteal area to differentiate among a popliteal cyst, aneurysm, and deep vein thrombosis. The size, depth, and extent of a soft-tissue neoplasm, hematoma, or abscess can readily be determined, and an ultrasound-guided percutaneous needle biopsy can easily be performed.

References

1. Lodwick GS: Solitary malignant tumors of bone: The application of predictor variables in diagnosis. Semin Roentgenol 1:293–313, 1966
2. Johnson LC: A general theory of bone tumors. Bull N Y Acad Med 29:164–171, 1953
2a. Tsai JC, Dalinka MK, Fallon MD, et al: Fluid-fluid level: A nonspecific finding in tumors of bone and soft tissue. Radiology 175:779–782, 1990
3. Mirowitz SA: Hematopoietic bone marrow within the proximal humeral epiphysis in normal adults: Investigation with MR imaging. Radiology 188:689–693, 1993
4. Fishman EK, Wyatt SH, Bluemke DA, et al: Spiral CT of musculoskeletal pathology: Preliminary observations. Skelet Radiol 22:253–256, 1993
5. Brown KT, Kattapuram SV, Rosenthal DI: Computed tomography analysis of bone tumors: Patterns of cortical destruction and soft tissue extension. Skeletal Radiol 15:448–451, 1986
6. Kirchner PT, Simor MA: Current concepts review: Radioisotopic evaluation of skeletal disease. J Bone Joint Surg [Am] 63:673–681, 1981
7. Greenfield GB: Conventional imaging of bone tumors: Its role in the age of CT, MRI, and radionuclide scanning. Contemp Diagn Radiol 13:1–6, 1990
8. Berquist TH, Ehman RL, Richardson ML: Magnetic Resonance of the Musculoskeletal System. 2nd ed. New York, Raven Press, 1990
9. Stoller DW: Magnetic Resonance Imaging in Orthopedics and Sports Medicine. Philadelphia, JB Lippincott, 1993
10. Sartoris DJ, Resnick D: MR imaging of the musculoskeletal system: Current and future status. AJR Am J Roentgenol 149:457–467, 1987
11. Stark DD, Bradley WG: Magnetic Resonance Imaging. 2nd ed. St. Louis, Mosby-Year Book, 1992
12. Greenfield GB, Warren DL, Clark RA: MR imaging of periosteal and cortical changes of bone. Radiographics 11:611–623, 1991
13. Yaghmai I: Angiography of Bone and Soft Tissue Lesions. New York, Springer-Verlag, 1979
14. Braunstein NM, Silver TM, Martel W et al: Ultrasonographic diagnosis of extremity masses. Skeletal Radiol 6:157–163, 1981
15. Yiu-Chiu VS, Chiu LE: Complementary values of ultrasound and computer tomography in the evaluation of musculoskeletal masses. Radiographics 3:46–82, 1983

Pathology

Kenneth R. Schroer

Neoplasms of bone represent some of the most challenging diagnostic problems faced by surgical pathologists. A lack of experience with these tumors because of their rarity and the lack of a specific histopathologic picture contribute difficulties to the diagnosis. To make an accurate bone tumor diagnosis, the radiologist must play an essential role.

The reparative reaction patterns of bone to injury are limited, and the dynamic metabolic changes of bone reactions are radiographically and pathologically similar despite different causes of injury. Trauma, infection, metabolic alterations, anoxia, and adjacent tumors can contribute to reaction patterns that mimic neoplasms.[1] Radiographic and clinical correlation are essential elements, and more than with other tumors, the diagnosis of bone tumors is a clinical-radiologic-pathologic diagnosis, not just a histologic diagnosis. This concept was presented by Ewing in 1922.[2]

At the time of biopsy, the radiographic picture is the gross pathology, and the histologic features complement the radiographic and clinical findings to give a complete picture of the tumor.[3] The radiologist, surgeon, and pathologist each contribute essential information that together constitutes a consultation rather than just a histologic opinion.[3]

Five items contribute to accurate diagnosis of bone tumors: the age of the patient, the bone involved, the area or areas of bone involved, the radiographic appearance of the bone and adjacent tissues, and the microscopic appearance.[4]

DIAGNOSTIC APPROACH

The finding of a diaphyseal tibial tumor in a 15-year-old patient in contrast to an epiphyseal tumor in a 20-year-old patient generates a different differential diagnosis because of the age and location differences, although the histopathology may appear similar, as with numerous giant cells in an early nonossifying fibroma and a giant cell tumor. The radiographic features may show the origin of the lesion from the cortex, medulla, or adjacent soft tissue. The degree of mineralization helps predict the histologic appearance and aids in deciding the type and site of representative biopsy and whether the biopsy is adequate. Actively destructive areas are preferred for biopsy to avoid reparative bone.

The pathologist when informed of age, site, area involved, and radiographic appearance can anticipate special studies that may be helpful in evaluation of the tumor.[5] These special studies include cytogenetics (e.g., for Ewing sarcoma and peripheral neuroepithelioma), electron microscopy (e.g., for eosinophilic granuloma, Ewing sarcoma, neuroepithelioma, neuroblastoma, and other metastatic round cell tumors), and frozen tissue banking of samples for molecular studies of gene expression and mutation of oncogenes (e.g., *MYC*, *RAS*) and tumor suppressor genes (e.g., the retinoblastoma *RB1* and *P53* genes).

Radiologic and Pathologic Correlations of Bone Lesions

Radiologic-pathologic correlation of solitary bone lesions is described for margins,[6] periosteal reactions,[7] and matrix patterns.[8] Margins are classified as type I, geographic, with slow growth; type II, permeative, with intermediate growth; and type III, permeative with rapid growth. The degree of osteolysis depends on the location in cancellous-rich bone of the metaphysis, cancellous-poor bone of the diaphysis, or cortical-dense bone. This is illustrated in the radiographic finding of endosteal bone scalloping of diaphyseal lesions that may be much better visualized by MRI than ordinary films because of the lack of margin between the tumor and the marrow of the diaphysis. In contrast, metaphyseal lucencies are outlined by the abundant adjacent cancellous bone.[6]

Periosteal reactions may be continuous or interrupted. If continuous, the reaction should be defined as having a cortical shell or a destroyed cortex. Bone is continuously destroyed endosteally as new bone is applied at the periosteal surface. This process is probably influenced by vascularity and diffusable cytokines originating from the tumor. As the rate of tumor growth correlates with periosteal new bone formation, the thickness of the shell predicts the aggressiveness of underlying tumor.[7] But exceptions may occur. Florid reactive periostitis of the small bones of the hands and feet is frequently mistaken for osteosarcoma or parosteal osteosarcoma, but it is a benign lesion similar to nodular fasciitis of the soft tissues.[9]

Matrix formation includes osteoid, chondroid, myxoid, and collagenous interstitial acellular accretions. Radiographically, however, mineralization of the matrix is required for visualization of tumor. For practical purposes, only chondroid and osteoid matrices calcify. The pattern of mineralization is more important than the mere presence of calcium. Tumors are often heterogenous, and even though the rings and arcs of radiographically recognizable enchondromas may be seen, coexistent chondrosarcoma cannot be excluded until the entire tumor is examined. Preoperative consultation with the surgeon is necessary to determine the site of the biopsy to minimize discrepancies with the final pathologic findings.[8] The rare event of a malignant tumor developing in a preexisting bone condition, such as infarct, enchondroma, osteomyelitis, or Paget disease, requires sampling of the radiographically different appearing areas to establish the diagnosis.[10]

Frozen Section and Tissue Handling

Frozen section analysis of the soft-tissue or lightly mineralized areas of tumor is useful for triage of limited tissue for special studies. Important information is gained regarding the adequacy of the biopsy, presence of areas requiring bacteriologic culture, and margins of resection. These are more important goals than immediate intraoperative diagnosis. Frozen section may be diagnostic in a minority of bone tumors, but the pathologist should not attempt definitive diagnosis if the intraoperative procedure will not be affected. Frozen sections are technically of poorer quality than permanent sections, hampering accurate diagnosis. Although frozen section is accurate with common epithelial tumors, the experience level with these tumors is higher than that with bone tumors, technical problems are less severe, and tumor sampling can be completed intraoperatively. Bone tumors are rare lesions, require more information than the slide alone provides, and usually cannot be fully sampled by frozen section because of mineralization. Frozen-section diagnoses should not be made without complete clinical and radiologic consultation before the biopsy, following the same rules of assessment given above for making a final histologic diagnosis.

Another procedure that may help in tumor evaluation is specimen fine-detail radiography.[11] Sectioned large bones may be inspected for the best areas (i.e., areas of active destruction) to sample histologically to improve the radiologic-pathologic correlation. Selection of material for electron microscopy may be helped by correlation with specimen radiographs to avoid areas of heavy mineralization or reparative changes.

TYPES AND DISTRIBUTION OF BONE TUMORS

The most common malignant tumor of bone is metastatic carcinoma. Primary malignant bone tumors are listed according to the WHO classification (Table 1-7). The frequency of the tumor types is estimated from the extensive experience with 8542 bone tumors at the Mayo Clinic for more than 40 years.[12] Multiple myeloma and lymphoma comprised 3401 (40%) cases, and most were diagnosed by marrow aspiration. Obviously important because of its frequency, multiple myeloma seldom enters the differential of the usual solitary bone lesion, and it is not dealt with here. Of the remaining 5141 primary nonmarrow bone tumors, 3113 (61%)

TABLE 1-7.
World Health Organization Classification of Primary Malignant Bone Tumors

Classification	Approximate Frequency (%)*
I. Bone-forming tumors	
1. Osteosarcoma	19
2. Juxtacortical (parosteal) osteosarcoma	<1
3. Dedifferentiated (parosteal) osteosarcoma	Rare
4. Periosteal osteosarcoma	
II. Cartilage-forming tumors	
1. Chondrosarcoma	10
2. Mesenchymal chondrosarcoma	<1
3. Dedifferentiated chondrosarcoma	<1
4. Myxoid chondrosarcoma	<1
5. Clear cell chondrosarcoma	<1
III. Giant cell tumors	<1
IV. Marrow tumors	
1. Ewing sarcoma	6
2. Peripheral neuroepithelioma	
3. Lymphoma of bone	6
4. Myeloma	34
V. Vascular tumors	
A. Intermediate malignancy	
1. Hemangioendothelioma	1
2. Hemangiopericytoma	<1
B. Malignant	
1. Angiosarcoma	<1
VI. Other connective tissue tumors	
1. Fibrosarcoma	3
2. Liposarcoma	<1
3. Malignant mesenchymoma	<1
4. Malignant fibrous histiocytoma	<1
5. Undifferentiated sarcoma	<1
VII. Other tumors	
1. Chordoma	4
2. Adamantinoma	<1
3. Parachordoma	Rare
VIII. Unclassified tumors	Rare

*The frequencies were estimated from a Mayo Clinic series of 8542 cases.[12]

were malignant and 2078 (39%) were benign. The malignant tumors consisted of 1330 (43%) osteosarcomas, 732 (23%) malignant cartilage tumors, 402 (13%) Ewing sarcoma cases, 262 (8%) chordomas, 207 (7%) fibrosarcomas, and 187 (6%) miscellaneous tumors. The benign lesions consisted of 1090 (52%) benign cartilage tumors, 425 (20%) giant cell tumors, 308 (15%) benign osteogenic tumors, and 142 (13%) miscellaneous tumor types.

Osteosarcoma

Osteosarcoma is the most frequent primary malignant bone tumor, after exclusion of hematopoietic bone tu-

mors, especially multiple myeloma. The peak incidence is between 10 and 25 years of age, and tumors in patients younger than 5 years of age are rare. Secondary osteosarcomas arise in Paget disease,[13] associated with foreign bodies; in precursor bone lesions such as fibrous dysplasia, enchondromatosis, osteochondromas, and nonossifying fibroma; and after radiation exposure in the older age group. Huvos stated that secondary osteosarcomas comprise 27% of all osteosarcomas occurring in patients older than 21 years of age, but only 3% of secondary osteosarcomas occur in young patients.[14] Of all secondary osteosarcomas, more than half occur in association with Paget disease. A distinctive association with heritable forms of retinoblastoma is also established. Osteosarcoma is the second malignancy in 80% of retinoblastoma survivors with second neoplasms.[15] Abramson reported a 15% to 20% incidence of second tumors occurring, with a mean latent interval of 11 years after treatment. In such patients, 71% of the second tumors occurred in the radiation field, and 19% occurred outside the field.[16] Among nonirradiated patients, 14% developed second tumors.[17]

The retinoblastoma gene (*RB1*) is a tumor-suppressor gene that appears to have an important role in development of sarcomas, especially osteosarcoma, and in the development of primary eye tumors. Deletions of the *RB1* gene have also been found in 3 of 9 nonfamilial osteosarcomas not associated with retinoblastoma,[18] and homozygous deletions have been found in osteosarcoma cells from the familial form of retinoblastoma.[19] This strongly indicates a genetic predisposition to osteosarcoma in retinoblastoma survivors, but a role for administered radiation and chemotherapy as cofactors is suggested from the Late Effect Study Group (LESG) findings. These researchers also observed that the occurrence of osteosarcoma was not limited to retinoblastoma survivors, but it also occurred in survivors of Ewing sarcoma, Hodgkin disease, Wilms tumor, neuroblastoma, and rhabdomyosarcoma.[20] The LESG found 28 of 91 bone sarcomas that occurred as second neoplasms were in retinoblastoma patients, but the remainder were in other pediatric tumor patients who had received radiation or combined irradiation and chemotherapy. The estimated relative risk of osteosarcoma after more than 6000 cGy of radiation was 38.3, and after chemotherapy, it was 8.5 for administration of three or more alkylating agents.[20]

Most osteosarcomas arise in the metaphyseal area of the long bones, with the distal femur and proximal tibia representing sites of high incidence. The diaphysis is a much less common site. Multicentricity may occur, predominantly in children, and it is associated with bone sclerosis. These tumors are highly aggressive. Predominantly intramedullary in origin, expansile growth with cortical breakthrough is common. Intracortical osteosarcoma is rare and occurs mainly in the diaphysis.

An important role of the radiologist is to help the surgeon determine the best site for the biopsy. Areas containing normal bone or adjacent normal soft-tissue components and tumor bone elements should be selected. A common error in the biopsy of chondroblastic osteosarcoma is a superficial biopsy demonstrating only the cartilaginous component and not the tumor osteoid that is essential for diagnosis. Erroneous diagnosis of chondrosarcoma, which has better survival than osteosarcoma, may be avoided by appropriate site selection. Triage of limited biopsy material may require frozen section to determine the adequacy of the biopsy and selection of tissue for electron microscopy in difficult cases or flow cytometry for aneuploidy determination. A specific diagnosis of osteosarcoma cannot be made reliably unless the pathologist is familiar with osteosarcomas and has reviewed the case with the radiologist and surgeon before the biopsy.

Types of Osteosarcoma

Raymond and his colleagues[21] at M.D. Anderson proposed an alternate classification of osteosarcoma into four clinicopathologic groups (Table 1-8).

CONVENTIONAL OSTEOSARCOMA. The gross features of large, lobulated masses of cartilage, solid masses of dense bone, and hemorrhagic cysts reflect the relative contribution of chondroblastic, osteoblastic, vascular, and fibrous elements that may comprise the tumor. These predominant elements give rise to the subclassifications of chondroblastic, osteoblastic, telangiectatic, and fibrohistiocytic osteosarcoma. Sampling of the tumor by the pathologist should focus on demonstrating local patterns of spread. Thorough examination of the proximal margin of resection, marrow space, cortex where ruptured, adjacent soft-tissue margins, and epiphyseal invasion or involvement of the joint spaces allows proper staging.

The microscopic pathology (see Color Fig. 1-1) and the gross pathology depend on the relative components of cartilage, small cells, bone-forming elements, and vascular and fibrous tissues. The essential feature for the diagnosis of osteosarcoma is the formation of malignant stroma with tumor osteoid away from the cartilaginous components of the neoplasm. Osteoid is type I collagen undergoing provisional calcification. With heavily decalcified bone, it becomes impossible to differentiate from ordinary hyalinized collagen, but it may be easily seen in electron micrographs (Fig. 1-18). The intimate relation to cytologically atypical tumor cells and the homogeneous appearance of the collagen favor interpretation as probable osteoid even without calci-

TABLE 1-8.
Clinicopathologic Classification of Osteosarcoma

Conventional osteosarcoma
  Chondroblastic
  Fibroblastic
  Osteoblastic
Histologically special types
  High-grade types
    Small cell osteosarcoma
    Telangiectatic osteosarcoma
  Low-grade types
    Well-differentiated osteosarcoma
    Osteoblastoma-like osteosarcoma
Surface types
  Periosteal osteosarcoma
  Parosteal osteosarcoma
  Dedifferentiated parosteal osteosarcoma
  High-grade surface osteosarcoma
Special clinical settings
  Associated benign lesions
  Paget disease or bone infarct
  Jaw location
  Multifocality
  Postirradiation

From Raymond AK, Chawla S, Carrasco CH et al: Osteosarcoma chemotherapy effect: A prognostic factor. Semin Diagn Pathol 4:212, 1987

fication. Tumor cells are pleomorphic and hyperchromatic. Hypercellularity and necrosis are common findings.

Whole-bone mapping shows areas of contiguous spread, identifies satellite nodules, multifocality, and skip metastases and estimates the effect of chemotherapy given before resection of the bone.[21,22] Areas of necrosis, fibrosis, and dense ossification in response to therapy (see Color Fig. 1-2) and residual intact tumor are quantified and have been correlated with prognosis.[23] Abundant necrosis is associated with improved outcome and is correlated with angiographic changes after preoperative chemotherapy.[21,24] Giant cells are a variable finding but important in confounding the differential diagnosis (see Color Fig. 1-1B). These patterns of tumor do not differ greatly in their prognoses.

HISTOLOGICALLY SPECIAL TYPES OF OSTEOSARCOMA. Microscopic variations may give rise to diagnostic difficulties because they simulate other lesions.

Small cell osteosarcoma should be differentiated from Ewing sarcoma, mesenchymal chondrosarcoma, lymphoma, neuroblastoma, spindle cell tumors, and metastatic small cell carcinoma.[25] Minute areas of osteoid are the clue to the correct diagnosis. Other tumors have little matrix, and these tumors occur in older patients.[26]

For determining *anaplastic osteosarcoma*, special

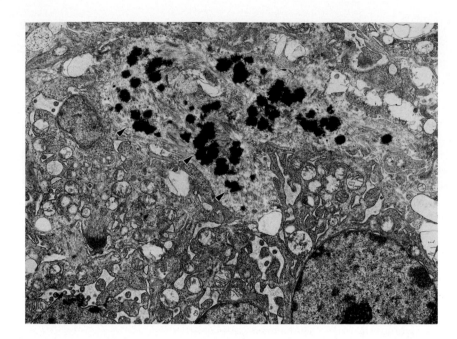

FIGURE 1-18. The electron-microscopic appearance of the provisionally calcified collagen matrix of osteoid adjacent to an osteoblast in osteosarcoma.

immunohistochemical stains are useful for ruling out lymphoma (i.e., CD45 or leukocyte common antigen positive), carcinoma (i.e., keratin positive), and melanoma (i.e., S100 and HMB45 positive).

Telangiectatic osteosarcoma should be differentiated from aneurysmal bone cyst, which may be truly cystic (95% of cases)[27,28] or solid (5%).[29] The solid variant of aneurysmal bone cyst is histologically identical to giant cell reparative granuloma of the small bones of the hands and feet.[27] Telangiectatic osteosarcoma has lace-like or filigree-type osteoid, mitotic figures, and atypical stromal cells. The stromal atypical cells are the essential finding to differentiate osteosarcoma from aneurysmal bone cyst (see Color Fig. 1-3), because the latter may also have lace-like osteoid and as many as 10 mitotic figures per 10 high-power fields (not atypical mitotic figures), but they lack cytologic atypia of the stromal component that is seen in osteosarcoma.[27] According to De Dios and colleagues, the diagnosis of aneurysmal bone cyst with atypical stromal cells should be viewed with skepticism.[27] Septate spaces are usually present, and multinucleated giant cells are abundant in both lesions.

Fibrohistiocytic osteosarcoma is differentiated from malignant fibrous histiocytoma by the presence of tumor osteoid and the lack of a storiform architecture.

Well-differentiated osteosarcoma must be differentiated from fibrous dysplasia, osteofibrous dysplasia, osteoblastoma,[30] and the solid variant of aneurysmal bone cyst.[27] These tumors lack the highly destructive appearance of conventional high-grade osteosarcoma, and microscopically, mitoses are scarce. Solid aneurysmal bone cyst is mitotically much more active and worrisome appearing to the pathologist. Differentiation of aneurysmal bone cyst from low-grade central osteosarcoma may be difficult.[29] The criteria for this differential diagnosis are based on architectural findings of regular trabecular osteoid with prominent osteoblastic rimming and more cellular but looser stroma in aneurysmal bone cyst.[27] Osteosarcoma produces irregular, disorganized trabeculae and compact, collagenized stroma. Recurrences of low-grade central osteosarcoma may show increased anaplasia, but metastasis and death are unusual.[30]

Intracortical osteosarcoma is an indolent, less-aggressive tumor but must be differentiated from metaphyseal fibrous defect, osteoid osteoma, and a Brodie abscess.[31,32]

Osteoblastoma-like osteosarcoma represents a difficult differential diagnosis in the exclusion of low-grade osteosarcoma.[33] The location of osteoblastic benign lesions, osteoid osteoma, and osteoblastoma may be cortical, periosteal, or medullary. Clinical and radiographic differentiation by size (i.e., 1 cm or 2 cm in diameter[34,35,37]), location, sclerosis, and pain patterns are essential. However, some tumors overlap in their features and some have borderline features that defy classification.[37] Some osteoblastomas have been described as malignant by Schajowicz, but because they are not associated with metastasis and lack abnormal mitotic activity, Dorfman considers these aggressive osteoblastomas.[35–37] These tumors are different from the lesions described by Bertoni as "osteosarcoma resembling osteoblastoma" that behave as osteosarcoma.[38] Associated aneurysmal bone cyst may lead to rapid enlargement,[33] and systemic symptoms of fever, periostitis, clubbing, and high output cardiac failure may be seen rarely.[39]

Microscopically, the lesions called *osteoid osteoma* have minimal or no atypia, have no mitoses, lack lace-like osteoid, but have irregular cement lines.

Osteoblastoma is larger (>2 cm) and appears similar to osteoid osteoma by light and electron microscopy, with no bizarre cells, sheet-like osteoid, or atypical mitoses but with occasional normal mitoses (average, 1 mitotic figure per 20 high-power fields), lace-like osteoid, and spindly storiform or hemangiopericytoma-like stroma.[40] The designation of *aggressive osteoblastoma* describes a larger tumor, usually in older patients, and it contains diagnostic epithelioid osteoblasts, sheet-like osteoid that is more than just focal, a low mitotic rate (1–4 mitoses per 20 high-power fields), but no atypical mitoses. None of these lesions have metastasized, and this lesion is not synonymous with low-grade osteosarcoma. Other problems in the differential diagnosis are the underdiagnosis of low-grade osteosarcoma as osteoblastoma[38] and overdiagnosis of cancer in osteoblastomas that have degenerative changes simulating malignancy.[37,41]

SURFACE TYPES. The three types of surface osteosarcoma are fairly uncommon.[12]

Juxtacortical (parosteal) osteosarcoma (see Color Fig. 1-4) is a metaphyseal, slow growing, radiographically dense, lobulated mass that may encircle the posterior lower femur and is attached with a broad base.[42] Other sites of development are the proximal humerus and proximal tibia. Microscopically, the stroma is cellular, atypical, and fibrous, with disorderly trabeculae. The diagnosis must exclude myositis ossificans, which shows zonal maturation. The tumor is prognostically favorable, but penetration into the medullary cavity is an ominous finding. Dedifferentiated parosteal osteosarcoma describes progression to a high-grade spindle sarcoma in the background of a parosteal osteosarcoma.

High-grade surface osteosarcoma is an aggressive tumor and may be indistinguishable from dedifferentiated juxtacortical osteosarcoma or conventional medullary osteosarcoma with juxtacortical spread. The histologic features are similar to conventional osteosarcoma.[43]

Periosteal osteosarcoma occurs commonly in the upper tibial shaft or femur. It is a lucent tumor because of the cartilaginous component with perpendicular or radial striations and saucerization of the cortex, often connected by a narrow pedicle. This tumor has a good prognosis. Periosteal osteosarcoma is part of the differential diagnosis for cartilaginous lesions of the bone surface and for osteosarcoma. Controversially, several investigators have suggested that a pure periosteal chondrosarcoma is distinguishable from periosteal osteosarcoma as described by Unni.[44,45] Bertoni and colleagues presented the case for differentiating periosteal

chondrosarcoma from periosteal osteosarcoma.[46] The former lesion differs histologically by lacking the minute areas of osteoid that define osteosarcoma.[47] Surface chondrosarcomas occur in slightly older patients, are more likely to be metaphyseal, and are less commonly painful. Microscopically, periosteal osteosarcoma is also prominently cartilaginous but has focal mineralization and osteoid production by definition. Peripheral condensation of spindle cells may occur. Atypia is usually mild, and mitoses are infrequent.

The prognosis of the periosteal chondrosarcoma is apparently better than that of periosteal osteosarcoma. The differential diagnosis should also consider periosteal chondroma,[48] which has reactive lamellar bone at the tumor bone interface, and high-grade or conventional osteosarcoma demonstrating a prominent surface component.

SPECIAL CLINICAL PRESENTATIONS. *Osteosarcoma of the jaws* constitutes about 6% of all osteosarcomas, but it occurs in older patients, tends to be chondroblastic, and has a better prognosis than conventional osteosarcoma. Difficulties may arise in demonstrating osteoid in the predominantly chondroblastic, low-grade tumors, giving rise to their misclassification as chondrosarcomas. Attention to the adequacy of the biopsy is important to avoid this difficulty.[49]

Osteosarcoma arising in patients who have Paget disease of bone tends to occur in the pelvis and humerus in older patients (mean age, 64 years). Microscopically, numerous osteoclastic giant cells may be present. The prognosis is poor, and most reported cases are fatal.[14]

Osteosarcoma after irradiation is histologically similar to conventional osteosarcoma but most common in the ilium, proximal femur, and proximal humerus.[50]

Lesions Simulating Osteosarcoma

The nonmalignant lesions that simulate osteosarcoma include fracture callus, myositis ossificans, fibrous dysplasia, osteoblastoma, and giant cell tumor. Radiographic correlation is often the most important step in the evaluation of the patient. Exuberant callus especially may closely mimic osteosarcoma when the chondro-osteoid matrix blends together haphazardly with some mitotic activity but without atypical mitoses or the obvious cellular anaplasia of osteosarcoma.[51] Careful radiologic, pathologic, and clinical evaluation is required to avoid serious mistakes in diagnosis.

Prognosis

Poor prognosis for patients with osteosarcoma has been associated with Paget disease, craniofacial sites other than the jaws, vertebral sites, multifocality, elevation of alkaline phosphatase, and hyperploidy.[52] Good prognosis correlates with jaw sites, fibroblastic morphology (i.e., small effect), surface growth in pure parosteal and periosteal types, well-differentiated medullary types, and if abundant necrosis follows neoadjuvant chemotherapy.

Cartilaginous Tumors

In one referral practice reviewing 1187 cartilage tumors, osteochondroma was the most common type, constituting 61% of such tumors.[53] The enchondroma comprised 29%, other benign cartilage tumors about 5%, and chondrosarcoma about 5% of tumors. Most of the other types of malignant cartilage tumors were rare and were absent in this series.

Osteochondroma

The solitary osteochondroma is the most common benign bone tumor occurring in bones formed from cartilage. Most commonly affected are the distal femoral metaphysis, proximal tibia, tibial metaphysis, and pelvis. Chondrosarcoma rarely develops in osteochondroma, but when present, it has a cap greater than 2 cm, extends into soft tissues, and shows greater atypia than seen in benign osteochondroma.[54] The important distinction is the thickness of the cartilaginous cap, which rarely exceeds 1 cm in osteochondroma. Cancellous bone usually underlies the cap. An important finding is flaring of the cortex into the base of a benign tumor. The cartilage often shows a jig-saw pattern of calcification. Atypia of the cartilage with binucleate chondrocytes should not be interpreted as evidence of malignancy using histologic analysis alone. Parosteal osteosarcoma with rounded contours may simulate osteochondroma. Complications such as fracture can make diagnosis extremely difficult.

Enchondroma

Enchondromatosis (i.e., Ollier disease) is a rare, nonhereditary, multisite cartilaginous dysplasia that may affect any bone with cartilaginous antecedent other than those formed by intramembranous ossification. Affected bones, commonly in the small bones of the hands, are malformed and shortened. Histologically, the curetted lesions contain cellular hyaline cartilage that may reveal a myxoid change (see Color Fig. 1-5). Anaplasia is not present, but binucleation and atypia are often features. Because the gross lesion is not present in curetted tissue, a radiologic-pathologic correlation is essential to correct interpretation of the atypical cartilage changes. Fibrous dysplasia and osteochondroma are considered in the differential diagnosis. Fibrous dysplasia may also have variable cartilage nodules in the polyostotic form of disease (14% of cases) but not the monostotic form.[55]

Malignant transformation, especially to chondrosarcoma, occurs in almost one fourth of cases of enchondromatosis. The radiologic findings of a larger lesion, cortical destruction, and soft-tissue mass and the clinical finding of pain favor chondrosarcoma. However, the diagnosis of malignancy may be difficult or impossible because of similar degrees of histologic atypia in the benign and malignant processes. Fracture in an enchondroma may be particularly treacherous diagnostically, with extravasation of cartilage into the soft-tissue simulating invasion and exuberant callus formation that simulates a high-grade sarcoma. Correlation with a history of trauma and comparison temporally with the radiographic appearance are important to avoid this pitfall. Mirra described histologic patterns that favor enchondroma, including the presence of islands of cartilage or a lamellar encasement pattern, but chondrosarcoma is permeative, marrow infiltrative, or has bands of fibrosis.[56] Liu and colleagues[57] regarded the presence of myxoid stroma as the most important single histologic finding, present in 100% of malignant tumors arising in enchondromatosis in their series. They found comparison with the underlying enchondroma useful for direct cytologic contrast, and they suggested that the surgeon be advised to biopsy benign- and malignant-appearing areas. Recurrence alone should not be considered definite evidence of malignant change.[57]

Other associated malignancies are osteosarcoma, dedifferentiated chondrosarcoma, and dedifferentiated chordoma.[57] Patients with the Maffucci syndrome (i.e., multiple enchondromas with associated cutaneous and visceral hemangiomas) have a high risk of extraskeletal malignancies.[58] Ollier disease is proposed to be a generalized mesodermal dysplasia, supported by the occurrence of three patients that have had associated ovarian sex cord tumors (two with Maffucci syndrome).[59,60]

Chondroblastoma

The incidence of benign chondroblastoma peaks in young patients, distinguishing it clinically from the older patients with giant cell tumor. The commonly affected long bones are the proximal humerus, femoral head, and proximal tibial epiphysis, and rarely, the metaphysis is involved. Rarely, chondroblastoma involves the skull and facial bones (6%–7% of cases), but the peak occurrence is at an older age (43.5 years).[61] Older patients often have involvement of the pelvic bones. The radiographic differential diagnosis may include epiphyseal osteosarcoma, epiphyseal enchondroma, and clear cell chondrosarcoma.[62]

The lesions often grossly resemble granulation tissue, but they may be cystic and simulate or contain areas of aneurysmal bone cyst evident grossly and microscopically.[63] Aneurysmal bone cyst is a component of chondroblastoma in 38% of patients, more commonly occurring in the bones of the hands and feet.[64] Chondroblastoma (see Color Fig. 1-6A) has a cellular mononuclear or spindle cell proliferation with giant cells and immature chondrocytes with some mitotic activity,[61] along with lacy, chicken-wire calcification (see Color Fig. 1-6B) or coarse calcification. Necrosis (30%), aneurysmal bone cyst-like areas (38%), epithelioid areas, and mitotic activity (77%) are more common in head and neck lesions than in the long bones.[61] Most cases have 1 to 4 mitotic figures per 10 high-power fields, but about 4% have more than 4 mitoses per 10 fields. Increased mitoses are not associated with an increased risk of metastasis.[64] Metastases have been described, usually after surgical curetting of the tumor.[65]

The differential diagnosis should include chondromyxoid fibroma, giant cell tumor, histiocytosis X, aneurysmal bone cyst, clear cell chondrosarcoma, and chondroblastic osteosarcoma. An S100 stain may help define the cartilaginous nature of the cellular proliferation, but the physician should remember that Langerhans cells of histiocytosis X are also S100 positive. Chondroblastoma cells are individually surrounded with stainable reticulin fibers and contain stainable glycogen. Giant cell tumor is cytologically different with the nuclei of the giant cells resembling those of the interspersed mononuclear cells. Matrix is absent in giant cell tumor, unless associated with fracture, in contrast to chondroblastoma. Clear cell chondrosarcoma and chondromyxoid fibroma are often lobulated, and the former shows areas of atypia and mitotic activity.

Periosteal Chondroma

Lesions are well circumscribed, sclerotic, and occur in the tubular long bones (especially the humerus) and phalanges, peaking in incidence in the first two decades. The lesions are 1 to 6 cm in diameter. Atypical chondrocytes may be found but do not predict malignant behavior; pleomorphism does favor chondrosarcoma. Often the key to the diagnosis is the radiographic appearance of the tumor.[48]

Chondromyxoid Fibroma

Chondromyxoid fibroma is an unusual tumor of bone that is sometimes confused with chondrosarcoma.[66] Occurring in the metaphyseal portion of the long bones and small bones of the hands and feet, chondromyxoid fibroma usually shows sharp scalloped margins with sclerosis and rare or absent calcifications of matrix. Microscopically, distinct lobulation with peripheral hypercellularity of the lobules is seen. The stroma is less mature than hyaline cartilage, with a

myxoid appearance and characteristic biphasic sudden transition from hyaline-like areas to more cellular tumor. Bizarre nuclei may be seen that are worrisome if interpreted without radiographic or clinical correlation. Some areas reminiscent of chondroblastoma are seen.[67] Aggressive recurrences in 10% of patients were reported from one series.[66]

Chondrosarcoma

Chondrosarcoma may arise as a primary tumor or in a preexisting bone lesion, such as enchondromatosis, Paget disease, or fibrous dysplasia, or in a patient with multiple osteochondromas. Site is an important predictor of malignancy. Chondrosarcomas are common in the pelvis, ribs, scapula, femur, and humerus but rare in the short, tubular bones of the hands and feet.[68] With the exception of clear cell chondrosarcoma[69] and mesenchymal chondrosarcoma,[70] which peak in the third decade, older patients are usually affected.

Chondrosarcomas can be divided into central, peripheral, and juxtacortical types. The central lesions involve the medullary cavity, usually of a long bone, and must be differentiated from enchondromas. Peripheral chondrosarcomas may arise in an osteochondroma or de novo. Surface periosteal chondrosarcoma is separated from periosteal osteosarcoma by Bertoni[46] and differs in presentation in several clinical features (see Periosteal Osteosarcoma).

The histologic characteristics of central and peripheral chondrosarcomas are similar. Clinical and radiographic correlation, rather than histologic analysis, often determines the final diagnosis. For example, the finding of clinical pain in an axial tumor with radiographic aggressive features points to a malignant tumor even if the cytoarchitectural features of the lesion are bland. Slight cytologic atypia, consisting of binucleation, mild hypercellularity, and slight nuclear enlargement, substantiates the radiographic impression of malignancy. Because atypicality may be quite focal, extensive sampling may be required. Promising ancillary methods to detect aneuploidy or oncogene activation may help with difficult cases, but the radiographic studies are pivotal in the final decision about low-grade cartilage lesions. The radiologist can help the surgeon decide about the site and type of biopsy. Because soft-tissue implantation in chondrosarcoma is a known complication, care should be taken to prevent compromise of any subsequent attempt at resection.

All cartilaginous tumors should be carefully examined for osteoid production to exclude chondroblastic osteosarcoma. Before diagnosis, consideration should be given to obtaining fresh tissue for cytophotometric image analysis by Feulgen staining of the nuclei to assess ploidy, although these analyses may also be performed retrospectively from paraffin-embedded tissue. Aneuploidy appears to be prognostically important.[71]

The microscopic diagnosis of chondrosarcoma relies on the combination of architectural and cytologic features (see Color Fig. 1-7). Atypia of chondrocytes, binucleation, myxoid matrix with variable staining, cellular pleomorphism, mitotic activity, and high cellularity are features favoring chondrosarcoma. Cytoarchitectural or nuclear-grading schemes give similar results.[72–74] Many reported series show clear differences in prognosis correlated with the grade of malignancy.[75–78] The following is the M.D. Anderson grading scheme:

> Grade I tumors show small dark nuclei, low cellularity, and no mitotic activity.
> Grade II tumors have medium-sized nuclei, increased cellularity and mitoses.
> Grade III tumors have hyperchromatism, high cellularity, and more than 2 mitoses per 10 high-power fields.

In cartilaginous lesions of the small bones of the hands and feet, the degree of atypia and cytologically aggressive features may be greater than tolerated at other sites. The diagnosis of chondrosarcoma depends on radiographic evidence of permeation through the cortex. Tumors in these sites are rare.[68]

DEDIFFERENTIATED CHONDROSARCOMA. A form of high-grade progression in chondrosarcoma is the dedifferentiated chondrosarcoma.[78] Clinically, the dedifferentiated chondrosarcoma peaks in incidence in the sixth decade of life, as is typical of cartilaginous tumors. This is a biphasic, high-grade tumor with typical chondrosarcoma and areas of storiform, high-grade spindle cell tumor, similar to malignant fibrous histiocytoma. Some tumors contain osteoid-like matrix in the spindle component. In tissue culture, BUdR- or retinoic acid-dedifferentiated chondrocytes cease producing the type II collagen that is characteristic of chondrocytes[79] and assume a fibroblastic appearance, providing a laboratory model for the clinical occurrence of this type of tumor change, arguably called "dedifferentiation." Clinically, obvious difficulties may arise in determining whether the tumor is chondroblastic osteosarcoma, dedifferentiated chondrosarcoma,[80] or malignant fibrous histiocytoma.[81] Malignant fibrous histiocytoma arising in a bone infarct has a better prognosis and should be diagnosed by thorough sampling of the tumor.[82] Immunohistochemical studies have shown that other forms of mesenchymal differentiation may be found with various tumors showing positive staining with α_1-antitrypsin, desmin, and myoglobin-specific antibodies.[83]

MESENCHYMAL CHONDROSARCOMA. These tumors may arise in ribs, vertebrae, pelvis, jaw, calvar-

ium, including the meninges, and appendicular soft tissues, usually in young patients.[84] Histologically, the tumors consist of a cartilaginous and undifferentiated stromal component revealed by light and electron microscopy.[85] Jacobson proposed that mesenchymal chondrosarcoma is one of a spectrum of bone tumors that he designated polyhistioma.[86]

The mitotic activity and pleomorphism are low,[70,84,87] but because of this blandness, it may be confused with chondromyxoid fibroma, which is also biphasic in its microscopic appearance. However, chondromyxoid fibroma is cytologically even more bland and presents with a different clinical and radiographic picture. Other patterns that are recognized in mesenchymal chondrosarcoma may simulate other entities, including a Ewing-like, small, round cell pattern; a lymphoma-like pattern; or a hemangiopericytoma pattern with delicate staghorn branching vascularity.[85] Osteoid-like areas may be seen, reflecting a possible relation to small cell osteosarcoma. Immunohistochemical stains can help in the differential diagnosis. In mesenchymal chondrosarcoma, the small cell component is Leu-7 positive, and the chondroid foci are S100 positive. Ewing sarcoma and hemangiopericytoma are negative for both. Staining for leukocyte common antigen excludes lymphoma in most cases. Calcified chondroid areas should be sought to help classify lesions with unusual patterns. Specimen radiography may help the pathologist locate areas of calcification for sampling.

MYXOID CHONDROSARCOMA. Myxoid chondrosarcoma (i.e., chordoid sarcoma) is a rare tumor considered on the basis of immunohistochemical and electron microscopic studies to be a variant of chondrosarcoma, although it may be confused with chordoma because of the similar appearance of columns of cells in a myxoid background.[88] The tumor is more common in soft tissues than bone and differs in these sites in immunohistochemical staining for epithelial membrane antigen (i.e., EMA positive in soft-tissue chordoid sarcoma and negative in the skeletal variety). Other immunochemical markers may be helpful in the differential diagnosis of these tumors.[89] As with chordoma, myxoid chondrosarcomas express Leu-7, S100, and vimentin, but they do not stain with anti-keratin or anti-lysozyme.[90]

CLEAR CELL CHONDROSARCOMA. The clear cell chondrosarcoma is a variant of chondrosarcoma that is lobular, has a ground glass or clear cytoplasm and sharp cell borders, contains calcifications, and resembles chondroblastoma in appearance and epiphyseal location. However, clear cell chondrosarcoma peaks in incidence in the fourth decade in contrast to a peak age in the second decade for chondroblastoma.[69] The early lesions may also mimic chondroblastoma radiographically with epiphyseal location and sclerotic margins, but larger lesions are more destructive. Microscopically, similar findings to chondroblastoma (see Color Fig. 1-8), including numerous mononuclear cells and multinucleated giant cells, are seen. S100 stains are positive as in other cartilaginous tumors, and this may help in differentiating this tumor from giant cell tumor.[91] Foci of trabecular woven bone or hemorrhagic cyst formation may be seen within the lesion, presenting the additional pathologic differential diagnoses of chondroblastic osteosarcoma, aneurysmal bone cyst, and ordinary chondrosarcoma. Ultrastructural studies have revealed chondrocytic and chondroblastic cells.[92] Areas of ordinary chondrosarcoma are sometimes identified within the lesion, which may lead to erroneous diagnosis if needle or small biopsies are performed.

The lesion is considered a low-grade malignant form of chondroblastoma,[91,93] and its distinction from chondroblastoma rests on clinical presentation, radiographic appearance of the lesion, and histopathology. Lung metastases occur in about 20% of patients, and the mortality rate is almost 30%.[93]

Chordoma

Chordomas constitute 1% to 4% of all bone tumors in most published series and are uncommon in patients younger than 30 years of age, except for those that occur in the spheno-occipital region. Sacrococcygeal chordomas typically arise in the fifth and sixth decades of life in bone from notochordal remnants. Most tumors in this location are distal to S3, unlike chondrosarcoma, giant cell tumor, and osteosarcoma. Fifty percent are sacrococcygeal, and 35% are spheno-occipital in origin; the latter tumors are common in children.[94,95] The sacrococcygeal neoplasms develop slowly and may be blastic but are more often lytic. Local symptoms may result from cord compression, bowel or bladder involvement, or spread to the retroperitoneum. The spheno-occipital lesions may present with cranial nerve involvement, with bone destruction, or as an asymptomatic mass.[96,97]

The gross appearance of chordoma is a lobular tumor with gelatinous degeneration with hemorrhage, occasional foci of necrosis, and cystic degeneration. Microscopically, as in myxoid chondrosarcoma (i.e., chordoid sarcoma), the tumor grows in cellular cords in a mucinous matrix. Four variants—the physaliferous cell type, the syncytial type, pink-cell variant, and mixed types—are found (see Color Fig. 1-9).[47] Rarely, a spindle cell variant is seen. The pink-cell variant resembles metastatic carcinoma, and keratin staining may not help to resolve this problem, but few carcinomas are S100 positive as is chordoma. Lobular architecture with nodules of tumor surrounded by bands of fibrosis are typical. These subtypes do not differ in prognosis.[98] Diagnostic physaliferous cells have large vesicular nu-

clei and cytoplasmic vacuolation, resembling lipoblasts to some extent, but they may be hard to find in the syncytial variant. Nucleoli are inconspicuous, and mitoses are rare. Cartilage and bone may be present and may prompt the differential diagnosis of other bone-forming neoplasms.

A cartilaginous type of tumor in the spheno-occipital region[95] and rarely the sacrococcygeal region[99] is often designated chondroid chordoma, and it may have a better prognosis than the nonchondroid tumors of that site.[95] This tumor, because of its immunohistochemical similarity to chondrocytic tumors and lack of dual epithelial-mesenchymal staining pattern, is considered a variant of chondrosarcoma, rather than chordoma, by Brooks.[100] Differing with this opinion, Hruban and colleagues have shown that sacrococcygeal chondroid chordomas with a typical microscopic appearance and the biphenotypic immunostaining pattern of chordoma may exist as well.[99]

The clear cell features with glycogen accumulation and occasional signet-ring cells may suggest renal cell carcinoma or metastatic signet-ring carcinoma. Pink cells may resemble metastatic prostate carcinoma, but metastatic carcinoma usually lacks the lobular features of chordoma. Positive immunostaining (see Color Fig. 1-10) for S100,[89] EMA, and cytokeratin[101] in chordoma are useful to rule out carcinoma (i.e., keratin positive, S100 negative), chondrosarcoma (i.e., S100 positive, negative for other stains), and myxopapillary ependymoma (i.e., glial fibrillary acidic protein and lysozyme positive,[100] S100 and keratin negative). A rare tumor called parachordoma or chordoma periphericum (i.e., Dabska tumor) resembles chordoma microscopically, immunologically, and ultrastructurally but occurs in the long bones as a juxtacortical or soft-tissue tumor.[102,103]

Distant metastasis in chordoma has been reported in as many as 43% of patients, most commonly to skin and bone[104] or to lung.[105] Analogous to dedifferentiated chondrosarcoma, dedifferentiated chordoma (i.e., chordoma with a malignant spindle cell component) is an aggressive neoplasm with features of malignant fibrous histiocytoma or osteosarcoma, and its presence portends an accelerated clinical course.[99] Loss of immunostaining for keratin and S100 in the high-grade malignant areas is typical.[106]

Giant Cell Tumor

The classical benign giant cell tumor occurs in the epiphysis of a long bone, commonly the distal femur, proximal tibia, lower radius, or sacrum. Small bones of the hands and feet[107–109] and vertebrae[110] are rare sites and should suggest another diagnosis. Rarely, a giant cell tumor may be multicentric.[111–113] Eighty-five percent of the patients are 20 years of age or older, and the lesion rarely occurs in children. Giant cell tumor has been associated with Paget disease,[114] especially in the jaws,[61] a rare site otherwise for giant cell tumor. Involvement of the sphenoid and temporal bones is rare,[115] and tumors of the temporal bone with giant cells are usually chondroblastomas.[61] Giant cell tumors may appear as very aggressive tumors with cortical breakthrough, soft-tissue invasion, and crossing of joint spaces.[116] However, none of these findings necessarily indicate that the giant cell tumor is malignant. The separation of benign from malignant tumors may be difficult to determine because as many as half of the benign tumors recur locally, and 5% to 10% metastasize, usually limited to the lungs. This criterion otherwise would be characteristic of malignancy.

Grossly, the tumors may be necrotic or hemorrhagic with cyst formation. Microscopically, giant cell tumor shows very large giant cells (see Color Fig. 1-11) and mononuclear stromal cells without the matrix that is seen in osteogenic, cartilaginous, and fibrogenic tumors. Giant cells may be seen in a large number of other neoplasms, including metaphyseal fibrous defect (i.e., nonossifying fibroma), giant cell reparative granuloma, chondromyxoid fibroma, chondroblastoma, eosinophilic granuloma, hyperparathyroid bone disease, solitary bone cyst, aneurysmal bone cyst, osteoid osteoma, and osteoblastoma.[4] Of these, only chondroblastoma is commonly in the radiologic differential diagnosis. Other radiographically considered malignant tumors such as chondrosarcoma, osteosarcoma, and malignant fibrous histiocytoma are excluded microscopically. Chondroblastoma may be difficult to differentiate from giant cell tumor, but it immunohisto-

chemically stains for S100 protein,[117] like eosinophilic granuloma.[118] Electron microscopy is helpful in the diagnosis of eosinophilic granuloma in which diagnostic Birbeck granules are found ultrastructurally (Fig. 1-19). The distribution of giant cells is usually uniform, unlike the uneven appearance in other giant cell-containing lesions.

The essential finding that favors malignant giant cell tumor is found in the microscopic examination of the stroma of the tumor, but grading of the stromal component has little value.[119] Increasing cellularity and mitotic activity correlate with malignant behavior, but even completely benign-appearing tumors may metastasize (usually after curetting), and the metastases may also appear benign.[120] Histologically, malignancy cannot be predicted with certainty,[121] and attempts to correlate ploidy with metastatic tendency have shown no correlation.[122] Malignant giant cell tumor may have an osteoid stroma, but most are fibrosarcomatous.[123] Tumors with this appearance require the presence of current or previous ordinary giant cell tumor. Typically, these patients have poor survival rates. A history of irradiation is common in patients with malignant giant cell tumor. Dahlin reported one malignant giant cell tumor for every 15 benign giant cell tumors.[12]

Ewing Sarcoma and Related Lesions

Ewing sarcoma, a tumor of unknown histologic origin, occurs predominantly in children, peaking in the second decade. Ninety percent of patients are younger than 30 years of age.[124] Usually a diaphyseal tumor of the medullary cavity, it may be predominantly perios-

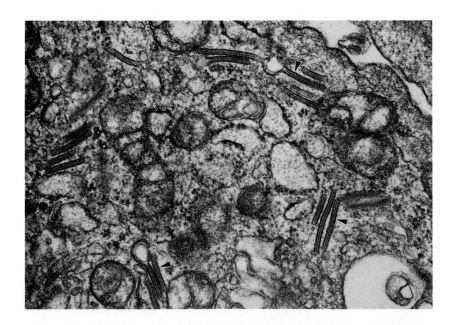

FIGURE 1-19. An electron micrograph of eosinophilic granuloma reveals diagnostic tennis-racket–shaped inclusions (*arrowheads*), the Birbeck granules of Langerhans cells.

teal or entirely outside of bone (i.e., soft-tissue Ewing sarcoma). The radiographs often show permeative destruction of bone, commonly in the femur, humerus, ilium, or rib. The tumor spreads to the lung, pleura, lymph nodes, and brain. Bone involvement may be multicentric with visceral involvement at presentation in as many as 25% of patients.[125] Soft-tissue involvement is prognostically unfavorable.[126]

Microscopically, Ewing sarcoma (Fig. 1-20A; see Color Fig. 1-12) is a round, small cell sarcoma (originally called "diffuse endothelioma of bone" by Ewing in 1921). Ewing sarcoma typically has an organoid appearance, with biphasic tumor cell populations of light and dark pyknotic cells but may show predominantly large cells, which is designated atypical Ewing sarcoma.[127] The differential diagnosis of typical Ewing

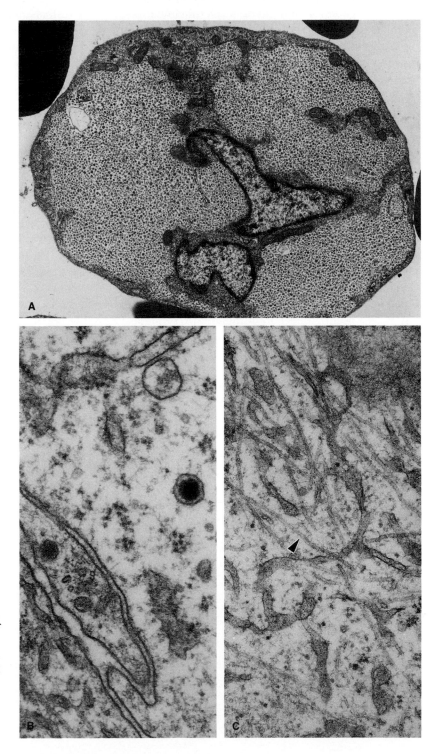

FIGURE 1-20. Peripheral neuroepithelioma or Ewing sarcoma of bone, is a small, round, blue cell tumor requiring electron microscopy, cytogenetics, and immunohistochemistry for the definitive exclusion of other similar-appearing tumors. **(A)** Electron micrographs show glycogen pools and an absence of organelles in a typical Ewing sarcoma. **(B)** A peripheral neuroepithelioma with neuritic processes. **(C)** A peripheral neuroepithelial tumor shows differentiated cytoplasmic microtubules. (See Color Figure 1-12.)

sarcoma is that of small, round, blue cell tumors.[128] Tumors that should be considered are lymphoma, metastatic rhabdomyosarcoma, metastatic medulloblastoma, metastatic carcinoma, neuroblastoma, and peripheral neuroepithelial tumor (PNET).[129] In these tumors, microscopic diagnosis is usually definitive for malignancy, but the exact differentiation of the cell type of the tumor often requires special studies, including histochemical and immunohistochemical stains, cytogenetics, and electron microscopy, if possible. The radiologist may aid the diagnosis by giving a radiographic differential diagnosis that includes Ewing sarcoma and suggesting to the pathologist that tissue be saved for cytogenetic studies, molecular diagnostic studies, and electron microscopy. Frozen-section preparations may confirm the differential diagnosis problem of the small, blue cell tumor and verify that nonnecrotic tissue has been obtained. Notable in the differential diagnosis is medulloblastoma, the commonest tumor of the central nervous system to give rise to extracranial metastasis.[130] Medulloblastoma bone metastasis may be osteoblastic, lytic, or mixed.[131]

The differential findings by histochemical staining in these tumors are summarized in Table 1-9. Ewing sarcoma is typically a glycogen-rich tumor, demonstrable in 80% of cases with periodic acid-Schiff (PAS) staining, and is poor in reticulin formation. The absence of PAS staining should suggest another diagnosis, but it may occur, especially if therapy precedes histochemical study.[23] Important antigenic differentiation markers may now be demonstrated by immunoperoxidase staining and can distinguish these otherwise morphologically similar tumors. Immunohistochemical stains may show myogenic, neural, or lymphoid differentiation that excludes Ewing sarcoma. Ewing sarcoma may exhibit epithelial differentiation that mimics metastatic carcinoma or may exhibit neural differentiation, pointing to a diagnosis of PNET. Two newer immunohistochemical studies of the expression of neural cell adhesion molecules (NCAM) with the antibody 5.1H11[132] and a Ewing-associated antigen HBA71 (see Color Fig. 1-12B)[133] are promising for differentiating the two classes of neural tumors, neuroblastoma, and Ewing or PNET (see Table 1-9).

Considerable evidence is mounting that Ewing sarcoma, PNET, and the thoracopulmonary tumor of Askin are part of a spectrum of tumors that may have overt neural differentiation by ultrastructure, as in the latter two, or no evident differentiation by ultrastructure, as in the Ewing tumor.[134] The thoracopulmonary tumor of Askin also shares features of Ewing and PNET by light and electron microscopy[135] and by staining with HBA71.

Cytogenetics may be useful in confirming Ewing sarcoma or PNET through the demonstration of a characteristic chromosomal abnormality, a translocation (t:11;22) that is found in Ewing sarcoma, PNET, and the Askin tumor.[136] Neuroblastoma differs in the pres-

TABLE 1-9.
Differential Diagnosis for Ewing Sarcoma

Tumor Type	Reaction to Stain								
	Glycogen	Reticulin	Keratin	Desmin	Leu-7	Neuron-Specific Enolase	Leukocyte Common Antigen (CD45)	Neural Cell Adhesion Molecules§	Ewing Sarcoma Antigen (HBA71)‖
Ewing sarcoma or PNET*	+	−	+	−	+	−	−	−	+
Lymphoma†	−	+	−	−	−	−	+	−	−/+
Rhabdomyosarcoma	+	−	−	+	+	−	−	+	−/+
Medulloblastoma	−	−	−	−	+	+	−	+	−
Carcinoma‡	−	−	+	−	±	±	−	±	−/+
Neuroblastoma†	−	−	−	−	+	+	−	+	−/+

+, positive; −, negative; ±, sometimes positive; −/+, usually negative.
*Cytokeratins are sometimes detected in Ewing sarcoma or peripheral neuroepithelioma (PNET) samples.[194]
†Some lymphomas and neuroblastomas[195] may be glycogen positive, but Ewing sarcoma is uncommonly glycogen negative. Glycogen is demonstrated by periodic acid-Schiff staining that is sensitive to prior diastase digestion.
‡Anti-neuron specific enolase (NSE) may also stain 20% of carcinomas with or without confirmed neuroendocrine differentiation.[196] Rhabdomyosarcoma rarely may be NSE positive.[197] Leu-7 positivity is described for prostatic carcinomas,[198] small cell lung carcinomas,[199] and thymomas,[200] but these are exceptions to the general findings for carcinomas.[201]
§The results of neural cell adhesion molecule (NCAM) tagging, identified with the antibody 5.1H11, are positive in 10% of samples of Ewing sarcoma or PNET.
‖Monoclonal antibody HBA71 (i.e., equivalent antibody is 013, Sigma Chemical, St. Louis, MO) reacts with the p30/32^{mic2} (i.e., Ewing sarcoma) antigen with a frequency of 95%. Twenty percent of lymphomas stain positively, and in 20% of rhabdomyosarcomas and 3% of carcinomas, 10% to 40% of the tumor cells stain positively (i.e., heterogeneous staining).[133]

ence of chromosome 1 deletions or rearrangements in stage III and IV disease, lack of the t:11;22 translocation, and presence of elevated levels of catecholamines that are not seen in PNETs.

The differential diagnosis may be clarified by ultrastructural examination (see Fig. 1-20). Electron microscopy identifies morphologic tumor markers through the recognition of differentiation specific organelles.[137] Tumors with neural differentiation, such as medulloblastoma, variants of primitive neuroectodermal tumors of the central nervous system, peripheral neuroectodermal tumors of bone, and neuroblastoma, may exhibit dense core neurosecretory granules and complex cytoplasmic dendritic processes (see Fig. 1-20C) or microtubules (see Fig. 1-20D). Rarely, ependymal differentiation is seen.[138] Rhabdomyosarcomas may show characteristic thick and thin filaments or Z-bands of myogenic differentiation. Carcinomas may show cell attachment structures, desmosomes, basement membrane investment, mucin, or tonofilaments. These features are not seen in Ewing sarcoma, for which the only finding is usually pools of glycogen (see Table 1-9) and microtubules (10% of cases).[139] For the latter finding, the distinction of Ewing sarcoma from PNET is blurred ultrastructurally and may represent the variable expression of neural differentiation in these related tumors. Caution is warranted in poorly differentiated tumors that may lack specific organelles. The pathologist should resist the temptation to lump these as Ewing sarcoma without the correlative clinical and radiographic findings typical of Ewing sarcoma.

Melanotic Neuroectodermal Tumor of Infancy

This small, round, blue cell tumor with melanin pigmentation reveals melanocytic and neuroblastic differentiation by electron microscopy and must be differentiated from metastatic neuroblastoma and Ewing sarcoma. Most (95%) are benign. Children younger than 1 year of age are predominantly affected, and 70% of the tumors are located in the maxilla. Only one case was described in a long bone.[140]

Malignant Lymphoma

Lymphomas of bone are classified by their morphologic appearance as non-Hodgkin lymphoma or Hodgkin disease. Malignant lymphomas may present as primary tumors of bone. These tumors occur at all ages but are distinctly more common after the age of 30. Patients present with pain and swelling or nerve involvement if tumors are located in the vertebrae. In one large series, 42% (179 of 422) of tumors were primary, 38% (161 of 442) had soft-tissue or lymph node involvement, and 19% (82 of 422) were multifocal.[141] Radiographically, the diaphysis (or metaphysis) of the long bone shows permeative destruction, but pure lytic, sclerotic, or mixed lesions may occur. The radiographic features have no diagnostic specificity.[142]

The differential diagnosis may include osteosarcoma, Ewing sarcoma, carcinoma, or osteomyelitis. Frozen-section examination usually narrows the differential considerably and helps determine the types of studies necessary for diagnosis. Most lymphomas of bone are the large cell type,[142] larger than the cells of Ewing sarcoma (except for the atypical Ewing tumors), and lymphoma may be strongly suspected at frozen section. As with nodal lymphomas, frozen section should not be used for immediate diagnosis, because the intraoperative procedure is not affected. However, assessment of the adequacy of the tissue obtained by biopsy for diagnosis and research studies and tissue triage for the often numerous studies requested are reasons to ask for a frozen section. Most useful are immunohistochemical stains for B-cell and T-cell markers (also possible on touch preparations, avoiding the problems of decalcified tissue). Other studies may consist of cytogenetic chromosomal analysis, DNA preparations for polymerase chain reaction (PCR) amplification, or Southern blots to examine T-cell and B-cell receptor rearrangements, and bacteriologic culture.

Typical microscopic findings in non-Hodgkin lymphomas are a sheet-like growth of noncohesive cells devoid of matrix. Diffuse, large cell lymphoma of the B-cell type is the most common type in Western countries, but T-cell lymphomas comprise 10% of bone lymphomas in Japan.[143] Some studies have shown a significant effect of the cytologic presence of cleaved or noncleaved large cells in patients with disease limited to one site.

In one study, patients with large cleaved and multilobated lymphomas had better survival rates than those with large noncleaved and immunoblastic lymphomas.[142,144] However, other studies have shown no significant prognostic value for the histologic grade of the lymphoma (i.e., low, intermediate, or high grade in the Working Formulation), while noting significant effects of stage of disease, site (i.e., spine and pelvis worse than jaws and femur), and age (i.e., poor prognosis for patients younger than 19 years of age).[141]

The pattern of lymphoma may be mimicked in Ewing sarcoma, small cell osteosarcoma, and other small, round, blue cell tumors (discussed with Ewing sarcoma). The larger nuclei of large cell lymphoma, presence of nucleoli, eosinophilic cytoplasm, and reticulin staining between individual cells favor lymphoma, because these findings are absent in ordinary Ewing sarcoma. Specific immunohistochemical staining for CD45 and the B-cell marker L26 (CD20) or T-cell marker UCHL-1 are found in lymphomas and not in the other small, round, blue cell tumors.[145] Burkitt lymphoma (i.e., small noncleaved cell type in the Working Formulation) may involve the long bones or pelvis.[146] Because of the small cell appearance of this neoplasm microscopically, confusion with Ewing sarcoma may occur, but attention to the cytologic features should allow differentiation. Other diagnostic pitfalls are the presence of signet-ring lymphoma, simulating metastatic mucinous carcinoma, and alveolar or single file growth that simulates carcinoma.[141] Special stains for keratin and CD45 usually resolve this problem. Other subtypes of lymphoma are possible with bone involvement. Their classification follows the Working Formulation for malignant lymphomas,[147] but as many as 18% may be unclassifiable.[141] Hodgkin disease comprised 3.1% of bone lymphomas in one large series.[141] Ordinary nodal Hodgkin disease commonly has bone changes, but the bone lesions may occur as the first manifestation of disease.[148]

Hemangiopericytoma

Hemangiopericytoma is a rare tumor, with only 7 cases in the Mayo Clinic series of 8542 bone tumors[12,149] and another 41 described in the literature.[150,151] The tumor usually occurs in persons older than 30 years of age. About one third of patients develop metastases, usually to the lungs, but malignant behavior is difficult to predict. One form of giant cell-containing hemangiopericytoma-like tumor is associated with osteomalacia, phosphate depletion, and production of renal phospha-turic substance. This phosphaturic mesenchymal tumor is usually benign.[152] Hemangiopericytoma is most common in the pelvis, presenting as a tender mass.[149] The radiographic appearance is usually purely lytic, but occasionally, it is honeycombed. Microscopically, the tumor contains cellular spindle areas with branched staghorn-shaped vessels. Grading is based on mitotic rate, cellularity, atypicality, and vascular architectural pattern.[150] The differential diagnosis includes other vascular tumors, mesenchymal chondrosarcoma with hemangiopericytoma-like areas, and small cell osteosarcoma. Immunocytochemical stains for factor VIII-related antigen and *Ulex europaeus* distinguishes vascular tumors, and Leu-7 and S100 are stainable in mesenchymal chondrosarcoma. Osteoid should be found for the diagnosis of small cell osteosarcoma.[25]

Hemangioendothelioma and Related Lesions

The group of vasoformative tumors includes epithelioid hemangioendothelioma (Fig. 1-21; see Color Fig. 1-13),[153–155] histiocytoid hemangioma,[156] and angiosarcoma.[154,157] These tumors vary from intermediate malignancy and low-grade malignancy to high-grade, fully malignant tumors. About 10 times more common than hemangiopericytoma, they may occur in almost any site, and in about 25% of patients, they are multicentric. The lesions are usually lytic and without periosteal reaction. The radiographic differential diagnosis usually includes osteosarcoma, fibrosarcoma, malignant fibrous histiocytoma, and malignant lymphoma. Metastatic carcinoma is often suspected when multicentric disease is seen.

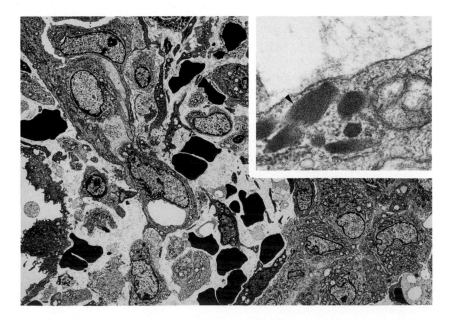

FIGURE 1-21. An electron micrograph of epithelioid hemangioma, or histiocytoid hemangioma. Endothelial Weible-Palade body (*inset*). (See Color Figure 1-13.)

Grossly, the lesions are bloody, dark red, and soft. Bone destruction may be evident. Microscopically, the low-grade tumors often show histiocytoid features with abundant eosinophilic cytoplasm and vesicular nuclei, low mitotic rates, and often grooved nuclei. Architecturally, they have anastomosing vascular channels, often with papillary folds in the vessels, hemorrhage, and stromal eosinophils or inflammatory cells. Metastases are unusual, but the patients often have a protracted course and may have associated soft-tissue lesions.[158,159] If associated with myxoid change, cartilaginous differentiation may occur, which was designated myxoid angioblastomatosis by Mirra.[160] A reticulin stain is useful for showing the clusters of tumor cells that have vasoformative tendency within the reticulin outlines. *Ulex europaeus* and factor VIII-related antigen staining also allow definition of the vascular cells (see Color Fig. 1-13).

High-grade neoplasms demonstrate pleomorphism, mitotic activity, enlarged nuclei, and necrosis. They often show little vasoformative tendency, exhibiting a predominance of solid spindle cell areas. The clinical behavior reflects the grade of tumor,[161] and metastases to the lungs are common. The differential diagnosis should include vascularized osteogenic sarcoma and metastatic carcinoma,[162] especially the well-vascularized renal cell carcinoma.[163] Correct interpretation should consider a panel of immunohistochemical stains, including those for vascular markers (factor VIII-related antigen and *Ulex europaeus*), and cytokeratins. Electron microscopy may be helpful in showing endothelial cell cytoplasmic differentiation (see Fig. 1-21).

Two related angiomatous lesions that may show skeletal destruction are skeletal angiomatosis[164] and massive osteolysis (i.e., Gorham disease).[165] Both are benign but may be associated with marked morbidity, including a hyperdynamic circulation, microangiopathic, hemolytic anemia, and respiratory impairment from thoracic fractures. These diseases are defined by their clinicoradiologic features, and pathologic examination shows hemangioma-like features, unlike the malignant changes described earlier.

Fibrosarcoma

Fibrosarcomas of bone occur commonly near the knee with about one fourth arising in the femur. Usually purely lytic without sclerosis, tumors may be poorly marginated and involve adjacent soft tissues, but the periosteal reaction is scant. Almost one third arise in preexisting lesions. Because the age distribution is older than that for osteosarcoma, myeloma and metastatic carcinoma are usually in the differential diagnosis, but giant cell tumor and osteosarcoma are also considerations radiologically.

Grossly, the lesions show firm tissue that may have hemorrhage, necrosis, myxoid changes, and cortical breakthrough. Microscopically, the presence of spindle cells evokes considerations of desmoplastic fibroma, malignant fibrous histiocytoma, fibroblastic osteosarcoma, and spindle cell carcinoma. Myeloma and giant cell tumor are excluded by the microscopic examination. Fibrosarcoma is characteristically defined by a herringbone pattern of the spindle cells. Collagenization of the tumor correlates with lower histologic grade and may be extensive. High nuclear grade, mitotic activity, necrosis, and pleomorphism are features of high-grade fibrosarcoma.

The pathologic differential diagnosis may include benign tumors that are clearly excluded by the radiographic findings. The radiologist plays an important role in directing the pathologist to the correct interpretation. Histologically, the pathologist may confuse fibrous dysplasia or osteofibrous dysplasia with fibrosarcoma. The correct interpretation requires recognition of the associated bone trabecular changes in these benign lesions. Fibrous dysplasia is a common asymptomatic bone lesion that affects the femoral neck or rib and less commonly affects the tibia or fibula, predominantly in children and young adults, and it is often discovered incidentally in radiographs. A polyostotic form is associated with skin pigmentation, isosexual precocity, thyroid abnormalities, and unilateral skeletal lesions. Gross examinations of resected lesions reveals fusiform lesions with dusky, gritty tissue in the medullary cavity and a thinned cortex. Polarized light microscopy reveals immature woven bone that forms thin and irregular trabeculae appearing as O, C, and Y shapes in two-dimensional profiles (see Color Fig. 1-14), unlike the lamellar trabeculae of normal mature bone. The stroma may be moderately cellular and mistaken for fibrosarcoma, but it is not atypical. Secondary changes may complicate the histologic picture with islands of atypical cartilage, cyst formation, giant cell or foam cell reactions, or pathologic fractures that evoke callus formation. Malignant tumors have occurred in fibrous dysplasia only rarely.

Osteofibrous dysplasia of long bones is a lesion that is also called intracortical fibrous dysplasia, ossifying fibroma, congenital fibrous defect of the tibia, or congenital and infantile pseudoarthrosis of the tibia. The lesion in children and adolescents is intracortical in the tibia, may involve the adjacent fibula, and is associated with anterior bowing. The similar-appearing lesion of the jaws (i.e., ossifying fibroma) is considered by some to be densely ossified fibrous dysplasia. In the tibia, the lesion may be multifocal and shows microscopically marked rimming of woven and lamellar trabeculae lined by osteoblasts (see Color Fig. 1-15), unlike fibrous dysplasia.[166] Campanacci[170] described the zonal architecture of osteofibrous dysplasia, characterized by gradual change from a loose fibrous zone in the center to dense cancellous bone at the periphery of the lesion. If this fibrous zone is biopsied, confusion with fibrosarcoma may occur. The cessation of the growth of the lesion with skeletal maturation is common, but recurrences may follow curetting or subperiosteal resection.

This lesion must be differentiated from adamantinoma of the tibia, which it may mimic radiologically and pathologically and which may occur with osteofibrous dysplasia.[167,168] The relation of these lesions is demonstrated by the finding of keratin-positive cells in osteofibrous dysplasia that occurs without adamantinoma.[169] Adamantinoma, unlike osteofibrous dysplasia, is unusual in children younger than 10 years of age.

Nonossifying fibroma is also called metaphyseal fibrous defect. The nonossifying fibroma is common in children and adolescents and represents a mature stage in the evolution of the cortical defect. Lesions commonly involve the tibia, fibula, and lower femur. Easily diagnosed radiographically, these lesions may be quite difficult to determine histopathologically, especially if complicated by fractures. Early lesions contain abundant, scattered or clustered giant cells, hemorrhage, and storiform architecture of the fibrous element, evoking differential considerations of giant cell tumor, hyperparathyroid brown tumors, and fibrous histiocytoma. The bone involved (e.g., ribs and vertebrae for fibrous histiocytoma), location in the bone (e.g., epiphyseal location of giant cell tumor) and clinical features (e.g., serum calcium abnormalities in hyperparathyroidism) with characteristic histopathologic findings can establish the diagnosis. Mature lesions are scarred with foam cell accumulation, hemosiderin deposits, and ossification (see Color Fig. 1-16). Careful attention to the cytologic features of the fibrous proliferation is important to rule out the rare intracortical osteosarcoma,[31,32] fibroblastic osteosarcoma, and fibrosarcoma.

A form of multiple nonossifying fibromas with extraskeletal abnormalities was described in 1978 as the Jaffe-Campanacci syndrome, consisting of café au lait spots, retardation, cataracts, and hypogonadism.[47,170,171] One instance of familial nonossifying fibromas has been described.[172] No definite association with neurofibromatosis has been demonstrated.[47]

Desmoplastic fibroma, a rare benign tumor that may be purely lytic, usually occurs in patients younger than 30 years of age. Microscopically, the lesion resembles extraskeletal aggressive fibromatosis, with low cellularity and a cytologically bland appearance. The herringbone pattern of fibrosarcoma is not evident, but the lesion may overlap histologically with low-grade fibrosarcoma in some cases that are more cellular.

Desmoplastic fibroma, although locally aggressive and prone to local recurrence, does not metastasize.[173] Microscopic exclusion of malignant fibrous histiocytoma depends on the absence of malignant features or the storiform pattern that defines the architectural appearance of this tumor. Areas of malignant fibrous histiocytoma may be found in otherwise typical fibrosarcoma, a finding that does not alter the prognosis of the fibrosarcoma.[174] The diagnosis of fibroblastic osteosarcoma requires diligent searching for areas of malignant osteoid that may be small. The diagnosis of spindle cell carcinoma is facilitated by positive immunohistochemical staining for appropriate keratin peptides.

Malignant Fibrous Histiocytoma

Malignant fibrous histiocytoma of bone appears similar to its soft-tissue counterpart. Predominantly a tumor of the long bones[175] or jaws,[176] it affects patients of all ages. Malignant fibrous histiocytoma occurs as a secondary bone tumor arising in the setting of a bone infarct,[82,177] foreign body,[178] after irradiation,[179] Paget disease,[175] or as the spindle cell high-grade component of dedifferentiated chondrosarcoma[78] or chordoma.[180,181] Malignant fibrous histiocytoma presents as a secondary tumor in 30% of cases. It may appear as the poorly differentiated component of a chondrosarcoma (i.e., dedifferentiated chondrosarcoma), chordoma (i.e., dedifferentiated chordoma), or as an isolated finding in otherwise typical osteosarcoma. Convention dictates that tumors without an associated component of cartilage or notochordal elements are called malignant fibrous histiocytoma. The other biphasic tumors are designated "dedifferentiated" by pathologists, even with the awareness that no dedifferentiation of cellular elements has been shown biologically.

Controversy exists over whether malignant fibrous histiocytoma exists.[182] Some researchers consider malignant fibrous histiocytoma as a common final morphologic expression of a high-grade tumor of mesenchyme regardless of the cell of origin. Similar arguments have been put forth for soft-tissue pleomorphic sarcomas classified as malignant fibrous histiocytoma initially. These tumors have been reclassified in 63% of cases after extensive immunohistochemical and ultrastructural examinations were performed to identify a specific line of differentiation.[183]

Grossly, malignant fibrous histiocytoma is a soft or fibrotic tumor that may exhibit necrosis and hemorrhage if it is high grade. In the dedifferentiated forms of chondrosarcoma, a cartilaginous component is evident. Microscopically, the lesions show a storiform or cartwheel pattern of spindle cell proliferation and may have a variable content of multinucleated giant cells, pleomorphic large cells, necrosis, and mitotic activity. Lipid-laden macrophages (i.e., xanthoma cells) may occur. The different histologic subtypes of malignant fibrous histiocytoma of bone do not differ in prognosis.[175]

The pathologic differential diagnosis usually includes benign fibrous lesions such as fibroma, benign histiocytoma, giant cell tumors of bone or synovium, and giant cell reparative granuloma. Malignant lesions such as carcinoma and fibroblastic osteosarcoma or fibrosarcoma should also be considered. Malignant fibrous histiocytoma may occur as a component of fibrosarcoma.[174] Useful in the diagnosis is the finding of muscle-specific actin (HHF-35) immunostaining in about half of malignant fibrous histiocytoma cases, correlating with the contractile properties of the myofibroblast cell, the presumed cell of origin of malignant fibrous histiocytoma. A lack of keratin immunostaining is useful for exclusion of metastatic carcinoma, but staining may occur focally in malignant fibrous histiocytoma.

Adamantinoma

Adamantinoma, a rare tumor, is located predominantly in the tibia (90% of patients) but also occurs in the femur, ulna, fibula, and the pretibial soft tissue.[184] An association with osteofibrous dysplasia has been observed.[167] The tumor is a low-grade malignancy, with metastases occurring, usually to the lungs, in as many as 20% of patients. It often consists microscopically of loose basaloid nests (i.e., stellate reticulum) with peripheral palisading. Campanacci described four types: basaloid, squamoid, spindle, and tubular. No difference in prognosis is correlated with any subtype. Mesenchymal differentiation may also accompany epithelial nests in a fibrous dysplastic pattern.[185] Lesions may be confused with vascular tumors and fibrosarcomas, but immunocytochemical stains for keratins (positive) and factor VIII-associated antigen (negative) are helpful in arriving at the correct diagnosis. Ultrastructural studies have demonstrated the epithelial nature of the tumor.[186] Metastatic squamous carcinoma is more problematic in older patients, but the typical radiographic appearance of adamantinoma is helpful in making the correct diagnosis.

Miscellaneous Rare Malignant Tumors

Myxoid liposarcoma is a rare primary bone tumor. Myxoid changes, however, are common in many bone lesions, including benign myxoma of bone, ganglia, neurilemoma, fibrous dysplasia, fibrosarcoma, chondrosarcoma, chondroma, and chondromyxoid fi-

broma.[187] Primary leiomyosarcoma of bone is so rare as to be a curiosity. About a dozen well-documented cases have appeared in the literature.[188,189] Malignant mesenchymoma is a neoplasm with two or more unrelated, differentiated tissue elements other than a fibrosarcomatous component, originally described by Stout in the soft tissues.[190] Differentiated elements may consist of rhabdomyosarcoma, liposarcoma, or leiomyosarcoma. Mixed components of only cartilage, fibrosarcomatous stroma, and malignant osteoid should not be categorized as mesenchymoma unless other differentiated neoplastic components are seen.[191] This may become a semantic problem; for example, in dedifferentiated chondrosarcoma, areas of rhabdomyosarcoma may be seen.[83,192]

References

1. Ackerman LV: Common errors made by pathologists in the diagnosis of bone tumors. Recent Results Cancer Res 54:120, 1976
2. Ewing JA: A review and classification of bone sarcomas. Arch Surg 4:485, 1922
3. Ragsdale BD, Sween DE, Vinh TN: Radiology as gross pathology in evaluating chondroid lesions. Hum Pathol 20:930, 1989
4. Rosai J: Ackerman's Surgical Pathology. St. Louis, CV Mosby, 1989:1472
5. Weatherby RP, Unni KK: Practical aspects of handling orthopaedic specimens in the surgical pathology laboratory. Pathol Annu 17:1, 1982
6. Madewell JE, Ragsdale BD, Sweet DE: Radiologic and pathologic analysis of solitary bone lesions. Part I: Internal margins. Radiol Clin North Am 19:715, 1981
7. Ragsdale BD, Madewell JE, Sweet DE: Radiologic and pathologic analysis of solitary bone lesions. Part II: Periosteal reactions. Radiol Clin North Am 19:749, 1981
8. Sweet DE, Madewell JE, Ragsdale BD: Radiologic and pathologic analysis of solitary bone lesions. Part III: Matrix pattern. Radiol Clin North Am 19:785, 1981
9. Spjut HJ, Dorfman HD: Florid reactive periostitis of the tubular bones of the hands and feet. A benign lesion which may simulate osteosarcoma. Am J Surg Pathol 5:423, 1981
10. Unni KK, Dahlin DC: Premalignant tumors and conditions of bone. Am J Surg Pathol 3:47, 1979
11. Fornasier VL: Fine detail radiography in the examination of tissue. Hum Pathol 6:623, 1975
12. Dahlin DC, Unni KK: Bone Tumors. General Aspects and Data on 8542 Cases. 4th ed. Springfield, IL, Charles C. Thomas, 1986
13. Wick MR, McLeod RA, Siegal GP, Greditzer HG, Unni KK: Sarcomas of bone complicating osteitis deformans (Paget's disease). Fifty years' experience. Am J Surg Pathol 5:47, 1981
14. Huvos AG, Butler A, Bretsky SS: Osteogenic sarcoma associated with Paget's disease of bone: A clinicopathologic study of 65 patients. Cancer 52:1489, 1983
15. Meadows A, D'Angio G, Mike V et al: Patterns of second malignant neoplasms in children. Cancer 40:1903, 1977
16. Abramson D, Ellsworth R, Kitchin F: Osteogenic sarcoma of the humerus after cobalt plaque treatment for retinoblastoma. Am J Ophthalmol 90:374, 1980
17. Abramson D, Ronner H, Ellsworth R: Second tumors in nonirradiated bilateral retinoblastoma. Am J Ophthalmol 87:624, 1979

18. Reissmann PT, Simon MA, Lee WH, Slamon DJ: Studies of the retinoblastoma gene in human sarcomas. Oncogene 4:839, 1989

19. Scholz RB, Kabisch H, Delling G, Winkler K: Homozygous deletion within the retinoblastoma gene in a native osteosarcoma specimen of a patient cured of a retinoblastoma of both eyes. Pediatr Hematol Oncol 7:265, 1990

20. Newton WA, Meadows AT, Shimada H et al: Bone sarcomas as second malignant neoplasms following childhood cancer. Cancer 67:193, 1991

21. Raymond AK, Chawla S, Carrasco CH et al: Osteosarcoma chemotherapy effect: A prognostic factor. Semin Diagn Pathol 4:212, 1987

22. Picci P, Bacci G, Campanacci M et al: Histologic evaluation of necrosis in osteosarcoma induced by chemotherapy. Regional mapping of viable and nonviable tumor. Cancer 56:1515, 1985

23. Ayala AG, Raymond AK, Jaffe N: The pathologist's role in the diagnosis and treatment of osteosarcoma in children. Hum Pathol 15:258, 1984

24. Carrasco CH, Charnsangavij C, Raymond AK et al: Osteosarcoma. Angiographic assessment of response to preoperative chemotherapy. Radiology 170:839, 1989

25. Martin SE, Dwyer A, Kissane JM, Costa J: Small-cell osteosarcoma. Cancer 50:990, 1982

26. Sim FH, Unni KK, Beabout JW, Dahlin DC: Osteosarcoma with small cells simulating Ewing's tumor. J Bone Joint Surg [Am] 61:207, 1979

27. De Dios AMV, Bond JR, Shives TC et al: Aneurysmal bone cyst: A clinicopathologic study of 238 cases. Cancer 69:2921, 1992

28. Martinez V, Sissons HA: Aneurysmal bone cyst: A review of 123 cases including primary lesions and those secondary to other bone pathology. Cancer 61:2291, 1988

29. Sanerkin NG, Mott MG, Roylance J: An unusual intraosseous lesion with fibroblastic, osteoclastic, osteoblastic, aneurysmal, and fibromyxoid elements: "Solid" variant of aneurysmal bone cyst. Cancer 51:2278, 1983

30. Unni KK, Dahlin DC, McLeod RA, Pritchard DJ: Intraosseous well differentiated osteosarcoma. Cancer 40:1337, 1977

31. Vigorita VJ, Jones JK, Ghelman B et al: Intracortical osteosarcoma. Am J Surg Pathol 8:65, 1984

32. Picci P, Gherlinzoni F, Guerra A: Intracortical osteosarcoma: Rare entity or early manifestation of classical osteosarcoma? Skeletal Radiol 9:255, 1983

33. Dorfman HD: Case records of the Massachusetts General Hospital, case 40. N Engl J Med 303:866, 1980

34. Byers PD: Solitary benign osteoblastic lesions of bone. Osteoid osteoma and benign osteoblastoma. Cancer 22:43, 1968

35. Schajowicz F, Lemos C: Osteoid osteoma and osteoblastoma. Acta Orthop Scand 41:272, 1970

36. Schajowicz F, Lemos C: Malignant osteoblastoma. J Bone Joint Surg [Br] 58:202, 1976

37. Dorfman HD, Weiss SW: Borderline osteoblastic tumors: Problems in the differential diagnosis of aggressive osteoblastoma and low-grade osteosarcoma. Semin Diagn Pathol 1:215, 1984

38. Bertoni F, Unni KK, McLeod RA et al: Osteosarcoma resembling osteoblastoma. Cancer 55:416, 1985

39. Mirra JM, Theros E, Smasson J et al: A case of osteoblastoma associated with severe systemic toxicity. Am J Surg Pathol 3:464, 1979

40. Steiner GC: Ultrastructure of osteoid osteoma. Hum Pathol 7:309, 1976

41. Mirra JM, Kendrick RA, Kendrick RE: Pseudomalignant osteoblastoma versus arrested osteosarcoma. A case report. Cancer 37:2005, 1976

42. Unni KK, Dahlin DC, Beabout JW, Ivins JC: Parosteal osteogenic sarcoma. Cancer 37:2466, 1976

43. Wold LE, Beabout JW, Unni KK, Dahlin DC: High-grade surface osteosarcomas. Am J Surg Pathol 8:181, 1984

44. Mirra J: Bone Tumors: Diagnosis and Treatment. Philadelphia, JB Lippincott, 1980

45. Unni KK, Dahlin DC, Beabout JW: Periosteal osteosarcoma. Cancer 37:2476, 1976

46. Bertoni F, Boriani S, Laus M, Campanacci M: Periosteal chondrosarcoma and periosteal osteosarcoma: Two distinct entities. J Bone Joint Surg [Br] 64:370, 1982

47. Mirra J: Bone tumors: Clinical, radiologic and pathologic correlations. Philadelphia, Lea & Febiger, 1989

48. Bauer T, Dorfman HD, Latham JT Jr: Periosteal chondroma: A clinicopathologic study of 23 cases. Am J Surg Pathol 6:631, 1982

49. Clark JL, Unni KK, Dahlin DC, Devine KD: Osteosarcoma of the jaw. Cancer 51:2311, 1983

50. Weatherby RP, Dahlin DC, Ivins JC: Postradiation sarcoma of bone. Review of 78 Mayo Clinic cases. Mayo Clin Proc 56:294, 1981

51. Kahn LB, Wood FW, Ackerman LV: Fracture callus associated with benign and malignant bone lesions and mimicking osteosarcoma. Am J Clin Pathol 52:14, 1969

52. Bauer HCF, Kreicbergs A, Silfversward C, Tribukait B: DNA analysis in the differential diagnosis of osteosarcoma. Cancer 61:1430, 1988

53. Adler C-P: Differential diagnosis of cartilage tumors. Pathol Res Pract 166:45, 1979

54. Garrison RC, Unni KK, McLeod RA et al: Chondrosarcoma arising in osteochondroma. Cancer 49:1890, 1982

55. Harris WH, Dudley HR, Barry RJ: The natural history of fibrous dysplasia. An orthopaedic, pathological, and roentgenographic study. J Bone Joint Surg [Am] 44:207, 1962

56. Mirra JM, Gold R, Downs J, Eckardt JJ: A new histologic approach to the differentiation of enchondroma from chondrosarcoma of the bones. A clinico-pathologic analysis of 51 cases. Clin Orthop 201:214, 1985

57. Liu J, Hudkins PG, Swee RF, Unni KK: Bone sarcomas associated with Ollier's disease. Cancer 59:1376, 1987

58. Schwartz HS, Zimmerman NB, Simon MA et al: The malignant potential of enchondromatosis. J Bone Joint Surg [Am] 69:269, 1987

59. Tamimi HK, Bolen JW: Enchondromatosis (Ollier's disease) and ovarian juvenile granulosa cell tumor. A case report and review of the literature. Cancer 53:1605, 1984

60. Lewis RJ, Ketcham AS: Maffucci's syndrome. Functional and neoplastic significance. Case report and review of the literature. J Bone Joint Surg [Am] 55:1465, 1973

61. Bertoni F, Unni KK, Beabout JW et al: Chondroblastoma of the skull and facial bones. Am J Clin Pathol 88:1, 1987

62. Tsuneyoshi M, Dorfman HD: Epiphyseal osteosarcoma. Distinguishing features from clear cell chondrosarcoma, chondroblastoma, and epiphyseal enchondroma. Hum Pathol 18:644, 1987

63. Dahlin DC, Ivins JC: Benign chondroblastoma. A study of 125 cases. Cancer 30:401, 1972

64. Kurt A-M, Unni KK, Sim FH, McLeod RA: Chondroblastoma of bone. Hum Pathol 20:965, 1989

65. Kyriakos M, Land VJ, Penning HL, Parker SG: Metastatic chondroblastoma. Report of a fatal case with a review of the literature on atypical, aggressive, and malignant chondroblastoma. Cancer 55:1770, 1985

66. Zillmer DA, Dorfman HD: Chondromyxoid fibroma of bone: Thirty-six cases with clinicopathologic correlation. Hum Pathol 20:952, 1989

67. Rahimi A, Beabout JW, Ivins JC, Dahlin DC: Chondromyxoid fibroma: A clinicopathologic study of 76 cases. Cancer 30:726, 1972

68. Dahlin DC, Salvador AH: Chondrosarcoma of the bones of the hands and feet: A study of 30 cases. Cancer 34:755, 1974

69. Bjornsson J, Unni KK, Dahlin DC et al: Clear cell chondrosarcoma of bone. Observations in 47 cases. Am J Surg Pathol 8:223, 1984

70. Huvos AG, Rosen G, Dabska M, Marcove, RC: Mesenchymal chondrosarcoma: A clinicopathologic analysis of 35 patients with emphasis on treatment. Cancer 51:1230, 1983

71. Kreicbergs A, Bosquist L, Borssen B, Larsson S-E: Prognostic factors in chondrosarcoma. A comparative study of cellular DNA content and clinicopathologic features. Cancer 50:577, 1982
72. O'Neal LW, Ackerman LV: Chondrosarcoma of bone. Cancer 5:551, 1951
73. Evans HL, Ayala AG, Romsdahl MM: Prognostic factors in chondrosarcoma of bone. A clinicopathologic analysis with emphasis on histologic grading. Cancer 40:818, 1977
74. Kreicbergs A, Slezak E, Soderberg G: The prognostic significance of different histomorphologic features in chondrosarcoma. Virchows Arch A Pathol Anat Histopathol 390:1, 1981
75. Gitelis S, Bertoni F, Picci P, Campanacci M: Chondrosarcoma of bone. The experience at the Istituto Ortopedico Rizzoli. J Bone Joint Surg [Am] 63:1248, 1981
76. Healey JH, Lane JM: Chondrosarcoma. Clin Orthop 204: 119, 1986
77. Pritchard DJ, Lunke RJ, Taylor WF et al: Chondrosarcoma. A clinicopathologic and statistical analysis. Cancer 45:149, 1980
78. Sanerkin NG, Gallagher P: A review of the behaviour of chondrosarcoma of bone. J Bone Joint Surg [Br] 61:395, 1979
79. Fernandez MP, Young MF, Sobel ME: Methylation of type II and type I collagen genes in differentiated and dedifferentiated chondrocytes. J Biol Chem 260:2374, 1985
80. Johnson S, Tetu B, Ayala AG, Chawla SP: Chondrosarcoma with additional mesenchymal component (dedifferentiated chondrosarcoma). I. A clinicopathologic study of 26 cases. Cancer 58:278, 1986
81. McCarthy EF, Dorfman HD: Chondrosarcoma of bone with dedifferentiation: A study of eighteen cases. Hum Pathol 13:36, 1982
82. McCarthy EF, Matsuno T, Dorfman HD: Malignant fibrous histiocytoma of bone: A study of 35 cases. Hum Pathol 10:57, 1979
83. Tetu B, Ordonez NG, Ayala AG, Mackay B: Chondrosarcoma with additional mesenchymal component (dedifferentiated chondrosarcoma). II. An immunohistochemical and electron microscopic study. Cancer 58:286, 1986
84. Nakashima Y, Unni KK, Shives TC, Swee RG, Dahlin DC: Mesenchymal chondrosarcoma of bone and soft tissue. A review of 111 cases. Cancer 57:2444, 1986
85. Steiner GC, Mirra JM, Bullough PG: Mesenchymal chondrosarcoma: A study of the ultrastructure Cancer 32:926, 1973
86. Jacobson SA: Polyhistioma. A malignant tumor of bone and extraskeletal tissues. Cancer 40:2116, 1977
87. Bertoni F, Picci P, Bacchine P et al: Mesenchymal chondrosarcoma of bone and soft tissues. Cancer 52:533, 1983
88. Martin RF, Melnick PJ, Warner NE et al: Chordoid sarcoma. Am J Clin Pathol 59:623, 1972
89. Wick MR, Burgess JH, Manivel JC: A reassessment of "chordoid sarcoma" ultrastructural and immunohistochemical comparison with chordoma and skeletal myxoid chondrosarcoma. Mod Pathol 1:433, 1988
90. Miettinen M, Lehto V-P, Dahl D, Virtanen I: Differential diagnosis of chordoma, chondroid, and ependymal tumors as aided by anti-intermediate filament antibodies. Am J Pathol 112:160, 1983
91. Weiss A-P, Dorfman HD: Clear-cell chondrosarcoma: A report of ten cases and review of the literature. Surg Pathol 1:123, 1988
92. Faraggiana T, Sender B, Glicksman P: Light- and electron-microscopic study of clear cell chondrosarcoma. Am J Clin Pathol 75:117, 1981
93. Unni KK, Dahlin DC, Beabout JW, Sim FH: Chondrosarcoma. Clear-cell variant. A report of sixteen cases. J Bone Joint Surg [Am] 58:676, 1976
94. Kaiser TE, Pritchard DJ, Unni KK: Clinicopathologic study of sacrococcygeal chordoma. Cancer 54:2574, 1984
95. Heffelfinger MJ, Dahlin DC, MacCarty CS, Beabout JW: Chordomas and cartilaginous tumors at the skull base. Cancer 32:410, 1973
96. Campbell WM, Mcdonald TJ, Unni KK, Laws ER Jr: Nasal and paranasal presentations of chordoma. Laryngoscope 90:612, 1980
97. Richter HJ, Batsakis JG, Bole R: Chordomas: Nasopharyngeal presentation and atypical long survival. Ann Otol Rhinol Laryngol 84:327, 1975
98. Azzarelli A, Quagliuolo V, Cerasoli S et al: Chordoma: Natural history and treatment results in 33 cases. J Surg Oncol 37:185, 1988
99. Hruban RH, May M, Marcove RC, Huvos AG: Lumbosacral chordoma with high-grade malignant cartilaginous and spindle cell components. Am J Surg Pathol 14:384, 1990
100. Brooks JJ, Troganowski JQ, LiVolsi VA: Chondroid chordoma: A low grade chondrosarcoma and its differential diagnosis. Curr Top Pathol 80:165, 1989
101. Salisbury J, Isaacson P: Demonstration of cytokeratins and epithelial membrane antigen in chordomas and human fetal notochord. Am J Surg Pathol 9:791, 1985
102. Dabska M: Parachordoma. A new clinicopathologic entity. Cancer 40:1586, 1977
103. Povysil C, Matejovsky Z: A comparative ultrastructural study of chondrosarcoma, chordoid sarcoma, chordoma, and chordoma periphericum. Pathol Res Pract 179:546, 1985
104. Chambers PW, Schwinn CP: Chordoma: A clinicopathologic study of metastasis. Am J Clin Pathol 72:765, 1979
105. Dehner LP: Pediatric Surgical Pathology. 2nd ed, p. 991. Williams & Wilkins, Baltimore, 1987
106. Meis JM, Raymond AK, Evans HL et al: Dedifferentiated chordoma. A clinicopathologic and immunohistochemical study of three cases. Am J Surg Pathol 11:516, 1987
107. Lorenzo JC, Dorfman HD: Giant cell reparative granuloma of short tubular bones of the hands and feet. Am J Surg Pathol 4:551, 1980
108. Wold LE, Swee RG: Giant cell tumor of the small bones of the hands and feet. Semin Diagn Pathol 1:173, 1984
109. Picci P, Baldini N, Sudanese A et al: Giant cell reparative granuloma and other giant cell lesions of the bones of the hands and feet. Skeletal Radiol 15:415, 1986
110. Savini R, Gherlinzoni F, Morandi M et al: Surgical treatment of giant cell tumor of the spine, Istituto Ortopedico Rizzoli. J Bone Joint Surg [Am] 65:1283, 1983
111. Sybrandy S, di la Fuente AA: Multiple giant cell tumor of bone. Report of a case. J Bone Joint Surg [Br] 55:350, 1973
112. Singson R, Feldman F: Multiple (multicentric) giant cell tumors of bone. Skeletal Radiol 9:276, 1983
113. Peimer CA, Schiller AL, Mankin JH, Smith RJ: Multicentric giant cell tumor of bone. J Bone Joint Surg [Am] 62:652, 1980
114. Jacobs TP, Michelsen J, Polay JS et al: Giant cell tumor in Paget's disease of bone. Familial and geographic clustering. Cancer 44:742, 1979
115. Wolfe JT III, Scheithauer BW, Dahlin DC: Giant cell tumor of the sphenoid bone: Review of 10 cases. J Neurosurg 59:322, 1983
116. Bertoni F, Present D, Enneking WF: Giant cell tumor of bone with pulmonary metastases. J Bone Joint Surg [Am] 67:890, 1985
117. Regezi JA, Zarbo RJ, Lloyd RV: Muramidase, alpha-1-antitrypsin, alpha-1-antichymotrypsin and S-100 protein immunoreactivity in giant cell lesions. Cancer 59:64, 1987
118. Beckstead JH, Wood G, Turner RR: Histiocytosis X cells and Langerhans cells: Enzyme histochemical and immunologic similarities. Hum Pathol 15:826, 1984
119. Sanerkin NG: Malignancy, aggressiveness, and recurrence in giant cell tumor of bone. Cancer 46:1641, 1980
120. Rock MG, Pritchard DJ, Unni KK: Metastases from histologically benign giant cell tumor of bone. J Bone Joint Surg [Am] 66:269, 1984
121. McDonald DJ, Sim FH, McLeod RA, Dahlin DC: Giant cell tumor of bone. J Bone Joint Surg [Am] 68:235, 1986

122. Ladanyi M, Traganos F, Huvos AG: Benign metastasizing giant cell tumors of bone. A DNA flow cytometric study. Cancer 64:1521, 1989

123. Rock MG, Sim FH, Juun KK et al: Secondary malignant giant cell tumor of bone. J Bone Joint Surg [Am] 68:1073, 1986

124. Kissane JM, Askin FB, Foulkes M et al: Ewing's sarcoma of bone. Clinicopathologic aspects of 303 cases from the Intergroup Ewing's Sarcoma Study. Hum Pathol 14:773, 1983

125. Gasparini M, Barni S, Lattuada A et al: Ten years' experience with Ewing's sarcoma. Tumori 63:77, 1977

126. Marcus RB Jr, Cantor A, Heare TC et al: Local control and function after twice-a-day radiotherapy for Ewing's sarcoma of bone. Int J Radiat Oncol Biol Phys 21:1509, 1991

127. Nascimento AG, Cooper KL, Unni KK et al: A clinicopathologic study of 20 cases of large-cell (atypical) Ewing's sarcoma of bone. Am J Surg Pathol 4:29, 1980

128. Triche TJ: Diagnosis of small round cell tumors of childhood. Bull Cancer 75:297, 1988

129. Jaffe R, Agostini RM, Santamaria M et al: The neuroectodermal tumor of bone. Am J Surg Pathol 12:885, 1984

130. Campbell AN, Chan HSL, Becker LE et al: Extracranial metastases in childhood primary intracranial tumors. A report of 21 cases and review of the literature. Cancer 53:974, 1984

131. Banna M, Lassman LP, Pearce GW: Radiological study of skeletal metastases from cerebellar medulloblastoma. Br J Radiol 43:173, 1970

132. Garin-Chesa P, Fellinger EJ, Huvos AG et al: Immunhistochemical analysis of neural cell adhesion molecules. Am J Pathol 139:275, 1991

133. Fellinger EJ, Garin-Chesa P, Triche TJ et al: Immunohistochemical analysis of Ewing's sarcoma cell surface antigen p30/32^{mic2}. Am J Pathol 139:317, 1991

134. Cavazzana AO, Miser JS, Jefferson J, Triche TJ: Experimental evidence for a neural origin of Ewing's sarcoma of bone. Am J Pathol 127:507, 1987

135. Askin FB, Rosai J, Sibley RK et al: Malignant small cell tumor of the thoracopulmonary region in childhood. A distinctive clinicopathologic entity of uncertain histogenesis. Cancer 43:2438, 1979

136. Maletz N, McMorrow LE, Greco MA, Wolman SR: Ewing's sarcoma. Pathology, tissue culture and cytogenetics. Cancer 58:252, 1986

137. Triche T: Morphologic tumor markers. Semin Oncol 14:139, 1987

138. Parham DM, Thompson E, Fletcher B, Meyer WH: Metastatic small cell tumor of bone with "true" rosettes and glial fibrillary acidic protein positivity. Am J Clin Pathol 95:166, 1991

139. Mahoney JP, Alexander RW: Ewing's sarcoma. A light and electron-microscopic study of 21 cases. Am J Surg Pathol 2:283, 1978

140. Johnson RE, Scheithauer BW, Dahlin DC: Melanotic neuroectodermal tumor of infancy. A malignant tumor of the femur. Mayo Clin Proc 57:719, 1982

141. Ostrowski ML, Unni KK, Banks PM et al: Malignant lymphoma of bone. Cancer 58:2646, 1986

142. Clayton F, Butler JJ, Ayala AG et al: Non-Hodgkin's lymphoma in bone. Cancer 60:2494, 1987

143. Ueda T, Aozasa K, Ohsawa M et al: Malignant lymphomas of bone in Japan. Cancer 64:2387, 1989

144. Dosoretz DE, Raymond AK, Murphy GF et al: Primary lymphoma of bone. The relationship of morphologic diversity to clinical behavior. Cancer 50:1009, 1982

145. Falini B, Binazzi R, Pileri S et al: Large cell lymphoma of bone. A report of three cases of B-cell origin. Histopathology 12:177, 1988

146. Fowles JV, Olweny CLM, Katongole-Mfiddle E et al: Burkitt's lymphoma in the apppendicular skeleton. J Bone Joint Surg [Br] 65:464, 1983

147. The Non-Hodgkin's Lymphoma Pathologic Classification Project, National Cancer Institute-sponsored study of classification of non-Hodgkin's lymphomas: Summary and description of a working formulation for clinical usage. Cancer 49:2112, 1982

148. Chan K-W, Rosen G, Miller DR, Tan CTC: Hodgkin's disease in adolescents presenting as a primary bone lesion. A report of four cases and review of the literature. Am J Pediat Hematol Oncol 4:11, 1982

149. Wold LE, Unni KK, Cooper KL et al: Hemangiopericytoma of bone. Am J Surg Pathol 6:53, 1982

150. Tang JSH, Gold RH, Mirra JM, Eckardt J: Hemangiopericytoma of bone. Cancer 62:848, 1988

151. Kahn LB, Nunnery EW, Lipper S, Reddick RL: Case report 144. Primary hemangiopericytoma of the right radius. Skeletal Radiol 6:139, 1981

152. Weidner N, Santa Cruz D: Phosphaturic mesenchymal tumors. A polymorphous group causing osteomalacia or ricket. Cancer 59:1442, 1987

153. Campanacci M, Boriani S, Giunti A: Hemangioendothelioma of bone: A study of 29 cases. Cancer 46:804, 1980

154. Dorfman HD, Steiner GC, Jaffe HL: Vascular tumors of bone. Hum Pathol 2:349, 1971

155. Otis J, Hutter RVP, Foote FW Jr et al: Hemangioendothelioma of bone. Surg Gynecol Obstet 127:295, 1968

156. Rosai J, Gold J, Landy R: The histiocytoid hemangiomas: A unifying concept embracing several previously described entities of skin, soft tissue, large vessels, bone and hear. Hum Pathol 10:707, 1979

157. Larsson S-E, Lorentzon R, Boquist L: Malignant hemangioendothelioma of bone. J Bone Joint Surg [Am] 57:84, 1975

158. Tsuneyoshi M, Dorfman HD, Bauer TW: Epithelioid hemangioendothelioma of bone. A clinicopathologic, ultrastructural, and immunohistochemical study. Am J Surg Pathol 10:754, 1986

159. Ose D, Vollmer R, Shelburne J et al: Histiocytoid hemangioma of the skin and scapula. A case report with electron microscopy and immunohistochemistry. Cancer 51:1656, 1983

160. Mirra JM, Kameda N: Myxoid angioblastomatosis of bones. A case report of a rare, multifocal entity with light, ultramicroscopic and immunopathologic correlation. Am J Surg Pathol 9:450, 1985

161. Wold LE, Unni KK, Beabout JW: Hemangioendothelial sarcoma of bone. Am J Surg Pathol 6:59, 1982

162. Weiss SW, Enzinger FM: Epithelioid hemangioendothelioma: A vascular tumor often mistaken for a carcinoma. Cancer 50:970, 1982

163. Unni KK, Ivins JC, Beabout JW et al: Hemangioma, hemangiopericytoma, and hemangioendothelioma (angiosarcoma) of bone. Cancer 27:1403, 1971

164. Gutierrez R, Spjut HJ: Skeletal angiomatosis. Clin Orthop 85:82, 1972

165. Halliday DR, Dahlin DC, Pugh DG et al: Massive osteolysis and angiomatosis. Radiology 82:636, 1964

166. Kempson R: Ossifying fibroma of the long bones: A light and electron microscopic study. Arch Pathol 82:218, 1966

167. Markel SF: Ossifying fibroma of long bones, its distinction from fibrous dysplasia and its association with adamantinoma of long bone. Am J Clin Pathol 69:91, 1978

168. Alguacil-Garcia A, Alonso A, Pettigrew NM: Osteofibrous dysplasia (ossifying fibroma) of the tibia and fibula and adamantinoma. Am J Clin Pathol 82:470, 1984

169. Sweet DE, Vinh TN, Devaney K: Cortical osteofibrous dysplasia of long bone and its relationship to adamantinoma. Am J Surg Pathol 16:282, 1992

170. Campanacci M, Boriani LS: Multiple non-ossifying fibromas with extraskeletal anomalies: A new syndrome? J Bone Joint Surg [Br] 65:627, 1983

171. Mirra JM, Gold RH, Rand F: Disseminated non-ossifying fibromas in association with cafe au lait spots (Jaffe-Campanacci syndrome). Clin Orthop 168:192, 1982

172. Evans GA, Park WM: Familial non-osteogenic fibromata. J Bone Joint Surg [Br] 60:416, 1978

173. Whitesides TE Jr, Ackerman LV: Desmoplastic fibroma. A report of three cases. J Bone Joint Surg [Am] 42:1143, 1960

174. Taconis WK, van Rijssel TG: Fibrosarcoma of the long bones. A study of the significance of areas of malignant fibrous histiocytoma. J Bone Joint Surg [Br] 67:111, 1985

175. Huvos AG, Heilweil M, Bretshy SS: The pathology of malignant fibrous histiocytoma of bone. A study of 130 patients. Am J Surg Pathol 9:853, 1985

176. Abdul-Karim FW, Ayala AG, Chawla SP et al: Malignant fibrous histiocytoma of jaws. A clinicopathologic study of 11 cases. Cancer 56:1590, 1985

177. Frierson HF Jr, Fechner RE, Stallings RG, Wang G-J: Malignant fibrous histiocytoma in bone infarct: Association with sickle cell trait and alcohol abuse. Cancer 59:496, 1987

178. Lee Y-S, Pho RWH, Nather A: Malignant fibrous histiocytoma at site of metal implant. Cancer 54:2286, 1984

179. Huvos AG, Woodard HQ, Heilweil M: Postradiation malignant fibrous histiocytoma of bone. A clinicopathologic study of 20 patients. Am J Surg Pathol 10:9, 1986

180. Belza MG, Urich H: Chordoma and malignant fibrous histiocytoma. Evidence for transformation. Cancer 58:1082, 1986

181. Miettinen M, Lehto V-P, Virtanen I: Malignant fibrous histiocytoma within a recurrent chordoma. A light microscopic, electron microscopic, and immunohistochemical study. Am J Clin Pathol 82:738, 1984

182. Dahlin DC, Unni KK, Matsuno T: Malignant (fibrous) histiocytoma of bone—fact or fancy? Cancer 39:1508, 1977

183. Fletcher CDM: Pleomorphic malignant fibrous histiocytoma: Fact or fiction? Am J Surg Pathol 16:213, 1992

184. Mills SE, Rosai J: Adamantinoma of the pretibial soft tissue. Clinicopathologic features, differential diagnosis and possible relationship to intraosseous disease. Am J Clin Pathol 83:108, 1985

185. Weiss SW, Dorfman HD: Adamantinoma of the long bones: An analysis of nine new cases with emphasis on metastasizing lesions and fibrous dysplasia-like changes. Hum Pathol 8:141, 1977

186. Rosai J: Adamantinoma of the tibia. Electron microscopic evidence of its epithelial origin. Am J Clin Pathol 51:786, 1969

187. McClure DK, Dahlin DC: Myxoma of bone. Report of three cases. Mayo Clin Proc 52:249, 1977

188. Wang T-Y, Erlandson RA, Marcove RC, Huvos AG: Primary leiomyosarcoma of bone. Arch Pathol Lab Med 104:100, 1980

189. Von Hochstetter AR, Eberle H, Ruttner JR: Primary leiomyosarcoma of the extragnathic bones. Case report and review of literature. Cancer 53:2194, 1984

190. Stout AP: Mesenchymoma, the mixed tumor of mesenchymal derivatives. Ann Surg 127:278, 1948

191. Scheele PM, Von Kuster LC, Krivchenia G: Primary malignant mesenchymoma of bone. Arch Pathol 114:614, 1990

192. Astorino RN, Tesluk H: Dedifferentiated chondrosarcoma with a rhabdomyosarcomatous component. Hum Pathol 16:318, 1985

193. Schajowicz F, Ackerman LV, Sissons HA: Histologic typing of bone tumours. International Histological Classification of Tumours, No. 6. Geneva, World Health Organization, 1972

194. Shinoda M, Tsutsumi MD, Jun-ichi H, Yokoyama S: Peripheral neuroepithelioma in childhood. Immunohistochemical demonstration of epithelial differentiation. Arch Pathol Lab Med 112:1155, 1988

195. Triche TJ, Ross WG: Glycogen-containing neuroblastoma with clinical and histopathological features of Ewing's sarcoma. Cancer 41:1425, 1978

196. Thomas P, Battifora H, Manderino GL, Patrick J: A monoclonal antibody against neuron-specific enolase: Immunohistochemical comparison with a polyclonal antiserum. Am J Clin Pathol 88:146, 1987

197. Tsokos M, Linnoila RI, Chandra RS, Triche TJ: Neuron-specific enolase in the diagnosis of neuroblastoma and other small, round-cell tumors in children. Hum Pathol 15:575, 1984

198. Rusthoven JJ, Robinson JB, Kolin A, Pinkerton PH: The natural-killer-cell-associated HNK-1 (Leu-7) antibody reacts with hypertrophic and malignant prostatic epithelium. Cancer 56:289, 1985

199. Bunn PA Jr, Linnoila I, Minna JD et al: Small cell lung cancer, endocrine cells of the fetal bronchus, and other neuroendocrine cells express the Leu-7 antigenic determinant present on natural killer cells. Blood 65:764, 1985

200. Kodama T, Watanabe S, Sato Y et al: An immunohistochemical study of thymic epithelial tumors: I. Epithelial component. Am J Surg Pathol 10:26, 1986

201. Michels S, Swanson PE, Robb JA, Wick MR: Leu-7 in small cell neoplasms: An immunohistochemical study with ultrastructural correlation. Cancer 60:2958, 1987

Imaging of Bone Tumors: A Multimodality Approach,
edited by George B. Greenfield and John A. Arrington,
J. B. Lippincott Company, Philadelphia © 1995.

c h a p t e r

TWO

PRIMARY MALIGNANT BONE TUMORS

IMAGING ANALYSIS OF THE SOLITARY BONE LESION

In the diagnosis of a solitary bone lesion, as in any other area, the advantages and limitations of the various imaging modalities must be well understood. Images alone often do not allow a definitive diagnosis, because they reflect only of the gross pathology. The close cooperation between the radiologist, the clinician, and the pathologist is essential. Each must understand the basis of the other's discipline to be able to arrive at a meaningful diagnosis. If the imaging picture fits a typical pattern (e.g., nonossifying fibroma), a definitive diagnosis can be made.

Although the conventional radiographic examination remains the mainstay of diagnosis in the peripheral skeleton, high-tech modalities have added another dimension to diagnosis. These techniques include computed tomography (CT), radionuclide bone scan, conventional and arterial digital angiography, ultrasound, magnetic resonance imaging (MRI), and needle biopsy.

Imaging Techniques

Computed Tomography

CT is particularly useful for viewing the central skeleton. It has the ability to show the anatomic detail of bone and soft tissue in the axial plane. Multiplanar reconstructions are less detailed on ordinary CT scans than on MR images employing sagittal and coronal planes, but CT can show calcific patterns and bone to better advantage. It has greater contrast sensitivity than conventional x-ray films, can show marrow attenuation, and can assess the vascularity of a tumor on postinfusion studies. Spiral CT shows promise of depicting detailed multiplanar reconstruction of bone. Three-dimensional CT reconstructions can show a lesion in perspective.

Radionuclide Bone Scanning

Radionuclide bone scanning is most useful for detection of an early lesion, determining whether a lesion is solitary, and screening for metastases. Depending on various factors, as much as 40% of bone must be destroyed before the changes can be visualized on conventional radiographs.[1]

An important indication for a radionuclide bone scan is the detection of metastases. The incidence of skeletal metastases at autopsy in patients with primary osteosarcoma is about 25%. In Ewing sarcoma, about 60% of patients have bone metastases at autopsy.[2]

One pitfall is that a larger abnormality on the radionuclide bone scan than on the radiograph is not necessarily indicative of tumor extension.[2] This is an extended response and may be caused by hyperemia, edema, or periosteal reaction. MRI can clearly define tumor margins and extent.

In benign bone tumors, an increase in radioisotope uptake may be the first sign of malignant change and is an indication for biopsy. Benign cartilaginous tumors can give rise to a positive scan. The absence of isotope accumulation is a reasonable assurance of benignity,[1] but certain anaplastic metastatic tumors and myeloma may not cause increased uptake and may even be photopenic.

Arteriography

Arteriography of bone lesions is useful in the investigation of cases that present with atypical radiographs.[3] The arteriographic pattern can yield much information, particularly in follow-up examinations. The response of a bone tumor to chemotherapy can best be judged not by a reduction in tumor size, but by a reduction in vascularity. The extent of a tumor and its vascular supply can be accurately determined. This method is also useful in the diagnosis of benign bone tumors.[4]

Percutaneous Needle Biopsy

Percutaneous needle biopsy of bone tumors is a radiologic-dependent procedure that is important in the diagnosis and follow-up of bone lesions. In a reported series, the overall accuracy of needle biopsy in diagnosis of benign and malignant tumors was 78.6%. The major tumor categories included osteosarcoma, giant cell tumor, Ewing sarcoma, and spindle cell sarcoma. The accuracy of needle biopsy in diagnosing these tumors was 78%, 88%, 95%, and 87%, respectively. To ensure adequate tissue for diagnosis, the investigators suggest that biopsy specimens of osteoblastic tumors should be obtained from their soft-tissue components, lytic areas, or the least dense areas, and a smear of aspirate from cystic lesions should be prepared for cytologic examination, with the clot embedded in paraffin for histologic study.[5] Care must be taken that biopsy material is obtained from the central area of a bone tumor, because the histologic nature of invaded soft tissue may radically change.

Ultrasound

Ultrasound can be useful in defining the soft-tissue component of a bony lesion. The tumor extent can be assessed and any cystic components are clearly defined. Color flow Doppler is a helpful noninvasive tool that can determine whether a palpable mass is vascular (e.g., aneurysm, pseudoaneurysm, arteriovenous malformation) in origin. It can also determine the vascularity of a tumor and demonstrate vascular displacement or compression by a mass. Ultrasound is useful in localizing deep or difficult to palpate lesions for biopsy, which can be performed in the radiology department or operating room.

Magnetic Resonance Imaging

MRI has the unique ability to show bone marrow changes. The age of the patient with respect to the marrow signal is a most important consideration. In the infant, all marrow cavities are filled with red or hematopoietic marrow. Shortly after birth, red marrow begins to convert to yellow or fatty marrow. This progresses from the periphery centrally. The epiphyses convert to yellow marrow very early in life. The diaphysis of the femur changes its signal intensity beginning at the age of 5 years to high signal intensity at 10 years. The distal metaphysis follows an adult pattern, showing low signal intensity only in the proximal metaphysis at 24 years of age. This is earlier than fatty marrow conversion seen in macroscopic specimens, presumably because of the higher sensitivity of MRI to fat.[6] At maturity, the appendicular skeleton is composed of yellow marrow except for the proximal metaphyses of the humeri and femora. The femoral metaphysis progresses through a patchy appearance to fat replacement in old age. Yellow marrow exhibits a homogeneous high signal intensity on T1-weighted images. Bone marrow ischemia hastens the conversion of red marrow to yellow marrow. The physeal scar is seen as a dark line. The spine, pelvis, and sternum continue to have red marrow admixed with yellow marrow. This yields a T1-weighted signal intensity lower than pure fat but

higher than cellular tissue. Age-related changes in the central skeleton show a band-like and patchy pattern representing changes which lead to fat replacement in older age. The calvarium also shows progressive fat replacement. In the pelvis, high signal intensity may be seen about the acetabuli and sacroiliac joints, and bright patches are apparent in the iliac bones on T1-weighted images.[7]

Osteoporosis in the spine results in a mixed or patchy signal on T1-weighted images. Replacement of normal marrow by focal or general infiltrative conditions alter the MR signal. On T1-weighted images, a lower signal intensity is seen relative to marrow, and on T2-weighted images, the signal intensity is increased. Unfortunately, these signal characteristics are not specific for neoplasm. Bone marrow edema with an increase in the water content of the marrow also produces focal, patchy, or homogeneous low signal areas on T1-weighted images and high-signal-intensity areas with T2 weighting. This change can be caused by trauma, stress, reflex sympathetic dystrophy, or acute infarction.

Bone marrow infarction is seen as low signal intensity on T1-weighted images but can produce a variable picture on T2-weighted images, depending on the stage of infarction. An acute infarct with reactive edema and an older infarct with cystic degeneration show high signal intensities on T2-weighted images. A healing infarct may have intermediate signal, and a healed infarct may be sclerotic and produce low signal intensity on T2-weighted images. A bone infarct can always be detected by its low signal component on T1-weighted images.

Residual necrotic fat may remain as high signal intensity. Certain conditions, such as radiation therapy, chemotherapy, or aplastic anemia, cause myeloid depletion, resulting in complete fat replacement with a higher signal intensity on T1-weighted images than normal marrow and a greater decrease in signal intensity on T2-weighted images.

MRI is the most sensitive method for detecting bone tumors. Intramedullary and extraosseous components can be better defined than with conventional x-ray films or with CT scans.[8] MRI is inferior to plain radiographs or CT scans for evaluating the extent and pattern of calcification. It can show patterns of cortical destruction and periosteal reaction.[9] For bone tumors with soft-tissue invasion, MRI best defines the extent of involvement and the relation of tumor to the neurovascular structures. MRI also clearly demonstrates areas of necrosis or hemorrhage.[10]

Spin echo (SE) technique is the foundation for MRI of musculoskeletal neoplasms. A heavily T1-weighted SE sequence (TR < 550 msec; TE < 30 msec) maximizes contrast between normal high-signal-intensity marrow and low-signal-intensity tumor. T1-

weighted SE images are extremely sensitive to marrow involvement and give excellent depictions of osseous and soft-tissue compartmental anatomy. A double echo SE sequence is achieved with a long TR (> 2000 msec) and by acquiring two echoes: an early echo (20–30 msec) and a late echo (80–100 msec). The first echo is proton or spin density weighted (PD weighted), and the second echo is T2 weighted. The development of fast spin echo techniques has allowed scan times to be significantly reduced for T2-weighted images or the TR greatly lengthened (>5000 msec) without increasing scan times.

Soft-tissue involvement is best detected on T2-weighted images as high signal intensity, but the PD-weighted image also gives good contrast between tumor and muscle and delivers excellent images of soft-tissue anatomy.[11] T1 weighting shows the dark tumor mass contrasted against high-signal-intensity fat, and T2 weighting best shows the bright tumor mass contrasted against gray muscle. PD-weighted images display good osseous and soft tissue detail and show tumor as a lighter shade of gray than muscle.

The sensitivity of MRI to calcifications can be increased by using a T2* gradient echo sequence as part of the MR protocol. Gradient echo sequences have greater magnetic susceptibility than spin echo sequences and are therefore more sensitive to calcium detection; however, these sequences cannot yet duplicate or replace plain radiographs for the detection and characterization of calcifications. MR angiography (MRA) allows a noninvasive evaluation of the relation between tumor and vessels. It is more sensitive than CT or conventional or digital angiography for encasement of vessels by tumor and clearly shows vessel displacement. MRA does not show tumor blush or neovascularity well or accurately, but it does detect arteriovenous shunting. MRA shows blood flow, rather than the anatomy of the vascular walls.

The multiplanar capability of MRI should be used to show the entire bone along its long axis to determine the extent of the tumor and any skip areas. Gadolinium enhancement does not have a well-defined role in evaluating malignant neoplasms. Cystic or necrotic areas of bone tumors do not enhance with contrast, but solid tumor and reactive edema usually do. Enhanced MRI can be helpful in evaluating the response of a bone tumor to radiation or chemotherapy by being more sensitive to tumor necrosis.

Classification of Primary Bone Tumors

The World Health Organization (WHO) classification[12] of bone tumors and tumor-like lesions is based on histologic typing (Table 2-1).

Origin of the Lesion

Lent C. Johnson,[13] in his general theory of bone tumors, stressed that bone is an organ with varying functions in different parts of the skeleton. He pointed out that there is a metabolic gradient within each individual bone that is minimal in the midshaft, low in the epiphysis, high in the metaphysis, and maximal in the metaphysis of a rapidly growing end. This gradient can be correlated with fields of cell activity. A tumor of a specific cell type tends to originate in the field of maximal activity of homologous normal cells, although exceptions occur. The preferential sites and times of origin of the various tumors are determined in this manner and are of the greatest diagnostic significance. The following are preferential sites of origin for various tumors:

EPIPHYSIS
Aneurysmal bone cyst
Chondroblastoma
Clear cell
  chondrosarcoma
Giant cell tumor (after
  fusion of growth plate)

METAPHYSIS
Chondrosarcoma
Enchondroma
Fibrosarcoma
Giant cell tumor (before
  fusion of growth plate)
Osteosarcoma
Parosteal sarcoma
Unicameral bone cyst

DIAMETAPHYSIS
Chondromyxoid fibroma
Nonossifying fibroma
Osteoblastoma

DIAPHYSIS
Adamantinoma
Ewing tumor
Malignant fibrous
  histiocytoma
Myeloma
Primary lymphoma of
  bone.

A wide age span in most tumors is possible. A large number of bone tumors develop at the time of the growth spurt in late adolescence. Other tumors develop in childhood, and some occur in adult life. The preferential time of origin of the various bone tumors is summarized in the following list, which gives the decades of maximal frequency of occurrence:

Osteosarcoma: 2, 3, 7 (smaller peak)
Parosteal sarcoma: 4, 5
Chondrosarcoma: 4, 5, 6
Fibrosarcoma: 4
Malignant fibrous histiocytoma: 5
Giant cell tumor: 3, 4
Ewing tumor: 2
Primary lymphoma of bone: 3, 4
Multiple myeloma: 5, 6, 7
Chondroblastoma: 2
Chondromyxoid fibroma: 2, 3
Nonossifying fibroma: 2

TABLE 2-1.
The World Health Organization Classification of Primary Bone Tumors and Tumor-like Conditions

I. Bone-forming tumors
   A. Benign
      1. Osteoma
      2. Osteoid osteoma and osteoblastoma (i.e., benign osteoblastoma)
   B. Malignant
      1. Osteosarcoma (i.e., osteogenic sarcoma)
      2. Juxtacortical osteosarcoma (i.e., parosteal osteosarcoma)
II. Cartilage-forming tumors
   A. Benign
      1. Chondroma
      2. Osteochondroma (i.e., osteocartilaginous exostosis)
      3. Chondroblastoma (i.e., benign chondroblastoma, epiphyseal chondroblastoma)
      4. Chondromyxoid fibroma
   B. Malignant
      1. Chondrosarcoma
      2. Juxtacortical chondrosarcoma
      3. Mesenchymal chondrosarcoma
III. Giant cell tumors (i.e., osteoclastoma)
IV. Marrow tumors
   A. Ewing sarcoma
   B. Reticulosarcoma of bone
   C. Lymphosarcoma of bone
   D. Myeloma
V. Vascular tumors
   A. Benign
      1. Hemangioma
      2. Lymphangioma
      3. Glomus tumor (i.e., glomangioma)
   B. Intermediate or indeterminate
      1. Hemangioendothelioma
      2. Hemangiopericytoma
   C. Malignant
      1. Angiosarcoma
	VI. Other connective tissue tumors
	   A. Benign
	      1. Desmoplastic fibroma
	      2. Lipoma
	   B. Malignant
	      1. Fibrosarcoma
	      2. Liposarcoma
	      3. Malignant mesenchymoma
	      4. Undifferentiated sarcoma
	VII. Other tumors
	   A. Chordoma
	   B. Adamantinoma of long bones
	   C. Neurilemoma (i.e., schwannoma, neurinoma)
	   D. Neurofibroma
	VIII. Unclassified tumors
	IX. Tumor-like lesions
	   A. Solitary bone cyst (i.e., simple or unicameral bone cyst)
	   B. Aneurysmal bone cyst
	   C. Juxtaarticular bone cyst (i.e., intraosseous ganglion)
	   D. Metaphyseal fibrous defect (i.e., nonossifying fibroma)
	   E. Eosinophilic granuloma
	   F. Fibrous dysplasia
	   G. Myositis ossificans
	   H. Brown tumor of hyperparathyroidism

Osteoid osteoma: 2, 3
Unicameral bone cyst: 1, 2
Aneurysmal bone cyst: 2, 3.

In very young patients, malignant bone tumors are likely to be metastases from neuroblastoma or leukemia. In the first decade, the most likely primary bone tumors are Ewing tumors and later, they are osteosarcomas. In adolescence and early adult life, various primary bone tumors are probable. In older age groups, most bone tumors are metastatic carcinomas or multiple myeloma.

Biochemical Studies

Biochemical studies in the evaluation of primary bone tumors are not always helpful. All benign tumors of bone show normal serum values except, rarely, tumors associated with osteomalacia. Osteosarcoma is usually associated with an elevated serum alkaline phosphatase level. Other malignant tumors and giant cell tumors may produce slight elevations of serum alkaline phosphatase values. The chief value of serum calcium and phosphorus determinations in assessing solitary lesions is to exclude a brown tumor or cyst of hyperparathyroidism. The metabolites of catecholamine may indicate a neuroblastoma. Serum electrophoresis is valuable in the diagnosis of multiple myeloma. It may be normal in solitary myeloma.

Imaging Patterns

The basic features of cortical destruction and expansion, periosteal response, and bone production are discussed and illustrated in Chapter 1. The location, size, margination, trabeculation, shape, and pattern of matrix calcification or ossification are critical factors in the diagnosis of the solitary bone lesion.

The location of a lesion is important with respect to which bone is involved, which portion (e.g., epiphysis, metaphysis, diaphysis) is involved, whether the lesion is central or eccentric, or whether it involves the medulla, cortex, or periosteum. The size of a lesion is also of significance, because malignant tumors are rarely small when first seen. Lodwick speaks of a 6-cm rule, in which malignant tumors are not smaller than 6 cm when first seen. Margination and trabeculation are important considerations. Malignant tumors tend to have an indistinct margin or wide zone of transition, although there are exceptions. The entire circumference of any lesion must be carefully inspected to prevent overlooking a segmental wide zone. Some lesions, such as giant cell tumor, are characteristically lightly trabeculated. A round shape favors a rapidly growing neoplasm, and an elongated shape usually favors a bone cyst or a benign tumor.

The calcification pattern of the tumor is of highest significance. The matrix of a tumor is the intracellular material produced by tumor cells. Some tumors, such as Ewing tumor and giant cell tumor, do not produce a matrix. Others, such as the osteoid, chondroid, and fibrous series of tumors, produce the matrix of their classification. The bone-forming tumors produce a pattern that may be homogeneous and sclerotic. The cartilage-forming tumors produce a pattern of calcification that may be amorphous, stippled, flocculent, or show arc-like and ring-like features. A medullary bone infarct may simulate the latter, but it has a tendency to be circumscribed by a calcific margin. A lack of calcification does not exclude any particular tumor, because the matrix may or may not be mineralized. A transition from mineralized to nonmineralized matrix indicates activity and may represent malignant change. Conventional radiography and CT can be used to demonstrate these patterns. MRI shows bone cortex and dense calcification as a signal void, but spin echo techniques cannot depict the pattern or extent of calcifications.

MRI is most valuable in determining the extent of soft-tissue and bone marrow involvement.[14] CT can demonstrate the extent of tumor, including cortical destruction, marrow involvement, soft-tissue invasion, and matrix mineralization. Radionuclide bone scanning is extremely sensitive. Most bone tumors are positive on radionuclide scan, with the exception of multiple myeloma and certain anaplastic metastatic tumors. Angiography is useful for demonstrating tumor vessel patterns and critical vessel involvement adjacent to the tumor. The angiographic pattern is a good indicator of tumor response. MRI is a valuable method for monitoring treatment.[15,16]

OSTEOSARCOMA

Osteosarcomas are classified with respect to cell type and to central or surface location (Table 2-2).[17,18] Several central types have surface analogs.

Conventional Osteosarcoma

Osteosarcoma (i.e., central osteosarcoma) is a primary malignant tumor of bone in which tumor cells directly form osteoid matrix.[19,20,21] This is an entity distinct from fibrosarcoma of bone, which does not give rise to osteogenesis, and chondrosarcoma, which is a malignant tumor of cartilage. Conventional osteosarcomas have traditionally been divided into three groups: osteoblastic, chondroblastic, and fibroblastic. About one half are osteoblastic, in which large amounts of osteoid are formed and the appearance is usually osteosclerotic. About one quarter are chondroblastic, which is a misnomer, because the cells are not chondroblasts. These usually show a cartilaginous pattern of calcification. The rest are fibroblastic with minimal osteoid, giving an osteolytic appearance.

TABLE 2-2.
Classification of Osteosarcomas by Cell Type and Location

Centrally located types	Surface types
Conventional osteosarcoma	High-grade surface osteosarcoma
Osteoblastic type	Periosteal osteosarcoma
Fibroblastic type	Parosteal sarcoma
Chondroblastic type	Intracortical osteosarcoma
Low-grade central osteosarcoma	Extraosseous osteosarcoma
Small cell osteosarcoma	
Telangiectatic osteosarcoma	
Osteosarcoma of the jaw	
Multicentric osteosarcoma	
Osteosarcoma arising in abnormal bone	
Osteosarcoma arising from other bone tumors	

Osteosarcomas may be grouped by location into central osteosarcomas and surface osteosarcomas, which include parosteal sarcoma. There is also soft tissue osteosarcoma.

About 75% of the tumors are conventional osteosarcomas. The remainder are classified into subtypes. One group that arises from abnormal bone. Another variety arises in the jaws, which has a better prognosis. A small group of tumors results from the dedifferentiation of chondrosarcomas. These have the distribution of the latter tumor but a poorer prognosis. Some tumors have histologies similar to malignant fibrous histiocytoma, but osteoid is produced by malignant cells. Another group, called telangiectatic osteosarcoma, is lytic throughout and radiographically may simulate Ewing sarcoma. These tumors are bloody and necrotic, and the prognosis is poor. Multicentric osteosarcoma is a rare form.

Low-grade central osteosarcomas comprise a small group that is the central analog of parosteal osteosarcoma and may be mistaken for fibrous dysplasia. Periosteal osteosarcoma is another distinctive type of lesion. It characteristically is seen on the surface of the tibial shaft and is a chondroblastic tumor with periosteal spiculation initially without medullary involvement. High-grade surface osteosarcoma is an aggressive type with histology similar to conventional osteosarcoma, but it arises on the surface of the bone.

Osteosarcoma is the second most common primary sarcoma of bone, after multiple myeloma. The ratio of affected males to females is about 2 to 1. Most tumors arise in the 10- to 25-year age group. It can even occur in a 3-year-old child (Fig. 2-1). A smaller peak incidence occurs in older age groups. Osteosarcomas in older age groups may be associated with Paget disease, postirradiated bone, or osteochondromas. They may also arise de novo (Fig. 2-2). The incidence in association with fibrous dysplasia is very low. An association with osteogenesis imperfecta has been reported,[22] although often a spurious picture develops because of excess callus formation.[23]

In younger patients, osteosarcoma most often involves the tubular bones. When it occurs in older persons, the flat bones are often involved.

In most instances, the tumor metastasizes by way of the bloodstream. The most common site of metastasis is the lung. Nodular pulmonary densities, best seen on CT scans, may ossify or cavitate. Skeletal metastases, usually involving the spine or pelvis, may be seen. Skip metastases along the shaft in the long bones also occur and are best demonstrated by MRI. Calcified renal metastases have been reported.[24] In rare instances, metastases may spread by way of the lymphatics, in which case calcification or ossification is seen in a regional lymph node (Fig. 2-3). In lesions of the shoulder and pelvic girdles, lymphatic involvement is more common than in peripheral osteosarcomas. The mediastinal or paraaortic lymph nodes may be involved.[25] CT can best demonstrate this finding.

The chief symptom is pain at the tumor site, which begins insidiously and progresses to severe constancy. A palpable mass develops, with inflammation and local venous dilatation. Systemic symptoms follow. Effusion in a contiguous joint is common. Pathologic fracture may occur. The duration of symptoms before diagnosis averages several months. The serum alkaline phosphatase level is usually slightly elevated in the case of a large tumor.

The areas most frequently involved in conventional osteosarcoma are the distal femur and the proximal tibia. This occurs in about 75% of tubular bone involvement. The proximal humerus, the distal radius, and the pelvis are not uncommon sites, and there may be involvement of the femoral shaft, maxilla, sternum, ribs, pelvis, spine,[26] and skull,[27,28] or almost any bone in the body, including the patella.[29]

The plain film findings in early osteosarcoma are subtle. There may be only minimal increase in bone density. CT can show increased marrow attenuation and calcification and subtle cortical and periosteal changes.[30] Radionuclide bone scanning is more sensitive than CT, and MRI is most sensitive to early changes. Conventional x-ray films are the primary imaging means of diagnosis of a peripheral skeletal lesion. They are most accurate in demonstrating calcific patterns. Periosteal reaction and bone destructive patterns can also be shown with MRI.

In the tubular bones, osteosarcoma most often originates in the metaphysis. The epiphysis is commonly involved, with a reported incidence of 80%, and is more readily seen on MR images (Fig. 2-4). The patients with uninvolved epiphyses in one series were 9 years of age or younger.[31] The thickness of the epiphyseal cartilage plate is a factor in preventing transepiphyseal spread of tumor in younger patients (Fig. 2-5), because the tumor readily crosses the cartilage plate after or near the time of epiphyseal fusion. The joint cartilage forms an effective barrier against transarticular spread until the tumor becomes very large.

Diaphyseal osteosarcomas have been reported to occur in 9.5% of patient with long bone involvement. The clinical and histologic features are the same as those of metaphyseal osteosarcomas.[32]

Primary osteosarcoma of the spine occurs in less than 2% of patients.[33] The findings may include osteolytic, mixed, expansile, or sclerotic lesions, which progress to compression and destruction of the vertebral body, and involvement of the neural canal and arch. An adjacent soft-tissue mass, possibly containing

(text continues on page 54)

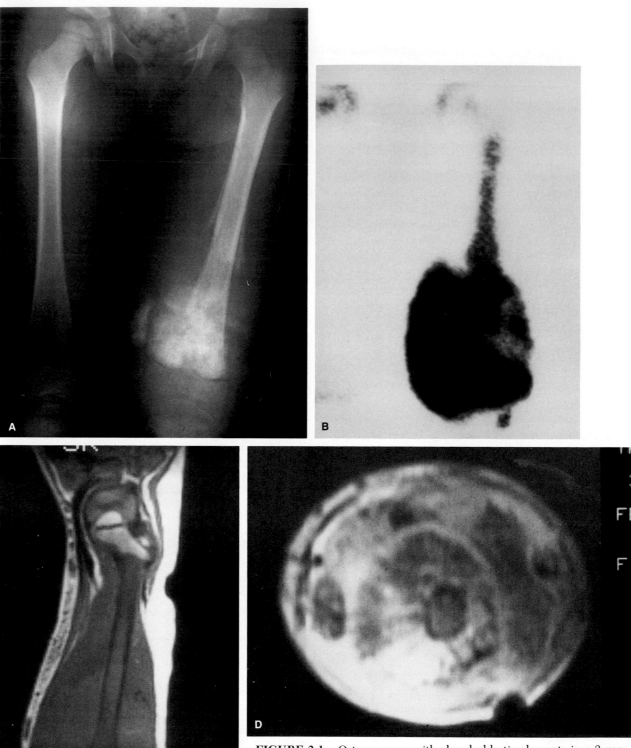

FIGURE 2-1. Osteosarcoma with chondroblastic elements in a 3-year-old girl. (**A**) The anteroposterior view of the femora reveals osteosarcoma of the distal left femoral metaphysis with extensive soft-tissue calcification. Bilateral Codman triangles are seen at the proximal end of the tumor. The tumor has only minimally involved the epiphyseal ossification center despite its large size. (**B**) Radionuclide bone scan. A large amount of increased activity in the distal left femur extends superiorly along the femoral shaft to the subtrochanteric region. A small focus of activity is seen at the lateral aspect of the epiphysis. (**C**) This T1-weighted MR (SE 500/20) image shows a large tumor mass and bone involvement to the intertrochanteric region. (**D**) The T2-weighted axial image shows a large tumor mass surrounding the partially destroyed cortex. Radiating low-signal-intensity spicules are evident.

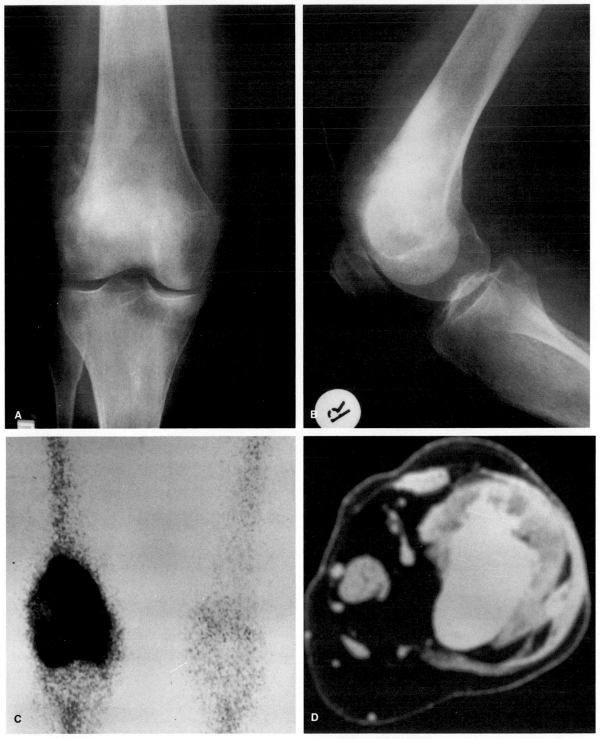

FIGURE 2-2.   Osteosarcoma in a 70-year-old woman without underlying bone disease. (**A**) Anteroposterior view of the right knee. Osteosarcoma involving the distal right femoral metaphysis is seen with a soft-tissue spiculated calcific pattern and bony sclerosis. (**B**) Lateral view. The tumor has destroyed the anterior cortex with soft-tissue invasion, bony sclerosis, and spiculated periosteal new bone formation. There is no evidence of underlying bone disease. (**C**) Radionuclide bone scan shows a large area of uptake involving the distal right femur and extending to the end of the bone. (**D**) CT scan shows a large tumor mass surrounding the bone, which shows destruction in its lateral aspect and soft-tissue calcifications.

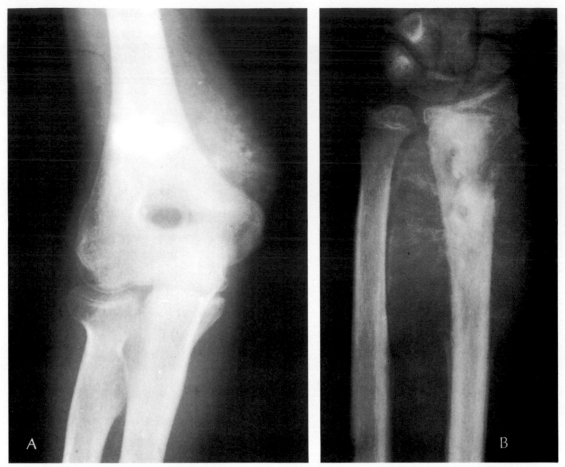

FIGURE 2-3. Osteosarcoma of the distal radius metastatic to a supratrochlear lymph node. (**A**) There is soft-tissue swelling containing streaky calcific densities. (**B**) The area of sclerosis at the distal radius involves the metaphysis and the diaphysis but not the epiphysis. The radiolucency is secondary to a biopsy. A large soft-tissue mass, perpendicular streaks of periosteal new bone formation, and a Codman triangle are also visible.

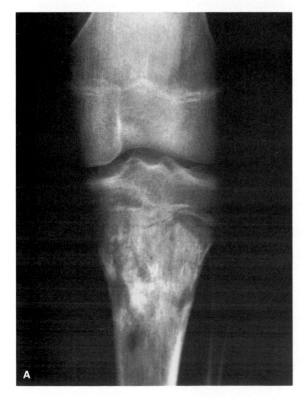

FIGURE 2-4. Osteosarcoma in a 15-year-old boy. (**A**) Anteroposterior view of the knee. Patchy osteosclerotic and destructive areas are evident in the proximal left tibial metaphysis. The epiphyseal cartilage plate is almost closed. The amount of epiphyseal involvement is not clear on this view. (**B**) The lateral view shows patchy destructive and osteosclerotic areas in the proximal tibial metaphysis. The tumor appears to have crossed the epiphyseal cartilage plate anteriorly. (**C**) The radionuclide bone scan shows increased activity in the proximal left tibial metaphysis and slight activity in the epiphysis. (**D**) MR image (SE 1700/35). The low-signal-intensity tumor replacing fatty marrow is seen in a patchy pattern in the metaphysis and involves the medial half of the epiphysis. (**E**) This T2-weighted MR (SE 1700/90) image shows a high-signal-intensity tumor involving the metaphysis in a patchy pattern and involving the entire medial half of the epiphysis.

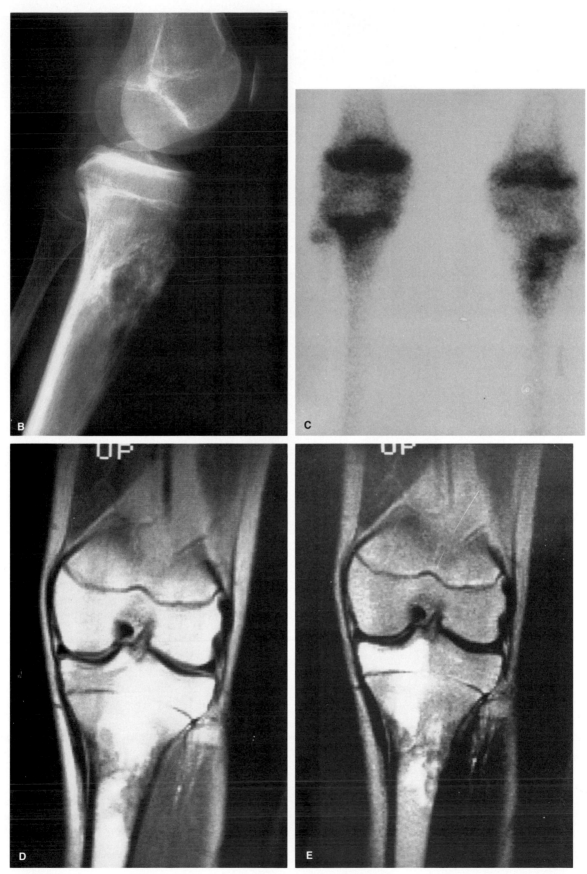

FIGURE 2-4.   *(Continued)*

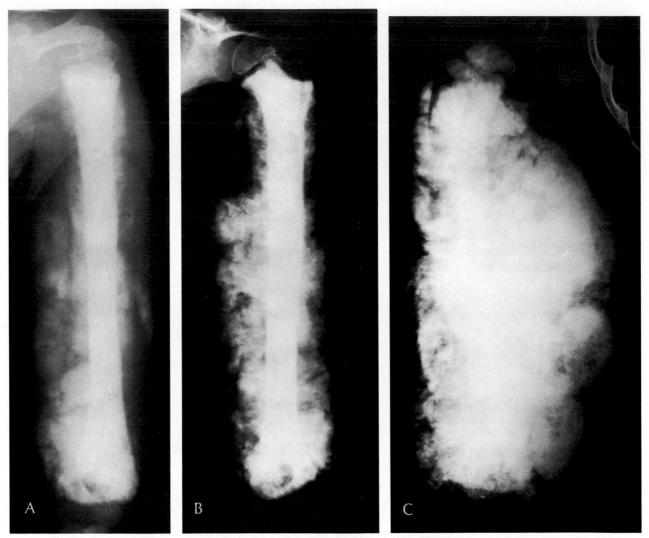

FIGURE 2-5. Osteosarcoma of the humerus. (**A**) The entire diaphysis is involved. The epiphyses at both ends of the humerus are spared. There is soft-tissue involvement, with extensive tumor bone formation and spiculated periosteal new bone formation. (**B**) One month after **A**, involvement of the humerus and soft tissues has progressed, and the bases of the epiphyseal ossification centers are starting to be invaded. (**C**) Four months after **B**, there is extreme soft-tissue ossification and complete involvement of the epiphyseal ossification centers. The sarcoma has not spread across the joints.

calcification, may result in neurologic symptoms.[34,35] A pleural effusion may be present if a thoracic vertebra is involved. Many of these cases may arise from Paget disease or previous irradiation to the spine. CT or MRI can show these changes. Metastatic osteosarcoma to the spine may also occur and is best shown by MRI (Fig. 2-6).

Osteosarcoma of the pelvis (Fig. 2-7) occurs less often than in the long bones, and this tumor is rare in the ribs. Rib involvement may be associated with an extrapleural mass. When it does involve sites other than the tubular bones, the radiographic findings are similar. They consist of various patterns of bone de-struction and sclerosis along with periosteal new bone formation and a soft-tissue mass. The calvarium usually has an osteolytic lesion. The flat bones are involved in about 5% of patients.

The tumor shows a dense sclerosis in about half of these patients (Fig. 2-8); a moderately ossifying appearance; a mixed productive and destructive appearance (Fig. 2-9); or a pure osteolytic lesion. These variations in density depend on the amount of calcified osteoid and vascularity. When the lesion is osteolytic, the pattern of bone destruction is usually geographic, with a wide zone of transition (Fig. 2-10).

Periosteal new bone formation classically is seen as

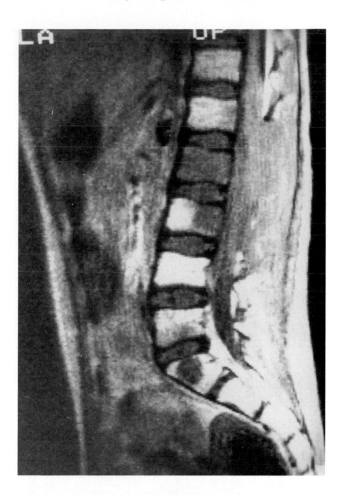

FIGURE 2-6. Osteosarcoma metastatic to the spine in a 13-year-old girl. The MR (SE 700/30) image shows the low-signal-intensity tumor replacing marrow in multiple vertebral bodies and the sacrum.

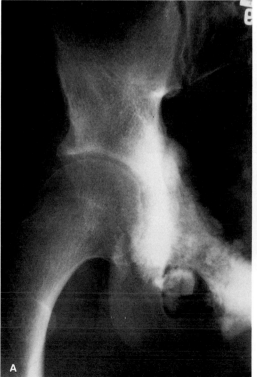

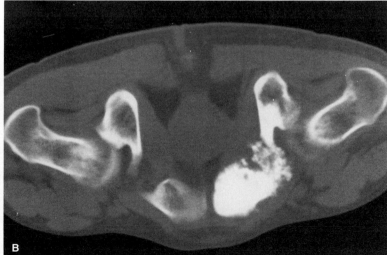

FIGURE 2-7. Osteosarcoma of the pubic bone in a 19-year-old man. (**A**) Anteroposterior view of the left hip shows bony sclerosis of the pubic bone, the ischium with spiculated periosteal new bone formation, and a large soft-tissue calcification projected over the obturator foramen. (**B**) The CT scan shows bony sclerosis and enlargement of the left pubic bone and extension into the ischium.

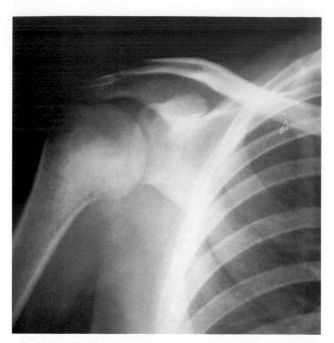

FIGURE 2-8. Osteosarcoma in an 18-year-old woman. The anteroposterior view of the shoulder shows dense sclerosis in the proximal humeral metaphysis with medial cortical destruction and soft-tissue calcification.

delicate filiform spicules radiating from a central point, called a sunburst pattern (Fig. 2-11). A long-segment pattern of parallel spiculation may occur in other cases. The angiographic appearance of a sunburst pattern is that of vessels running along and between the periosteal perpendicular spicules (Fig. 2-12).[36] Simple (Fig. 2-13), laminated (Fig. 2-14), and mixed types of periosteal reaction may occur, and there may be a transition from one type to another (Fig. 2-15).

A spiculated periosteal reaction may be seen in metastatic tumors, particularly carcinoma of the prostate (Fig. 2-16), and in benign conditions, such as healed fractures (Fig. 2-17), osteomyelitis, and thyroid acropachy (Fig. 2-18). Malignant spicules tend to be long, thin, filiform, and delicate, but benign spicules are short and squat.

A Codman triangle is often apparent (Fig. 2-19). This triangle may also be found in other malignant tumors and in aggressive benign conditions. Rarely, an expansile lesion may be seen. Pathologic fractures are common. Cortical destruction and invasion of the soft tissues is characteristic of osteosarcoma. The soft-tissue mass may be very large (Fig. 2-20). Areas of ossification

(*text continues on page 62*)

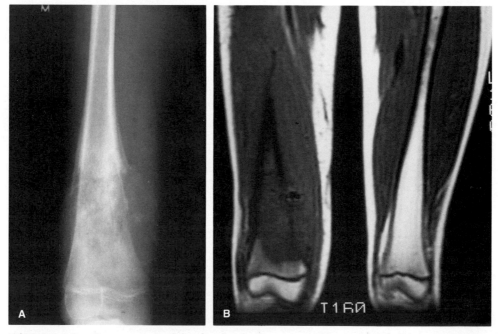

FIGURE 2-9. Osteosarcoma of the distal right femur in a 10-year-old girl. (**A**) An anteroposterior view of the right femur shows a mixed osteosclerotic and destructive tumor pattern of the distal femur with laminated periosteal new bone formation and Codman triangles proximally. The femoral metaphysis shows mixed sclerotic and destructive changes. There is a large, calcified, soft-tissue mass with denser calcifications medially. (**B**) The MR (SE 550/20) image shows marrow replacement at the extent of the tumor in the distal femur. The epiphysis is not involved. There is a signal void medially, corresponding to the calcifications seen on plain film. (**C**) This T2-weighted MR (SE 2000/80) image shows high and low signal intensities in the tumor and the surrounding soft-tissue mass. (**D**) The axial MR (SE 2000/80) image shows high and low signal intensities within the bone and a large surrounding soft-tissue mass. The low-signal-intensity areas in the soft-tissue mass correspond to the calcification seen on plain film radiographs.

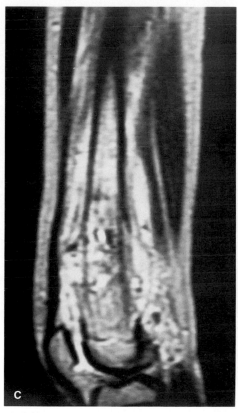

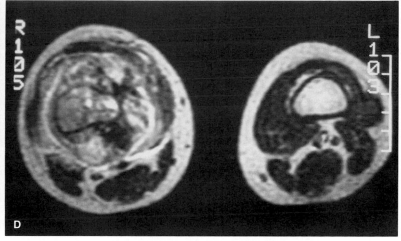

FIGURE 2-9.   *(Continued)*

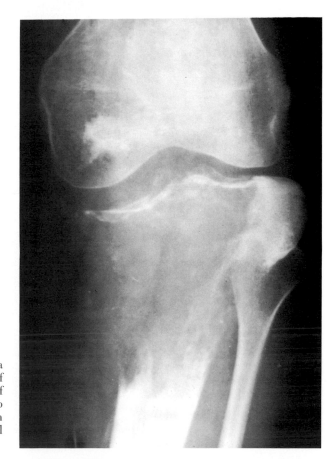

FIGURE 2-10.   Osteosarcoma in a 17-year-old girl. This is a purely destructive lesion of the proximal tibia. The margin of the destroyed area is irregular, and several moth-eaten areas of destruction can be seen extending down the shaft. There is no expansion of bone. The last two findings differentiate this from a giant cell tumor. Osteoporosis, not tumor invasion, of the distal femur causes a radiolucent appearance.

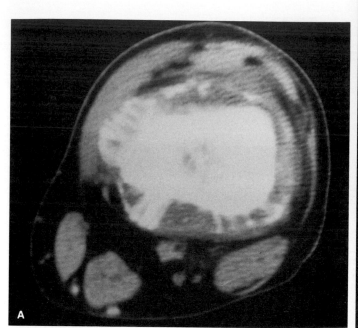

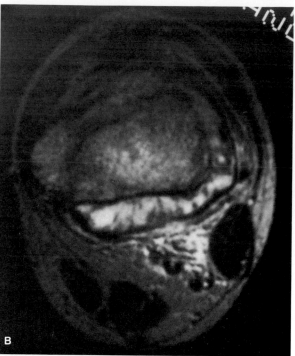

FIGURE 2-11. Osteosarcoma, showing spiculated periosteal new bone formation. (**A**) The CT scan shows that the central bone is osteosclerotic. A low-attenuation tumor surrounds the bone. Dense spicules radiate out from the bone into the tumor. (**B**) The T2-weighted MR image corresponds to the CT image. The medullary cavity shows low and high signal intensities surrounded by the low-signal-intensity cortex. The high-signal-intensity tumor surrounds the bone, showing low-signal-intensity radiating spicules that correspond to the high-density spicules in the CT image.

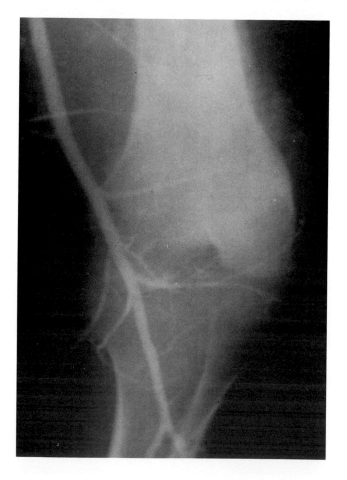

FIGURE 2-12. Osteosarcoma in a 60-year-old woman with spiculated periosteal new bone formation. Blood vessels are seen in a perpendicular pattern, running parallel to the periosteal spiculation.

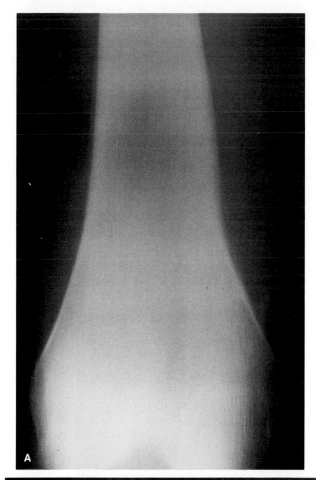

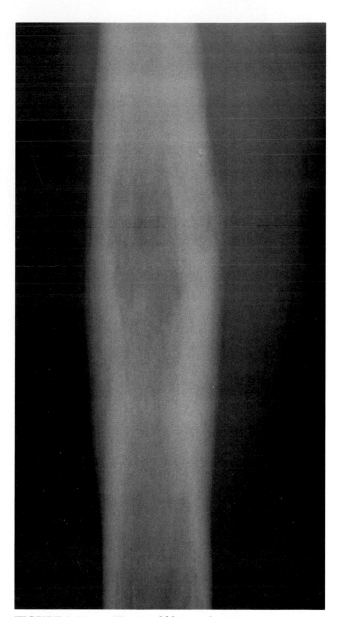

FIGURE 2-14.   A 15-year-old boy with osteosarcoma involving the diaphysis of the left femur. Bony sclerosis and laminated periosteal new bone formation can be seen.

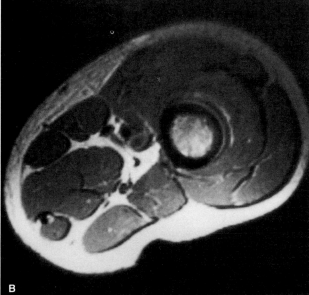

FIGURE 2-13.   Osteosarcoma with simple periosteal new bone formation. (**A**) A conventional tomogram shows simple periosteal new bone formation along the distal femoral shaft and a Codman triangle. (**B**) The MR proton density image shows a low-signal-intensity thin stripe around the cortex with high signal intensity within the marrow cavity and surrounding the periosteal new bone.

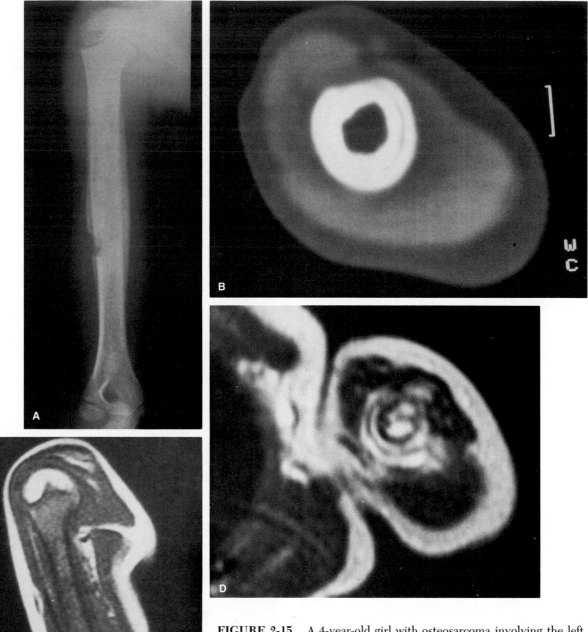

FIGURE 2-15. A 4-year-old girl with osteosarcoma involving the left humeral diaphysis. (**A**) Anteroposterior (AP) view of the humerus. Simple periosteal new bone formation with a greatest thickness of 2 mm is seen surrounding a mixed sclerotic and lytic osteosarcoma of the diaphysis. (**B**) In the CT scan, thick, simple periosteal new bone formation surrounds the cortex. (**C**) The MR (SE 600/20) sagittal section shows bone marrow replacement of almost the entire humerus with surrounding simple periosteal new bone formation. (**D**) The MR (SE 2700/80) scan shows high signal intensity in the marrow cavity, low-signal-intensity simple periosteal new bone formation, and high-signal-intensity soft tissue surrounding the periosteal new bone. (**E**) AP view of the humerus taken 4 months after the prior images. Mixed sclerotic and destructive changes in the humeral shaft are seen along with spiculated periosteal new bone formation superiorly and laminated periosteal new bone formation at the most distal aspect of the tumor. The spicules have a long, thin, filiform pattern. (**F**) In a CT scan obtained at the same time as **E**, a spiculated pattern of periosteal new bone formation is seen with long, thin, filiform spicules surrounding the cortex.

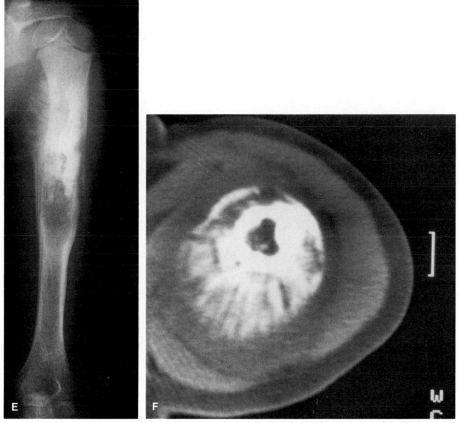

FIGURE 2-15. *(Continued)*

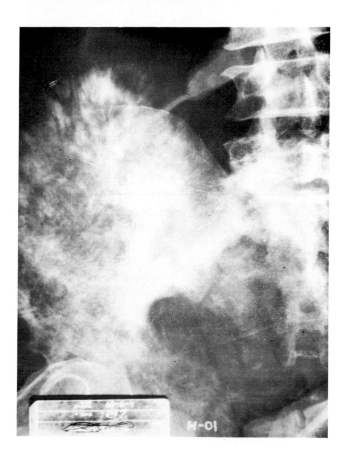

FIGURE 2-16. Osteoblastic metastasis to the ilium from carcinoma of the prostate. A marked spiculated type of periosteal new bone formation is seen, as are bone sclerosis and destructive areas.

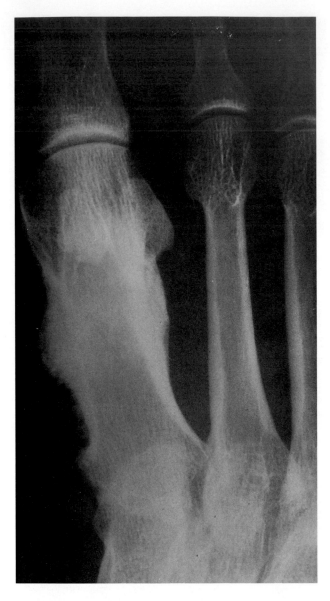

FIGURE 2-17. An old, healed fracture of the first metatarsal, showing spiculated periosteal new bone formation medially.

or amorphous calcification may be present in the mass, and there may be an apparent alignment of calcific densities radiating outward from the central tumor. The amount of new bone formation in the soft tissues may exceed that in the intraosseous component (Fig. 2-21).

Chondroblastic osteosarcoma has a predominant chondroid differentiation. This may be reflected as a cartilaginous pattern of calcification inside the medullary cavity or in the surrounding tumor mass. This pattern is composed of amorphous, stippled, linear, circular, or popcorn-like calcification. It can be seen on conventional films, CT scans, or MR images and can sometimes be extensive (Fig. 2-22).

Preoperative chemotherapy has increased 5-year survival, with a rate as high as 80% in at least one series.[37] Patients with a good response show medullary sclerosis, thick periosteal new bone formation, and some reduction of the soft-tissue mass. Peripheral and central calcification represent healing. This calcification appears more solid than that of tumorous new bone. The tumor mass is surrounded by a fibrous shell, which may calcify, resulting in an expansile appearance (see Fig. 2-20). Angiography reveals a decrease in tumor vascularity in favorably responding tumors.[38]

CT offers several imaging advantages, particularly in assessing the central skeleton.[39,40] It can determine the extent of the soft-tissue component, but not as accurately as MRI. Intravenous contrast enhancement is useful for determining the vascularity and the relation of the soft-tissue mass to major vessels. Calcification within the tumor can be detected more readily with CT than with conventional films. It can show bony detail in the central skeleton and calcification and new bone

(text continues on page 68)

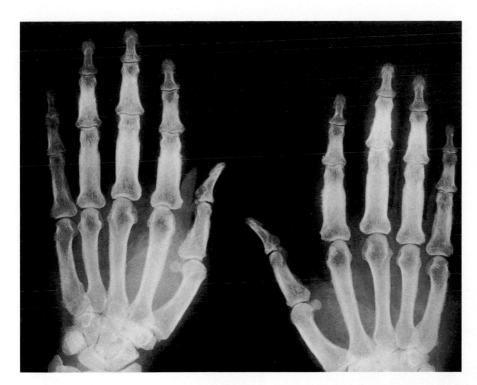

FIGURE 2-18. Thyroid acropachy of the hands. Spiculated periosteal new bone formation occurs bilaterally and symmetrically. The first and second rays show most pronounced changes at the radial side, and the fifth ray shows the most pronounced changes at the ulnar side. Soft-tissue masses are associated with the periosteal new bone formation. The spicules are short and squat, characteristic of a benign spiculative process. (From Greenfield GB, Escamilla CH, Schorsch HA: The hand as an indicator of generalized disease. AJR Am J Roentgenol 99:736–745, 1967)

FIGURE 2-19. Osteosarcoma of the distal femur. (**A**) The anteroposterior view of the distal femur shows mixed osteosclerotic and destructive areas with Codman triangles proximally. (**B**) In the T2-weighted MR image, the Codman triangles at the proximal aspect of the tumor, the heterogeneous signal intensity in the medullary cavity, and tumor extension into the soft tissues are seen.

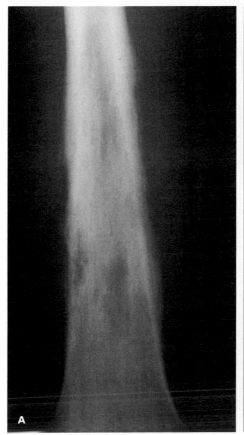

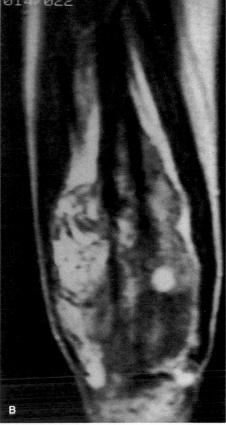

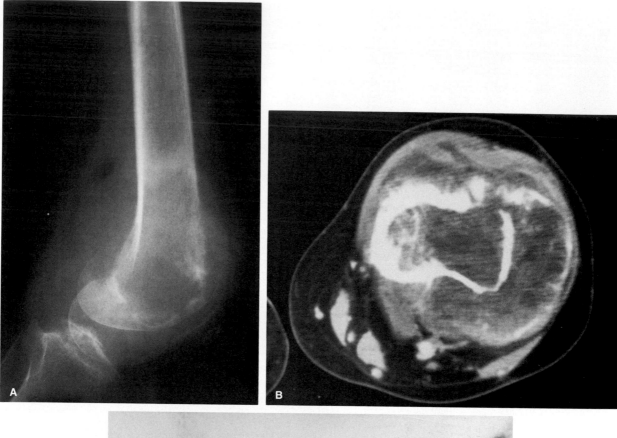

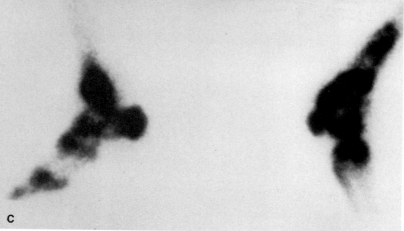

FIGURE 2-20. A 19-year-old woman with osteosarcoma of the left distal femur. (**A**) The lateral view shows destruction of the distal femoral metaphysis, a large adjacent soft-tissue mass, and spiculated periosteal new bone formation anteriorly along with cortical destruction. (**B**) The CT scan shows a large soft-tissue mass surrounding the bone on its lateral aspect along with cortical destruction. (**C**) In the radionuclide bone scan, increased activity in the distal femur is seen. There is also activity in the proximal tibia, the distal tibia, and the tarsal bones, although there is no tumor involvement at these sites. (**D**) MR (SE 800/20) sagittal section. The tumor is seen in the metaphysis with considerable soft-tissue extension into the popliteal fossa. A small skip area replaces the marrow signal posteriorly, proximal to the tumor. (**E**) On this T2-weighted MR image, the large soft-tissue mass involves the popliteal artery. (**F**) MR (SE 600/20) image taken after 3 months of treatment. The soft-tissue mass has a lobulated appearance, and it is marginated by a thin, low-signal-intensity shell. There is a small skip lesion proximal to the main tumor. (**G**) The postresection radiograph shows a calcific shell completely surrounding the entire tumor.

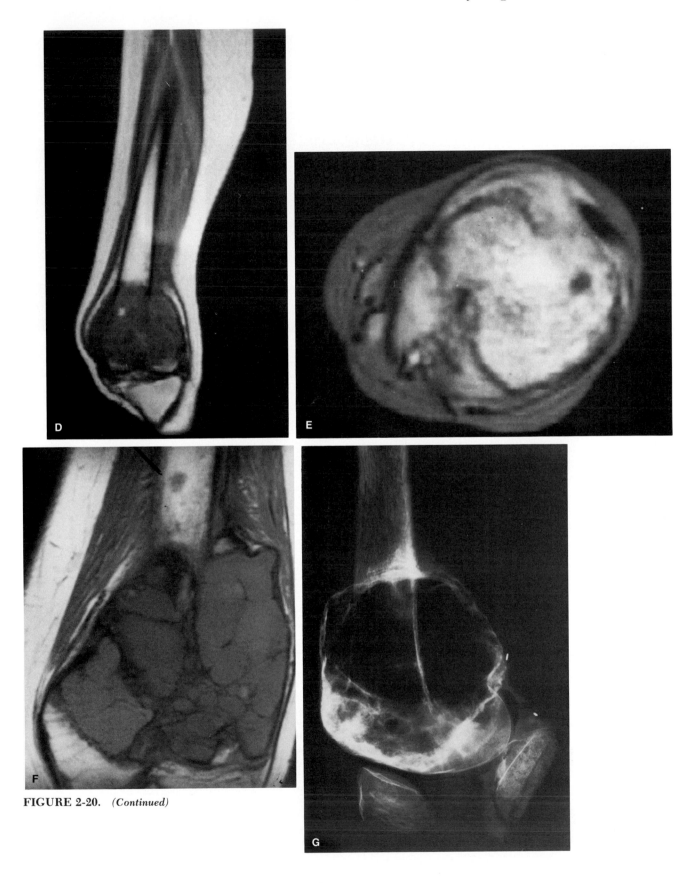

FIGURE 2-20.   *(Continued)*

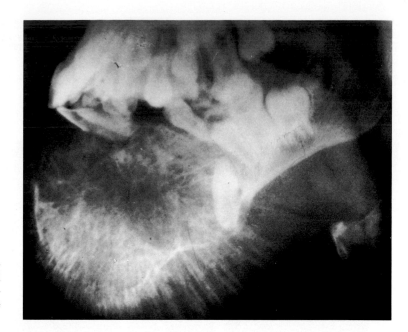

FIGURE 2-21. Osteosarcoma involves the mandible, with long, slender, spiculated, periosteal new bone formation, called the "sunburst" pattern. Destructive and sclerotic changes in the mandible represent a mixed type of osteosarcoma.

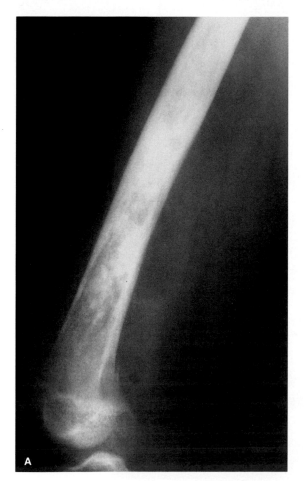

FIGURE 2-22. A 12-year-old girl with chondroblastic osteosarcoma involving the major portion of the right femur. (**A**) The lateral view shows amorphous calcification and osteosclerosis in the femoral shaft. (**B**) The CT scan shows dense, irregular calcification within the medullary cavity. (**C**) MR image (SE 500/15). The entire femoral bone marrow has been replaced to almost the articular surface. A low-signal-intensity, irregular pattern corresponds to the calcification seen on plain films and CT scans. Soft-tissue invasion can also be seen. (**D**) The MR (SE 2700/80) image shows high signal intensity within the marrow cavtiy and surrounding tumor and a signal void within the marrow cavity corresponding to the calcification previously seen.

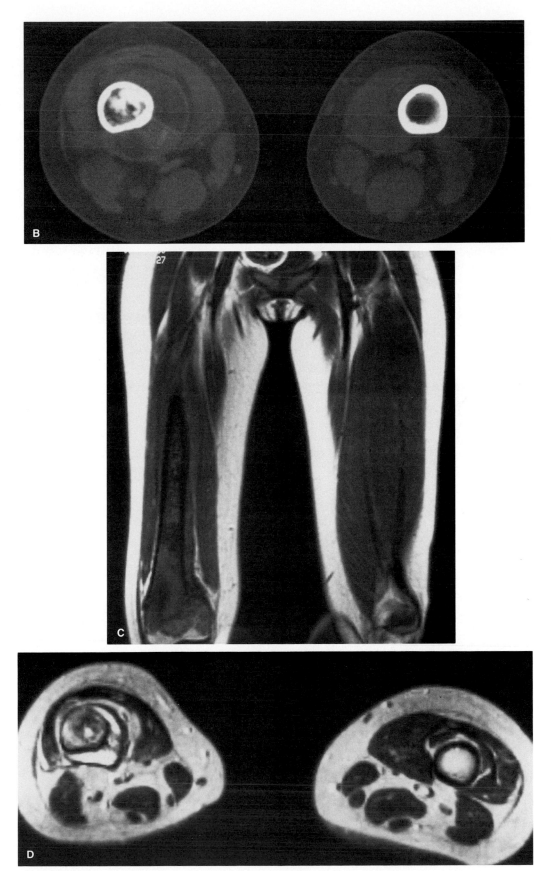

FIGURE 2-22.   *(Continued)*

formation in the marrow cavity and soft tissues that are not seen using MR spin echo techniques. CT can determine intramedullary extension and can best assess the response of the bony portion of the lesion to chemotherapy.[41]

CT shows the attenuation of the medullary cavity. The normal medullary cavity has a fat density of −50 to −80 Hounsfield units. With tumor involvement, this density is significantly increased. The CT scan can differentiate medullary from surface tumors. Surface osteosarcomas initially have no medullary involvement, only juxtacortical and soft-tissue components. Conventional osteosarcomas have soft-tissue and medullary involvement. Osteomyelitis can cause similar changes in marrow attenuation. CT can also show anatomic relations, but definitive staging is best achieved using MRI.

MRI is most important and is more accurate than CT in defining the extent of and in staging osteosarcoma.[42] Coronal and sagittal sections and axial T1-weighted and T2-weighted images are needed. Intra-medullary disease is best shown by coronal or sagittal T1-weighted images, and soft-tissue tumor extension is best demonstrated by T2-weighted axial images. High- or low-signal-intensity intramedullary lesions can be seen with T2 weighting; the former is caused by cellular tumor, and the latter is caused by osteosclerosis (Fig. 2-23). T1-weighted images show both types as low-signal-intensity areas replacing high-signal-intensity fatty marrow. Extraosseous and intramedullary tumors on T2-weighted images have a high signal intensity, except for heavily calcified regions. The tumor extent is sharply demarcated from normal muscle. Its relation to vessels, tendons, compartments, and other structures can be assessed. MRA may prove useful in assessing major vessels. MRI can best define both the intraosseous and extraosseous extent of the tumor, any skip areas, and response to therapy. Details of the pattern of cortical destruction and periosteal new bone formation can also be seen on MRI.[9] Marrow edema may simulate tumor involvement.

Radionuclide bone scans of osteosarcoma demon-

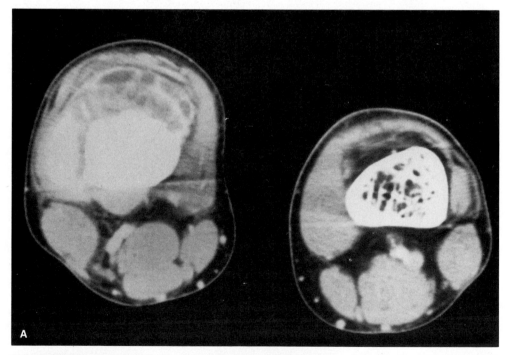

FIGURE 2-23. An 18-year-old man with osteosarcoma involving the right distal femur. (**A**) The CT scan shows sclerosis of the right distal femur with surrounding soft-tissue tumors containing dense calcification. (**B**) The radionuclide bone scan shows increased activity of the distal femur with a zone of lesser increase in the midportion of the tumor. (**C**) MR (SE 800/20) sagittal section. A mixed signal intensity in the distal femoral shaft, metaphysis, and epiphysis occurs with a surrounding soft-tissue tumor. The midportion of the tumor is of low signal intensity. (**D**) MR image (SE 2000/20). Low signal intensity in the midportion of the tumor corresponds to the area of sclerosis. A surrounding soft-tissue mass containing calcification is also seen. (**E**) MR image (SE 2000/80). The osteosclerotic area in the tumor remains of low signal intensity, and the more cellular portions increase in signal intensity, as does the soft-tissue component. The dense calcification in these soft tissues remains of low signal intensity. This sclerotic zone corresponds to the area of lower signal intensity seen on the radionuclide scan. (**F**) The digital subtraction arteriogram shows tumor stain throughout the entire tumor. (**G**) Plain film shows the sclerotic pattern.

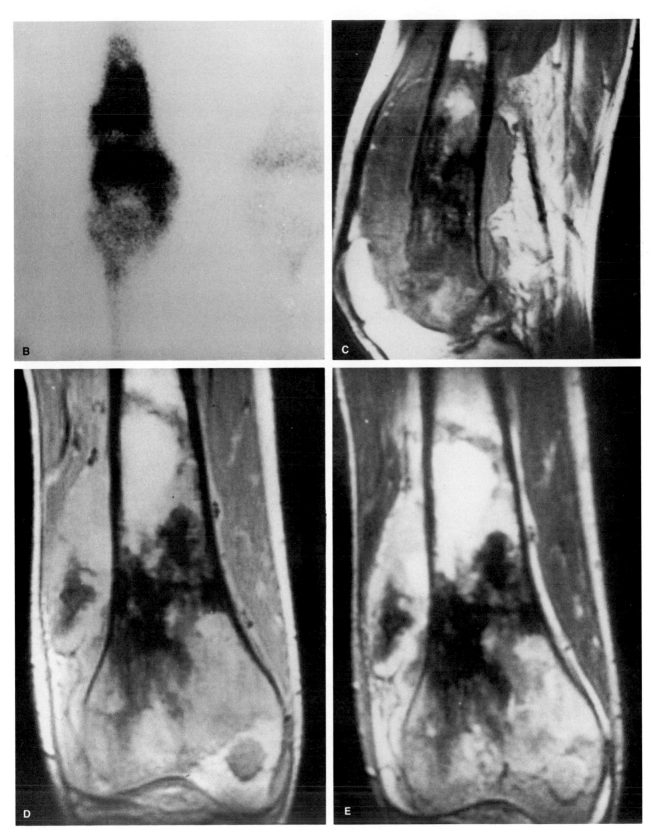

FIGURE 2-23.   *(Continued)*

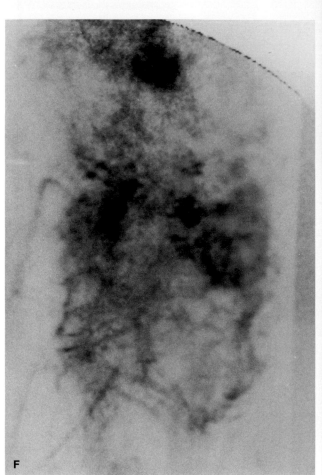

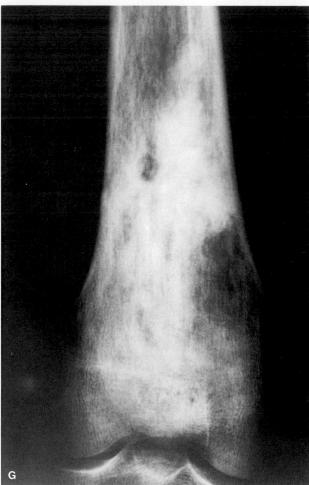

FIGURE 2-23. *(Continued)*

strate increased uptake by the tumor, but osteosarcoma is usually evident on conventional x-ray films at presentation. The chief uses of radionuclide bones scans are to detect bony metastases and in following patients during chemotherapy. However, the uptake pattern may not represent the true limits of the tumor, instead showing a false extended response, probably because of marrow hyperemia, medullary reactive bone, or periosteal new bone. Increased uptake may also be present within synovial fluid in an involved joint.[43] A photopenic lesion on ^{99m}Tc bone scan in a case of osteolytic-appearing osteosarcoma has been reported.[44] It is not uncommon to see a photopenic region within an area of increased uptake in an osteosarcoma because of interrupted blood supply, which may be from a variety of causes. A joint distal to a tumor in an extremity may show increased activity secondary to disuse osteoporosis or possibly stress (Fig. 2-24).

Angiography is used to determine the vascular pattern and the extent of the osteosarcoma and for the selection of a biopsy site.[45] Most osteosarcomas are vascular tumors. The vascular supply arises from surrounding tissues. An important use of angiography is assessing the response of osteosarcoma to chemotherapy.[46] A good local response produces a diminution of vascularity, which is more significant than diminution of size (Fig. 2-25).

Other Types of Osteosarcomas

Telangiectatic Osteosarcoma

Telangiectatic osteosarcoma is characterized by large cystic cavities filled with fresh and clotted blood, similar to an aneurysmal bone cyst.[47] Osteoid is scant. It is a rare, aggressive type of osteosarcoma. A conventional osteosarcoma may contain telangiectatic elements. Some pathologists consider only those tumors that completely contain telangiectatic tissue as true examples of this entity. The skeletal distribution is similar to conventional osteosarcoma, principally involving the

(text continues on page 74)

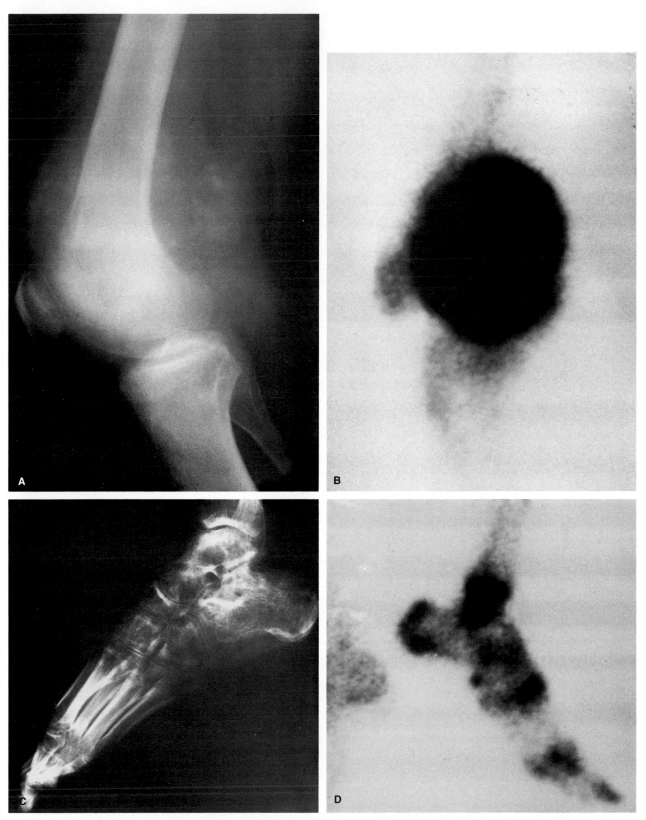

FIGURE 2-24.   Osteosarcoma of the distal femur in an 18-year-old woman. (**A**) The lateral view of the right femur shows sclerosis of the distal femoral metaphysis extending to the epiphysis with a large, calcified, adjacent soft-tissue mass representing an osteosarcoma. (**B**) The radionuclide bone scan shows increased uptake in the distal femur and in the soft-tissue component of the tumor. (**C**) Lateral view of the right foot and ankle 2 months after chemotherapy. Marked patchy osteoporosis is seen. (**D**) The radionuclide bone scan of the right foot and ankle shows multiple areas of increased activity. No tumor was evident.

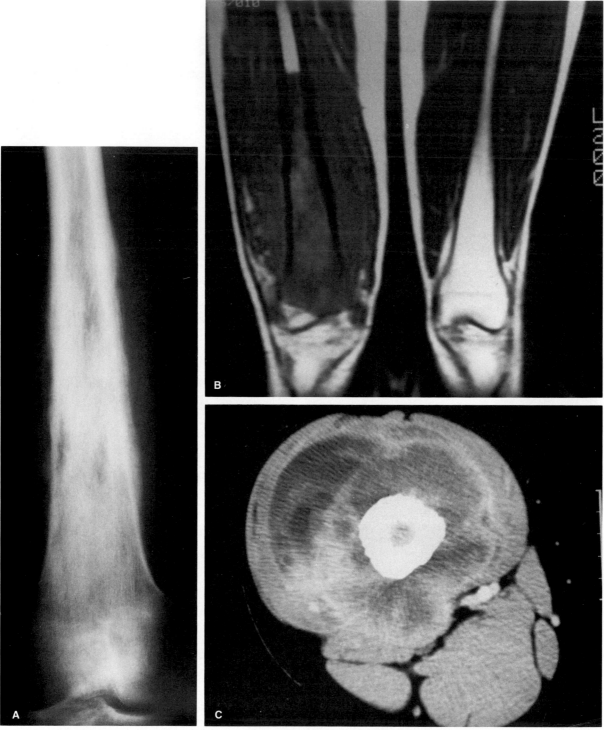

FIGURE 2-25. A 17-year-old man with osteosarcoma involving the distal half of the femur.
A) The anteroposterior view of the femur shows osteosclerosis of the distal diaphysis and metaphysis extending to the epiphysis. Periosteal new bone formation of the laminated type and a proximal Codman triangle are evident. (**B**) MR image (SE 600/25). The extent of the tumor replacing marrow fat and a large soft-tissue mass are seen. (**C**) Enhanced CT. Bony sclerosis and a large inhomogeneously enhancing soft-tissue mass, which displaces the femoral artery and vein posteriorly, are demonstrated. (**D**) The axial MR (SE 500/25) image shows a large, surrounding soft-tissue mass with cortical destruction. The femoral artery is displaced posteriorly. The profunda femoral artery is not seen. (**E**) Digital subtraction angiography (DSA) shows that the femoral artery is intact. Tumor stain in the intraosseous and extraosseous components of the tumor are seen. (**F**) One month later after chemotherapy, there has been a decrease in tumor vascularity. The extraosseous components of the tumor are only minimally diminished in size, on this DSA image.

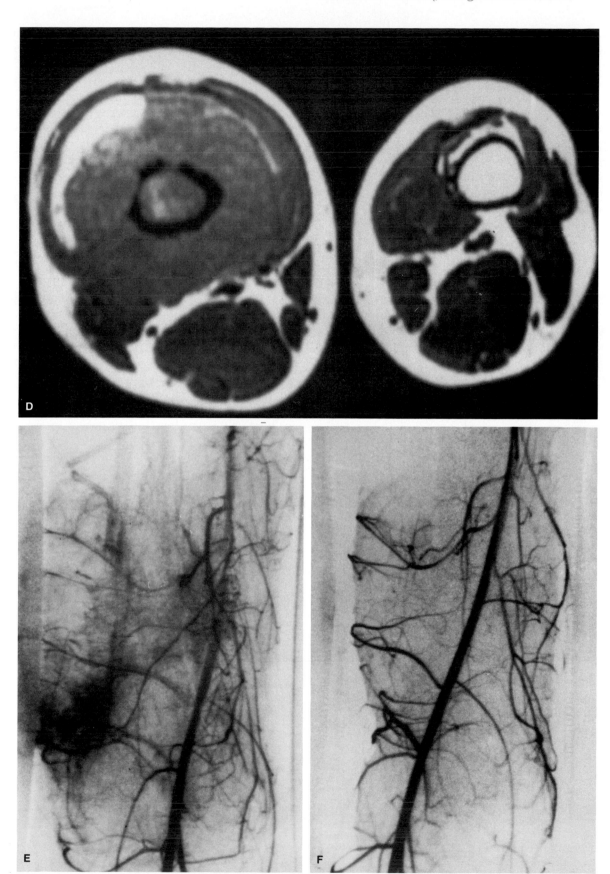

FIGURE 2-25. *(Continued)*

femur, tibia, and humerus at the metaphysis. Diaphyseal involvement is also possible. The age distribution is the same as that of conventional osteosarcoma. Most of these lesions are osteolytic or expansile or have a reticular pattern (Fig. 2-26) or a geographic pattern. Osteosclerosis mitigates against this diagnosis. The tumor margin maybe well defined or show a wide zone of transition. Periosteal new bone formation may exist in any pattern, or it may not be seen. Cortical destruction, sometimes with a geographic pattern (Fig. 2-27), pathologic fracture, and soft-tissue invasion, may occur (Fig. 2-28). It is not clear whether the prognosis is worse for this variant than for conventional osteosarcoma. The signal intensity pattern may be mixed on T1-weighted images. Fluid-fluid levels may occasionally be seen.

Osteoclast-Rich Osteosarcoma

Osteoclast-rich osteosarcoma is related to telangiectatic osteosarcoma.[48] Its imaging appearance is varies, and it is less aggressive than telangiectatic osteosarcoma.

Small Cell Osteosarcoma

Small cell osteosarcoma is characterized histologically by sheets of round cells that resemble Ewing tumor, but unlike the latter, produce an osteoid matrix.[49] The osteoid is sometimes hard to find histologically. It is a rare tumor that occurs usually in the second to fourth decades. It presents with pain and swelling of varying duration. The tumor usually involves the long bones, and the most frequent sites are the distal femur and humerus. Radiologically, the appearance is variable. Sclerotic or mixed osteoblastic and osteolytic appearances extending from the metaphysis to the shaft are seen with a geographic or permeative destructive pattern and Codman triangles (Fig. 2-29). Periosteal reaction is seen in many patients. Soft-tissue invasion occurs in most cases.

Low-Grade Central Osteosarcoma

Low-grade central osteosarcoma is a rare variant representing less than 2% of all osteosarcomas.[50] It can be considered as the central analog of parosteal sarcoma. It is a highly differentiated spindle cell tumor with only minimal atypia. This lesion may be histologically mistaken for fibrous dysplasia or osteoblastoma. Clinically, the tumor chiefly affects young adults, with a mean age at diagnosis of 28 years. The duration of symptoms may range from 2 weeks to 5 years. The prognosis is much better than in conventional osteosarcoma. Most tumors are located in the long bones, principally metaphyseal, but they also occur in the shaft. After epiphyseal fusion, the tumor may extend to the end of the bone. Radiologically, a large expansile, tra-

(text continues on page 80)

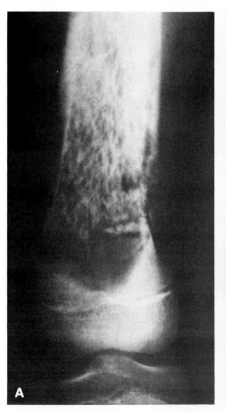 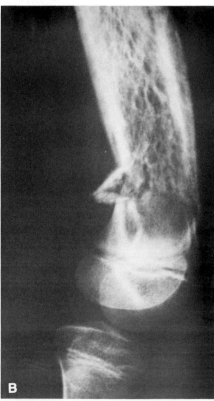

FIGURE 2-26. Telangiectatic osteosarcoma in a 6-year-old girl, showing the characteristic pattern of regular striation in the shaft. (**A**) Anteroposterior view and (**B**) lateral view. The bone is fractured. The tumor involves more than one half of the bone. (Courtesy of Dr. D. Vanel, Villejuif, France. Previously published in Skeletal Radiol 16:196–200, 1987)

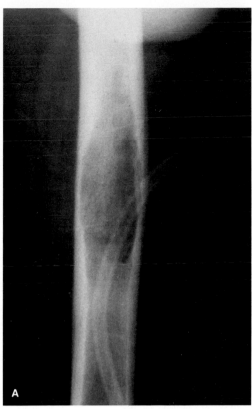

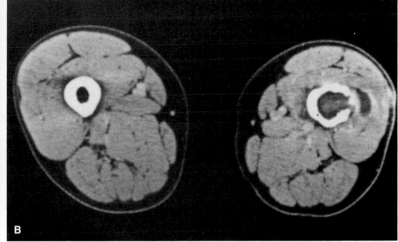

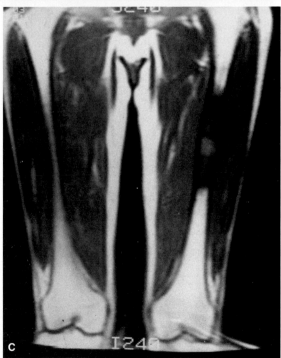

FIGURE 2-27. A 43-year-old man with telangiectatic osteosarcoma of the midfemoral shaft. (**A**) A well-circumscribed geographic destructive lesion with a reticular pattern is seen in the femoral shaft with a small amount of simple periosteal new bone formation. (**B**) A destructive focus in the lateral cortex with soft tissue invasion is seen on the CT scan. (**C**) MR image (SE 400/20). A zone of low signal intensity replaces the marrow. A high-signal-intensity focus, representing hemorrhage, is in its midportion.

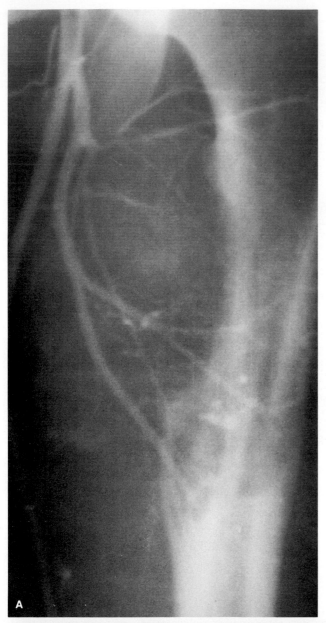

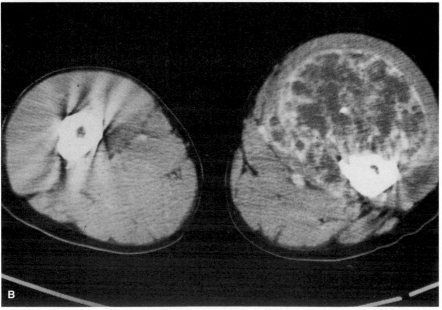

FIGURE 2-28. A 19-year-old man with telangiectatic osteosarcoma of the left proximal femur. (**A**) An angiogram shows eccentric cortical destruction and the extent of the large soft-tissue mass. (**B**) A CT scan shows a large, eccentric, calcified soft-tissue mass with a reticular pattern of calcifications and cortical destruction. The femoral artery is displaced but not invaded. This correlates with the angiogram. (**C**) Digital subtraction angiogram shows tumor stain, puddling of contrast material, and early venous fill. (**D**) The radionuclide bone scan shows increased activity in the large soft-tissue component. The uptake is inhomogeneous.

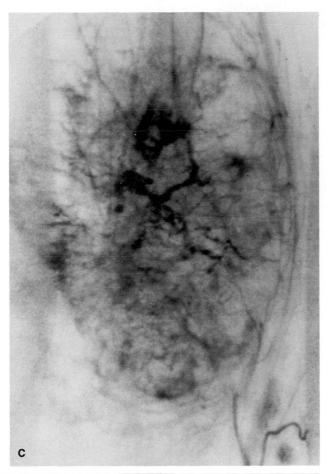

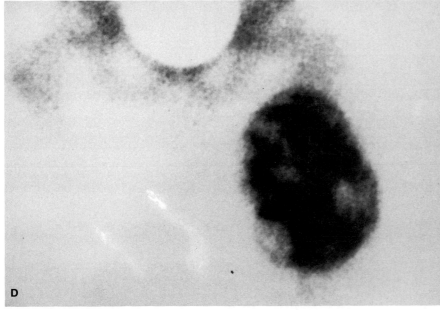

FIGURE 2-28.   *(Continued)*

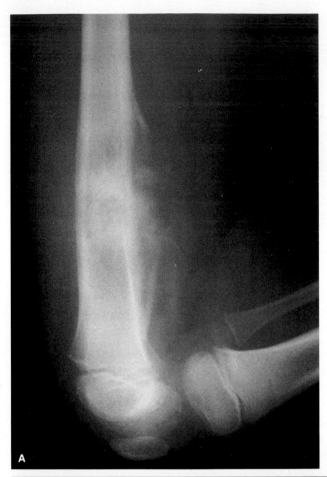

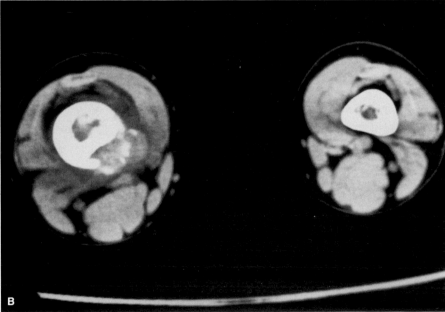

FIGURE 2-29. A 7-year-old boy with small cell osteosarcoma involving the distal femur. (**A**) The lateral view shows a mixed sclerotic and destructive tumor, principally in the diametaphyseal region of the right distal femur. Codman triangles, soft-tissue calcification, and spiculated periosteal new bone formation are seen. (**B**) The CT scan shows cortical destruction, spiculated periosteal new bone formation, and a low-density surrounding tumor mass. (**C**) MR coronal T1-weighted image. The tumor is replacing the marrow signal. The soft-tissue extent of the tumor can be seen. A low-signal-intensity Codman triangle is seen proximally. (**D**) The axial MR (SE 2500/90) image shows a high-signal-intensity tumor surrounding the bone. Low signal intensity corresponds to calcification and sclerosis.

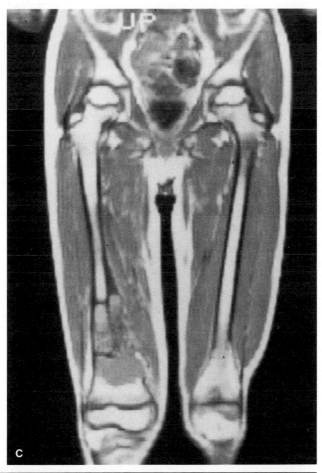

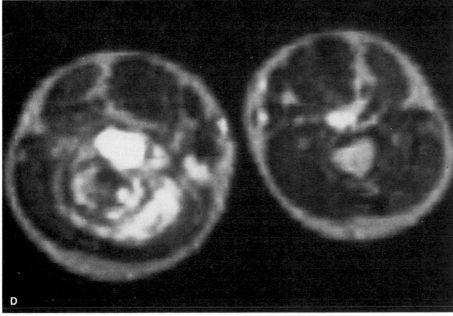

FIGURE 2-29.   *(Continued)*

beculated radiolucency is usually seen. Calcification and ossification (Fig. 2-30) or a ground glass appearance is occasionally observed. Poor margination or minimal cortical destruction offers the clue to malignancy, although many may have sharp, well-defined margins. Cortical destruction may become extensive with soft-tissue invasion. Periosteal new bone formation, affecting only a minority of cases, may be spiculated or laminated. Codman triangles may also be evident. Pathologic fractures rarely occur. The tumor may recur after surgery as a high-grade osteosarcoma.

Multicentric Osteosarcoma

Multicentric osteosarcoma (e.g., sclerosing osteosarcomatosis) is a rare entity consisting of osteosarcomas of synchronous multicentric origin at many sites.[51–55] In children, these tumors are high grade, but if they occur in adults, they are of lower grade. Some cases of multiple tumors may be metastatic osteosarcomatosis, with the lack of pulmonary metastases sometimes caused by tumor dissemination by means of the Batson vertebral vein plexus.

This condition can be classified by immature and mature skeletal involvement. Most cases occur in childhood. Bone pain is a constant feature, followed by general debility. Metastasis to the lungs occurs in most patients early in the course of the disease. The serum alkaline phosphatase level is elevated, and the serum calcium and phosphorus values are normal.

Radiologically, in synchronous disease, the lesions are distributed bilaterally and symmetrically, usually in the metaphyses of the long bones. They are osteosclerotic with any or all of the features of an individual osteosarcoma. They are all approximately the same size, indicating multicentricity. If a dominant lesion that is much larger than the others is seen, the case is a conventional osteosarcoma with bony metastases or a second primary tumor. The picture of multiple, small, sclerotic foci widely distributed in bone was called "miliary osteosarcomatosis" by Mirra.

They may also involve the pelvis, spine, sternum, ribs, and clavicles. The lesions invade the epiphyses, or multiple round sclerotic areas in the epiphyseal ossification centers may develop independently. In the early stages, the lesions may resemble multiple, well-circumscribed metaphyseal bone islands or may simulate the metaphyseal densities seen in heavy metal intoxication.

Surface Osteosarcomas

Three types of osteosarcomas arising on the surface of the bone are commonly described. Periosteal osteosarcoma is a well-differentiated chondroblastic type.

High-grade surface osteosarcoma is highly anaplastic and may be fibroblastic or osteoblastic. Parosteal sarcoma is the best known tumor at this location and is of low grade.

Periosteal Osteosarcoma

Periosteal osteosarcoma has an age-related incidence that is close to conventional osteosarcoma, with a 2 to 1 male predominance.[56,57] The most common location is the proximal third of the femur, and it usually occurs along the anterior diaphysis. It is a well-differentiated chondroblastic tumor. The cortex is always involved, showing thickening without initial medullary involvement. The radiographic appearance is that of a spiculated mass originating from the cortex and of variable length (Figs. 2-31 and 2-32). The tumor is denser at its cortical base, which it does not outgrow. There is no radiolucent line between the tumor and the cortex, as seen in a parosteal sarcoma. The periosteal spicules are perpendicular to the cortex and may vary from coarse to fine. Calcification is not as dense or solid as that seen in parosteal sarcoma. Areas may show the amorphous or stippled calcification pattern of cartilage. Periosteal new bone formation, sometimes laminated, and a Codman triangle may be seen. A soft-tissue mass may be uncalcified. Cortical thickening or destruction may occur, but the medullary cavity is spared before invasion.

High-Grade Surface Osteosarcoma

High-grade surface osteosarcoma is a rare, highly anaplastic tumor.[58] It may be fibroblastic or osteoblastic, analogous to a conventional central osteosarcoma. The age and skeletal distribution is similar to conventional central osteosarcoma. Radiologically, a destructive lesion occurs at the surface of the bone with spiculated periosteal new bone formation and a soft-tissue mass. It may radiologically resemble a periosteal osteosarcoma, but it is histologically high grade. High-grade surface osteosarcoma is similar in its course and histology to medullary osteosarcoma.[59]

Parosteal Sarcoma

Parosteal sarcoma originates in the periosteum or immediate parosteal connective tissue.[60–64] Fibrous, cartilaginous, and osseous elements are present. It is the surface analog of low-grade central osteosarcoma. Clinically, parosteal sarcoma is rare, comprising 4% to 5% of all osteosarcomas. It has an age range from childhood to the sixth decade, with most cases occurring in young adults. Females are more frequently affected than males with a 3 to 2 ratio.

The patient complains of a slowly growing mass

(text continues on page 84)

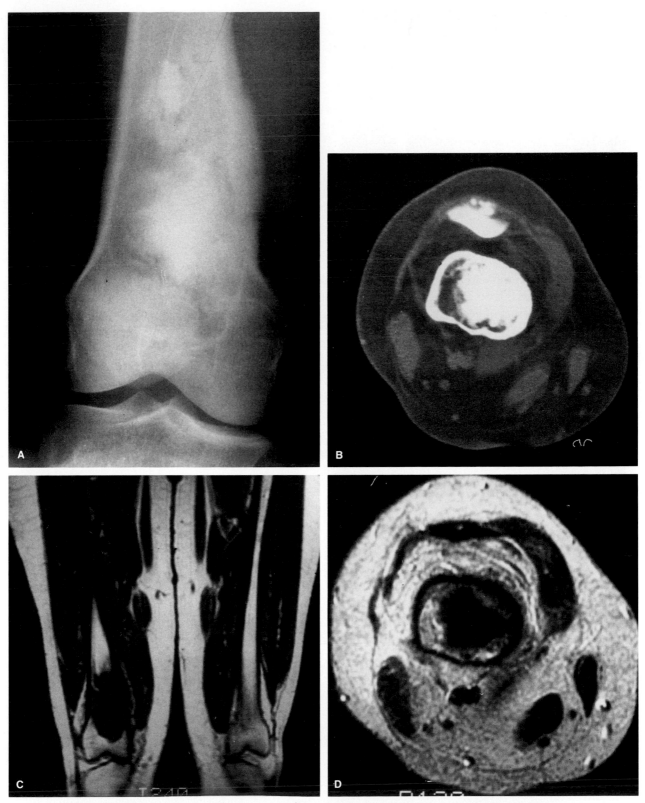

FIGURE 2-30.   A 30-year-old woman with low-grade central osteosarcoma. **(A)** The anteroposterior view of the distal right femur reveals a large, central osteosclerotic area and thickening of the cortex. **(B)** A large osteosclerotic area within the medullary cavity is seen on the CT scan. **(C)** MR image (SE 600/20). The tumor replaces marrow fat in the distal femoral metaphysis. An irregular signal void area represents the sclerotic portion. **(D)** The axial MR (SE 2700/80) section shows a large signal void area within the medullary cavity, corresponding to that seen as calcification on CT. The cortex is intact.

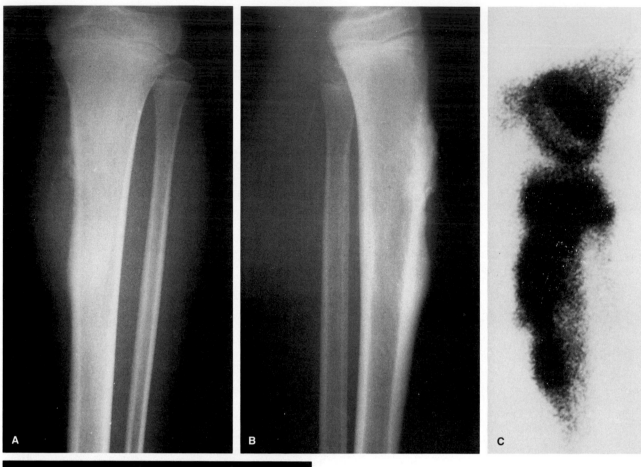

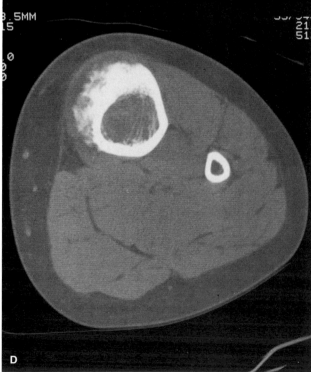

FIGURE 2-31. An 11-year-old girl with periosteal osteosarcoma involving principally the diametaphyseal area of the proximal left tibia. (**A**) In the anteroposterior view, the tumor eccentrically involves the proximal tibia with saucerization of the medial cortex and an adjacent calcified soft-tissue mass. (**B**) The lateral view shows thickening of the anterior cortex with sclerosis and calcifications within the adjacent soft-tissue mass. (**C**) A radionuclide bone scan shows increased activity in the proximal tibia, particularly at the anterior cortex and adjacent to soft tissue. (**D**) CT scan shows involvement of the anterior and medial cortex.

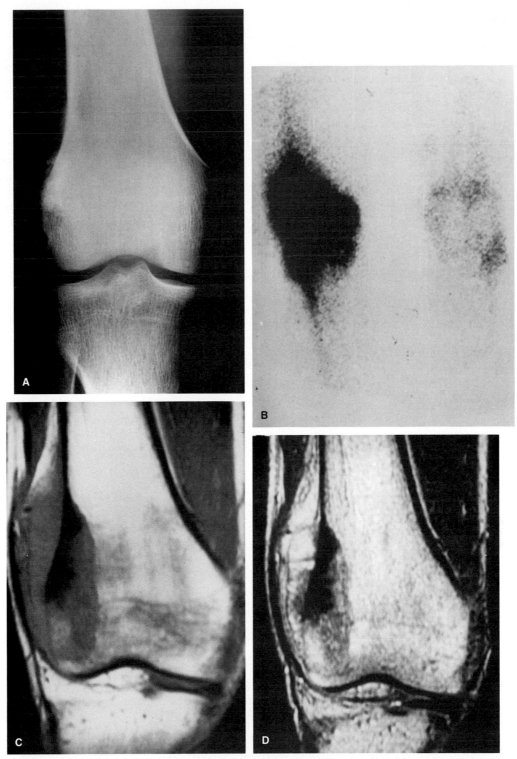

FIGURE 2-32. An 18-year-old man with periosteal osteosarcoma involving the right distal femoral metaphysis. (**A**) Spiculated periosteal new bone formation along the lateral aspect and a Codman triangle. (**B**) The radionuclide bone scan shows marked uptake at the distal right femur and increased uptake of the proximal tibia, which contains no tumor. (**C**) MR image (SE 500/20). The thickened cortex is seen as a signal void. The tumor is seen with low signal intensity. A small amount is intrinsic to bone and the larger component in the soft tissue. The proximal tibia shows normal marrow signal. (**D**) MR image (SE 2000/70). The osteosclerotic cortex is seen as a signal void. The soft-tissue component of the tumor has increased in signal intensity. The tumor extends to the epiphysis, with the major portion of the medullary cavity showing a normal marrow signal.

that interferes with articular motion if the tumor is located near a joint. Pain may or may not be a feature. The prognosis is better than in conventional osteosarcoma. The tumor may later dedifferentiate, invade the medullary cavity, and then metastasize to the lungs, particularly after local excision.[65]

Radiologically, most cases arise at the posterior aspect of the distal metaphysis of the femur, with the metaphyses of the proximal femur, proximal humerus, and tibia as other common sites. It may also arise along the shaft. The tumor may arise in the facial bones and rarely from the outer table of the skull.[66]

The size of the lesion ranges from a small juxtacortical mass limited to the site of attachment to the cortex to a bulky tumor completely surrounding the entire bone. As the tumor outgrows its base, a radiolucent line representing the periosteum remains between it and the cortex, except at the base. This has been called the string sign, and it can be well demonstrated with CT (Fig. 2-33). Later, this may be obliterated. The tumor may have a homogeneous ivory density, or it may show lobulated areas of calcification (Fig. 2-34). The density of the tumor is usually greatest near the cortex. Round, large, dense masses in the soft tissue, separate from the bulk of the tumor, may form. These may show more pronounced calcification at the periphery. The tumor may grow completely around the bone without invasion. A nonossified soft-tissue component may also be present, and rarely, there is a sunburst periosteal pattern.

Angiography helps to differentiate parosteal sarcoma from more aggressive tumors (Fig. 2-35) by their lack of hypervascularity. Parosteal sarcomas are low-grade tumors. In about 10% of patients, the tumor dedifferentiates and becomes invasive, usually as a recurrence after surgery. Osteolytic areas, a sparsely calcified soft-tissue component, and hypervascular foci are clues to this condition. Rarely, dedifferentiated parosteal osteosarcoma may be seen as an initial presentation. CT and MRI are particularly useful in this determination (Fig. 2-36). In these cases, the prognosis is similar to that for conventional osteosarcoma.[67]

Osteosarcomas Developing in Abnormal Bone

Osteosarcoma may rarely develop de novo in older age groups, where it usually arises from an underlying bone abnormality. One possibility is the malignant transformation of a previously benign tumor. The development of osteosarcoma in bone involved with Paget disease or in irradiated bone is well documented. Osteosarcoma rarely develops in fibrous dysplasia, and it has also been associated with enchondroma,[68] osteogenesis imperfecta, and bone infarction.[69,70] Dediffer-

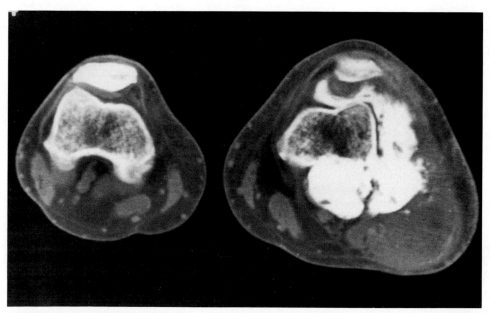

FIGURE 2-33. A 38-year-old man with parosteal sarcoma of the left distal femoral metaphysis. A densely calcified soft-tissue mass originates from the posterior cortex and extends around the anterior aspect of the bone. There is a radiolucency between the calcified mass and the cortex of the bone laterally and anteriorly. This corresponds to the periosteum and has been referred to as the "string sign." The medullary cavity is free of tumor.

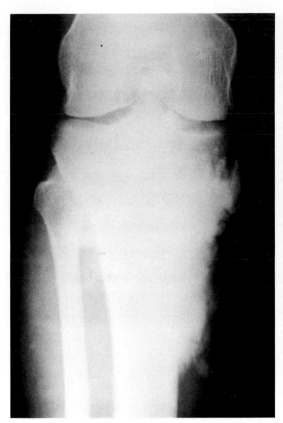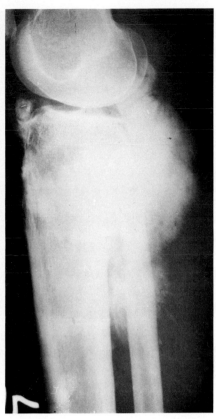

FIGURE 2-34. Parosteal sarcoma. A large, densely and uniformly calcific, lobulated soft-tissue mass is seen in relation to the dorsal and lateral aspect of the proximal tibia. The margins are lobulated. (Courtesy of Drs. A. Pizarro and J. F. Kurtz, Veterans Administration Hospital, Hines, IL.)

entiated chondrosarcoma may also occur as an osteosarcoma.

Osteosarcoma as a Complication of Paget Disease

The cause of Paget disease is unknown, but it is characterized by destructive and reparative changes in bone. Malignant transformation occurs in a small percentage of patients.[71] This disease may be limited in distribution and still be the site of a sarcoma.

The serum alkaline phosphatase level is elevated in Paget disease. A sudden rise in an already elevated alkaline phosphatase value may herald the development of an osteosarcoma. The presenting symptoms are pain or a mass.

The type of sarcoma developing in Paget disease is high-grade osteosarcoma in more than half of cases. Chondrosarcoma, fibrosarcoma, and malignant fibrous histiosarcoma account for most of the remainder. Giant cell tumor also rarely occurs. The tumors arise in bone involved with Paget disease.

The range of the patients' ages is 46 to 91 years.[72] The ratio of men to women is 2 to 1.

Radiologically, the pelvis, humerus, and femur are frequently involved.[73] The calvarium, scapula, mandible,[74] calcaneus, vertebral column, and other long bones may also be involved. Bone destruction with ill-defined margins and a wide zone of transition is usually seen (Figs. 2-37 and 2-38). Increased density (Fig. 2-39) and mixed or permeative patterns are rarely seen. Periosteal new bone formation is rare. Soft-tissue invasion may occur, and there is a high incidence of pathologic fractures. The lesions rarely are multiple. The tumor usually metastasizes by the hematogenous route.

Osteosarcoma in Previously Irradiated Bone

Exposure to ionizing radiation may lead to the formation of malignant bone tumors. These changes can result from internal[75] or external[76] radiation sources. Historically, internal radiation effects on humans were documented by Martland in watch-dial painters who had ingested radium and mesothorium by shaping the ends of their paintbrushes with their tongues. They developed anemia, bone necrosis, osteomyelitis, patho-

(text continues on page 89)

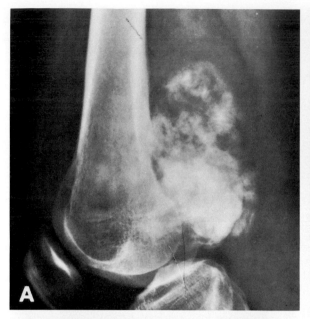

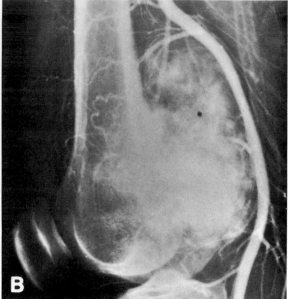

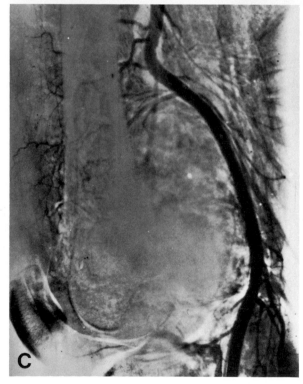

FIGURE 2-35. Parosteal sarcoma in a 38-year-old man with a 10-year history of tumefaction and pain. (**A**) Lateral roentgenogram of the knee reveals a sclerotic lesion attached to the posterior aspect of the distal femur, typical for parosteal sarcoma. (**B**) Angiogram of the arterial phase reveals displaced, but normal, vascularity in the tumor area. (**C**) Angiogram of the venous phase reveals normal veins with displacement. The lack of hypervascularity is a diagnostic sign for differentiating parosteal sarcoma from osteosarcomas and can explain less aggressive behavior of some of these tumors. (Courtesy of Dr. Issa Yaghmai, Medical College of Virginia, Richmond, VA.)

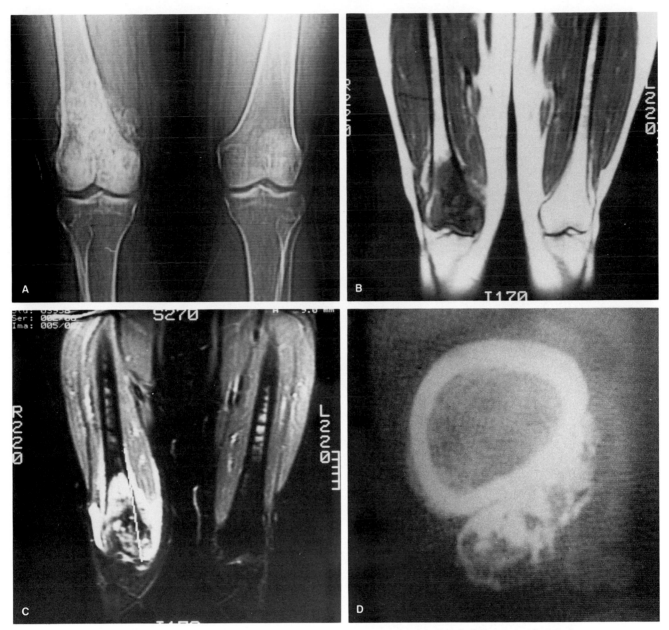

FIGURE 2-36. A 28-year-old woman with a parosteal sarcoma that has dedifferentiated. (**A**) The digital radiograph shows lobulated soft-tissue masses at the distal femoral metaphysis. (**B**) MR image (SE 600/20). A low-signal-intensity tumor involves the distal femoral metaphysis and epiphysis in this coronal section. (**C**) MR image (SE 2000/40). A high signal intensity is seen in the tumor, and a signal void represents calcification in the soft-tissue component and in the medullary cavity. (**D**) The CT scan demonstrates a well-formed soft-tissue mass posteriorly with dense calcifications. A thin, radiolucent line separates the mass from the cortex. (**E**) The CT scan at a lower level shows the well-formed calcified mass posteriorly. There has been invasion of the medullary cavity with sclerosis. The cortex is largely intact. A radiolucent line between the calcified tumor and cortex at the medial aspect is evident. (**F**) MR (SE 2000/20) axial section. The calcifications and osteosclerosis are seen as low signal intensity. The lightly calcified portions of the tumor produce low signal intensity. The calcified soft-tissue component can be seen as separate from the bony cortex. (**G**) Digital subtraction angiography shows the tumor to be relatively avascular, with one small focus of hypervascularity. *continued*

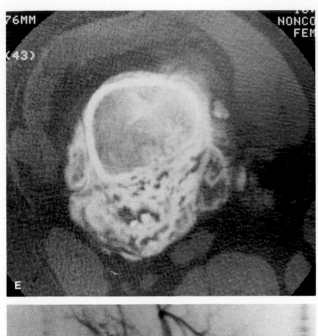

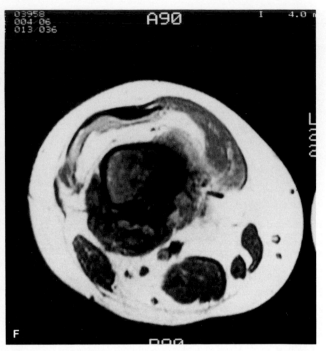

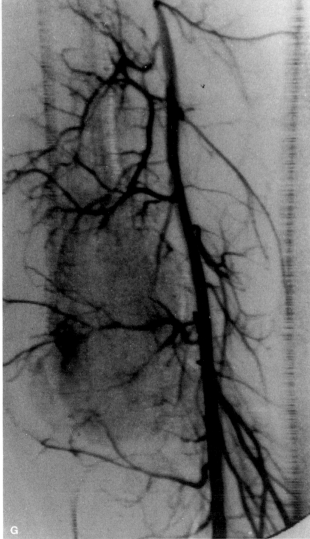

FIGURE 2-36. *(Continued)*

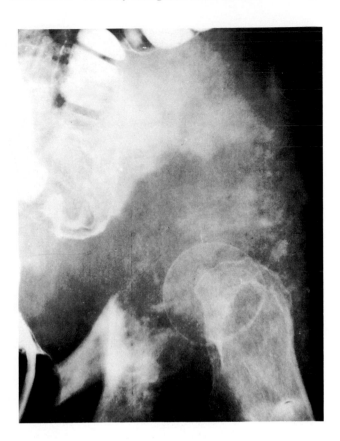

FIGURE 2-37. Osteosarcoma of the pelvis associated with Paget disease produces extensive destructive areas in the acetabulum and ilium. New bone formation in the tumor mass is apparent. The tumor does not cross the articular surface, and the femoral head is spared. The changes of Paget disease in the ischium and pubis are also visible. The associated soft-tissue mass may cause displacement of the barium-filled colon. This represents the radiologic osteolytic picture of osteosarcoma.

logic fractures, carcinomas of the paranasal sinuses and mastoids, and bone sarcomas. Ingested bone-seeking radioactive substances are metabolized and deposited in the body by the same pathway as calcium.

External sources, such as a radiation treatment field, can cause radiation osteitis, destruction, sclerosis, pathologic fracture, local inhibition of bone growth, and induce a sarcoma.

The latent period between exposure to a ionizing radiation and the diagnosis of a tumor ranges from 9 months to 50 years, with an average of 13 years. Sarcoma may develop in previously normal bone that was in the radiation field or at the site of a preexisting irradiated lesion. Sarcoma is rare after irradiation for metastatic bone carcinoma; high-grade osteosarcoma is usually seen. Fibrosarcoma, chondrosarcoma, and Ewing tumor may also occur. Malignant fibrous histiocytoma, malignant lymphoma, metastasizing chondroblastoma, and chondroblastic osteosarcoma have also been reported.[77–80] The age range of patients is from 8.5 to 77 years, with an average of 47 years. Benign bone tumors, particularly giant cell tumor, may show sarcomatous changes after irradiation.

Fibrous Dysplasia with Sarcomatous Change

The development of sarcoma in fibrous dysplasia is rare. The fibrous dysplasia may be polyostotic or monostotic. The gender-related incidence is approximately equal. The age range of patients is 11 to 54 years. The sites involved are the mandible, femur, pelvis, scapula, humerus, tibia, maxilla, and fibula. The cell types seen are osteosarcoma, fibrosarcoma, chondrosarcoma, and giant cell tumor.

Radiologically, an area of bone destruction is superimposed on the changes of fibrous dysplasia. There may be an expansile or trabeculated lesion. Bone sclerosis and a sunburst type of periosteal reaction may be seen.

Osteosarcoma in Osteogenesis Imperfecta

A fracture in osteogenesis imperfecta may be surrounded by a large soft-tissue mass containing very dense calcification, much more than in the usual healing fracture in normal bone. This is caused by hyperplastic callus formation and can simulate an osteosarcoma. Rarely, a true osteosarcoma is found.

Other Types

Osteosarcoma associated with a bone infarct is rare. Most infarct-associated bone sarcoma is malignant fibrous histiocytoma; only 18% are osteosarcomas. The long bones are chiefly affected.[81] A single case has been reported of osteosarcoma associated with osteopoikilosis.[82]

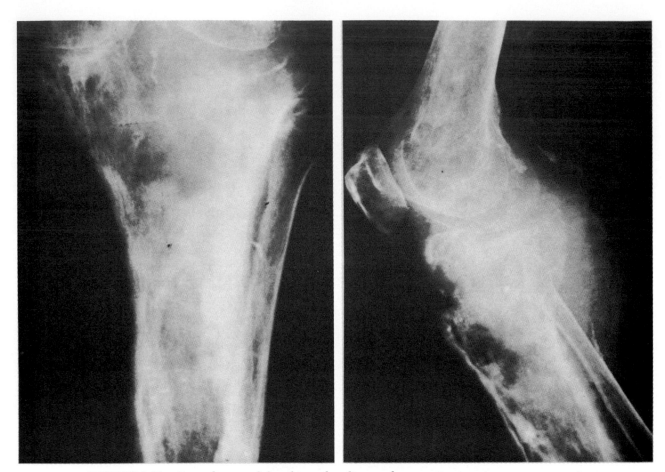

FIGURE 2-38. Paget disease of the tibia and malignant degeneration to osteosarcoma are evident in these arteroposterior and lateral views. The characteristics of the combined phase are cortical thickening and trabecular accentuation. There is also a destructive process involving the proximal tibia, and the midlateral and lateral aspects of the articular surface have been destroyed. There is an ill-defined margin at the distal aspect, representing osteosarcoma. The destructive tumor is situated anteriorly at the proximal tibia, and the margins of the tumor are poorly defined.

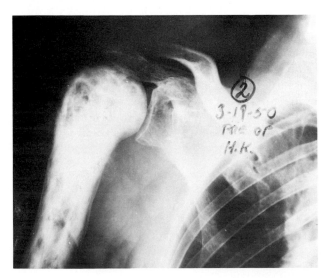

FIGURE 2-39. Osteosarcoma of the proximal humerus in Paget disease. The classic changes of Paget disease are present, with cortical thickening and accentuation of the trabecular pattern. A dense area of osteosclerosis involves the humeral head and neck and a portion of the shaft and proved to be osteosarcoma. A slight periosteal reaction suggests spiculation at the medial aspect. (Courtesy of Drs. A. Pizarro and J. F. Kurtz, Veterans Administration Hospital, Hines, IL.)

Osteosarcoma of the jaw occurs later in life than conventional osteosarcoma. It may be in the maxilla or the mandible. It is more differentiated than other forms and tends to be chondroblastic. The radiologic features are similar to the conventional type (Fig. 2-40).

Intracortical osteosarcoma is the rarest subtype of osteosarcoma.[83] The average age of patients is 24 years, with a range of 10 to 43 years. Radiologically, a well-marginated intracortical osteolytic lesion as large as 4 cm may be seen, with smooth thickening of the cortex. The lesion may simulate an osteoid osteoma. It may also present as an intracortical destructive lesion with indistinct margins.[84]

Staging

Staging is based on the concept that the tumor progresses from disease limited to the site of origin, to invasion of adjacent tissues, and then to distant metastases.[85] The classification system of the American Joint Committee Task Force on Staging of Bone Tumors is used to stage these tumors. Primary non-round cell sarcomas of bone are divided into low grade (I) and high grade (II). They are then separated according to whether cortical penetration has not occurred (A) or occurred (B). This classification system has a disadvantage in that over 90% of osteosarcomas without metastases fall into class IIB, regardless of tumor size or extent of soft-tissue invasion.

A further subclassification system has been proposed at the University of Florida for class IIB nonmetastatic osteosarcomas that depends on their relation to the periosteum and the number of soft-tissue structures involved. The researchers found a significantly greater 5-year disease-free survival for patients whose tumor did not invade two or more soft-tissue structures or spaces. These studies were based on pathology specimens of untreated tumors.[85]

For patients undergoing radiation therapy and or chemotherapy before limb-sparing surgery, the response of the sarcoma to this therapy can be evaluated by several modalities. The presurgical therapy may cause necrosis of tumor cells and shrink or sterilize the sarcoma. Tumor necrosis can be demonstrated by an interval decrease in activity on serial bone scans. However, if there is bone repair in response to tumor necrosis, it is seen as increased activity and can create a false-negative response on the bone scan. Gadolinium-enhanced MRI separates necrosis from tumor by the lack of enhancement in necrotic or cystic areas; tumor and necrosis show similar signal characteristics on non-contrast MR images. Digital angiography can demonstrate a response to therapy by showing a decrease in arterial supply and neovascularity of the sarcoma.

CHONDROSARCOMA

Chondrosarcoma is a primary malignant tumor of cartilage.[86–91] It retains its cartilaginous nature although it often contains enchondral ossification or calcification. It accounts for slightly more than 10% of all malignant bone tumors. It is slow growing and may range from small to large sizes. It is rare in the distal extremities. Most of these tumors are primary, but some may de-

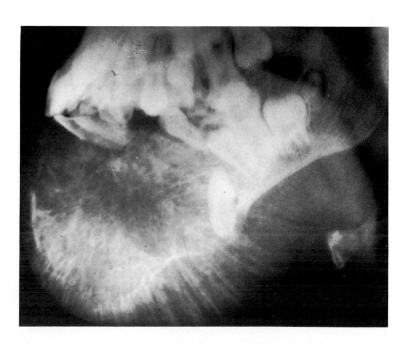

FIGURE 2-40. Osteosarcoma involves the mandible, with long, slender, spiculated, periosteal new bone formation in the "sunburst" pattern. Destructive and sclerotic changes in the mandible are also present, representing a mixed type of osteosarcoma.

velop in a preexisting osteochondroma or enchondroma. Rarely, chondrosarcomas may arise in Paget disease or in postirradiated bone. A chondrosarcoma has been reported to have developed in a unicameral bone cyst[92] and even in synovial osteochondromatosis.[91] Chondrosarcomas can secrete high levels of chorionic gonadotropin.[93] Low levels of this hormone have been reported with osteosarcomas. Chondrosarcomas show wide variations in their clinical, histologic, and behavioral features.[12] Classification of chondrosarcomas is presented in Table 2-3.

Chondrosarcomas originating within a bone are central chondrosarcomas. One originating outside of the cortex is either a peripheral or a juxtacortical chondrosarcoma. A central chondrosarcoma may be primary or secondary. Peripheral chondrosarcoma is a secondary lesion.[94]

Juxtacortical or periosteal chondrosarcoma is a rare malignant tumor arising from the external surface of bone, characterized by well-differentiated hyalin cartilage-containing areas of enchondral ossification. It is found most commonly in young adults, usually involving the diaphysis of a long bone, but it may also affect the metaphysis. The femur is most often involved. The prognosis is relatively favorable. It must be differentiated from periosteal osteosarcoma. Periosteal chondrosarcoma is less painful than periosteal osteosarcoma and runs a slower course. It contains granular opacities. Periosteal osteosarcoma more often affects the mid-diaphysis and shows osteolytic lesions with spicules of reactive bone perpendicular to the cortex.[95]

Chondrosarcomas have developed in children who were long-term survivors of treatment of unrelated tumors at sites other than where the chondrosarcoma arose. The children received radiation therapy, sur-

gery, and chemotherapy. The intervals were 5 to 10 years after the initial therapy.[96]

Central chondrosarcoma is more common than peripheral chondrosarcoma, and primary chondrosarcomas are much more common than secondary ones. Secondary chondrosarcomas occur in a younger age group.

Mesenchymal chondrosarcoma is a rare tumor that originates from primitive cartilage-forming mesenchymal cells. It has elements of well-differentiated cartilage and undifferentiated small round cells. It usually arises in soft tissues and may sometimes be multicentric. This is a highly lethal tumor with a predilection for young patients,[97,98] and it possibly has a higher incidence among females.[91]

Clear cell chondrosarcoma is a rare tumor that may not be recognized as being cartilaginous on inspection of the gross specimen.[99] It is slow growing, with a wide range of age distribution, from the second to the ninth decade of life. As a group, chondrosarcomas are the third most common primary malignant tumors of bone component tissue, after multiple myeloma and osteosarcoma.

The histologic distinction of high-grade and low-grade chondrosarcomas can be correlated with the radiographic and CT appearances.[89] Tumor margins and the pattern of cortical destruction, distribution and pattern of calcifications, soft-tissue involvement, and necrosis are significant features. High-grade tumors show large, concentric, soft-tissue masses with irregular calcifications and large uncalcified areas. Infiltrating margins and necrotic regions at times may be seen in high-grade lesions, which also may show hypervascularity on angiography. A wide zone of transition between the tumor and normal bone is characteristic of high-grade chondrosarcoma, whereas low-grade lesions show a sharp or sclerotic margins. Calcification in low-grade tumor is more uniformly distributed, denser, with ring or spicule formation. The soft-tissue masses are eccentric, reflecting slower growth within anatomic boundaries. Low-grade chondrosarcomas are often hypovascular on angiography and show no necrosis. MRI can define soft-tissue tumor extent and margination better than CT. Gadolinium-enhanced MR images show enhancement of fibrovascular septa, which correlates with a low-grade chondrosarcoma.[100]

Central Chondrosarcoma

The age distribution for patients with central chondrosarcoma is that of adulthood and old age, with more than half of the patients older than 40 years of age. Men are slightly more affected than women. The most frequent complaint is dull pain, with an average duration of several years. Local swelling without inflammatory signs and impairment of a contiguous joint may also be

TABLE 2-3.
Classification of Chondrosarcomas

I. Primary chondrosarcoma
    A. Central
        1. High grade
        2. Low grade
        3. Borderline
    B. Juxtacortical (i.e., periosteal)
    C. Mesenchymal
    D. Dedifferentiated
    E. Clear cell
    F. Malignant chondroblastoma
II. Secondary chondrosarcoma
    A. Central chondrosarcoma
        1. Chondroma (i.e., enchondroma)
        2. Multiple enchondromatosis, with or without Ollier or Maffucci syndrome
    B. Peripheral chondrosarcoma
        1. Osteochondroma (i.e., osteocartilaginous exostosis)
        2. Multiple hereditary exostoses
        3. Juxtacortical (i.e., periosteal)

present. The tumor is slow growing and usually metastasizes late hematogenously. It tends to invade the veins and may even propagate through venous channels to the heart and lungs. Lymphatic metastases are rare but may occur. Although a small percentage of chondrosarcomas follow a fulminant course, in the average case, the prognosis is much better than for osteosarcoma. The closer a cartilaginous lesion is to the central skeleton, the greater its malignant potential.

The most common site of involvement is the femur, most often at the ends, but also involving the midshaft. The proximal humerus is also commonly involved. The tibia, ribs, ilium (Fig. 2-41), scapula, spine, and sternum may be involved.

Cartilage is recognized on conventional x-ray films and CT scans by amorphous, punctate, small, linear, circular, flocculent, dense, or irregular calcifications, which range from sparse to heavy. This finding is seen in approximately two thirds of central chondrosarcomas. A large segment of the shaft of a long bone may be affected (Fig. 2-42).

The tumor may present as an osteolytic, well-marginated, expansile lesion with cortical thickening or thinning. It may not be possible to differentiate this appearance from an enchondroma, but a large size or a location in the proximal skeleton should raise the suspicion of malignancy. A focus of endosteal destruction or an area of endosteal scalloping may be seen. There may be simple periosteal elevation or, rarely, fine spiculation or lamination.

With rapid tumor growth, sharp margination is not seen, and there is a wide zone of transition (Fig. 2-43). The entire diaphysis may be involved. The lesion may progress to cortical destruction and soft-tissue invasion. A large, bulky, soft-tissue tumor mass containing calcifications associated with bone destruction is characteristic of advanced chondrosarcoma.

Cortical thickening along the medial femoral neck and intertrochanteric area, remote from where the tumor is, may sometimes be seen with a femoral tumor. Rarely, it may present as a sclerotic lesion (Fig. 2-44).[101]

It may present in the spine as a purely destructive process of the body with involvement of the lamina (Fig. 2-45)[102] or other portions of the neural arch. A

(text continues on page 96)

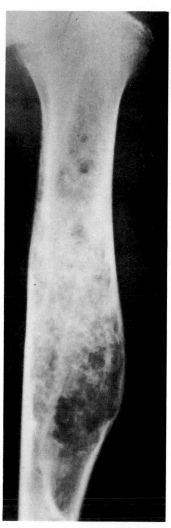

FIGURE 2-42. Chondrosarcoma of the humerus. The expansile lesion involves the proximal and middle third of the humeral shaft. Endosteal scalloping and thickening of the cortex at the medial margin of the lesion are apparent. The lesion is fairly well demarcated. The characteristic streaky and amorphous calcification can be seen within the matrix.

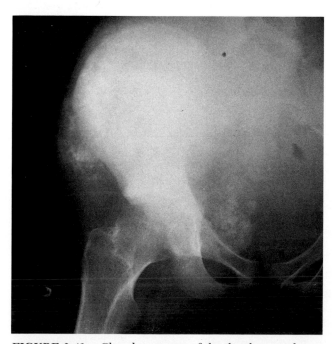

FIGURE 2-41. Chondrosarcoma of the iliac bone. A large, bulky soft-tissue mass containing linear, fine calcifications and reactive sclerosis of the iliac bone are apparent on anteroposterior view of the pelvis.

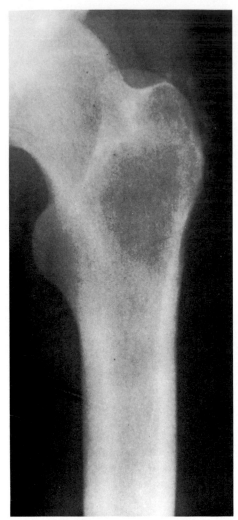

FIGURE 2-43. Chondrosarcoma of the femur. There is an ill-defined, poorly margin-ated area of radiolucency in the intertro-chanteric region of the femur. The outer cortex has been destroyed regionally, and a minimal amount of amorphous soft-tissue calcification can be seen. (Courtesy of Dr. Marion Magalotti, Chicago, IL.)

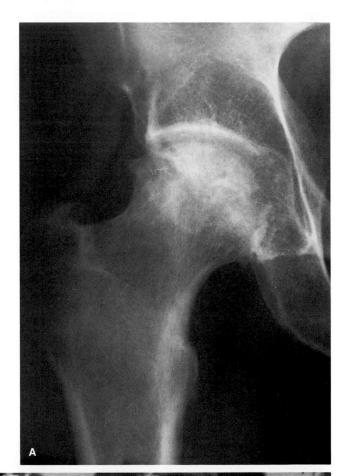

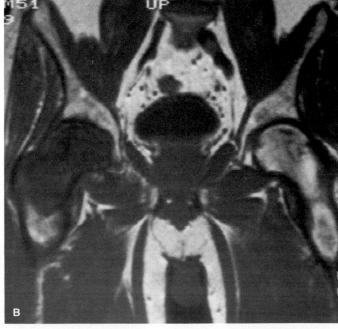

FIGURE 2-44. A 55-year-old man with chondrosarcoma involving the proximal right femur. (**A**) The anteroposte-rior view of the right hip shows the sclerotic appearance of the femoral head, simulating avascular necrosis. (**B**) MR image (SE 800/20). A marrow replacement pattern of low signal intensity involves the femoral head and neck through the subtrochanteric region, indicating the extent of the chondrosarcoma.

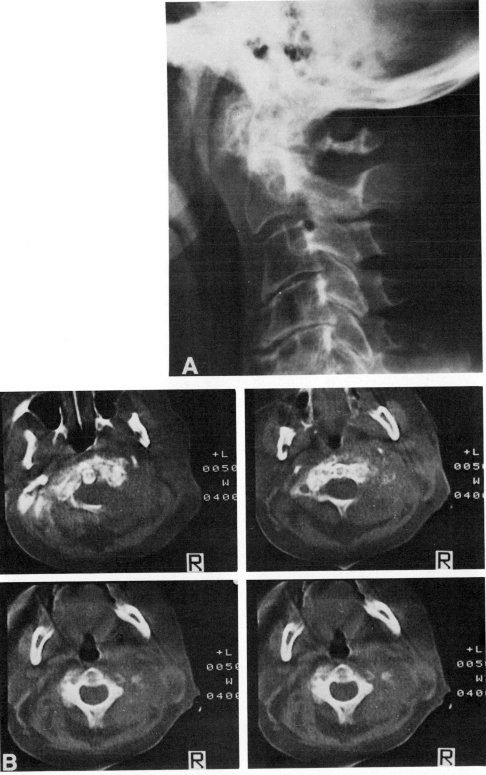

FIGURE 2-45. Chondrosarcoma of the first cervical vertebra. (**A**) The lateral view of the spine shows destruction at the C1 level associated with a large, calcified soft-tissue mass. Degenerative changes in the lower spine are incidentally present. (**B**) CT scan. The odontoid process is easily identified. Expansile, destructive, and calcific changes of the ring of C1 are evident. (Courtesy of Dr. J. P. Petasnick, Rush-Presbyterian St. Luke's Hospital, Chicago, IL.)

bulky tumor of the transverse process in the thoracic spine may simulate a pulmonary mass (Fig. 2-46).

Chondrosarcoma rarely occurs in the small bones of the foot, but it has been reported, with an average age of 38 years. Men are more often affected than women. In the short bones, this tumor must be differentiated from osteosarcoma and spina ventosa of tuberculosis or syphilis. Ewing tumor in the phalanges and myeloma may have an expansile appearance. Chondrosarcoma in the distal extremities is very rare.

A case of primary chondrosarcoma of the proximal tibia with transarticular spread to the distal femur has been reported.[103] A chondrosarcoma may dedifferentiate to a fibrosarcoma,[104] a malignant fibrous histiocytoma, or an osteosarcoma.

Borderline chondrosarcoma with histologic features intermediate between enchondroma and chondrosarcoma has been called grade ½ by Pritchard and Unni. It is most common in middle-aged women. A large, calcified, expansile lesion with cortical thickening may be seen. Surgery is curative.

Peripheral Chondrosarcoma

Peripheral chondrosarcoma refers to tumors resulting from the malignant change of multiple or solitary osteochondromas.[94,105] This transformation occurs much more frequently in multiple exostoses than in solitary exostosis. Peripheral chondrosarcoma is approximately one fifth as common as central chondrosarcoma. It may rarely occur secondary to synovial osteochondromatosis.[91]

The average age of patients with peripheral chondrosarcoma is lower than that of patients having the central type. Most cases occur in middle life, although it rarely may be seen in patients as young as 3 years of age. The patient complains of a slowly growing, painless mass, which may have reached large size at the time of presentation.

The most frequent areas of involvement are the pelvic and shoulder girdles, upper femur, and humerus. Occasionally, other sites are affected. The characteristic finding on plain x-ray films is flocculent, streaky, disorganized calcific densities extending from an osteochondroma into an adjacent soft-tissue mass (Fig. 2-47). The lesion is not marginated. The tumor may be large, but a benign osteochondroma may also be large. In the later stages, the underlying bone may be invaded and destroyed. The cartilaginous cap of an osteochondroma is not as thick as a secondary chondrosarcoma. A thickness of 2 cm should raise the suspicion of a malignancy. Ultrasound has been reported as an accurate means of measuring cap thickness.[106]

CT is useful in the evaluation of a chondrosarcoma. It can show the intraosseous and extraosseous extent of

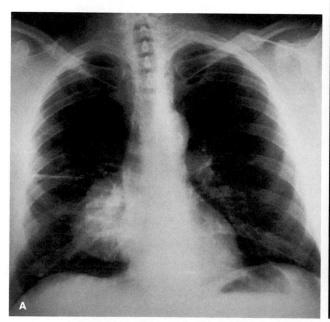
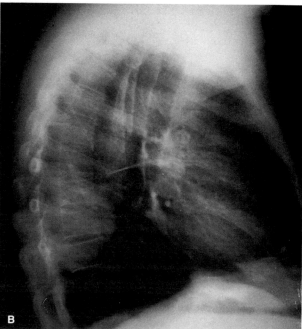

FIGURE 2-46. A 53-year-old man with chondrosarcoma of the right transverse process of the ninth thoracic vertebra. (**A**) Posteroanterior view of the chest. A large bulky mass is posterior to the heart, and there is a 1.0-cm pulmonary metastasis in the right upper lobe. (**B**) The lateral view of the chest shows an ovoid mass abutting the pleural surface projected over the eighth, ninth, and tenth vertebrae. This is a chondrosarcoma simulating a pulmonary mass.

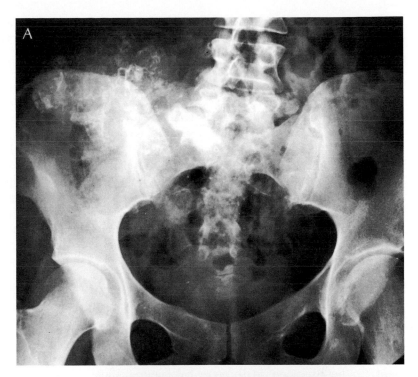

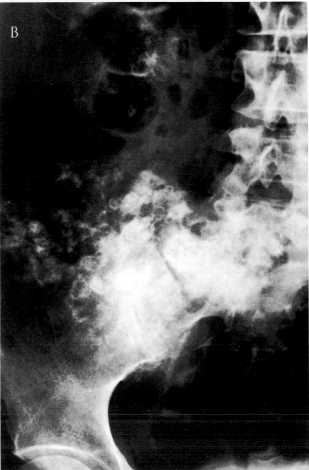

FIGURE 2-47. (**A**) Peripheral chondrosarcoma of the pelvis. There has been malignant degeneration caused by an osteochondroma. A large intrapelvic mass contains disoriented, streaky, and flocculent calcifications. The patient has multiple osteochondromatosis, visible at the left femoral neck and left pubis. (**B**) Recurrent chondrosarcoma in the same patient as in **A** 1 year after resection of tumor and iliac crest. There has been massive recurrence with formation of a large mass in the pelvis and on the right side of the abdomen, exhibiting flocculent and disorganized, linear, streaky calcification.

the tumor and any vascular involvement.[107] CT can define features that help correlate with histologic grade, such as morphology and distribution of calcifications within the lesion, the pattern of tumor growth within soft tissues, and the presence of necrosis.[89] It can show calcifications better than MRI, but CT does not show soft-tissue or bone marrow detail as well.

MRI is valuable in the diagnosis of chondrosarcoma, although current spin echo techniques cannot accurately show the pattern and extent of calcifications.[90,108,109] It can show a marrow replacement pattern to help differentiate this lesion from an infarct or avascular necrosis (see Fig. 2-44). The extent of the lesion in the marrow cavity (Fig. 2-48) and any soft-tissue involvement can be well demonstrated. The tumors show intermediate signal intensity on T1-weighted images and high signal intensity on T2-weighted images. They may be lobulated. Denser calcifications can be seen as scattered irregular signal void areas within the tumor. These may have a punctate, circular, linear, or irregular pattern. Endosteal erosion or cortical expansion may be seen (Fig. 2-49). Cortical destruction, if present, can be discerned. MRI can reveal a central chondrosarcoma that has invaded soft tissue or a peripheral tumor, a large soft-tissue mass containing or bounded by a low-signal-intensity calcification (Fig. 2-50), and the margination, shape, and precise location can be demonstrated (Fig. 2-51). Gadolinium-enhanced T1-weighted images show enhancement in a ring-and-arc pattern of septa, as well as scalloped margins reflecting the lobulated growth pattern of chondrosarcoma. This pattern has only been demonsrated for low-grade tumors and enchondromas.[109a]

Radionuclide bone scans are useful in chondrosarcoma but must be carefully interpreted. Increased uptake usually corresponds to the anatomic extent of the tumor, but some cases may display increased uptake beyond the true tumor margins.[110] This extended pattern of uptake is less common in medullary chondrosarcomas than in many other primary bone tumors. Therefore, increased uptake beyond the radiographic margin of the tumor suggests possible tumor spread. Diminished uptake in the center of the tumor does not necessarily indicate necrosis.[110] Benign enchondromas also show increased uptake.

Radionuclide bone scans to differentiate benign exostoses from peripheral chondrosarcomas are not reliable.[110] Increased uptake in benign exostoses occurs in areas of enchondral ossification. Uptake in chondrosarcomas occurs in areas of osteoblastic activity and hyperemia, not in amorphous cartilage calcification. Activity correlates with areas of ossification visible radiographically, and large masses of nonossifying cartilage may not be detected.

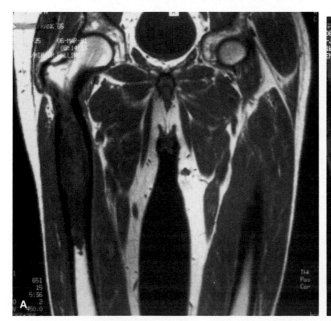
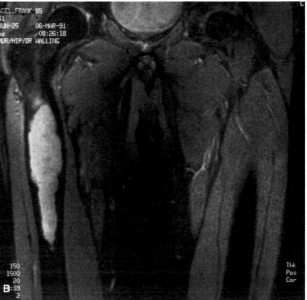

FIGURE 2-48. A 65-year-old man with chondrosarcoma of the right femur. (**A**) MR (SE 651/15) coronal section. Bone marrow replacement in the femoral diaphysis occurs with expansion of the cortex and a low to intermediate inhomogeneous signal intensity. A small nodular extension of the tumor is seen at its inferior aspect. (**B**) MR inversion recovery image. The inhomogeneous high signal intensity of the tumor contains low-signal-intensity foci representing calcifications. (**C**) MR (SE 2700/20) axial section. The tumor increases in signal intensity. An expanded cortex is intact, but there is some soft tissue invasion. (**D**) MR (SE 2700/80) axial section. The tumor now has high signal intensity. A low-signal-intensity central focus indicates calcification. There is no surrounding tumor invasion, and the cortex is intact.

The angiographic appearance of chondrosarcomas varies, because a large variety of vascularity exists in chondrosarcomatous tissue. Some high-grade chondrosarcomas are very vascular, but most chondrosarcomas show low to moderate vascularity (see Fig. 2-50). Low vascularity reflects the intracellular type of nutrition that exists in cartilaginous tumors. Hypovascularity in a malignant chondroid tumor does not necessarily rule out the presence of malignant cells.[3]

Yaghmai[3] classified the angiographic appearance of chondrosarcomas on the basis of angioarchitecture into three groups: hypervascular, moderately vascular, and hypovascular. The hypervascular group has typical malignant features, including pathologic vessels, arteriovenous shunts, rapid tumor circulation, vessel encasement, obstruction of large arteries and veins, abnormal venous lakes, and collateral veins. The moderate vascularity group shows some of the above features. The group with low vascularity correlates well with histologically well-differentiated chondrosarcomas. They present difficulty in diagnosing a malignancy. Some findings in this group include a few pathologic vessels and occasional encasement, encroachment, and obstruction of second- and third-degree arteries and veins.[3]

Periosteal Chondrosarcoma

Periosteal (i.e., juxtacortical) chondrosarcoma presents as flocculent soft-tissue calcifications within a soft-tissue mass, attached to bone without a preexisting osteochondroma. Pressure effects and sclerosis of underlying bone may be seen. It may show long-segment involvement of the diaphysis with a soft-tissue mass

(text continues on page 108)

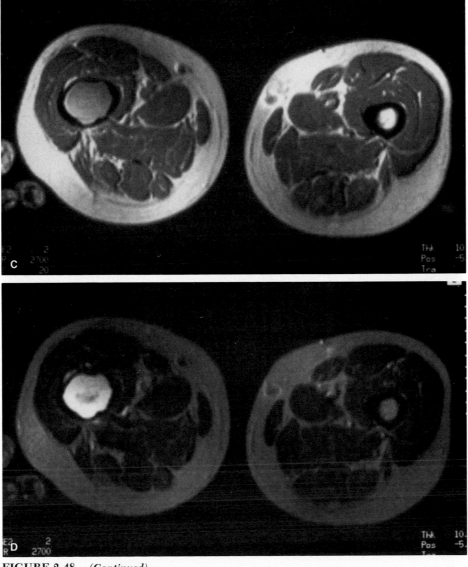

FIGURE 2-48.   *(Continued)*

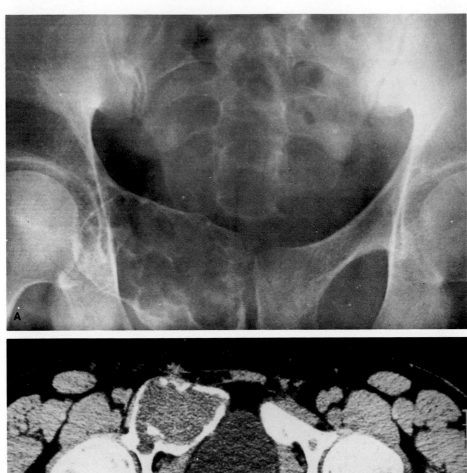

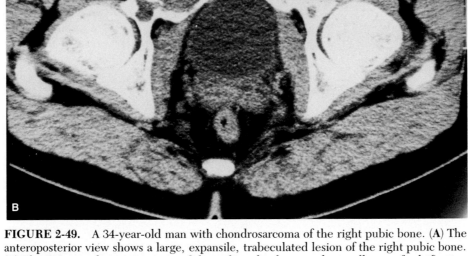

FIGURE 2-49. A 34-year-old man with chondrosarcoma of the right pubic bone. (**A**) The anteroposterior view shows a large, expansile, trabeculated lesion of the right pubic bone. (**B**) The CT scan shows expansion of the right pubic bone and a small area of calcification within the lesion. The cortex appears to be destroyed in several small areas, but there is no soft-tissue invasion. (**C**) MR (SE 800/20) coronal section. Expansion of the right pubic bone is apparent. A small focus of low signal intensity within the intermediate signal intensity lesion is seen corresponding to the internal calcification. There is no soft-tissue invasion. (**D**) The axial MR (SE 2700/20) section shows expansion of the symphysis pubis, corresponding to that seen on CT. There is no evidence of soft-tissue invasion. Small areas of cortical destruction can be seen. (**E**) MR image (SE 2700/80). The tumor shows inhomogeneous high signal intensity. The internal low-signal areas correspond to internal calcifications that were perhaps not visualized on CT images or sclerotic fibrous tissue within the lesion. There is no evidence of soft-tissue invasion.

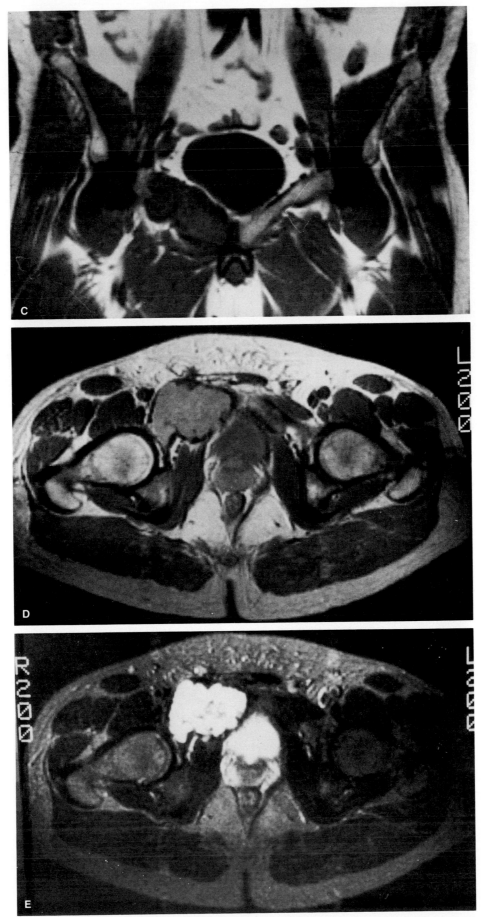

FIGURE 2-49. *(Continued)*

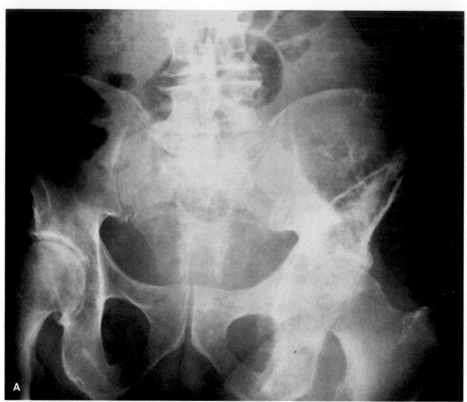

FIGURE 2-50.   Chondrosarcoma of the left iliac bone in a 73-year-old man. (**A**) The anteroposterior view of the pelvis shows a large soft-tissue mass on the left, bony destruction of the central portion of the iliac bone, and fine, linear soft-tissue calcifications. (**B**) MR (SE 700/17) coronal section of the pelvis corresponding to **A**. A large, bulky, soft-tissue mass surrounds the left iliac bone. Marrow replacement by tumor produces low signal intensity of the left iliac bone and acetabulum. (**C**) CT scan. A large, bulky, soft-tissue mass anterior to the left iliac bone contains multiple amorphous calcifications and is partially bounded by calcific margin. Osteosclerosis of the outer aspect of the iliac bone is also seen. (**D**) MR (SE 3000/70) axial section of the pelvis corresponding to **C**. A large, soft-tissue mass anterior to the left iliac bone is seen with a low-signal-intensity margin and containing low signal intensities within the tumor, corresponding to calcifications seen by CT. The full extent of the calcifications is not demonstrated. (**E**) CT scan of the pelvis at a lower level shows involvement of the ischium and an intrapelvic mass. (**F**) MR (SE 3000/70) axial section of the pelvis corresponding to **E**. The tumor including the intrapelvic component and a posterior component not clearly seen on CT scans is seen as high signal intensity. High signal intensity within the ischium indicates bony involvement. (**G**) Digital subtraction angiography of the left hypogastric artery shows the tumor to have low vascularity.

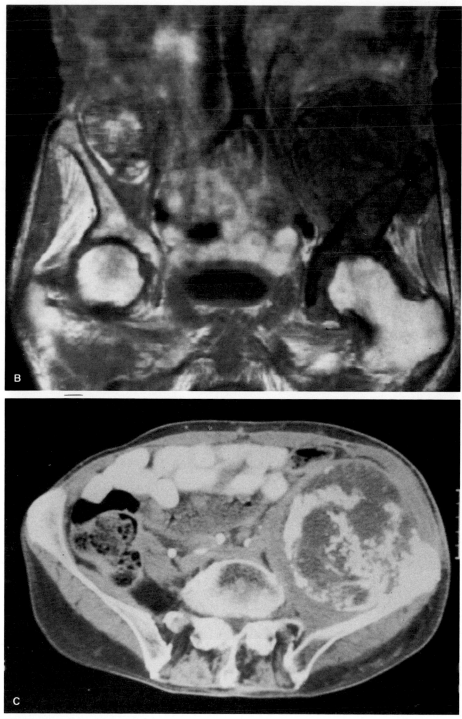

FIGURE 2-50. *(Continued)*

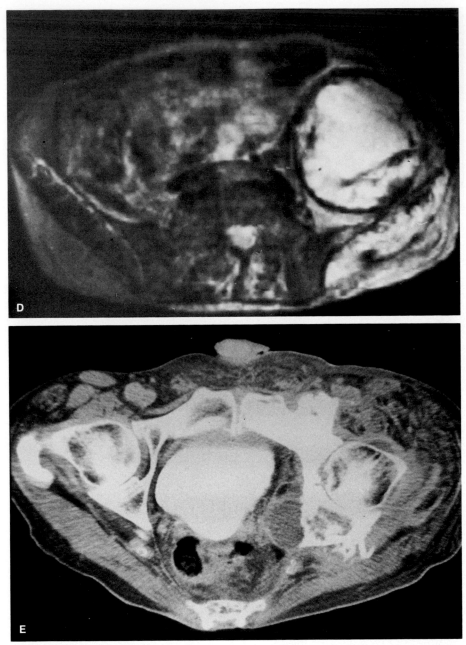

FIGURE 2-50. *(Continued)*

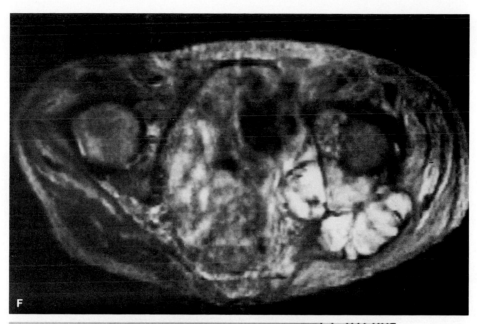

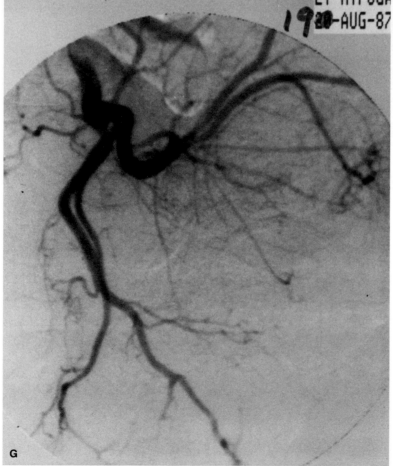

FIGURE 2-50. *(Continued)*

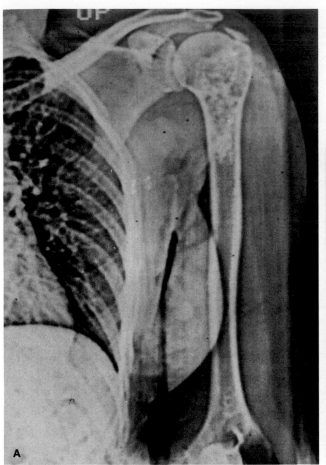

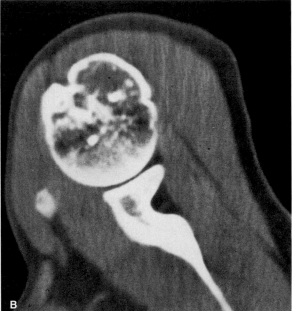

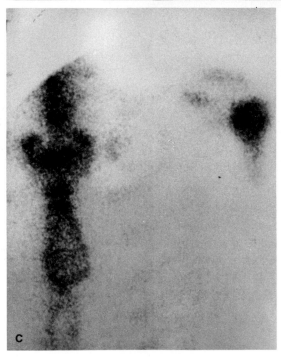

FIGURE 2-51. A 40-year-old woman with chondrosarcoma of the left proximal humerus. (**A**) The digital radiograph shows amorphous calcification within the humeral head and metaphysis. The proximal diaphysis is involved with a dense calcification. (**B**) The CT scan shows amorphous, spotty calcification within the medullary cavity. (**C**) On a radionuclide bone scan, an area of increased uptake in the humeral head is seen. The increased activity is not indicative of the entire extent of the tumor. (**D**) MR (SE 500/20) coronal section. A low-signal-intensity tumor replaces fatty marrow in the proximal humerus. The dense area of calcification seen at the distal aspect of the lesion is now seen as a signal void. (**E**) MR (SE 3000/20) axial section. Tumor is within the medullary cavity has a central area of low signal intensity representing calcification. (**F**) MR image (SE 3000/80). The tumor is seen as inhomogeneous high signal intensity in the medullary cavity with a central area of low-signal-intensity calcification. There is no invasion of the soft tissues, and the cortex is intact.

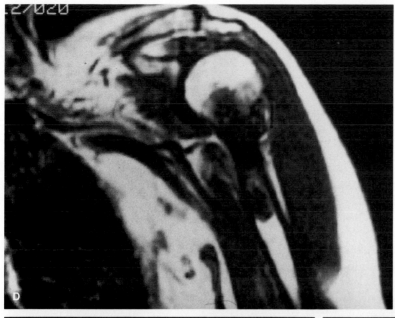

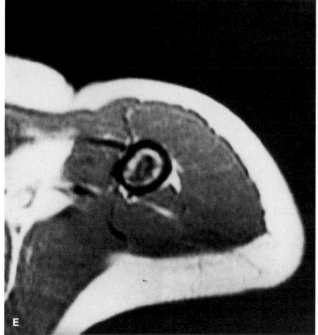

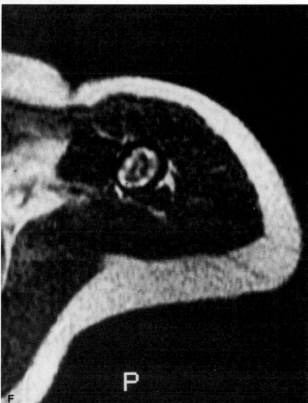

FIGURE 2-51.   *(Continued)*

containing striated calcifications (Fig. 2-52).[111] The long axis of the tumor is parallel to the long axis of the bone. The adjacent cortex may be eroded. Involvement of the medulla is usually not seen. Periosteal osteosarcoma with cartilage components also shows this type of calcification.

Clear Cell Chondrosarcoma

Clear cell chondrosarcoma is a low-grade malignant tumor of cartilage.[112,113,114] The tumor cells are distinctive, with a centrally placed vesicular nucleus surrounded by clear cytoplasm. The symptoms usually are mild, localized pain of long duration, possibly with a pathologic fracture. The usual age distribution for these lesions is the third to fifth decades. The location is most often in the proximal epiphysis of the femur and the humerus. Radiologically, the tumor may be mistaken for a chondroblastoma, with a well-defined osteolytic or expansile appearance. The margination and calcification pattern of this tumor varies. Some cases show cortical destruction and soft-tissue invasion. This is a slow-growing tumor with a better prognosis than conventional chondrosarcoma. It is usually curable with en bloc resection. Distant metastases may occur many years after resection. MRI shows intermediate-to-low signal intensity on T1-weighted images and increased signal intensity on T2-weighted images for clear cell chondrosarcoma (Fig. 2-53).[109]

Mesenchymal Chondrosarcoma

Mesenchymal chondrosarcoma is a rare, aggressive tumor with a poor prognosis. It may arise from bone or soft tissue and rarely may be multicentric.[97,98] It has a histologic appearance of elements of cartilage and undifferentiated stromal cells. This tumor occurs in patients younger than those with conventional chondrosarcoma. Long-standing pain and a soft-tissue mass are typical findings. Any site in the skeleton and any portion of a long bone may be involved. The radiologic pattern varies but is largely similar to that of a conventional chondrosarcoma. Expansion, cortical bone destruction, periosteal new bone formation, and calcification may all be seen. The younger age of the patient should suggest the diagnosis.

Dedifferentiated Chondrosarcoma

Dedifferentiated chondrosarcoma is a highly malignant tumor in which a low-grade chondrosarcoma is associated with high-grade sarcoma.[115,116] The associated

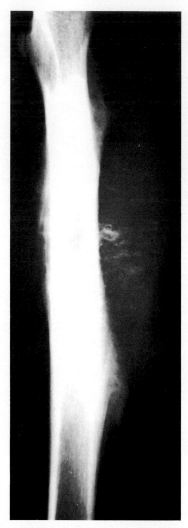

FIGURE 2-52. Chondrosarcoma of the femur. There is involvement of a long segment of the femoral shaft. Cortical destruction has occurred, with breakthrough and a large soft-tissue mass. Fine, long, spiculated calcifications can be seen perpendicular to the shaft of the bone in the central portions and at the periphery. Laminated periosteal new bone formation and a large Codman triangle formed at the distal outer aspect are also visible.

component may be osteosarcoma, fibrosarcoma, or malignant fibrous histiocytoma. This occurs in approximately 10% of chondrosarcomas and affects older patients who present with pain and a soft-tissue mass. Pathologic fracture may occur. The skeletal distribution is similar to that of conventional chondrosarcoma. Radiologically, bony destruction and a soft-tissue mass without calcifications are associated with an area containing calcifications. The latter represents the low-grade portion of the tumor. The aggressive portion may show permeative or moth-eaten destructive patterns, soft-tissue invasion, and pathologic fracture. This is a highly malignant tumor with a tendency toward distant metastasis and a poor prognosis.

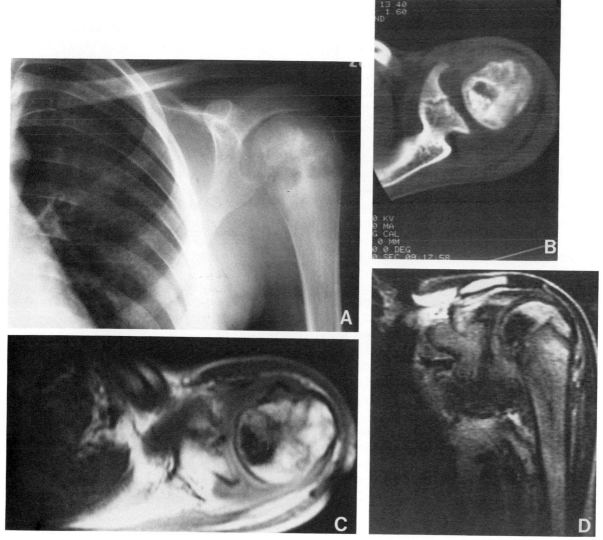

FIGURE 2-53. Clear cell chondrosarcoma of the humerus. (**A**) Anteroposterior film of a lytic, eccentric, epiphyseal lesion in the humerus. (**B**) Computed tomography shows a lytic, calcified lesion. (**C**) Axial image (SE 600/20, 2 Nex, 128 × 256 matrix), showing an intermediate-signal-intensity lesion containing areas of lower intensity. (**D**) Axial image (SE 2500/40, 2 Nex, 128 × 256 matrix) demonstrates a high-signal-intensity lesion. A joint effusion is visible. (Courtesy of Dr. M. K. Dalinka, Philadelphia, PA. Previously published in Fobben ES, Dalinka MK, et al: Skeletal Radiol 16:647–651, 1987)

Enchondroma Protuberans

Enchondroma protuberans is a rare variant of enchondroma that forms a prominent exophytic mass.[117] A broad-based, eccentric, expansile lesion containing calcifications associated with a central tumor that has a cartilage pattern of calcifications is seen. Of the four reported cases, three were in the proximal humerus, and one was in a rib. The intact bony margin of the protruding mass, lack of bone destruction, and lack of a soft-tissue component all help to differentiate this lesion from a chondrosarcoma.

FIBROSARCOMA OF BONE

Fibrosarcoma of bone is a rare, spindle cell, primary malignant tumor that does not form neoplastic osteoid or cartilage.[118,119] It is much less common than osteosarcoma. It usually arises de novo, but fibrosarcoma complicating ameloblastic fibroma, bone damaged by radiation, bone infarcts,[120] chronic osteomyelitis,[121] desmoplastic fibroma, fibrous dysplasia (rare), multicentric fibrosarcomatosis, Paget disease, and irradiated and nonirradiated giant cell tumor have been reported. The tumor may contain hemorrhage and necrosis. Periosteal fibrosarcoma also rarely occurs. Another fibro-genic malignant bone tumor, malignant fibrous histio-cytoma (MFH), is rare in bone but common in the soft tissues. Many tumors called fibrosarcomas in the past meet the modern histologic criteria for MFH. Fibro-sarcoma may also be somewhat difficult to differentiate histologically from some fibroblastic osteosarcomas.

The age distribution for patients ranges from 8 to 88 years, with median age of 41 years. The tubular bones are more often involved in the younger patients, and older patients tend toward flat bone involvement. The chief complaints are progressive local pain and swelling. The tumor metastasizes hematogenously to the lungs and central skeleton in a large percentage of cases.[122] This tumor shows a tendency for lymphatic metastasis. The prognosis in aggressive fibrosarcoma is poor. Pathologic fractures and soft-tissue invasion are common. Fibrosarcoma of the jaws has a more favor-able prognosis than fibrosarcoma in other locations.[123]

The tumor usually originates in the medullary cav-ity but, less often, occurs periosteally. A periosteal fi-brosarcoma may be associated with a large soft-tissue mass. The most common sites of origin are the distal femur and proximal tibia. It usually is seen eccentri-cally in the metaphysis of a long bone and may extend into the epiphysis. A central location has a poorer prog-nosis than an eccentric one. There is a wide zone of transition. Other sites of involvement are the mandi-ble, upper limbs, ribs, scapula, sacrum, and pelvis. The lesion is usually larger than 6 cm. The chief finding is an osteolytic lesion that may assume any destructive pattern (Fig. 2-54). A permeative pattern indicates a more aggressive tumor with a much lower survival rate than one with a geographic pattern.[124] There is no neo-plastic new bone formation nor a chondritic pattern of calcifications. A bone sequestrum of any size may fre-quently be seen within the tumor (Fig. 2-55). The le-sion may cause endosteal erosion and progress to a large, expansile appearance with a thin cortical shell. Trabeculation is not prominent. There may be break-through of the expanded shell or complete cortical de-struction. This may involve only one side of the cortex in an eccentric lesion. Reactive bone formation is sparse. The periosteal reaction, rarely present, may display lamination, spiculation, or a Codman triangle. Pathologic fractures may occur. Periosteal fibrosarcoma may show thickening, erosion, or invasion of the cor-tex. Soft-tissue invasion occurs in advanced cases of both forms of the tumor.

The radionuclide bone scan may show increased uptake around the periphery of the tumor, with less uptake centrally because of a lack of uptake within tu-mor tissue. Angiography of fibrosarcomas reveals vari-able vascularity (Fig. 2-56). The most vascular site should be selected for a biopsy.[125]

MALIGNANT FIBROUS HISTIOCYTOMA OF BONE

MFH is a malignant tumor arising in bone or soft tissue of fibroblastic and histiocytic origin. These cells are considered by some to arise from a common precursor. It is much more common in the soft tissues and is rare

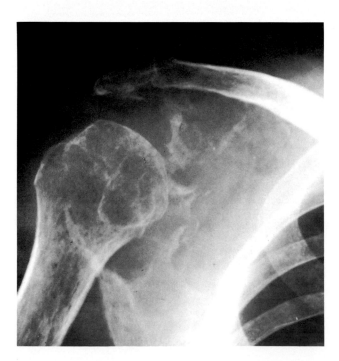

FIGURE 2-54. Fibrosarcoma of the scapula. There is marked destruction of the scapula, including the glenoid fossa, coracoid process, and base of the acromion. The margins are irregular. Residual bone spicules, which do not represent neoplastic new bone formation, can be seen within the destroyed area.

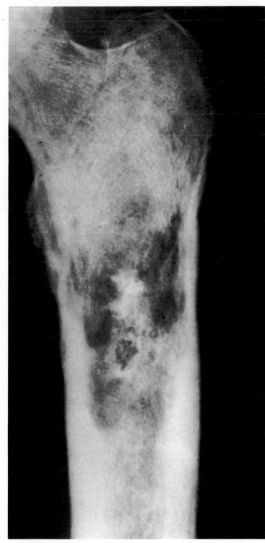

FIGURE 2-55. Fibrosarcoma of the proximal femur. Notice the localized but poorly marginated destructive area at the proximal femoral shaft containing a small segment of increased density, which represents a sequestrum. Scalloping of the endosteum at the lateral aspect of the lesion is also apparent.

in bone. It has wide latitude in histologic differentiation and pleomorphic appearance.[126,127]

The age distribution of patients ranges from the first through the eighth decades, with an average age of 50 years. The male to female ratio is 1.5 to 1. Clinical features and survival statistics are similar to those of fibrosarcoma.[124] Pain of variable duration and a mass occur. Pathologic fractures are common. The most frequent sites of involvement are the femur, tibia, humerus, ribs, pelvis, and craniofacial bones. The tumor may arise in areas of abnormal bone, such as bone infarct,[128] enchondroma, irradiated bone,[79,129] or Paget disease. One case has been reported of two tumors arising in bone infarcts in the same patient.[130]

The lesions may be as large as 10 cm in diameter (Fig. 2-57) with a moth-eaten or permeative destructive pattern. A sequestrum may be seen. The most frequent location in the long bones is in the metaphysis, and it can extend into the epiphysis or diaphysis. The femur is the most common location, followed by the tibia, humerus, and pelvis. Sclerosis, calcification, and periosteal new bone formation are rarely seen. An increased trabecular pattern within the tumor is caused by partial destruction of the underlying bone trabeculae. Invasion by means of cortical permeation or complete cortical destruction may result in a soft-tissue mass, which may be expansile in the flat bones. Massive osteolysis of the skull of the skull has been reported in one case of MFH.[131]

The imaging signs useful for prognosis are the same as those for fibrosarcoma. Favorable signs include geographic rather than permeative bone destruction, eccentric location, and cortical destruction involving no more than two quadrants of the bone circumference as seen on CT scans.[124] Ultrasonography is useful for evaluating the soft-tissue component and demonstrates a mass of mixed echogenicity.

CT can accurately define the location and extent of tumor. The radionuclide bone scan shows increased uptake in the MFH and is useful for detecting metastases. It sometimes shows an "extended-uptake" pattern with increased activity beyond the true limits of the tumor. Plain radiographs are unreliable for depicting the actual limits of the tumor.

MRI can best define the intraosseous and extraosseous components of the tumor. T1-weighted images may show a low to intermediate heterogenous signal intensity. T2-weighted images may not show a uniform increase in signal intensity.

Benign fibrous histiocytoma with fibroblastic and histiocytic elements microscopically has been reported.[127] The lesions in the long bones radiologically resembled giant cell tumors with an epiphyseal-metaphyseal location, osteolysis, trabeculation, and cortical thinning. No periosteal reaction or soft-tissue invasion occurred. This lesion has also been reported in the cervical spine.[132]

EWING TUMOR

Ewing tumor is a distinctive small, round cell, primary sarcoma, probably arising from undifferentiated mesenchyme.[91,133–136] It is in the group of round cell tumors with primary non-Hodgkin lymphoma (i.e., reticulum cell sarcoma). These tumors have some imaging similarities but differ in age-related incidence. A related entity in the histologic differential diagnosis is primitive neuroectodermal tumor (PNET).[137,138]

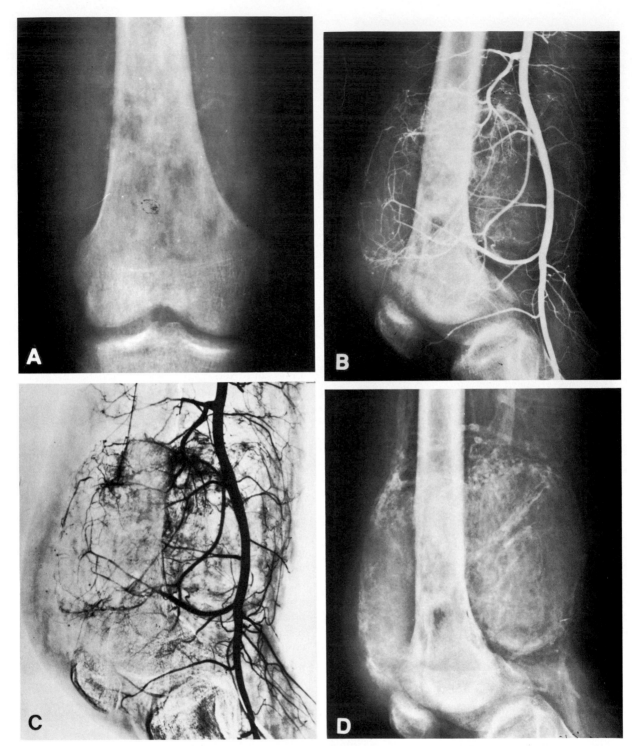

FIGURE 2-56. Fibrosarcoma in a 22-year-old man who complained of soft-tissue swelling for a few months. (**A**) Anteroposterior radiograph of the knee reveals a permeative lesion involving the distal femur with questionable sequestration, suggestive of a fast-growing lesion, possibly osteomyelitis. (**B**) Early arterial phase, (**C**) subtraction of early arterial phase, and (**D**) venous phase views reveal considerable hypervascularity, abnormal arteries and veins, encasement of second-degree arteries, and a large soft-tissue component around the lesion, diagnostic of a neoplastic lesion rather than infection. The biopsy specimen of the lesion was diagnosed as grade IV fibrosarcoma. (Courtesy of Dr. Issa Yaghmai, Medical College of Virginia, Richmond, VA.)

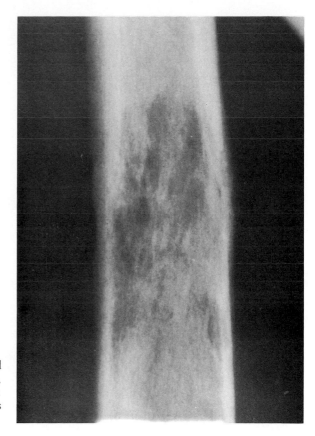

FIGURE 2-57. Malignant fibrous histiocytoma. A destructive and slightly expansile, ill-defined lesion is in the distal femoral shaft, with cortical thickening and a slight periosteal reaction medially. An increased trabecular appearance within a destructive area occurs centrally.

Ewing tumor occurs less frequently than myeloma, osteosarcoma, or chondrosarcoma. The peak age incidence is 15 years, with a usual range between 5 and 30 years. It is rare in African Americans. Males are more often affected than females.

Local pain occurs, usually of several months' duration, which increases in severity. The duration of the pain is important in differentiating this tumor from osteomyelitis, which may present with similar clinical and imaging findings but with a history of pain of only a few weeks duration. A soft-tissue mass, tender but not warm, and dilated veins are usually present. Malaise, fever as high as 105°F, leukocytosis, anemia, and a rapid erythrocyte sedimentation rate are seen. The tumor spreads to the surrounding soft tissues by permeating through the cortex. It produces early hematogenous metastases to the lungs and other bones.

The site of involvement varies with the age of the patient because of the different sites of red marrow conversion at various ages. The tubular bones are most often involved in younger patients, but in patients older than 20 years of age, the flat bones are the most common sites. Of the long bones, the femur followed by the tibia are affected most commonly. The most frequent site in the flat bones is the innominate bone. Tu-

mors may develop in the hands[139,139a] and feet.[140] The os calcis may also be involved.

The classic appearance of this tumor in the long bones probably accounts for much less than half of cases. This pattern consists of a permeative area of bone destruction involving a large segment of the diaphysis, associated with delicate laminated periosteal new bone formation (Fig. 2-58). Typically, the tumor cells permeate the haversian canals and invade the soft tissues, leaving an intact cortex, cortical sequestration, or a cortex destroyed only segmentally (Figs. 2-59 and 2-60), unlike most other primary malignant bone tumors. This mechanism allows the formation of a large soft-tissue component with a relatively intact cortex. There is no tumor bone, only reactive bone formation or debris.

Ewing tumor in the flat bones has a characteristic imaging appearance of mottled destruction and patchy reactive bone sclerosis (Fig. 2-61). The cortex may be destroyed, with thin delicate laminations present (Fig. 2-62), or be thickened rather than destroyed (Fig. 2-63). The os calcis has a similar appearance when involved with this tumor. This appearance resembles osteomyelitis.

(text continues on page 118)

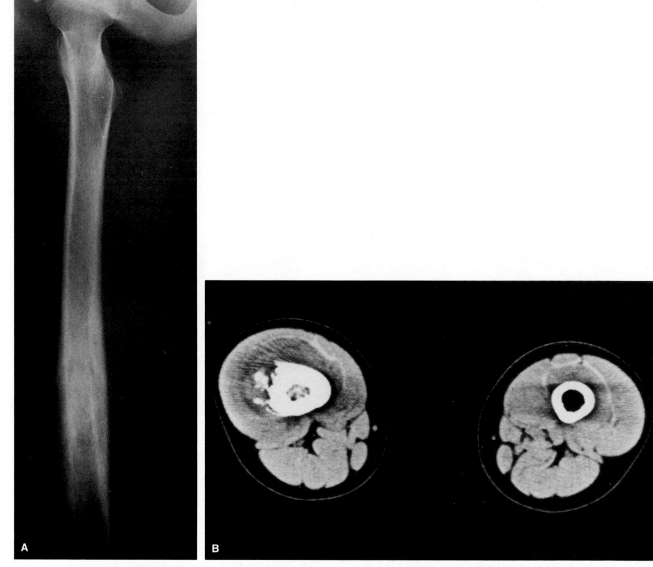

FIGURE 2-58.   Ewing tumor of the right femoral diaphysis in a 10-year-old girl presenting as a classic pattern. (**A**) The lateral view of the right femur shows a diaphyseal lesion with reactive sclerosis and laminated periosteal new bone formation. (**B**) The CT scan shows high-density reactive bone in the medullary cavity, in the soft-tissue component, and reactive cortical thickening. (**C**) The radionuclide bone scan shows increased activity in the intraosseous and soft-tissue components of the tumor. (**D**) MR image (SE 600/20) shows low-signal-intensity marrow replacement by the tumor in the diaphysis. A small hemorrhagic area secondary to biopsy is in its midportion. A small satellite lesion is seen at the inferior aspect of the tumor. (**E**) The axial MR (SE 1800/80) section shows high-signal-intensity soft-tissue tumor surrounding an intact cortex. The low signal intensity within the soft-tissue component corresponds to the reactive calcification seen on CT scans.

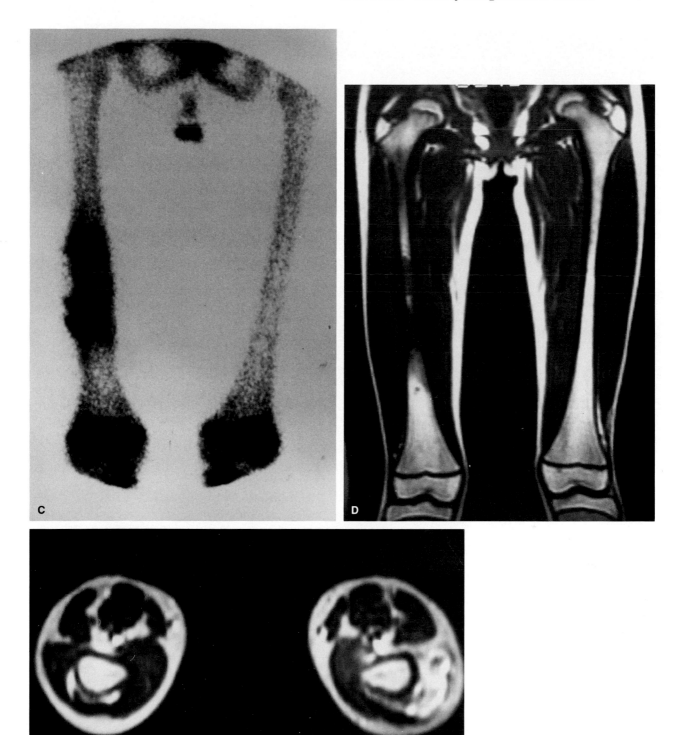

FIGURE 2-58.   *(Continued)*

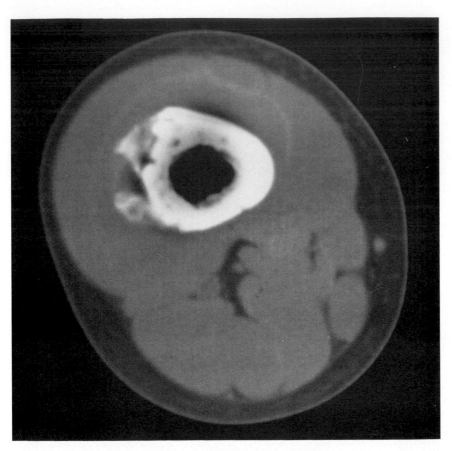

FIGURE 2-59. Ewing tumor. The CT scan shows permeated cortex with multiple, low-density foci. Reactive bony changes are also seen.

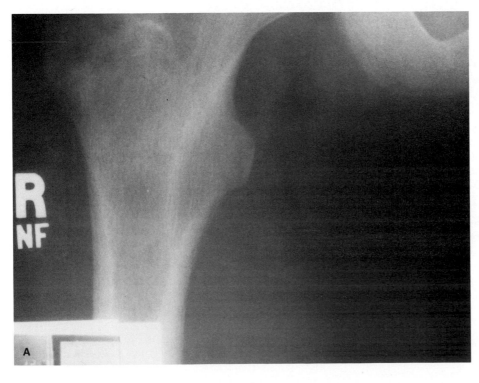

FIGURE 2-60. A 15-year-old boy with Ewing tumor of the right femur. **(A)** The anteroposterior view of the proximal femur shows patchy radiolucency and cortical destruction inferior to the greater trochanter. Periosteal new bone formation is seen inferior to the lesser trochanter. **(B)** MR image (SE 600/20) shows marrow replacement of the femoral neck and diaphysis. An area of periosteal new bone formation laterally and a large, bulky, soft-tissue tumor surrounding the bone are visible. Cortical destruction occurs at the proximal lateral aspect, but the cortex is intact in the major portion of tumor involvement. **(C)** The T2-weighted axial image shows high-signal-intensity foci permeating the cortex, which is not segmentally destroyed. A large, high-signal-intensity tumor mass surrounds the bone.

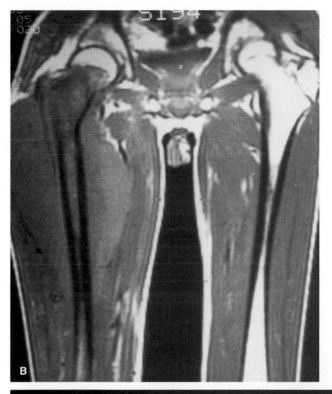

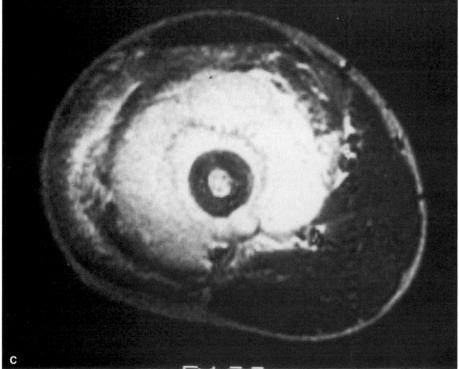

FIGURE 2-60. *(Continued)*

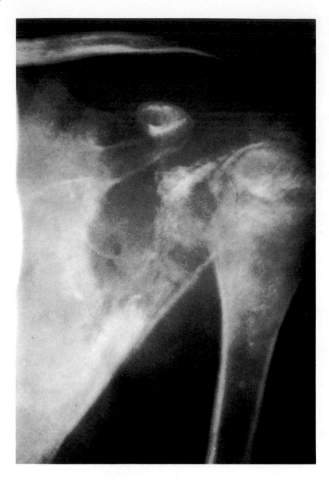

FIGURE 2-61. Ewing tumor of the scapula. An ill-defined area of destruction involves the body of the scapula, the glenoid, and the acromion process, with several small areas of reactive bone sclerosis.

Variations in the classic pattern occur in most cases. The tumor may atypically develop in the metaphysis (Fig. 2-64), intracortically in the diaphysis or metaphysis, or involve the epiphysis before or after fusion. The rate of growth may be slower, leading to expansion (Fig. 2-65) or a geographic zone of destruction. An expansile lesion in the short tubular bones of the hands or feet with a thinned cortex but without periosteal new bone formation is a common appearance when these sites are involved (Fig 2-66).[107,141] Bone sclerosis may range from minimal to prominent, and it may be patchy or take the form of thickened trabeculae. No neoplastic new bone is formed. Because the tumor forms no osteoid or chondroid, the soft-tissue mass is free of calcifications except for reactive periosteal new bone formation or debris, which may be considerable (Fig. 2-67). Cortical thickening may occur.

A laminated periosteal reaction is often present and is a good indicator of Ewing tumor. It is, however, not pathognomonic of Ewing tumor and need not be present. A simple periosteal elevation may be seen, as well as a Codman triangle. A spiculated periosteal response may sometimes be seen. The tumor may rarely have an eccentric or cortical location. Pathologic frac-

tures occur in 5% to 10% of patients. In the spine, vertebral body collapse, sclerotic reaction,[142] and a paraspinal or extradural soft-tissue mass may be present. More than one segment may be involved with spread to the intervertebral spaces and contiguous vertebral bodies. Expansion of the neural arch and a calcified paravertebral mass have been reported.[143] The vertebrae may initially present as a metastatic site with a subtle lesion in a long bone as the primary site, which can only be seen on an MR image or radionuclide bone scan (Fig. 2-68). Sacral involvement has been reported as presenting with spondylolisthesis.[144] The ribs are involved in about 10% of patients.[145] They usually show a fusiform, expansile lesion without periosteal reaction but may be sclerotic. An extrapleural soft-tissue mass and pleural effusion are frequently observed.[146]

Angiography is most useful when the lesion involves the flat bones or the spine where the imaging appearances of Ewing tumor and osteomyelitis are quite similar. Ewing sarcoma has the typical angiographic features of malignant hypervascular bone lesions. Hypervascularity and pathologic vessels are evident. Numerous feeding arteries arise from the soft

(*text continues on page 126*)

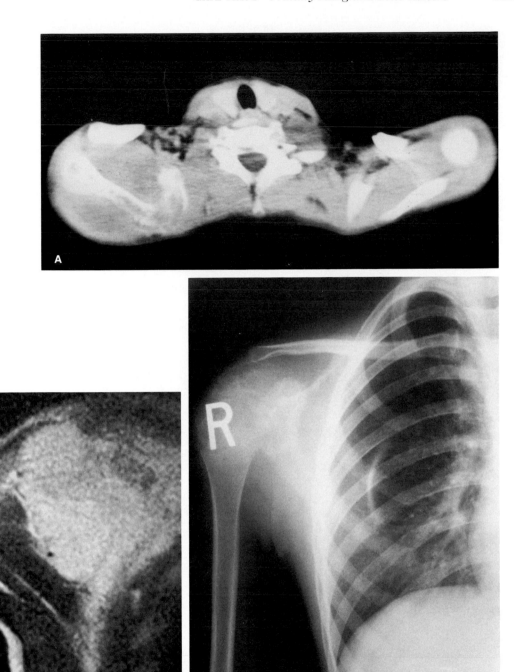

FIGURE 2-62. An 8-year-old boy with Ewing tumor involving the right scapula. (**A**) The CT scan shows a large, low-density tumor mass surrounding the scapula, which is expanded with a thin cortex. (**B**) MR image (SE 2000/80) shows a high-signal-intensity soft-tissue component of the tumor about the scapula. (**C**) The anteroposterior view of the right shoulder shows bony destruction and a soft-tissue mass.

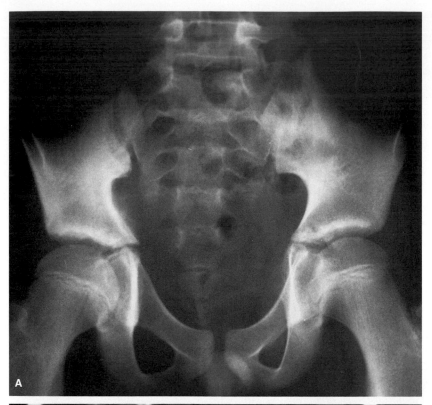

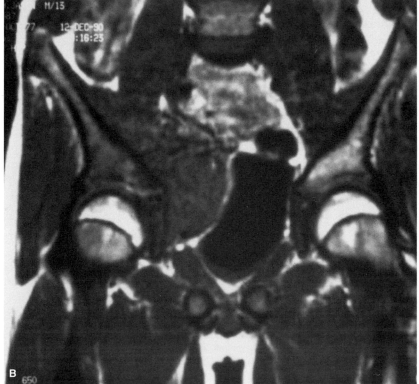

FIGURE 2-63. A 15-year-old boy with Ewing tumor involving the right iliac bone. (**A**) The anteroposterior view of the pelvis shows cortical thickening of the right iliac bone and reactive periosteal new bone formation. This film does not show involvement of the medulla of the bone. (**B**) T1-weighted MR image shows a large, low-signal-intensity tumor mass displacing the pelvic viscera and marrow replacement of the entire iliac bone and acetabulum. (**C**) The CT scan shows a large, intrapelvic soft-tissue mass displacing the bladder, bony sclerosis of the iliac bone, and reactive bone in the soft tissues. (**D**) T1-weighted MR image corresponding to **C**. A large, mixed-signal-intensity soft-tissue mass displaces the bladder, and there is cortical thickening. Marrow replacement in the iliac bone is seen as low signal intensity.

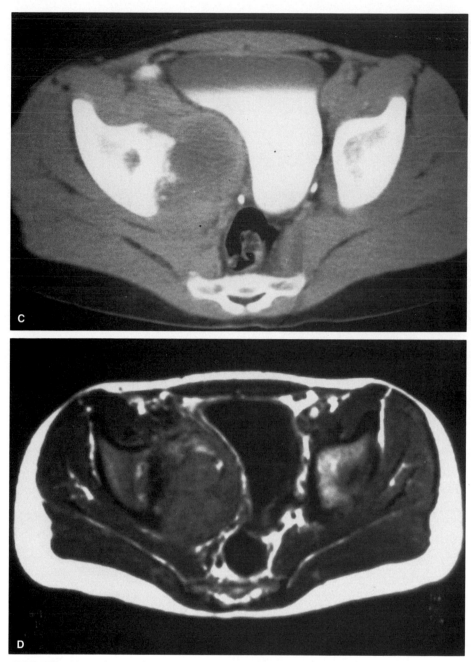

FIGURE 2-63. *(Continued)*

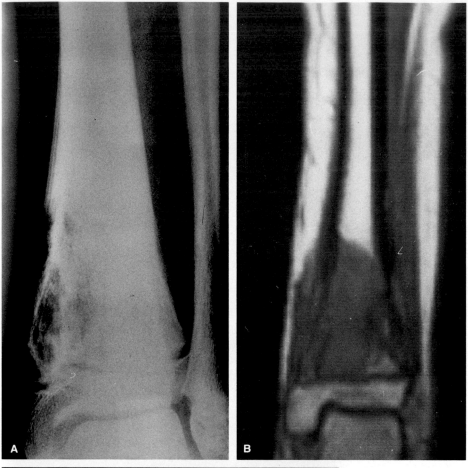

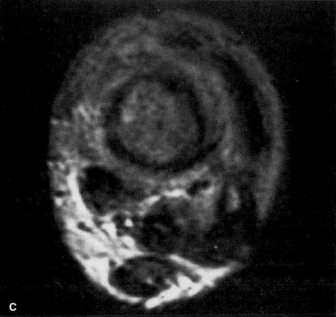

FIGURE 2-64. A 12-year-old girl with Ewing tumor of the distal tibial metaphysis. This patient is of African descent, which is a rare factor for involvement with this tumor. (**A**) The anteroposterior view of the distal tibia shows an area of patchy destruction in the metaphysis. Laminated periosteal new bone formation proximally at the medial aspect is also seen. (**B**) The T1-weighted MR image shows a well-defined region of marrow replacement in the metaphysis and laminated periosteal new bone formation medially. (**C**) The T2-weighted MR image, axial section, shows delicate periosteal laminations.

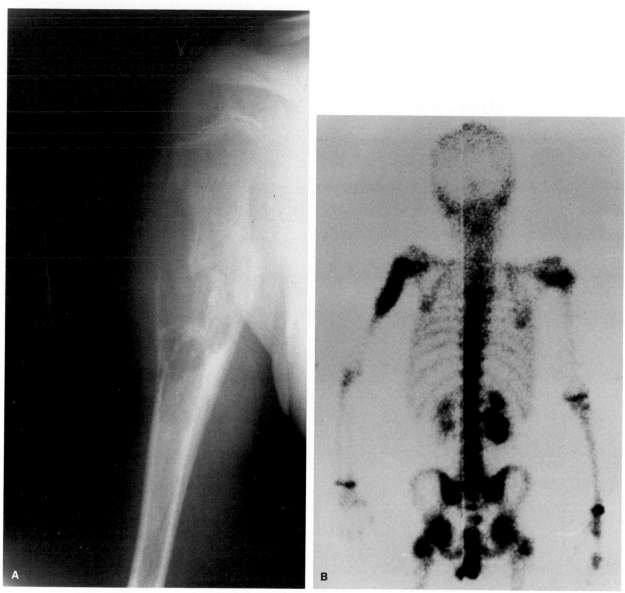

FIGURE 2-65.   A 6-year-old girl with Ewing tumor involving the proximal humerus. (**A**) An expansial lesion in the diametaphyseal region of the humerus is seen with a segment of lateral cortical destruction and medial laminated periosteal new bone formation. (**B**) The radionuclide bone scan shows increased uptake in the proximal half of the humerus.

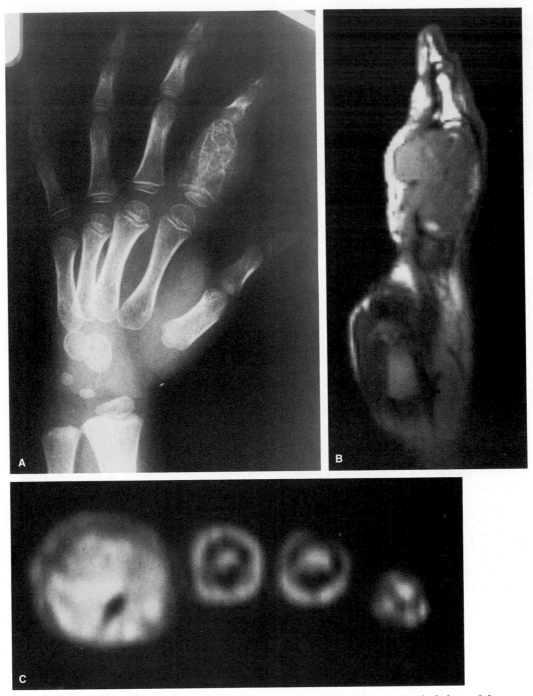

FIGURE 2-66.   A 3-year-old girl with Ewing tumor involving the proximal phalanx of the index finger. (**A**) The anteroposterior view of the hand shows an expansile trabeculated proximal phalanx with an intact cortex. (**B**) T1-weighted MR image. The soft-tissue component is seen at the palmar aspect in this sagittal image. (**C**) The T2-weighted axial image shows a high-signal-intensity tumor involving the soft tissue surrounding the bone.

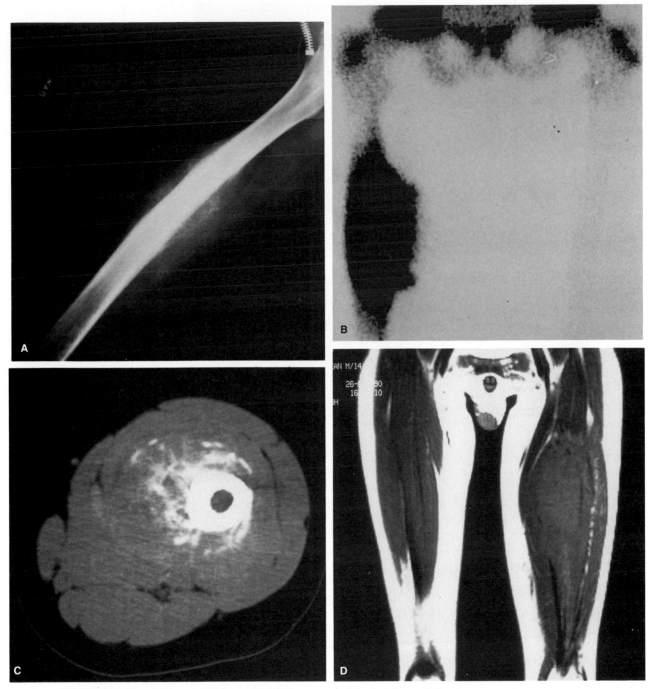

FIGURE 2-67. A 14-year-old boy with Ewing tumor of the left femoral diaphysis. (**A**) The lateral view of the femur reveals involvement of the femoral diaphysis with reactive sclerosis. Periosteal reactive new bone formation in the soft tissues and Codman triangles are evident. (**B**) The radionuclide bone scan shows increased activity in the bone and the soft-tissue component of the tumor. (**C**) The CT scan shows thickening of the cortex, the surrounding low-density soft-tissue mass, and extensive calcification, which is reactive bone, within the soft-tissue tumor. (**D**) The T1-weighted MR image shows a large soft-tissue mass of intermediate signal intensity with multiple low-signal-intensity foci representing calcification. (**E**) The T2-weighted axial image shows high-signal-intensity tumor surrounding the bone and high signal intensity within the medullary cavity. Low-signal-intensity areas within the tumor represent the calcification corresponding to that seen in **C**. High-signal-intensity foci in the cortex represent tumor permeation.

continued

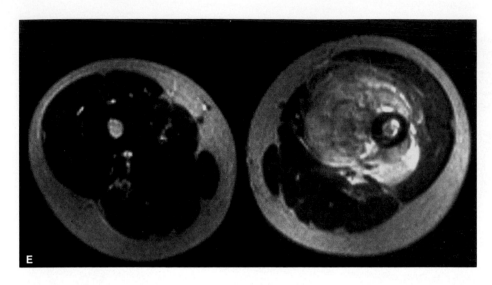

E

FIGURE 2-67. *(Continued)*

tissues around the lesion (Fig. 2-69). About 12% of cases show poorly circumscribed areas of avascularity due to tumor necrosis.[3]

MRI is the method of choice for demonstrating soft-tissue and bone marrow involvement. It can precisely define tumor extent in bone (Fig. 2-70). It can show cortical permeation by small, high-signal-intensity foci in the cortex on T2-weighted and PD-weighted images (see Fig. 2-60).

Plain-radiographic predictors of survival after treatment include a central location and large size as unfavorable and a honeycomb appearance as favorable.[147] On MR images after chemotherapy, a high signal intensity on T2-weighted images may be seen with recurrence, necrosis, reactive lesions, or a hematoma. The value of MRI in excluding active disease is controversial.[148–150]

PRIMARY NON-HODGKIN LYMPHOMA OF BONE

Primary non-Hodgkin lymphoma (NHL) of bone is a rare, round cell malignant tumor.[151–153] This is considered by many investigators to be a separate entity distinct from generalized lymphoma involving bone. It previously was called reticulum cell sarcoma, a name which is still used by some. The criteria for primary NHL include initial involvement of a single bone and at least 6 months before the appearance of distant metastases, without generalized NHL.

The latest generally accepted clinical classification of NHL is the Working Formulation, in which low-, intermediate-, and high-grade tumors are based on descriptions of histologic morphology (see Chap. 5).[154]

Pain and swelling of long duration at the tumor site are usually present, while systemic symptoms are usu-

ally absent. Pathologic fractures occur. The usual age range of patients is between 25 and 40 years. The ratio of male to female involvement is 2 to 1. About half of the lesions occur in the lower extremities, especially the femora, with the remainder in the humeri, scapulae, vertebrae, pelvis, and other bones. In the long bones, the shaft or the metaphysis may be involved.

The principle imaging finding is permeative bone destruction in separate areas that coalesce to a motheaten appearance (Fig. 2-71). The cortex is broken through, and pathologic fracture frequently occurs (Fig. 2-72). Periosteal reaction of a simple or laminated type and cortical expansion (Fig. 2-73) may rarely be seen. Cortical thickening and reactive bone sclerosis may be present, as well as a geographic destructive area. Sequestration, single or multiple, has been reported in 11% of cases in one series of 246 primary bone lymphomas.[155] A localized osteolytic lesion in the epiphysis with surrounding sclerosis has been reported.[156] An associated soft-tissue mass may be present. CT or MRI can demonstrate the extent of the mass. Synovitis and effusion may occur with a tumor near a joint.

MULTIPLE MYELOMA AND OTHER DISEASES WITH ALTERED IMMUNOGLOBULINS

There are five distinct classes of immunoglobulins normally present in human serum: IgG, IgA, IgM, IgD, and IgE.[157] Their molecular structure comprises four polypeptide chains: two identical heavy chains (i.e., H chains) and two identical light chains (i.e., L chains), linked by disulfide bonds and covalent interactions.

The heavy chain has a molecular weight of about

(text continues on page 130)

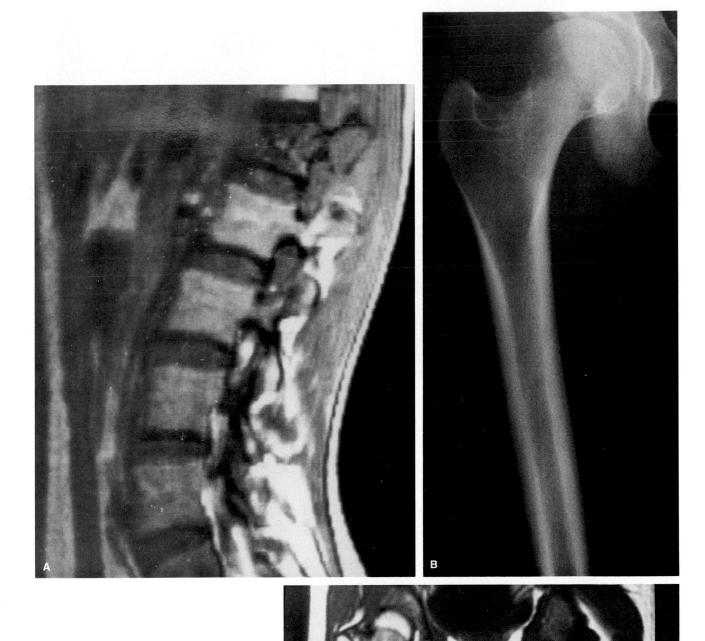

FIGURE 2-68. A 15-year-old girl who presented with metastatic Ewing tumor to her first lumbar vertebra. The primary tumor in her right femoral shaft was subsequently found and proven by biopsy. (**A**) The T1-weighted MR image shows low signal intensity and partial collapse of the first lumbar vertebra. (**B**) The anteroposterior view of the femur shows the normal, plain film appearance. (**C**) The T1-weighted MR coronal section shows marrow replacement in the diaphysis, which on biopsy proved to be a Ewing tumor.

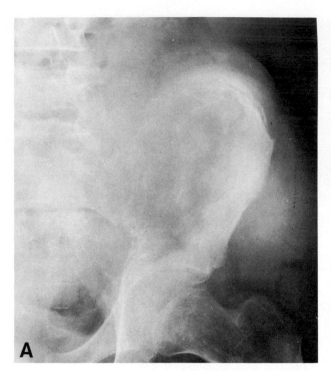

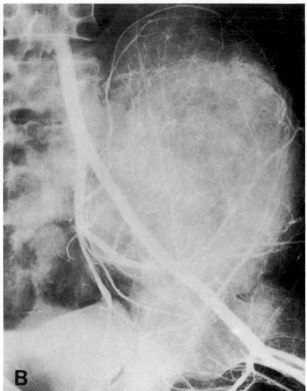

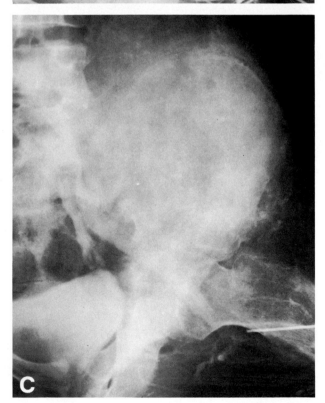

FIGURE 2-69. Ewing sarcoma in a 12-year-old boy. (**A**) Conventional anteroposterior radiograph of the pelvis reveals a radiolucent permeative lesion involving the upper part of the iliac bone. (**B**) Early arterial and (**C**) late venous phases reveal hypervascularity and abnormal veins and arteries with a moderate degree of tumor stain, suggestive of round cell tumor. Notice the exact soft-tissue component of the tumor in **B**. (Courtesy of Dr. Issa Yaghmai, Medical College of Virginia, Richmond, VA.)

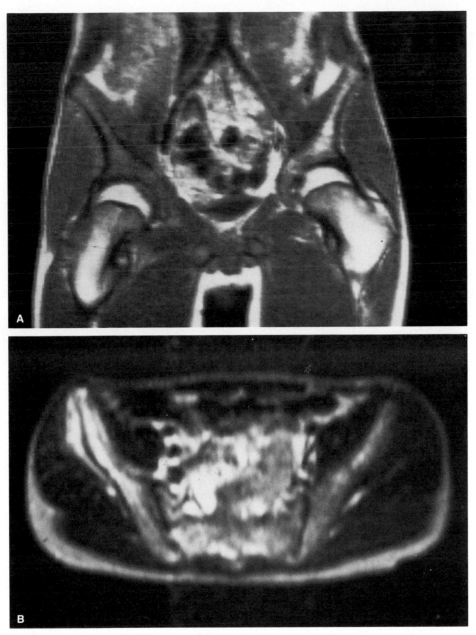

FIGURE 2-70.   Ewing tumor involving the right iliac bone. (**A**) MR image (SE 500/30). Marrow replaces the entire right iliac bone, but the cortex appears intact. (**B**) MR image (SE 2100/100). The right iliac bone shows the high signal intensity of the tumor, with the soft-tissue component of the tumor surrounding the bone also showing high signal intensity. The cortex appears intact.

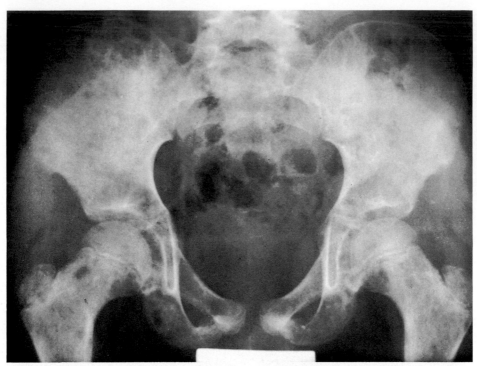

FIGURE 2-71. Primary reticulum cell sarcoma of the pelvic bone. Multiple, small, destructive areas are in the ischia and femoral heads and necks. There is no reactive bone sclerosis and no periosteal new bone formation in this case. (Courtesy of Dr. Harvey White, Chicago, IL.)

55,000, and the light chain has a molecular weight of about 22,000. The heavy chain determines the different immunoglobulin classes. The heavy chains of IgG, IgA, IgM, IgD, and IgE have been denoted, respectively, by Greek letters: γ, α, μ, δ, and ε. Two types of light chains, called κ and λ, have been identified. Combinations of these make up the various types of human immunoglobulins.

The two main components derived from proteolytic cleavage of an IgG molecule are the Fc (i.e., crystallizable fragment) and Fab (i.e., antibody-combining fragment). The Fc fragment consists of the major portions of the heavy chain, and the Fab fragment consists of the light chain and the remainder of the heavy chain.

The major disease characterized by altered immunoglobulins is multiple myeloma. Much less common are heavy chain disease and macroglobulinemia.

Multiple Myeloma

Multiple myeloma is a primary malignant tumor of bone marrow, characterized by malignant proliferation of a single clone of plasma cells.[159] It is the most common primary malignant neoplasm involving bone. The annual incidence is 3 per 100,000 members of the population. The tumors tend to remain confined to bone.

Involvement of other organs may follow later, and primary tumors of extraskeletal origin may rarely occur. The disease is most often generalized but may be localized to a single osseous focus, called a solitary myeloma or solitary plasmacytoma. Most of these lesions subsequently disseminate throughout the skeleton or arise in multicentric sites; however, a few plasmacytomas may remain localized.

About three fourths of patients are between the ages of 50 and 70 years at the time of diagnosis. Multiple myeloma is rare in patients younger than 30 years of age. It may, however, occur in the young,[160] and a 13-year-old patient has been reported.[161] The male-to-female ratio is 2 to 1. The symptoms are initially vague complaints, fever, and symptoms resulting from the accompanying anemia. Bone pain is progressive in severity and usually occurs in the lower back. This can be complicated by pathologic compression fracture of the vertebral bodies, resulting in severe pain and paraplegia. This is most difficult to differentiate from acute vertebral compression due to osteoporosis, even with MRI. Both occur in the same age group. Pain in other bones and soft-tissue masses from extraskeletal invasion of myeloma eventually occur.

Renal failure in multiple myeloma, usually not accompanied by hypertension, is second to pneumonia as the most frequent cause of death. Hepatosplenomeg-

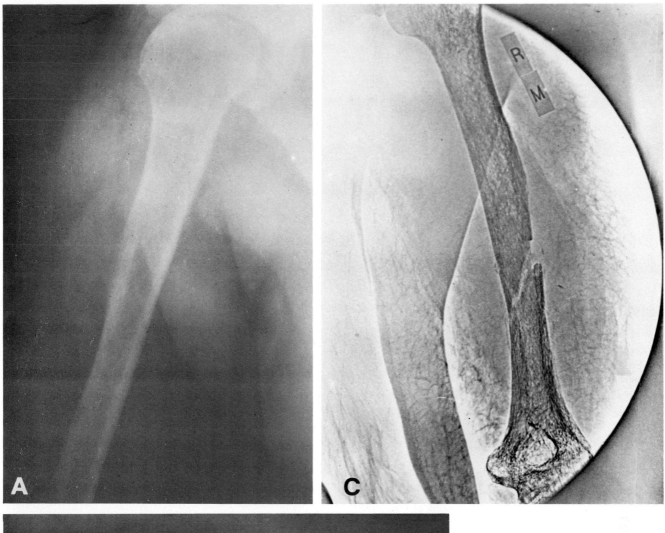

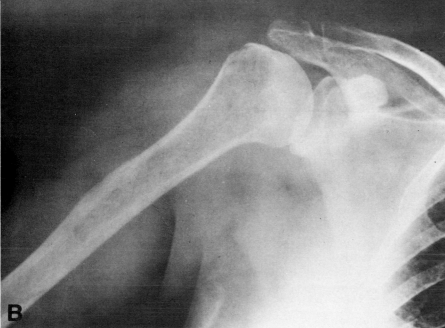

FIGURE 2-72. Reticulum cell sarcoma of the humerus. (**A**) Film taken at initial complaint shows minimal permeative destructive areas in the midhumeral shaft. (**B**) Film taken after a short interval shows extensive permeative destruction of humeral diaphysis. (**C**) Xeroradiograph shows that the destruction has progressed to a pathologic fracture.

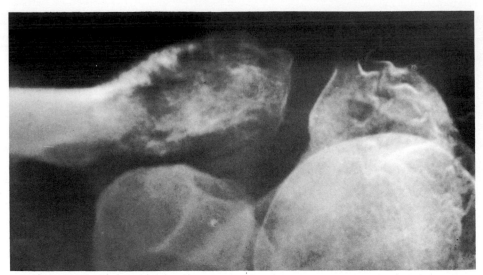

FIGURE 2-73. Reticulum cell sarcoma of the distal clavicle. Small, ill-defined destructive areas occur with expansion of the superior aspect of the distal clavicle and slight cortical thickening.

aly, lymphadenopathy, and amyloid or paramyloid deposits are common. Metastatic calcifications due to hypercalcemia and renal failure, particularly in the kidneys but occasionally in the lungs and other organs, sometimes occur.

The blood picture is a normochromic, normocytic anemia that may be mild to severe. Marked rouleaux formation can be seen in blood smears. The leukocyte count is usually within normal limits, although numerous plasma cells are occasionally found in the blood, a condition referred to as plasma cell leukemia. Thrombocytopenia is partially responsible for the common bleeding tendency.

The diagnosis of multiple myeloma can be established by bone marrow smears when the proportion of plasma cells is greater than 10%. Increased numbers of plasma cells can also be found in Waldenström macroglobulinemia and heavy chain (i.e., Fc fragment) disease.

The serum calcium level is usually elevated because of mobilization of calcium from bones. Hypercalcemia may occur with or without hyperproteinemia. The serum phosphorus level becomes elevated in cases of renal glomerular insufficiency. The serum alkaline phosphatase level is within normal limits, except in advanced disease with pathologic fractures. The serum uric acid level may be elevated, leading to secondary gout.[162]

The serum proteins show several changes. Most patients have hyperglobulinemia with reversal of the albumin-globulin ratio. In the presence of proteinuria, the serum proteins may not be elevated. The albumin level is normal or slightly low.

Multiple myeloma is characteristically associated with a monoclonal increase of immunoglobulins, arising from a single clone of antibody-forming cells. This finding is also present in certain lymphoproliferative diseases and has been found in the serum of some patients with nonreticular neoplasms or inflammatory diseases. The monoclonal proteins are designated as M components. They are normal immunoglobulins present in abnormal quantities. Most patients have IgG myeloma. In the case of a solitary plasmacytoma or of a solitary myeloma that has metastasized, the serum electrophoresis may not show an M protein peak.

Bence Jones protein is the light chain of the immunoglobulin molecule. It has a peculiar thermal behavior; it first coagulates and then dissolves at temperatures above 60°C. About 40% of myeloma patients show detectable Bence Jones proteinuria by the heating method, and a higher percentage may be detected by electrophoresis. A 5% incidence of Bence Jones proteinuria is found for conditions such as malignant lymphomas, metastatic bone tumors, idiopathic hemolytic disease, and essential cryoglobulinemia. The protein abnormalities in myeloma may precede visible bony lesions by several years.

A staging system of 1 to 3 has been proposed, based on blood chemistries, hemoglobin levels, and skeletal lesions.[163]

Radiologically, the findings of myeloma vary widely. The following appearances, alone or in any combination, may occur:

- change of bone texture
- diffuse bone destruction
- expansile lesions
- loss of bone density

- osteosclerosis (rare in untreated cases)[164]
- punched-out lesions
- soft-tissue masses.

Loss of bone density results from diffuse marrow involvement causing loss of bone trabeculae and thinning of the cortices. The imaging picture mimics that of advanced osteoporosis. The spine is principally involved, and the vertebral bodies may show a greater radiolucency than the intervertebral spaces. The bony trabecular pattern is accentuated by a similar mechanism. The central skeleton is most often affected because of the primary involvement of red marrow. The vertebral bodies, pelvis, sacrum, ribs, skull, and mandible are most often involved. The pedicles are involved much less frequently than the bodies of the vertebrae because of the proportion of red marrow

between the two. This finding is called the pedicle sign and is a relative differential point between myeloma and osteolytic metastases (Fig. 2-74).[165] However, destruction of the pedicle (Fig. 2-75) or an entire posterior vertebral arch may also occur in myeloma.

The hallmark of this disease is the sharply circumscribed, punched-out lesion. These lesions are multiple, round, sharply marginated, and purely osteolytic, without a sclerotic rim. They may involve the endosteal surface of the cortex, causing scalloping (Fig. 2-76), or involve both surfaces. They vary in size and may coalesce, destroying large segments of bone. The bones most commonly involved are the skull (Fig. 2-77) and the long bones (Figs. 2-78 and 2-79). The distal clavicle and the acromion are frequently involved, as are the ribs, glenoid, and pelvis (Fig. 2-80). Pathologic frac-

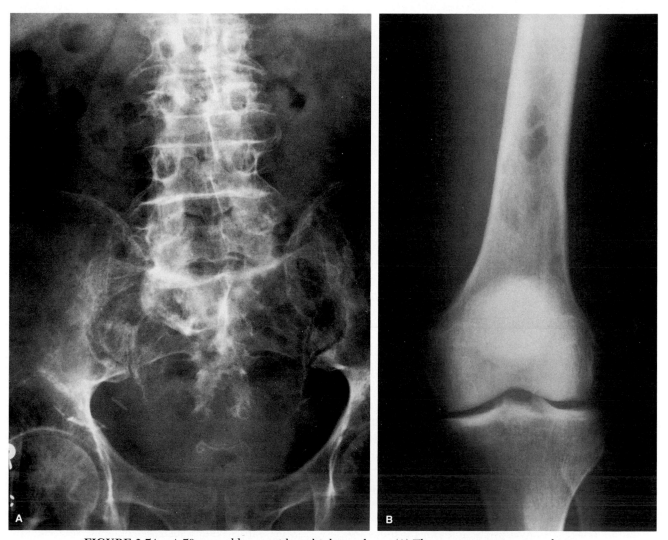

FIGURE 2-74. A 70-year-old man with multiple myeloma. (**A**) The anteroposterior view shows multiple destructive lesions in the spine and the pelvis with collapse of the third lumbar vertebra. All pedicles appear intact. (**B**) Destructive lesions are seen in the distal femur. There is no sclerotic margin surrounding the radiolucent foci.

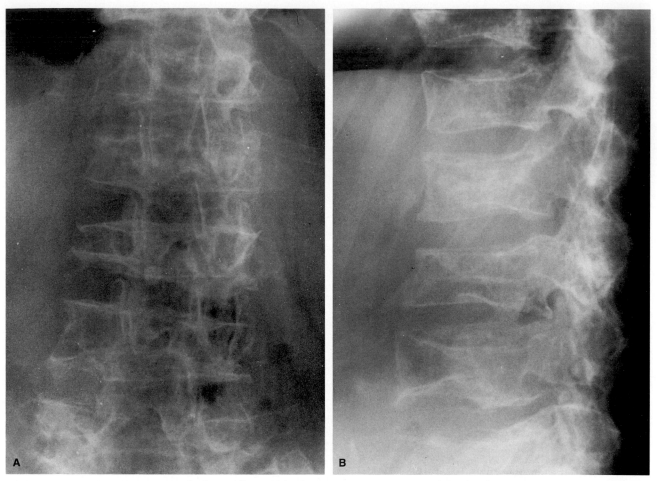

FIGURE 2-75. Multiple myeloma. (**A**) The anteroposterior view of the lumbar spine reveals collapse of all of the lumbar vertebral bodies with osteopenia. The right pedicle of L4 is also involved. (**B**) The lateral view of the lumbar spine shows wafer-like collapse of the lumbar vertebral bodies with marked osteopenia. The intervertebral spaces are preserved.

tures are common (Fig. 2-81). The skull base may be involved.[166]

Severe diffuse bone destruction, particularly of the pelvis and sacrum, is common and can resemble osteolytic metastases. The terminal phalanges may rarely be involved (Fig. 2-82).

Expansion of bone is a common feature and may occur in the ribs, long bones (Fig. 2-83), or pelvis (Fig. 2-84). A solitary myeloma may present with expansion. Periosteal reaction is sparse.

MRI is more sensitive than plain radiographs or CT in detecting lesions in myeloma (Fig. 2-85). MRI of the spine in myeloma shows diffuse or focal areas of low to intermediate signal intensity on T1-weighted images and increased signal intensity on T2-weighted images because of marrow replacement by tumor. The signal intensity may not be markedly increased on T2-weighted images. Bony destruction can be more obvious on CT than on MRI (Fig. 2-86). Compression fractures are associated with tumor signal changes

in about half of these patients. Signal intensity on T2-weighted images may appear after treatment. If fatty replacement of red marrow has occurred, then high signal patterns on T1-weighted images will be seen.[163,167] MR spinal imaging in early cases, including asymptomatic patients, shows three distinct patterns which correlate with marrow involvement and hemoglobin levels. Diffuse and focal patterns indicate more severe involvement. An inhomogenous appearance of tiny lesions on a background of normal marrow correlates with a lower percentage of marrow plasmacytosis.[168]

Radionuclide bone scanning in myeloma is unreliable, because many lesions do not provoke enough bone repair to cause uptake. Focal uptake may also occur in associated amyloid lesions and in some tumor sites. The scintigram may show photopenic lesions.

Most rarely, bone sclerosis may be seen in untreated cases. There may be a thin, sclerotic margin

(text continues on page 143)

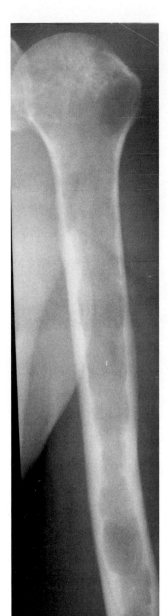

FIGURE 2-76. Multiple myeloma. The anteroposterior view of the humerus shows extensive destruction with endosteal scalloping.

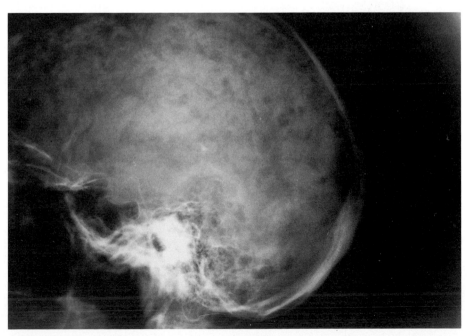

FIGURE 2-77. The lateral view of the skull shows extensive, punched-out, radiolucent lesions without any reactive sclerosis.

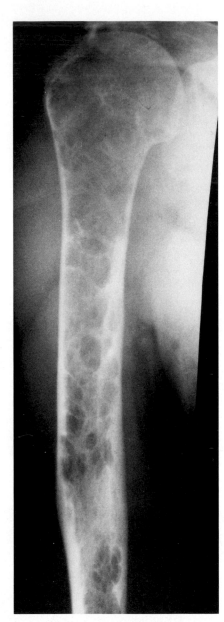

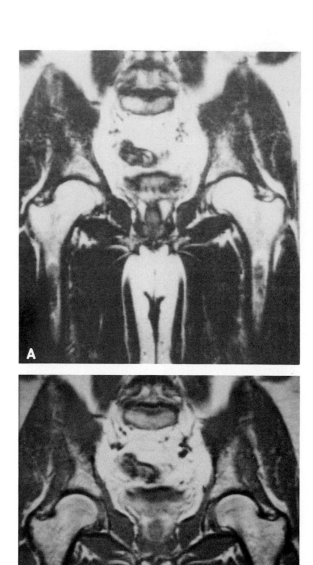

FIGURE 2-78. Multiple myeloma in a 71-year-old man. The anteroposterior view of the humerus shows extensive destructive changes involving the entire humeral shaft, but the cortex is intact.

FIGURE 2-79. (**A**) Plasmacytoma—shown on a T1-weighted MR image. Multiple destructive lesions occur in both proximal femora. (**B**) Inversion-recovery sequence (TR 2 sec/T1 400 msec/TE 30 msec). The bony destructive changes are more clearly seen. (Courtesy of Dr. Werner Von Dewes, Bonn, Germany. Previously published in Fortschr Geb Rontgenstr 147:654–661, 1987)

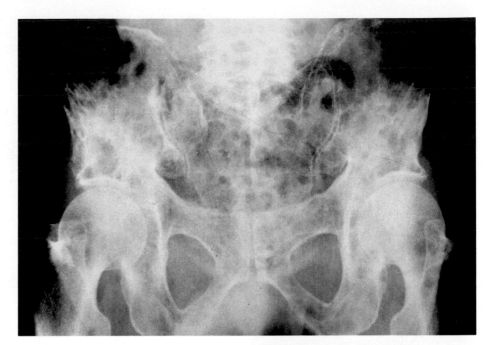

FIGURE 2-80. Multiple myeloma. The anteroposterior view of the pelvis shows extensive destructive lesions in the pelvis and proximal femora, with an expansile area superior to the right acetabulum.

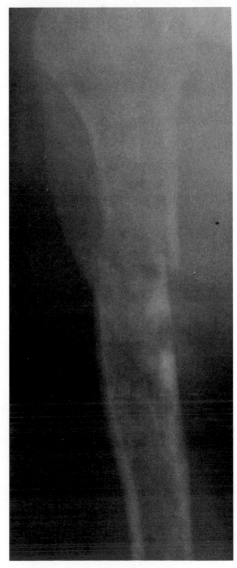

FIGURE 2-81. Multiple myeloma, showing a pathologic fracture of the proximal humerus. Multiple destructive lesions are seen throughout.

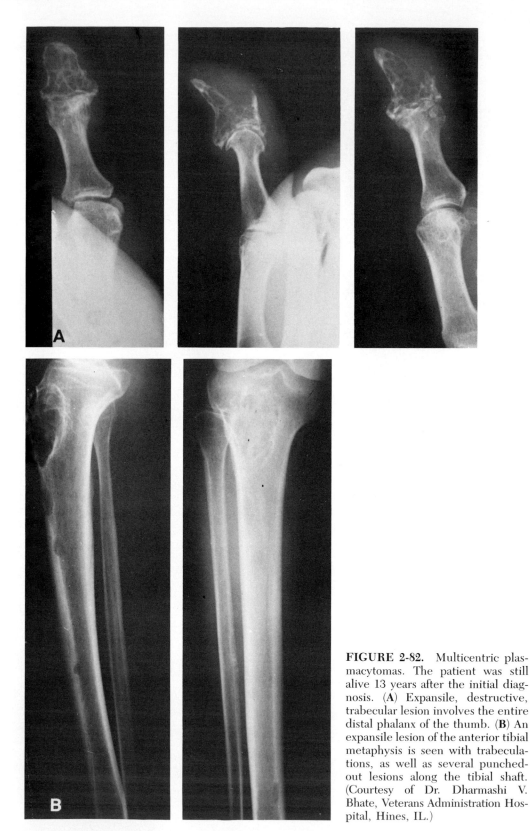

FIGURE 2-82. Multicentric plasmacytomas. The patient was still alive 13 years after the initial diagnosis. **(A)** Expansile, destructive, trabecular lesion involves the entire distal phalanx of the thumb. **(B)** An expansile lesion of the anterior tibial metaphysis is seen with trabeculations, as well as several punched-out lesions along the tibial shaft. (Courtesy of Dr. Dharmashi V. Bhate, Veterans Administration Hospital, Hines, IL.)

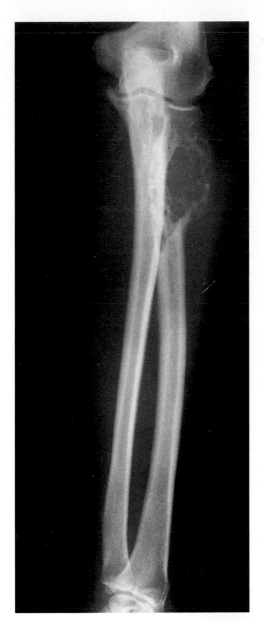

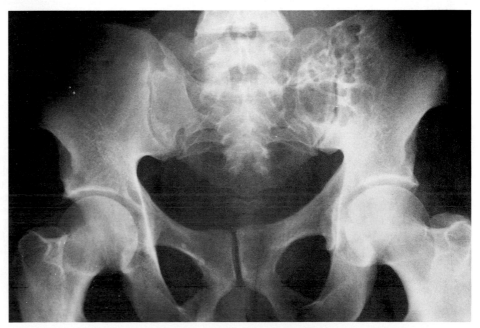

FIGURE 2-83. Multiple myeloma. A large, expansile, destructive lesion occurs in the proximal radius.

FIGURE 2-84. Multiple myeloma. The anteroposterior view of the pelvis shows a large, multilocular, expansile lesion in the left sacroiliac region.

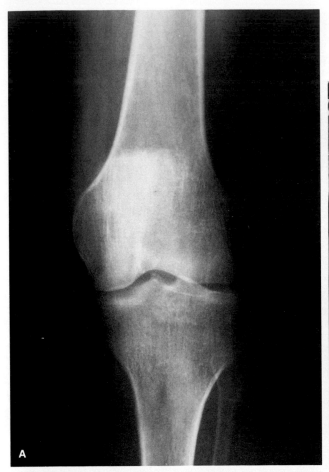

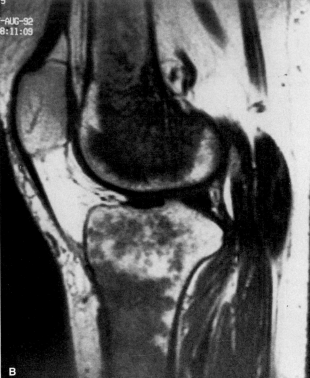

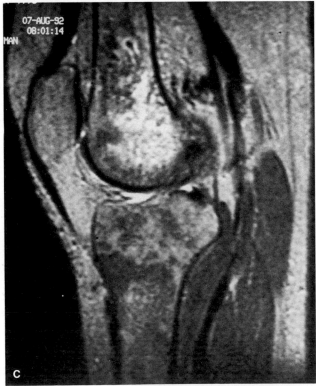

FIGURE 2-85. A 73-year-old woman with multiple myeloma. (**A**) The anteroposterior view of the left knee shows diffuse osteopenia and a radiolucency in the midproximal tibia. (**B**) MR (SE 400/15) sagittal section of the knee. Marrow replacement in the distal femur and in the proximal tibial metaphysis by tumor is seen. A patchy appearance of fatty marrow in the proximal tibial epiphysis is also seen. (**C**) MR image (SE 2700/80). The tumor in the distal femur increases in signal intensity, but the tumor in the proximal tibia does not. (**D**) The lateral view of the lumbar spine shows a partial collapse of the third lumbar vertebral body and osteopenia in all of the vertebral bodies. (**E**) MR image (SE 650/15). Collapse of the third lumbar vertebra is seen with a spotty marrow pattern in all of the vertebral bodies. (**F**) T2-weighted MR image. Partial collapse of the third lumbar vertebral body has occurred with a slightly higher signal intensity than the remainder of the vertebral bodies. There has been no general increase in signal intensity in the vertebral bodies.

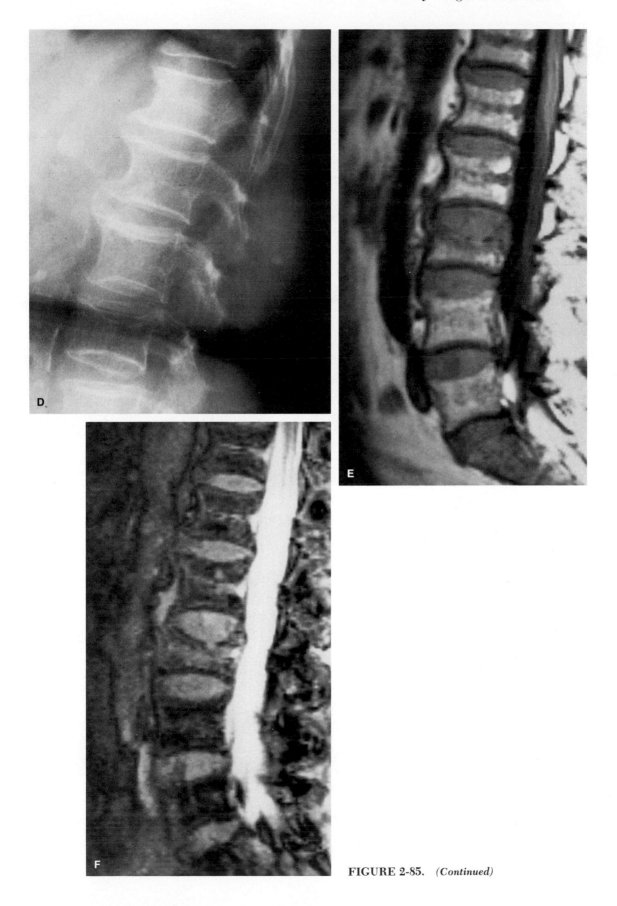

FIGURE 2-85.   *(Continued)*

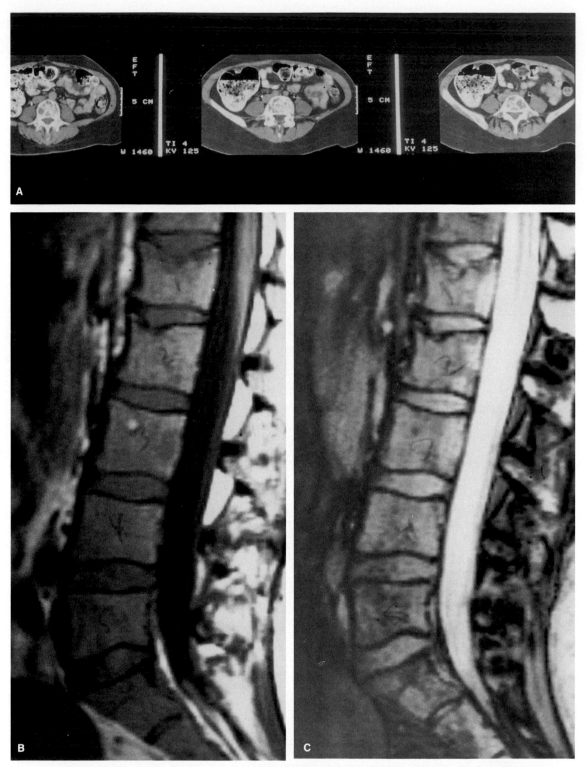

FIGURE 2-86. A 45-year-old woman with multiple myeloma. (**A**) The CT scan shows extensive destructive changes in the lower lumbar spine and in the iliac bones. (**B**) MRI (SE 600/15). All of the marrow fat has been replaced by tumor in the lumbar spine. Partial collapse of L1 and L2 are seen. There is no evidence of the marked bony destruction that is seen on CT. (**C**) T2-weighted MR image. The lumbar vertebral bodies do not increase in signal intensity. Low-signal-intensity foci are seen in the lower lumbar spine and sacrum.

completely or partially surrounding an osteolytic lesion. Spiculated periosteal new bone formation may rarely be present. Focal sclerosis of a vertebral body or generalized patchy (Fig. 2-87) or uniform bone sclerosis (Fig. 2-88), may be seen. A solitary ivory vertebra has been reported.[169]

Amyloid lesions of bone may coexist with myelomas and be lytic or expansile. These do not regress with radiation therapy, as does myeloma.[170] Rarely, chondro-osseous metaplasia in amyloid masses may occur, showing scattered calcifications.

Soft-tissue invasion commonly occurs and can often be seen as a paraspinal or extrapleural mass. The most common sites of palpable tumor are the ribs, ilium, clavicle, and sternum.

Slowly growing, scattered osteoblastic lesions associated with dense plasmacytic infiltrates have been reported with normal laboratory findings. This condition represents plasma cell granuloma rather than myeloma.[171]

Heavy Chain Disease

Heavy chain disease (HCD) is a group of syndromes characterized by the excess production of heavy chain fragments.[172] Three forms are recognized: α, γ, and μ chain disease.

The most common entity is αHCD, presenting with lymphoma-like progressive intestinal involvement. It occurs in younger age groups and does not involve the marrow, liver, or spleen.

The clinical picture of γHCD resembles that of a malignant lymphoma rather than multiple myeloma. The age range of patients is 18 to 76 years, and the disease occurs most often in elderly men. Lymphadenopathy and hepatosplenomegaly are common. Bone radiographs appear normal in most cases, but destructive changes may be seen (Fig. 2-89).

The μHCD is a rare abnormality associated with chronic lymphocytic leukemia.

Primary Macroglobulinemia

Primary macroglobulinemia (i.e., Waldenström macroglobulinemia) is associated with excessive production of monoclonal IgM globulins.[173–176] The clinical picture is variable, with anemia, bleeding tendency, hyperviscosity syndrome, and with symptoms related to the large amount of serum macroglobulin. Men and women are equally affected, most commonly in the fifth and sixth decades of life. Cholecystitis and other infections often occur. Lymphadenopathy and hepato-

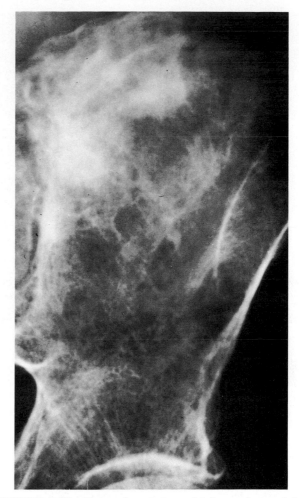

FIGURE 2-87. Osteosclerosis in multiple myeloma of the ilium. Patchy sclerotic areas of the ilium occur alongside wide-spread diffuse destruction. This is a rare finding in multiple myeloma.

splenomegaly may develop, resulting in a clinical picture of lymphoma or leukemia. Cryoglobulin-related symptoms are present, including cold sensitivity, vascular occlusion, gangrene, and the Raynaud phenomenon. Bence Jones proteinuria develops in some patients, but impairment of renal function is not as common as in multiple myeloma.

An increased number of abnormal lymphocytes and plasma cells are seen in the bone marrow. Osteolytic lesions may rarely be seen in primary macroglobulinemia (Fig. 2-90).

POEMS syndrome is a rare variety of plasma cell dyscrasia characterized by polyneuropathy, organomegaly (especially hepatosplenomegaly and lymphadenopathy), endocrine dysfunction, M-protein peak, and skin abnormalities. The imaging findings include single or multiple osteosclerotic lesions and bony pro-

(text continues on page 146)

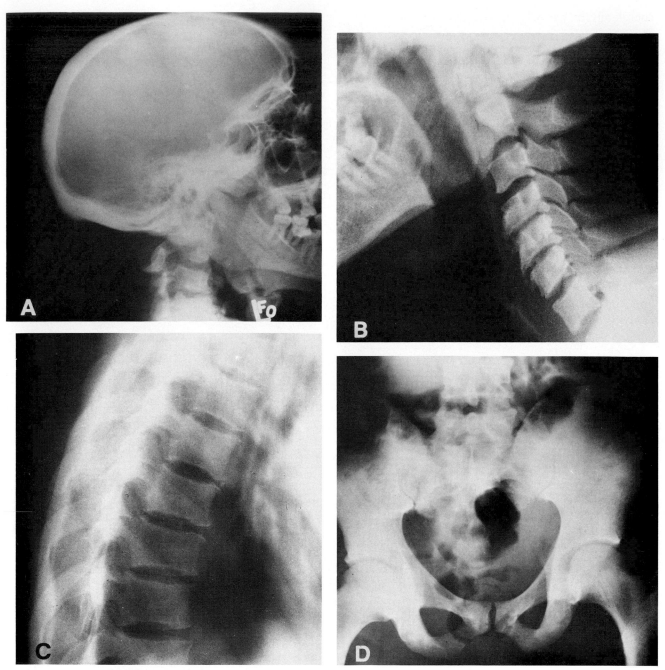

FIGURE 2-88. Multiple myeloma presenting as dense, uniform sclerosis. (**A**) Lateral view of the skull shows sclerosis about the base of the skull. (**B**) Lateral view of the cervical spine shows marked sclerosis of the bodies of the mid- and lower cervical region. (**C**) Lateral view of the dorsal spine shows uniform sclerosis of the bodies. (**D**) Uniform bony sclerosis is seen in the pelvis.

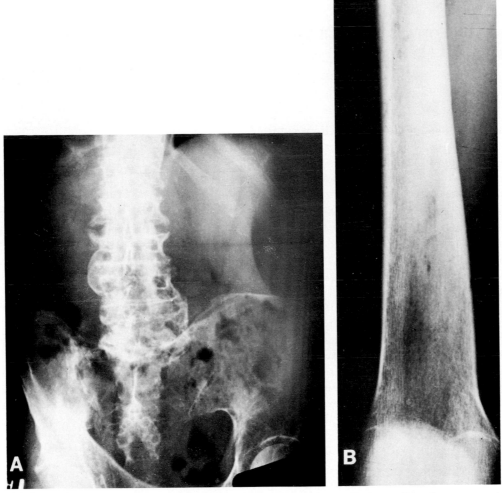

FIGURE 2-89. Heavy chain disease. (**A**) Extensive destructive changes affect the spine and pelvis. The pedicles are intact. (**B**) Permeative destructive changes occur along the femoral shaft.

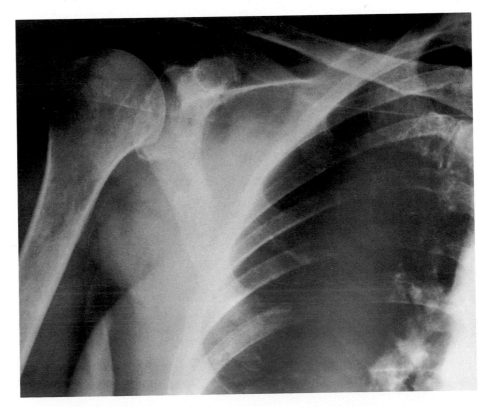

FIGURE 2-90. Primary macroglobulinemia. The anteroposterior view of the shoulder shows multiple small osteolytic lesions in the clavicle and the proximal humerus.

liferation. The relation of this disorder to multiple myeloma is obscure.[177,178]

CHORDOMA

Chordoma is an uncommon tumor derived from notochordal remnants or rests.[179–182] It is malignant, with local invasiveness, but distant metastases are rare. Most chordomas develop in the sacrum and at the base of the skull in the sphenoido-occipital area, with about 10% of cases occurring elsewhere along the spine. Men are affected more than women. The usual age distribution for patients is 30 to 70 years of age. Benign notochordal rests in the sphenoido-occipital region also occur and must be differentiated from malignant tumor. Chordomas are painful and are associated with neurologic symptoms and usually with a palpable mass. Distant metastases occur rarely, most commonly involving lymph nodes, liver, and lungs. Chordoma has also been reported in the posterior mediastinum.[183]

This tumor most often appears as a large midline mass, causing bone destruction at the base of the skull or in the caudal region, particularly the sacrum. It usually originates in the vertebral body. Bony destruction and cortical expansion may be seen, as well as a soft-tissue mass with flocculent calcifications. Osteosclerosis may be pronounced.[184]

Intracranial lesions may present as sella turcica tumors, with erosion of the clivus, calcification, or extensive destruction. A nasopharyngeal mass is present in one third of these cases (Fig. 2-91). It may rarely not be in the midline.

Sacral tumors are seen as midline destructive and expansile lesions, accompanied by a large soft-tissue mass, with or without calcification or osteosclerosis. In the later stages, the tumor need not be confined to the midline (Fig. 2-92). In spinal involvement, bone destruction with or without destruction of the intervertebral disk may occur, and two or more vertebrae may be affected. A paraspinal soft-tissue mass containing calcification is often present.[179] Chordoma of the cervical spine has been reported with intervertebral foramina enlargement resembling neurofibroma.[185]

CT is more accurate than conventional x-ray films, because it can better define an associated soft-tissue mass and calcific debris.[186] It can show better detail, providing cross-sectional anatomy at the base of the skull and in the sacrum. The extent of intrapelvic involvement can be ascertained.

MRI provides superior contrast with surrounding soft tissues and intrapelvic viscera, defining the precise extent of the tumor.[187] Chordoma may be seen as a low-signal-intensity (Fig. 2-93) or as a mixed-signal-intensity tumor (Fig. 2-94) on T1-weighted images, with increased or inhomogenous signal intensity seen on T2-weighted images. MRI and CT are equivalent in the detection of chordomas. MRI can better delineate the full extent of the tumor,[188] and intracranial lesions are best defined by MRI.

GIANT CELL TUMOR

Giant cell tumor (GCT; osteoclastoma) is an uncommon tumor derived from skeletal connective tissue, accounting for about 5% of all primary bone tumors.[94,189–195] It is not possible to predict histologically or radiologically the future behavior of most of these lesions. Even histologically benign-appearing GCT can metastasize to the lungs.[196] The incidence of malignancy has been estimated at about 20%.

Most of these lesions occur in patients between the ages of 20 and 40 years. It has rarely been reported in children and in one patient 80 years of age.[197] This is one of the very few bone tumors that have a female predominance. The patients complain of an intermittent dull ache, sometimes associated with a palpable, tender mass. Symptoms in a contiguous joint often develop, and pathologic fracture may occur. The tumor may recur after excision or metastasize to the lungs. Malignant transformation into fibrosarcoma or osteosarcoma after radiation therapy is also known to occur. GCT also may rarely be associated with Paget disease.

When the diagnosis of GCT is considered, it is imperative to determine the serum calcium, phosphorus, and alkaline phosphatase levels, because a brown tumor of hyperparathyroidism may simulate this lesion radiologically and histologically.

The most common locations are the distal femur, proximal tibia, and the distal radius. The lesion has been reported in almost all tubular bones, as well as a rib,[198] the patella, talus,[199] calcaneus, hamate, and ischium.[200] It extends to the articular cortex, and usually is eccentric with respect to the central axis. The true origin is metaphyseal, attested to by the principal metaphyseal location of the rare giant cell tumor that arises in a young patient before fusion of the epiphyseal cartilage plate.[201–203] The tumor may then be limited by the cartilage plate or extend into the epiphysis (Fig. 2-95). The epiphysis is not involved if the growth plate is still open. Epiphyseal involvement increases with age in children and adolescents.[204] This lesion in an adult may rarely not quite extend to the articular surface, extend down the shaft,[205] or be located in the shaft.[206] Locations other than the long bones occur in about 15% of patients. Mandibular involvement is rare. GCT of the spine is rare, except in the sacrum. It may involve the body, pedicle (Fig. 2-96), or the rest of the neural arch. The pelvis, ribs, or scapula may rarely be in-

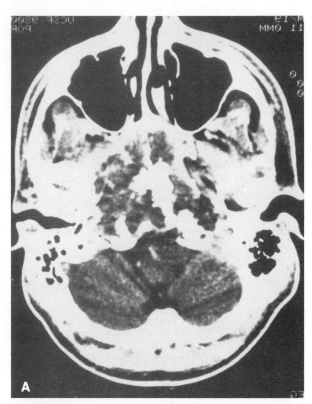

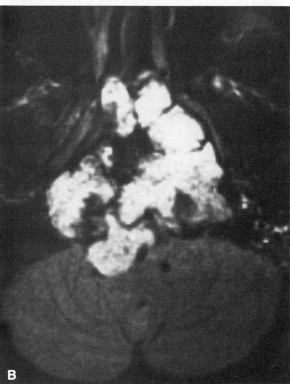

FIGURE 2-91.   Recurrent chordoma in a 20-year-old man. (**A**) Contrast material-enhanced CT scan and (**B**) MR image at the same level show that the MR image better delineates the tumor anteriorly into nasopharyngeal structures and posteriorly into the posterior fossa. It also gives an excellent depiction of the relation of the tumor to the vertebral-basilar system. Mastoiditis is probably secondary to occlusion of the eustachian tube by tumor (SE 2000/80). (Courtesy of Dr. Gordon Sze, San Francisco, CA. Previously published in Radiology 166:187–191, 1988)

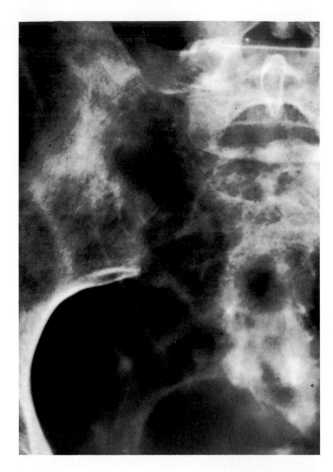

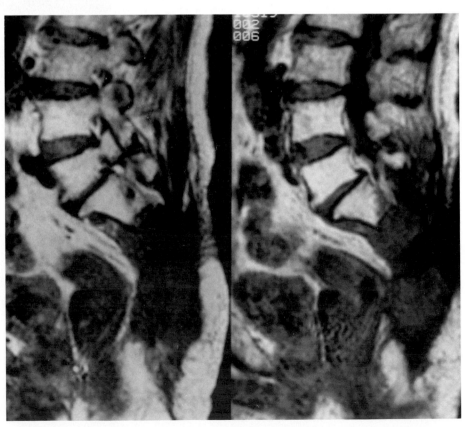

FIGURE 2-92. Chordoma. The ill-defined area of destruction involves the sacrum and extends to the right sacral wing.

FIGURE 2-93.

volved. Multicentric giant cell tumors are rare and difficult to differentiate from a primary giant cell tumor that has metastasized.

The classic appearance is a roundish, moderate-sized, expansile, radiolucent lesion off the central axis of the bone (Fig. 2-97), extending to the subarticular surface. Light trabeculation often occurs. The tumor may also involve the entire diameter of the bone (Fig. 2-98). Occasionally, no trabeculations are seen. Heavy

trabeculation suggests posttreatment change or recurrence. The tumor margin is fairly well defined. There is usually neither a sclerotic rim nor a wide zone of transition. The cortex is expanded and thinned, and segments may not be seen on plain x-ray films because it is too thin to be visible. There is typically no periosteal new bone formation, even with a pathologic fracture. The cortex may be destroyed with soft-tissue in-

(text continues on page 153)

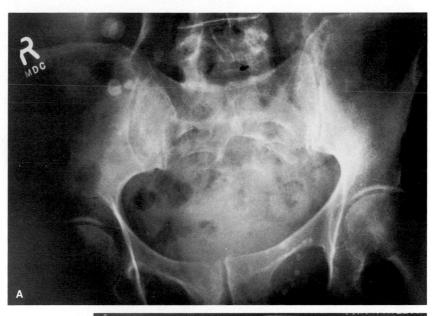

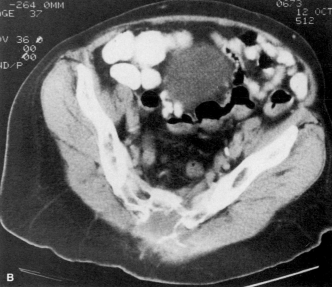

FIGURE 2-94.   A 68-year-old woman with a chordoma involving the sacrum. (**A**) The anteroposterior view of the sacrum reveals destruction of its middle and lower portions with a large tumor mass. (**B**) The CT scan shows bony destruction of the sacrum at the upper aspect of the tumor. (**C**) The axial MR (SE 600/20) section of the pelvis at a slightly lower level shows a large, inhomogeneous tumor mass with loculated high signal intensity, which may represent hemorrhage. (**D**) The sagittal MR (650/20) section shows the entire intrapelvic and extrapelvic extent of the tumor. (**E**) MR image (SE 2000/90). The tumor increases in signal intensity and shows greater heterogeneity in this T2-weighted image.   *continued*

◀ **FIGURE 2-93.**   MR image (SE 700/20) of a chordoma. A large tumor is destroying a major portion of the sacrum. The tumor is of low signal intensity.

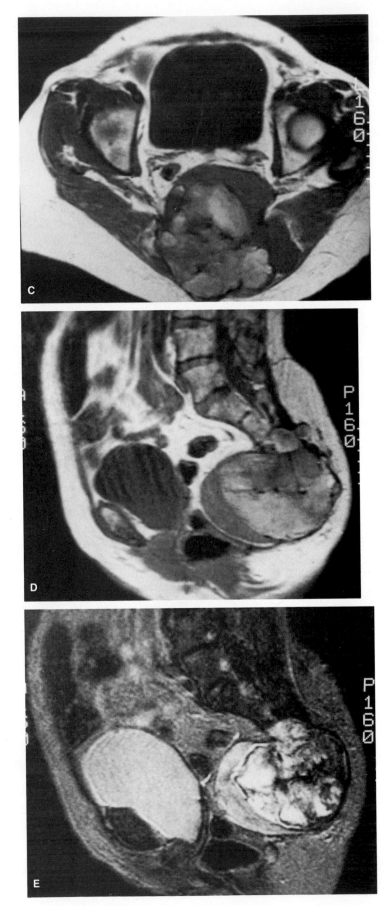

FIGURE 2-94. *(Continued)*

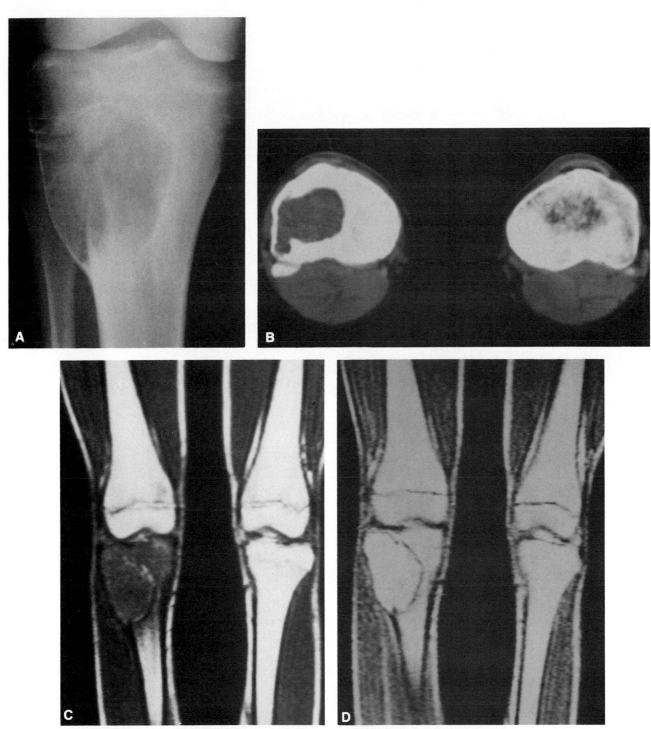

FIGURE 2-95. Giant cell tumor of the proximal tibia in a 16-year-old boy. (**A**) Conventional anteroposterior view. An expansile lesion involves the epiphysis and metaphysis. The lateral half of the bone is involved. Solid periosteal buttressing at the inferior aspect of the tumor is seen. A sharp line of demarcation surrounds the tumor except at its inferior aspect. (**B**) CT scan. The lesion involves the lateral aspect of the tibial plateau on the right. It is well demarcated and has a thin lateral shell. The proximal fibula is seen posteriorly. (**C**) Coronal T1-weighted MR image. The tumor is seen as a region of low signal intensity replacing the bright marrow fat. Involvement of the marrow beyond the tumor capsule is also shown. This may be due to edema, but extension should not be ruled out. (**D**) T2-weighted coronal image. The tumor shows high signal intensity. It extends up to the articular surface laterally. The low-signal capsule is clearly visible. The age of this patient is below the usual 20-year minimum. In addition, the metaphysis is principally involved. (Courtesy of Dr. J. P. Petasnick, Rush-Presbyterian St. Luke's Hospital, Chicago, IL.)

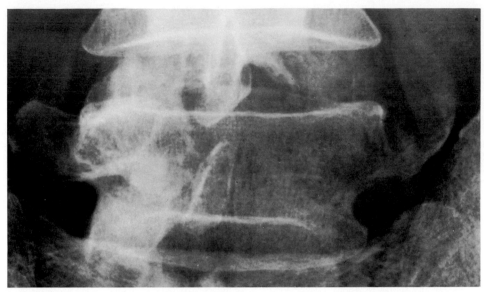

FIGURE 2-96. Giant cell tumor involving the left pedicle of the fifth lumbar vertebra, causing destruction and partial destruction of the superior aspect of the transverse process.

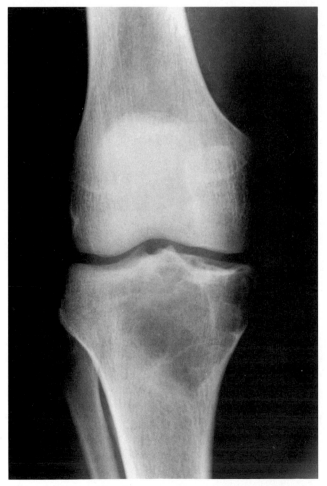

FIGURE 2-97. The classic appearance of a giant cell tumor is a rounded, medium-size, expansile, radiolucent lesion off the central axis of the bone.

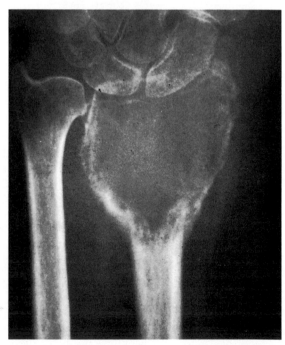

FIGURE 2-98. Giant cell tumor of the distal radius. There is a central radiolucent, destructive, and expansile lesion at the distal radius, extending to the articular surface. The expanded cortex is intact. Lack of definition of the proximal margin of the lesion and very light trabeculation can be seen. No periosteal new bone formation is present, a characteristic of this tumor.

vasion. Short tubular bone involvement shows changes similar to that of a long bone (Fig. 2-99).

CT is of value to determine any soft-tissue component, to assess the intraosseous extent (Fig. 2-100), to demonstrate the integrity of the cortex, and for postoperative evaluation.[207] Contrast-enhanced CT scans provide useful information about soft-tissue extent and relation to major vessels.

The angiographic features of giant cell tumor are similar to those of aneurysmal bone cyst.[3] The blood supply is from surrounding soft-tissue arteries. Many, small, corkscrew-shaped vessels are seen at the periphery. There is early visualization of variable-sized vascular spaces, along with an uneven and prolonged tumor stain. Early venous filling and abnormal veins are observed. There is no vascular encasement or invasion (Fig. 2-101). Avascular tumors are rare. Yaghmai divided aggressive giant cell tumors into two angiographic types. The first revealed cyst-like vascular spaces, vascular rims, and prolonged uneven tumor

stain; the second showed high to moderate degrees of vascularity without spaces, uniform tumor stain, and soft-tissue extension.[3]

MR images of giant cell tumor are superior to plain radiographs and CT scans in defining the extent of bone marrow replacement, inhomogeneity within the tumor, and soft-tissue invasion.[208,209] MRI provides the ability to evaluate tumor extension into the joint. It can show spread of tumor into the subchondral cortex and destruction of articular cartilage. T1-weighted images show diminished signal intensity, and T2-weighted images show isointense or hyperintense signal intensity of tumor compared with uninvolved marrow (Figs. 2-102 and 2-103). Irregular tumor margins may rarely be seen.[205] Fluid-fluid levels are occasionally detected.

Radioscintigraphy of giant cell tumors show increased uptake, usually more intense at the periphery than at the center. Intense uptake beyond the true tumor limits may be seen.[210] Scanning may not detect soft-tissue tumor extension. Gallium scans are unreliable in assessing this condition.[211]

A nonneoplastic osteolytic lesion containing giant cells, originally described in the jaw and called giant cell reaction or giant cell reparative granuloma, may also occur in the tubular (Fig. 2-104) and long bones. It usually occurs in association with Paget disease or fibrous dysplasia. One case has been reported in the femur without an underlying bone disorder.[212,213]

Benign giant cell tumor of bone may implanted into the surrounding soft tissues during surgery or pathologic fracture and may produce a peripheral rim of ossification.[214]

RARE MALIGNANT BONE TUMORS

Adamantinoma

Adamantinoma of the long bones is a rare malignant bone tumor with a histologic pattern resembling that of ameloblastoma of the jawbones.[215–217] It accounts for 0.1% of all primary bone tumors. There are also histologic and imaging patterns similar to fibrous dysplasia and osteofibrous dysplasia (Fig. 2-105).[218] Some of the latter cases may actually be adamantinomas. It occurs most often in the tibia and less often in the fibula. It is most common in adolescents and young adults. The typical appearance is a large, lobulated, expansile radiolucency in the midshaft of the tibia. Osteosclerosis may be widespread. The tumor may extend to the ends of the bone (Fig. 2-106). Cortical destruction and soft-tissue invasion occur in later stages. Simple and laminated periosteal new bone formation has been de-

(text continues on page 157)

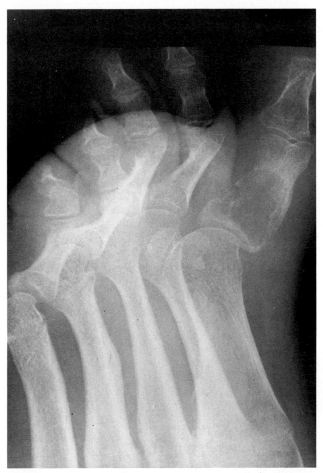

FIGURE 2-99. Giant cell tumor of the proximal phalanx of the great toe, showing expansion and extension to the articular surface. The cortex is interrupted at its inferior aspect. The tumor is well marginated.

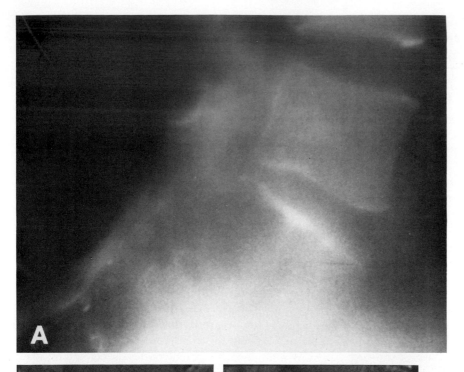

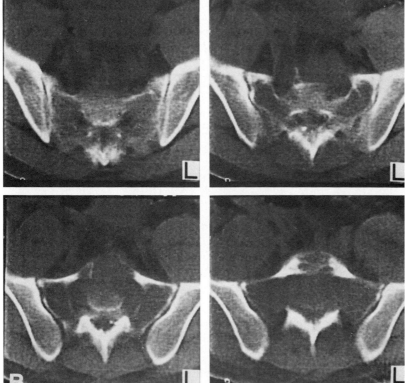

FIGURE 2-100. Giant cell tumor of the sacrum in a 25-year-old man who complained of sciatica. (**A**) Lateral tomogram of the sacrum shows a destructive lesion at the posterior aspect of the first sacral segment with cortical destruction. (**B**) CT scan shows destruction at the central aspect of the sacrum. (Courtesy of Dr. J. P. Petasnick, Rush-Presbyterian St. Luke's Hospital, Chicago, IL.)

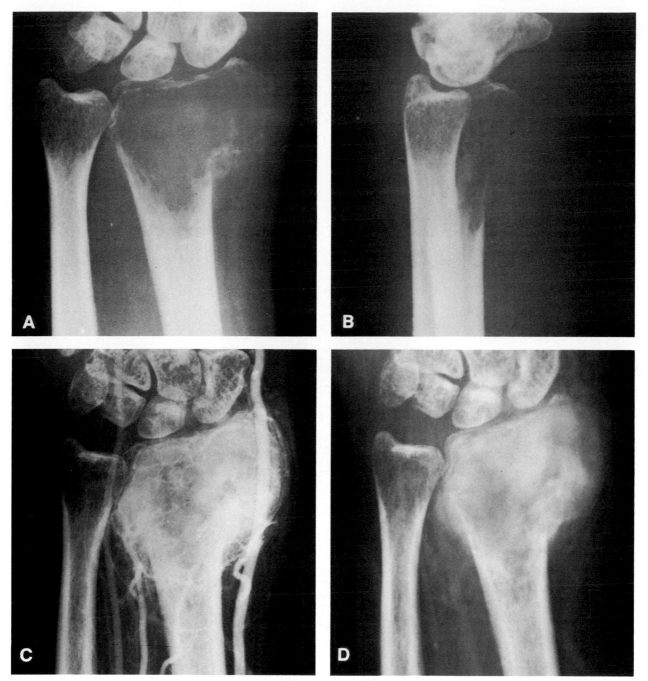

FIGURE 2-101. Giant cell tumor in a 21-year-old woman with pain and swelling for a few weeks and a recent history of trauma. Conventional (**A**) anteroposterior and (**B**) lateral views of the wrist reveal evidence of a pathologic fracture at the end of the radius with ill-defined margins and a very thin cortex laterally. Notice the elevated fat and cortical destruction in the lateral projection, suggestive of a fast-growing tumor. (**C**) Arteriograms in early arterial phase and (**D**) late venous phase reveal typical arteriographic findings of a giant cell tumor and aneurysmal bone cyst. Vascular spaces occur in the early venous phase with uneven tumor stain due to the absence of vascular spaces in the medial part of the tumor and opacification of vascular spaces after 60 seconds. (Courtesy of Dr. Issa Yaghmai, Medical College of Virginia, Richmond, VA.)

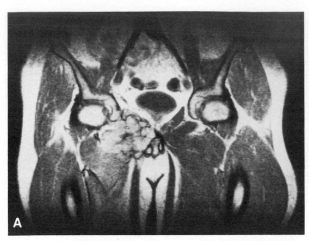
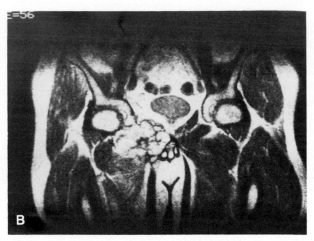

FIGURE 2-102. MR scans of a giant cell tumor of the right pubic bone. (**A**) T1-weighted MR image shows a lobulated tumor mass involving the pelvis and distorting the bladder on the right and an extrapelvic extension. High signal intensity of the femoral head is noted. (**B**) T2-weighted image. The lobulated tumor mass increases in signal intensity. The bladder contents have changed signal intensity from black to gray, and the femoral head has diminished somewhat in intensity. (Courtesy of Dr. Harry Genant, San Francisco, CA.)

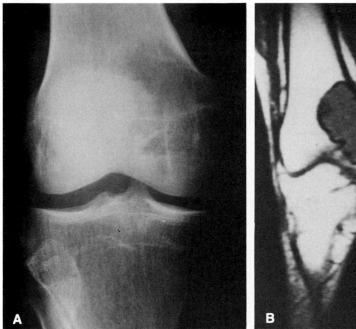
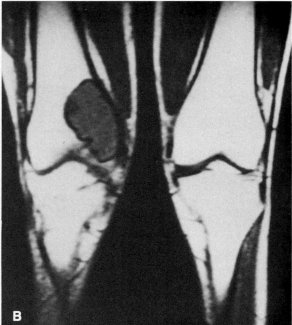

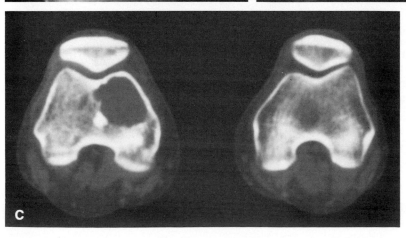

FIGURE 2-103. Giant cell tumor of the distal femur in a 26-year-old man. (**A**) Anteroposterior view. A radiolucent lesion involves the medial aspect of the distal femoral epiphysis and metaphysis. (**B**) CT scan. A well-circumscribed low-density lesion with a thin medial margin involves the tibial articular surface. (**C**) Coronal T1-weighted image. The tumor is seen as low signal intensity with a signal-void margin contrasted against the bright marrow fat. The epiphysis and metaphysis are involved. (Courtesy of Dr. J. P. Petasnick, Rush-Presbyterian St. Luke's Hospital, Chicago, IL.)

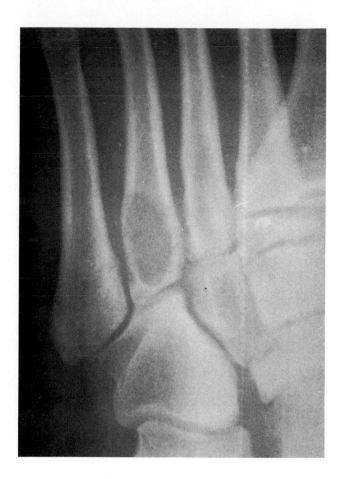

FIGURE 2-104. Giant cell reparative granuloma in a 17-year-old boy with an expansile lesion extending to the proximal articular surface of the fourth metacarpal. Biopsy proved this lesion to be a giant cell reparative granuloma.

scribed. The tumor may recur and metastasize. Metastases may present as spontaneous pneumothorax.[219]

Hemangioendothelioma

Hemangioendothelioma (i.e., angiosarcoma) is a rare malignant tumor that arises from endothelial cells of blood vessels.[220–225] It comprises less than 1% of all primary bone malignancies. The grade may range from low to high, with rapid growth and metastases. The ratio of affected males to females is 2 to 1. The peak incidence is in the third and fourth decades of life. It may occur at sites of chronic osteomyelitis or bone infarcts. The location is usually metaphyseal in a long bone.

The radiographic appearance is that of solitary or multiple destructive skeletal lesions, usually geographic, without a sclerotic margin. Multifocal tumors may be in the same bone or adjacent bones. Rarely, periosteal reaction, expansion, and a mild degree of peripheral sclerosis may occur, and a soft-tissue mass may be associated. The tumors may remain stable, or some may rapidly progress (Fig. 2-107). On MR images, the tumor is of low signal intensity on T1-weighted images and of high signal intensity on T2-weighted images, possibly with some hemorrhagic areas showing foci of mixed signal intensity (Fig. 2-108). A rare subtype is

epitheloid hemangioendothelioma.[226,227] This tumor usually affects men under the age of 30 years. The lesions are multifocal or polyostotic, most often purely osteolytic in a moth-eaten pattern, but they sometimes have a honeycomb appearance. The periosteal reaction is sparse, and soft-tissue invasion may occur.

Hemangiopericytoma

Hemangiopericytoma of bone is a rare tumor. The future behavior of these tumors is difficult to predict. Histologic diagnosis may depend on identification of pericytes by electron microscopy. Older patients are most often affected, and any bone may be involved. It is a solitary lesion. It may be expansile, trabeculated, or seen as a relatively well-marginated, destructive lesion (Fig. 2-109). Periosteal reaction is rare.

Liposarcoma and Leiomyosarcoma

Liposarcoma of bone is rare and may show extensive destruction of bone, with a periosteal reaction.[228–230] The most common site is the tibia. Other bones may be involved. This tumor rarely contains osteosarcoma-

(text continues on page 162)

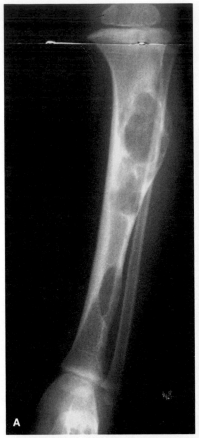

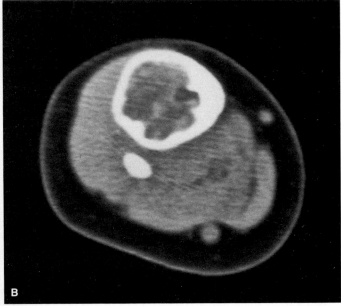

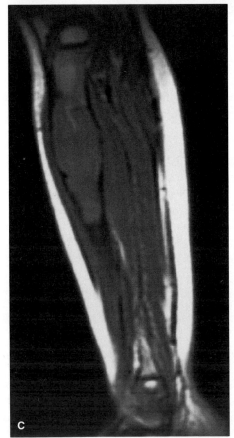

FIGURE 2-105. Osteofibrous dysplasia. (**A**) The lateral view of the tibia reveals an expansile, loculated appearance of the entire diaphysis. (**B**) The CT scan shows expansion of the bone with inhomogeneous density within the medullary cavity. (**C**) The sagittal MR (SE 600/20) section shows low signal intensity within the medullary cavity and expansion of bone at the proximal half of the tibial diaphysis. (**D**) The axial MR (SE 3000/20) section shows expansion of the bone with slight inhomogeneity corresponding to **B**. (**E**) MR image (SE 3000/80). The lesion in the medullary cavity increases in signal intensity and shows inhomogeneities. This increase in signal intensity is not expected in a purely dense fibrous lesion.

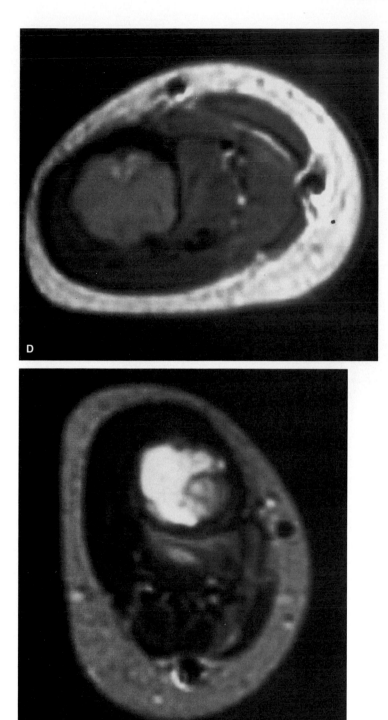

FIGURE 2-105. *(Continued)*

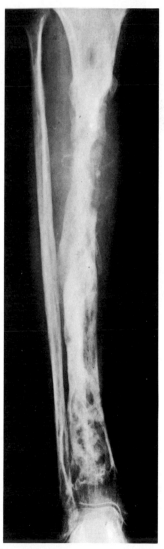

FIGURE 2-106. Adamantinoma of the tibia. There is extensive involvement of the entire shaft of the tibia, with a multilocular, expansile appearance at the distal aspect and a destructive appearance with periosteal new bone formation at the proximal aspect. Reactive sclerosis is visible in the midshaft.

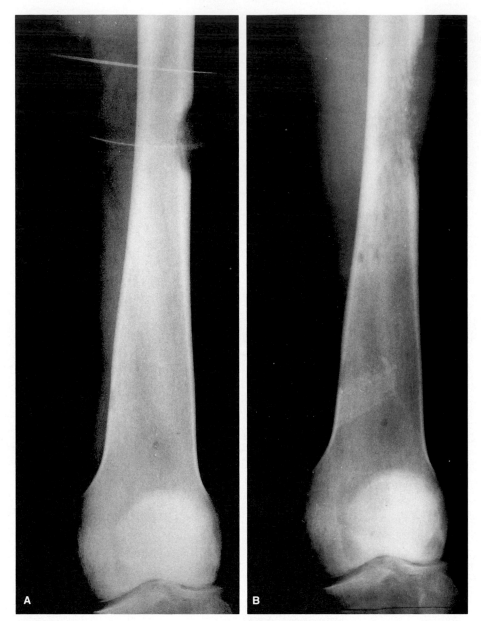

FIGURE 2-107. Hemangioendothelioma. Widespread osteolytic lesions were found in this patient. (**A**) The anteroposterior view of the femur shows a destructive cortical area proximally and a smaller radiolucency distally. (**B**) The anteroposterior view of the femur 6 months after **A**. The cortical destructive lesion has increased considerably, and a permeative destructive zone surrounds it. Multiple radiolucencies are seen in the femoral shaft. There is no bone sclerosis nor periosteal reaction.

FIGURE 2-108. Hemangioendothelioma. (**A**) The anteroposterior view of the tibia reveals a radiolucent, expansile lesion in the diametaphyseal area. (**B**) The T1-weighted MR image shows low-signal-intensity tumor replacing fatty marrow. Small foci of high signal intensity represent hemorrhagic areas. (**C**) The T2-weighted image shows an increase in the signal intensity of the tumor and an inhomogeneous appearance. (**D**) Digital subtraction angiography shows tumor stain in several distinct areas.

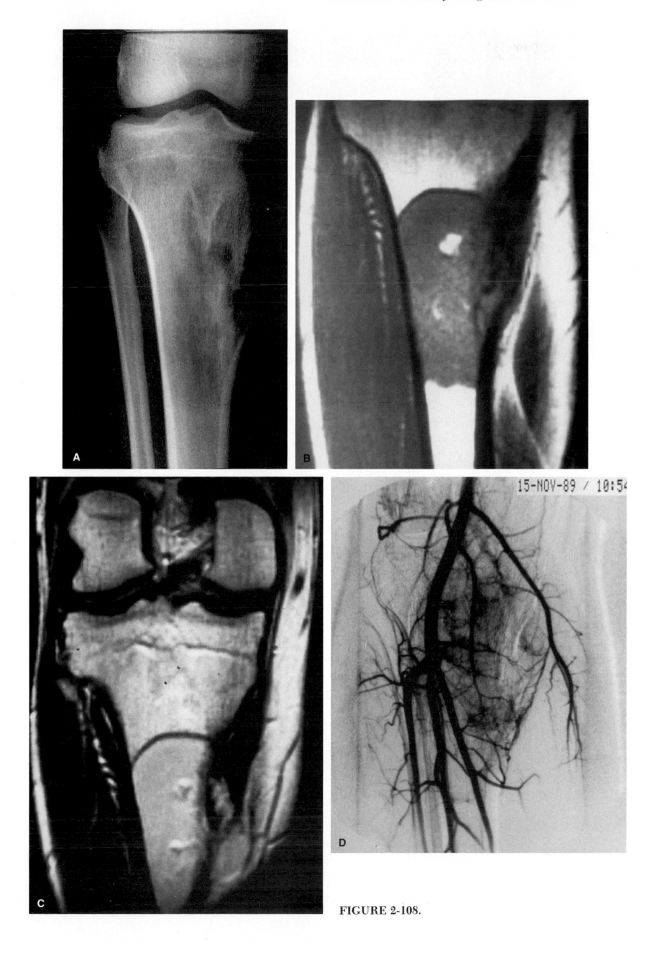

FIGURE 2-108.

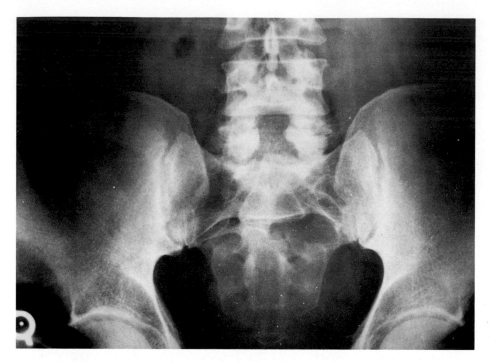

FIGURE 2-109. Hemangiopericytoma of the sacrum in a 45-year-old man. The anteroposterior view of the pelvis shows a destructive lesion in the body of the sacrum on the left. The sacral foraminal lines have been obliterated. The patient had a prior laminectomy at L5 for pain before the lesion became evident radiographically.

tous foci and metastasizes as an osteosarcoma.[231] The transformation of benign lipoma of bone to liposarcoma and malignant fibrous histiocytoma has been reported.[232] Primary leiomyosarcoma of bone has been reported. It had a purely destructive appearance and produced a pathologic fracture.[233]

References

1. Bassett LW, Gold RH, Webber MM: Radionuclide bone imaging. Radiol Clin North Am 19:675–702, 1981
2. Fordham EW, Ali A, Turner DA, Charters JR: Atlas of Total Body Radionuclide Imaging, vol 1. Philadelphia, Harper & Row, 1982
3. Yaghamai I: Angiography of Bone and Soft Tissue Lesions. New York, Springer-Verlag, 1979
4. Laurin S, Akerman M, Kindblom LG et al: Angiography in myeloma (plasmacytoma). Skeletal Radiol 4:8–18, 1979
5. Ayala AG, Zornosa J: Primary bone tumors: Percutaneous needle biopsy. Radiology 149:675–679, 1983
6. Moore SG, Dawson KL: Red and yellow marrow in the femur: Age-related changes in appearance after MR imaging. Radiology 175:219–223, 1990
7. Ricci C, Cova M et al: Normal Age-related patterns of cellular and fatty bone marrow distribution in the axial skeleton: MR imaging study. Radiology 177:83–88, 1990
8. Bohndrof K, Reiser M et al: Magnetic resonance imaging of primary tumors and tumor-like lesions of bone. Skeletal Radiol 15:511–517, 1986
9. Greenfield GB, Warren DL, Clark RA: MR imaging of periosteal and cortical changes of bone. Radiographics 11:611–623, 1991
10. Pettersson H, Gillespy T III et al: Primary musculoskeletal tumors: Examination with MR imaging compared with conventional modalities. Radiology 164:237–241, 1987
11. Boyko OB, Cory DA et al: MR imaging of osteogenic and Ewing's sarcoma. Am J Roentgenol 148:317–322, 1987
12. Schajowicz F: Tumors and Tumor-like Lesions of Bones and Joints. New York, Springer-Verlag, 1981
13. Johnson LC: A general theory of bone tumors. Bull N Y Acad Med 29:164–171, 1953
14. Redmond OM, Stack JP et al: Osteosarcoma: Use of MR imaging and MR spectroscopy in clinical decision making. Radiology 172:811–815, 1989
15. Just VM, Gutjahr P et al: Moeglichkeiten der MR: Tomographie in der Therapiekontrolle Maligner Knochtumoren. Fortschr Geb Rontgenstr 147:413–242, 1977
16. Pan G, Raymond AK et al: Osteosarcoma: MR imaging after preoperative chemotherapy. Radiology 174:517–526, 1990
17. Unni KK, Dahlin DC: Osteosarcoma: Pathology and classification. Semin Roentgenol 24:143–152, 1989
18. Edeiken-Monroe B, Edeiken J, Jacobson HG: Osteosarcoma. Semin Roentgenol 24:153–173, 1989
19. deSantos LA et al: Osteogenic sarcoma after the age of 50: A radiographic evaluation. AJR Am J Roentgenol 131:481–484, 1978
20. Lee ES: Osteosarcoma: A reconnaissance. Clin Radiol 26:5–25, 1975
21. Miller CW, McLaughlin RE: Osteosarcoma in siblings: Report of 2 cases. J Bone Joint Surg [Am] 59:261–262, 1977
22. Klenerman L, Ockenden BG, Townsend AC: Osteosarcoma occurring in osteogenesis imperfecta: Report of 2 cases. J Bone Joint Surg [Br] 49:314–323, 1967
23. Banta JV, Schreiber RR, Kulik WJ: Hyperplastic callus formation in osteogenesis imperfecta simulating osteosarcoma. J Bone Joint Surg [Am] 53:115–122, 1971
24. Nelson JA, Clark RE, Palubinskas AJ: Osteogenic sarcoma with calcified renal metastases. Br J Radiol 44:802–804, 1971
25. Caceres E, Zaharia M, Tantalean E: Lymph node metastasis in osteogenic sarcoma. Surgery 65:421–422, 1969
26. Fielding JW et al: Primary osteogenic sarcoma of the cervical spine. J Bone Joint Surg [Am] 58:892–894, 1977
27. Nora FE, Unni KK, Pritchard DJ et al: Osteosarcoma of extragnathic craniofacial bones. Mayo Clin Proc 58:268–272, 1983
28. Rao VRK, Rout D, Radhakrishnan V: Osteogenic sarcoma of the skull. Neuroradiology 25:51–53, 1983

29. Goodwin MA: Primary osteosarcoma of the patella: A case report. J Bone Joint Surg [Br] 43:338–341, 1961

30. deSantos LA, Edeiken BS: Subtle early osteosarcoma. Skeletal Radiol 13:44–48, 1985

31. Norton KI, Hermann G et al: Epiphyseal involvement in osteosarcoma. Radiology 180:813–816, 1991

32. Haworth JM, Watt I, Part WM et al: Diaphyseal osteosarcoma. Br J Radiol 54:932–938, 1981

33. Miller TT, Abdelwahab IF et al: Case report 735. Skeletal Radiol 21:277–279, 1992

34. Patel DV, Hammer RA et al: Primary osteogenic sarcoma of the spine. Skeletal Radiol 12:276–279, 1984

35. Shives TC, Dahlin DC et al: Osteosarcoma of the spine. J Bone Joint Surg 68:660–668, 1986

36. Rittenberg GM et al: The vascular "sunburst" appearance of osteosarcoma: A new angiographic finding. Skeletal Radiol 2:243–244, 1978

37. Smith J, Heelan RT, Huvos AG: Radiographic changes in primary osteogenic sarcoma following intensive chemotherapy. Radiology 143:355–360, 1982

38. Chuang VP, Benjamin R, Jaffe N et al: Radiographic and angiographic changes in osteosarcoma after intraarterial chemotherapy. Am J Roentgenol 139:1065–1069, 1982

39. Coffre C, Vanel D et al: Problems and pitfalls in the use of computed tomography for the local evaluation of long bone osteosarcoma: Report on 30 cases. Skeletal Radiol 13:147–153, 1985

40. Schreiman JS, Crass JR et al: Osteosarcoma: Role of CT in limb-sparing treatment. Radiology 161:485–488, 1986

41. Azouz ME, Esseltine DW, Chevalier L: Radiologic evaluation of osteosarcoma. J Can Assoc Radiol 33:167–171, 1982

42. Gillespy T III, Manfrini M et al: Staging of intraosseous extent of osteosarcoma: Correlation of preoperative CT and MR imaging with pathologic macroslides. Radiology 167:765–767, 1988

43. Sandler MS, Heyman S, Watts H: Localization of ^{132m}Tc methylene diphosphonate within synovial fluid in osteosarcoma. AJR Am J Roentgenol 143:349–350, 1984

44. Rossleigh MA, Smith J et al: Case reports: A photopenic lesion in osteosarcoma. Br J Radiol 60:497–499, 1987

45. Yaghmai I, Abdolmahmoud SZ, Shams S, Afshari R: Value of arteriography in the diagnosis of benign and malignant bone lesions. Cancer 27:1134–1147, 1971

46. Kumpan W, Lechner G et al: The angiographic response of osteosarcoma following pre-operative chemotherapy. Skeletal Radiol 15:96–102, 1986

47. Vanel D, Tcheng S et al: The radiological appearances of telangiectatic osteosarcoma. Skeletal Radiol 16:196–200, 1987

48. Bathurst N, Sanerkin N et al: Osteoclast-rich osteosarcoma. Br J Radiol 59:667–673, 1986

49. Edeiken J, Raymond AK et al: Small-cell osteosarcoma. Skeletal Radiol 16:621–628, 1987

50. Kurt AM, Unni KK et al: Low-grade Intraosseous osteosarcoma. Cancer 65:1418–1428, 1990

51. Cremin BJ, Heselson NG, Webber BL: The multiple sclerotic osteogenic sarcoma of early childhood. Br J Radiol 49:416–419, 1976

52. Davidson JW, Chacha PB, James W: Multiple osteosarcomata: Report of a case. J Bone Joint Surg [Br] 47:537–541, 1965

53. Grosswasser JR, Brunebaum M: Metaphyseal multifocal osteosarcoma. Br J Radiol 51:671–681, 1978

54. Hopper KD, Moser RP et al: Osteosarcomatosis. Radiology 175:233–239, 1990

55. Hopper KD, Haseman DB et al: Case report 634. Skeletal Radiol 19:535–537, 1990

56. deSantos LA et al: The radiographic spectrum of periosteal osteosarcoma. Radiology 127:123–129, 1978

57. Unni KK, Dahlin DC, Beabout JW: Periosteal osteogenic sarcoma. Cancer 37:2476–2485, 1976

58. Sonneland PRL, Unni KK: Case report 258. Skeletal Radiol 11:77–80, 1984

59. Levine E, DeSmet AA et al: Juxtacortical osteosarcoma: A radiologic and histologic spectrum. Skeletal Radiol 14:38–46, 1985

60. Ahuja SC et al: Juxtacortical (parosteal) osteogenic sarcoma. J Bone Joint Surg [Am] 59:632–647 1977

61. Edeiken J, Farrel C, Ackerman LV, Spjut HJ: Parosteal sarcoma. AJR Am J Roentgenol 111:579–583, 1971

62. Ranniger K, Altner PC: Parosteal osteoid sarcoma. Radiology 86:648–651, 1966

63. Stark HH, Jones FE, Jernstrom P: Parosteal osteogenic sarcoma of a metacarpal bone: A case report. J Bone Joint Surg [Am] 53:147–153, 1971

64. Hermann G, Abdelwahab IF et al: Case report 711. Skeletal Radiol 21:69–71, 1992

65. Sauer DD, Chase DR: Case report 461. Skeletal Radiol 17:72–76, 1988

66. Kumar R, Moser RP et al: Parosteal osteogenic sarcoma arising in cranial bones: Clinical and radiologic features in eight patients. AJR Am J Roentegenol 155:113–117, 1990

67. Wold LE, Unni KK, Beabout JW et al: Dedifferentiated parosteal osteosarcoma. J Bone Joint Surg [Am] 66:53–59, 1984

68. Smith GD, Chalmers J et al: Osteosarcoma arising in relation to an enchondroma. J Bone Joint Surg [Am] 68:315–319, 1986

69. Heater K, Collins PA: Osteosarcoma in association with infarction of bone. J Bone Joint Surg [Am] 69:300–302, 1987

70. Resnik CS, Aisner SC et al: Case report 767. Skeletal Radiol 22:58–61, 1993

71. Moore TE, King AR et al: Sarcoma in Paget disease of bone: Clinical, radiologic, and pathologic features in 22 cases. AJR Am J Roentgenol 156:1199–1203, 1991

72. Price CHG, Goldie W: Paget's sarcoma of bone: A study of 80 cases from the Bristol and Leeds bone tumour registries. J Bone Joint Surg [Br] 51:205–224, 1969

73. Greditzer HG, McLeod RA, Unni KK et al: Bone sarcomas in Paget's disease. Radiology 146:327–333, 1983

74. Rosenmertz SK, Schare HJ: Osteogenic sarcoma arising in Paget's disease of the mandible: Review of the literature and report of a case. Oral Surg Oral Med Oral Pathol 28:304–309, 1969

75. Aub JC, Evans RP, Hempelmann LH, Martland HS: The late effects of internally deposited radioactive materials in man. Medicine (Baltimore) 31:221, 1952

76. Yoneyama T, Greenlaw RH: Osteogenic sarcoma following radiotherapy for retinoblastoma. Radiology 93:1185–1186, 1969

77. Ironside JAD: Second malignant neoplasms after childhood cancer: A report of three cases of osteogenic sarcoma. Clin Radiol 38:195–199, 1987

78. Kofoed H, Lindenberg S: Postirradiation chondroblastic osteogenic sarcoma. J Bone Joint Surg [Br] 64:590–591, 1982

79. Smith J: Postradiation sarcoma of bone in Hodgkin disease. Skeletal Radiol 16:524–532, 1987

80. Weatherby RP, Dahlin DC, Ivins JC: Postradiation sarcoma of bone. Mayo Clin Proc 56:294–306, 1981

81. Torres FX, Kyriakos M: Bone infarct-associated osteosarcoma. Cancer 70:2418–2430, 1992

82. Mindell ER, Northrup CS, Douglass HO: Osteosarcoma associated with osteopoikilosis. J Bone Joint Surg [Am] 60:406–408, 1978

83. Mirra JM, Dodd L et al: Case report 700. Skeletal Radiol 20:613–616, 1991

84. Picci P, Gherlinzoni F, Guerra A: Intracortical osteosarcoma: Rare entity or early manifestation of classical osteosarcoma? Skeletal Radiol 9:255–258, 1983

85. Spanier SS, Shuster JJ et al: The effect of local extent of the tumor on prognosis in osteosarcoma. J Bone Joint Surg [Am] 72:643–653, 1990

86. Patel MR, Pearlman HS, Engler J, Wollowick BS: Chondrosarcoma of the proximal phalanx of the finger: Review

of the literature and report of a case. J Bone Joint Surg [Am] 59:401–403, 1977

87. Reiter FB, Ackerman LV, Staple TW: Central chondrosarcoma of the appendicular skeleton. Radiology 105:525–530, 1972
88. Roberts PH, Price CHG: Chondrosarcoma of the bones of the hand. J Bone Joint Surg [Br] 59:213–221, 1977
89. Rosenthal DI, Schiller AL, Mankin HJ: Chondrosarcoma: Correlation of radiological and histological grade. Radiology 150:21–26, 1984
90. Varma DGK, Ayala AG et al: Chondrosarcoma: MR imaging with pathologic correlation. Radiographics 12:687–704, 1992
91. Dahlin DC, Unni KK: Bone Tumors. 4th ed. Springfield, IL, Charles C Thomas, 1986
92. Grabias S, Mankin HJ: Chondrosarcoma arising in histologically proved unicameral bone cyst: A case report. J Bone Joint Surg [Am] 56:1501–1509, 1974
93. Mack GR, Robey DB, Kurman RJ: Chondrosarcoma secreting chorionic gonadotropin. J Bone Joint Surg [Am] 59:1107–1111, 1978
94. Jaffe HL: Tumors and Tumorous Conditions of the Bones and Joints. Philadelphia, Lea & Febiger, 1958
95. Bertoni F, Boriani S, Laus M et al: Periosteal chondrosarcoma and periosteal osteosarcoma. J Bone Joint Surg [Br] 64:370–376, 1982
96. Vanel D, Coffre C, Zemoura L et al: Chondrosarcoma in children subsequent to other malignant tumours in different locations. Skeletal Radiol 11:96–101, 1984
97. Pepe AJ, Kuhlmann RF, Miller DB: Mesenchymal chondrosarcoma: A case report. J Bone Joint Surg [Am] 59:256–258, 1977
98. Pirschel J: A mesenchymal chondrosarcoma of the sternum. Fortschr Geb Rontgenstr 124:91–93, 1976
99. Unni KK, Dahlin DC, Beabout JW, Sim FH: Chondrosarcoma: Clear-cell variant: A report of 16 cases. J Bone Joint Surg [Am] 58:676–683, 1976
100. Geirnaerdt MJA, Bloem JL et al: Cartilaginous tumors: Correlation of gadolinium-enhanced MR imaging and histopathologic findings. Radiology 186:813–817, 1993
101. Greenfield GB, Cardenas C et al: Case report 650. Skeletal Radiol 20:67–70, 1991
102. Hermann G, Sacher M et al: Chondrosarcoma of the spine: An unusual radiographic presentation. Skeletal Radiol 14:178–183, 1985
103. Pinstein ML, Sebes JI, Scott RL: Transarticular extension of chondrosarcoma. AJR Am J Roentgenol 142:779–780, 1984
104. Mirra JM, Marcove RC: Fibrosarcomatous dedifferentiation of primary and secondary chondrosarcoma: Review of 5 cases. J Bone Joint Surg [Am] 56:285–296, 1974
105. Norman A, Sissons HA: Radiographic hallmarks of peripheral chondrosarcoma. Radiology 151:589–596, 1984
106. Malghem J, Berg BV et al: Benign osteochondromas and exostotic chondrosarcomas: evaluation of cartilage cap thickness by ultrasound. Skeletal Radiol 21:33–37, 1992
107. Hudson TM, Manaster BJ, Springfield DS et al: Radiology of medullary chondrosarcoma: Preoperative treatment planning. Skeletal Radiol 10:69–78, 1983
108. Cohen EK, Kressel HY et al: Hyaline cartilage-origin bone and soft-tissue neoplasma: MR appearance and histologic correlation. Radiology 167:477–481, 1988
109. Fobben ES, Dalinka MK et al: The magnetic resonance imaging appearance at 1.5 Tesla of cartilaginous tumors involving the epiphysis. Skeletal Radiol 16:647–651, 1987
109a. Aoki JA, Sone S, Fujioka F et al: MR of enchondroma and chondrosarcoma: Rings and arcs of Gd-DPTA enhancement. J Comp Asst Tomogr 15:1011–1016, 1991
110. Hudson TM, Chew FS, Manaster BJ: Radionuclide bone scanning of medullary chondrosarcoma. AJR Am J Roentgenol 138:1071–1076, 1982
111. Schajowicz F: Juxtacortical chondrosarcoma. J Bone Joint Surg [Br] 59:473–480, 1977
112. Kumar R, David R et al: Clear cell chondrosarcoma. Radiology 154:45–48, 1985
113. Present D, Bacchini P et al: Clear cell chondrosarcoma of bone. A report of 8 cases. Skeletal Radiol 20:187–191, 1991
114. Bagley L, Kneeland JB et al: Unusual behavior of clear cell chondrosarcoma. Skeletal Radiol 22:279–282, 1993
115. de Lange EE, Pope TL Jr et al: Dedifferentiated chondrosarcoma: Radiographic features. Radiology 160:489–492, 1986
116. Frassica JF, Unni KK et al: Dedifferentiated chondrosarcoma. J Bone Joint Surg 68:1197–1205, 1986
117. Crim JR, Mirra JM: Enchondroma protuberans. Report of a case and its distinction from chondrosarcoma and osteochondroma adjacent to an enchondroma. Skeletal Radiol 19:431–434, 1990
118. Eyre-Brook AL, Price CHG: Fibrosarcoma of bone. J Bone Joint Surg [Br] 51:20–37, 1969
119. Larsson SE, Lorentzon R, Roquist L: Fibrosarcoma of bone. J Bone Joint Surg [Br] 58:412–417, 1976
120. Dorfman HD, Norman A, Wolff H: Fibrosarcoma complicating bone infarction in a caisson worker: A case report. J Bone Joint Surg [Am] 48:528–532, 1966
121. Akbarnia BA, Wirth CK, Colman N: Fibrosarcoma arising from chronic osteomyelitis. Case report and review of the literature. J Bone Joint Surg [Am] 58:123–125, 1976
122. Jeffree GM, Price CHG: Metastatic spread of fibrosarcoma of bone. J Bone Joint Surg [Br] 58:418–425, 1976
123. Taconis WK, Rijssel TGV: Fibrosarcoma of the jaws. Skeletal Radiol 15:10–13, 1986
124. Taconis WK, Mulder JD: Fibrosarcoma and malignant fibrous histiocytoma of long bones: Radiographic features and grading. Skeletal Radiol 11:237–245, 1984
125. Yaghmai I: Angiographic features of fibromas and fibrosarcomas. Radiology 124:57–64, 1977
126. Turculet V: Aspects radiologiques des tumeurs histiocytaires malignes des parties molles et osseuses. J Radiol 62:429–436, 1981
127. Matsuno T: Benign fibrous histiocytoma involving the ends of long bone. Skeletal Radiol 19:561–566, 1990
128. Gaucher AA, Regent DM et al: Case report 656. Skeletal Radiol 20:137–140, 1991
129. Vanel D, Hagay C, Rebibo G et al: Study of three radio-induced malignant fibrohistiocytomas of bone. Skeletal Radiol 9:174–178, 1983
130. Heselson NG, Price SK, Path MRC et al: Two malignant fibrous histiocytomas in bone infarcts. J Bone Joint Surg [Am] 65:1166–1171, 1983
131. Akai M, Ohno T et al: Case report 601. Skeletal Radiol 19:154–157, 1990
132. Destouet JM, Kyriakos M, Gilula LA: Fibrous histiocytoma (fibroxanthoma) of a cervical vertebra. Skeletal Radiol 5:241–246, 1980
133. Dahlin DC, Coventry MB, Scanlon PW: Ewing's sarcoma: A critical analysis of 165 cases. J Bone Joint Surg [Am] 43:185–192, 1961
134. deSantos LA, Jing BS: Radiographic findings of Ewing's sarcoma of the jaws. Br J Radiol 51:682–687, 1978
135. Kittredge RD: Arteriography in Ewing's tumor. Radiology 97:609–610, 1970
136. Whitehouse GH, Griffiths GJ: Roentgenologic aspects of spinal involvement by primary and metastatic Ewing's tumor. J Can Assoc Radiol 27:290–297, 1976
137. Varma DGK, Moulopoulos A et al: Case report 682. Skeletal Radiol 20:391–393, 1991
138. Rousselin B, Vanel D et al: Clinical and radiologic analysis of 13 cases of primary neuroectodermal tumors of bone. Skeletal Radiol 18:115–120, 1989
139. Lacey SH, Danish EH et al: Ewing's sarcoma of the proximal phalanx of a finger. J Bone Joint Surg 69:931–934, 1987
139a. Dick HM, Francis KC, Johnston AD: Ewing's sarcoma of the hand. J Bone Joint Surg [Am] 53:345–348, 1971
140. Reinus WR, Gilula LA et al: Radiographic appearance of

Ewing's sarcoma of the hands and feet. AJR Am J Roentgenol 144:331–336, 1985

141. Escobedo EM, Bjorkengren AG, Moore SG: Case report. Ewing's sarcoma of the hand. AJR Am J Roentgenal 159:101–102, 1992

142. Vacher H, Lavenu MCV, Sauvegrain J: Etude anatomo-radio-clinique des sarcomes d'Ewing's du rachis lombaire. J Radiol 62:425–428, 1981

143. Weinstein JB, Siegel MJ, Griffith RC: Spinal Ewing's sarcoma: Misleading appearances. Skeletal Radiol 11:262–265, 1984

144. Klaassen MA, Hoffman G: Ewing's sarcoma presenting as spondylolisthesis: Report of a case. J Bone Joint Surg 69:1089–1092

145. Levine E, Levine C: Ewing's tumor of rib: Radiologic findings and computed tomography contribution. Skeletal Radiol 9:227–233, 1983

146. Azouz ME: Masse intrathoracique dans le sarcome d'Ewing des cotes. J Radiol 64:391–395, 1983

147. Reinus WR, Gehan EA et al: Plain radiographic predictors of survival in treated Ewing's sarcoma. Skeletal Radiol 21:287–291, 1992

148. MacVicar AD, Olliff JFC et al: Ewing sarcoma: MR imaging of chemotherapy-induced changes with histologic correlation. Radiology 184:859–864, 1992

149. Erlemann R, Sciuk J et al: Response of osteosarcoma and Ewing sarcoma to preoperative chemotherapy: Assessment with dynamic and static MR imaging and skeletal scintigraphy. Radiology 175:791–796, 1990

150. Fletcher BD: Review article. Response of osteosarcoma and Ewing sarcoma to chemotherapy: Imaging evaluation. AJR Am J Roentgenol 157:825–833, 1991

151. Griffiths HJ: Marrow tumors. *In* Bone Tumors, vol 5, part 6. Berlin, Springer-Verlag, 1977

152. Ivins JC, Dahlin DC: Reticulum-cell sarcoma of bone. J Bone Joint Surg [Am] 35:835–842, 1953

153. Parker F, Jackson H: Primary reticulum-cell sarcoma of bone. Surg Gynecol Obstet 68:45–51, 1939

154. Osborne BM: Contextual diagnosis of Hodgkin's disease and non-Hodgkin's lymphoma. Radiol Clin North Am 28:669–682, 1990

155. Mulligan ME, Kransdorf MJ: Sequestra in primary lymphoma of bone: Prevalence and radiologic features. AJR Am J Roentgenol 160:1245–1248, 1993

156. Beatty PT, Bjorkengren AG et al: Case report 764. Skeletal Radiol 21:559–561, 1992

157. Solomon A, McLaughlin CL: Immunoglobulin structure determined from products of plasma cell neoplasms. Semin Hematol 10:3–17, 1973

159. Gompels BM, Vataw ML, Martel W: Correlation of radiological manifestations of multiple myeloma with immunoglobulin abnormalities and prognosis. Radiology 104:509–514, 1972

160. Hermann G, Abdelwahab IF et al: Case report 621. Skeletal Radiol 19:379–381, 1990

161. Jaffe HL: Tumors and Tumorous Conditions of the Bones and Joints. Philadelphia, Lea & Febiger, 1958

162. Bronsky D, Bernstein A: Acute gout secondary to multiple myeloma: A case report. Ann Intern Med 41:820–822, 1954

163. Libshitz HI, Malthouse SR et al: Multiple myeloma: Appearance at MR imaging. Radiology 182:833–837, 1992

164. Engels EP, Smith RC, Krantz S: Bone sclerosis in multiple myeloma. Radiology 75:242–247, 1960

165. Jacobson HG, Poppel MH, Shapiro JH, Grossberger S: The vertebral pedicle sign: A roentgen finding to differentiate metastatic carcinoma from multiple myeloma. AJR Am J Roentgenol 80:817–821, 1958

166. Toland J, Phelps PDD: Plasmacytoma of the skull base. Clin Radiol 22:93–96, 1971

167. Fruehwald FJ, Tscholakoff T et al: Magnetic resonance imaging of the lower vertebral column in patients with multiple myeloma. Invest Radiol 23:193–199, 1988

168. Moulopoulos LA, Varma DGK, Dimopoulos MA, et al: Multiple myeloma: Spinal MR imaging in patients with untreated newly diagnosed disease. Radiology 185:833–840, 1992

169. Sundaram M, McGuire MH et al: Magnetic resonance imaging of osteosarcoma. Skeletal Radiol 16:23–29, 1987

170. Himmelfarb E, Sebes J, Rainowitz J: Unusual roentgenographic presentations of multiple myeloma: Report of 3 cases. J Bone Joint Surg [Am] 56:1723–1728, 1974

171. Theros E: Plasma cell granuloma of pelvis and femora: RPC case of the month from AFIP. Radiology 95:679–686, 1970

172. Frangione B, Franklin EC: Heavy chain diseases: Clinical features and molecular significance of the disordered immunoglobulin structure. Semin Hematol 10:53–64, 1973

173. Bottomly JP, Bradley J, Whitehouse GH: Waldenstrom's macroglobulinemia and amyloidosis with subcutaneous calcification and lymphographic appearances. Br J Radiol 47:232–235, 1974

174. Renner RR, Nelson DA, Lozner EL: Roentgenological manifestations of primary macroglobulinemia (Waldenström). AJR Am J Roentgenol 113:499–508, 1971

175. Vermess M, Pearson KD, Einstein AB, Fahey JL: Osseous manifestations of Waldenstrom's macroglobulinemia. Radiology 102:497–504, 1972

176. Whitehouse GH, Bottomley JP, Bradley J: Lymphangiographic appearances in Waldenstrom's macroglobulinemia. Br J Radiol 47:226–229, 1974

177. Resnick D, Greenway GD, Bardwick PA et al: Plasma-cell dyscrasia with polyneuropathy, organomegaly, endocinopathy, M-protein, and skin changes: The POEMS syndrome. Radiology 140:17–22, 1981

178. Aggarwal S, Goulatia RK et al: Case Report. POEMS syndrome: A rare variety of plasma cell dyscrasia. AJR Am J Roentgenol 155:339–341, 1990

179. Firooznia H et al: Chordoma: Radiologic evaluation of 20 cases. AJR Am J Roentgenol 127:797–805, 1976

180. Fox JE, Batsakis JG, Owano LR: Unusual manifestations of chordoma. J Bone Joint Surg [Am] 50:1618–1628, 1968

181. Hagenlocher HU, Ciba K: The radiological aspects of cervical chordomas. Fortschr Geb Rontgenstr 125:228–232, 1976

182. Yuh WTC, Flickinger FW et al: MR imaging of unusual chordomas. J Comput Assist Tomogr 12:30–35, 1988

183. Stratt B, Steiner RM: The radiologic findings in posterior mediastinal chordoma. Skeletal Radiol 5:171–173, 1980

184. deBruine FT, Kroon HM: Spinal chordoma: Radiologic features in 14 cases. AJR Am J Roentgenol 150:861–863, 1988

185. Wang AM, Joachim CL, Shillito J et al: Cervical chordoma presenting with intervertebral foramen enlargement mimicking neurofibroma: CT findings. J Comput Assist Tomogr 8:529–535, 1984

186. Smith J, Ludwig RL et al: Sacrococcygeal chordoma. Skeletal Radiol 16:37–44, 1987

187. Rosenthal DI, Scott JA et al: Sacrococcygeal chordoma: Magnetic resonance imaging and computed tomography. AJR Am J Roentgenol 145:143–147, 1985

188. Sze G, Uichanco LS III et al: Chordomas: MR imaging. Radiology 166:187–191, 1988

189. Campanacci M, Baldini N et al: Giant-cell tumor of bone. J Bone Joint Surg 69:106–114, 1987

190. Dahlin DC: Giant cell tumor of bone: Highlights of 407 cases. AJR Am J Roentgenol 144:955–960, 1985

191. Jacobs P: The diagnosis of osteoclastoma (giant-cell tumour): A radiological and pathological correlation. Br J Radiol 45:121–136, 1972

192. McInerney DP, Middlemiss JH: Giant-cell tumor of bone. Skeletal Radiol 2:195–204, 1978

193. Mnaymneh WA, Dudley HR, Mnaymneh LG: Giant-cell tumor of bone: An analysis and follow-up study of the 41 cases observed at the Massachusetts General Hospital between 1925 and 1960. J Bone Joint Surg [Am] 46:63–75, 1964

194. Murray JA, Schlafly B: Giant-cell tumors in the distal end of the radius. J Bone Joint Surg 68:687–694, 1986

195. Wilkerson JA, Cracchiolo A: Giant-cell tumor of the tibial diaphysis. J Bone Joint Surg [Am] 51:1205–1209, 1969
196. Tubbs WS, Brown LR et al: Benign giant-cell tumor of bone with pulmonary metastases: Clinical findings and radiologic appearance of metastases in 13 cases. AJR Am J Roentgenol 158:331–334, 1992
197. Gould ES, Cooper JM et al: Case report 740. Skeletal Radiol 21:335–338, 1992
198. Hanna RM, Kyriakos M, Quinn SF: Case report 757. Skeletal Radiol 21:482–488, 1992
199. Mechlin MB, Kricun ME, Stead J et al: Giant cell tumor of tarsal bones. Skeletal Radiol 11:266–270, 1984
200. Shankman S, Greenspan A et al: Giant cell tumor of the ischium: A report of two cases and review of the literature. Skeletal Radiol 17:46–51, 1988
201. Peison B, Feigenbaum J: Metaphyseal giant-cell tumor in a girl of 14 years. Radiology 118:145–146, 1976
202. Sherman M, Fabricus R: Giant-cell tumor in the metaphysis of a child: Report of an unusual case. J Bone Joint Surg [Am] 43:1225–1229, 1961
203. Kransdorf MJ, Sweet DE et al: Giant cell tumor in skeletally immature patients. Radiology 184:233–237, 1992
204. Schutte HE, Taconis WK: Giant cell tumor in children and adolescents. Skeletal Radiol 22:173–176, 1993
205. Yao L, Mirra JM et al: Case report 715. Skeletal Radiol 21:124–127, 1992
206. Shaw JA, Mosher JF: A giant-cell tumor in the hand presenting as an expansile diaphyseal lesion. J Bone Joint Surg [Am] 65:692–695, 1983
207. deSantos LA, Murray JA: Evaluation of giant-cell tumor by computerized tomography. Skeletal Radiol 2:205–212, 1978
208. Brady TJ, Gebhardt MC, Pykett IL et al: NMR imaging of forearms in healthy volunteers and patients with giant-cell tumor of bone. Radiology 144:549–552, 1982
209. Herman SD, Mesgarzadeh M et al: The role of magnetic resonance imaging in giant cell tumor of bone. Skeletal Radiol 16:635–643, 1987
210. Hudson TM, Schiebler M, Springfield I et al: Radiology of giant cell tumors of bone: Computed tomography, arthrotomography, and scintigraphy. Skeletal Radiol 11:85–95, 1984
211. Levin E, DeSmet AA, Neff JR et al: Scintigraphic evaluation of giant cell tumor of bone. AJR Am J Roentgenol 143:343–348, 1984
212. Jernstrom P, Stark HH: Giant-cell reaction of a metacarpal. Am J Clin Pathol 55:77–81, 1971
213. Hermann G, Abdelwahab IF et al: Case report 603. Skeletal Radiol 19:367–369, 1990
214. Cooper KL, Beabout JW et al: Giant cell tumor: Ossification in soft-tissue implants. Radiology 153:597–602, 1984
215. Besemann EF, Perez MA: Malignant angioblastoma, so-called adamantinoma, involving the humerus: A case report. AJR Am J Roentgenol 100:538–541, 1967
216. Donner R, Dickland R: Adamantinoma of the tibia: A long-standing case with unusual histological features. J Bone Joint Surg [Br] 48:139–144, 1966
217. Bloem JL, van der Heul RO et al: Fibrous dysplasia vs adamantinoma of the tibia: Differentiation based on discriminant analysis of clinical and plain film findings. AJR Am J Roentgenol 156:1017–1023, 1991
218. Ishida T, Iijima T et al: A clinicopathological and immunohistochemical study of osteofibrous dysplasia, differentiated adamantinoma, and adamantinoma of long bones. Skeletal Radiol 21:493–502, 1992
219. Winter WG: Spontaneous pneumothorax heralding metastases of adamantinoma of the tibia: Report of 2 cases. J Bone Joint Surg [Am] 58:416–417, 1976
220. Bundens WD, Brighton CT: Malignant hemangioendothelioma of bone: Report of 2 cases and review of the literature. J Bone Joint Surg [Am] 47:762–772, 1965
221. Srinivasan CK et al: Malignant hemangioendothelioma of bone. J Bone Joint Surg [Am] 60:696–700, 1978
222. Sweterlitsch PR, Torg JS, Watts H: Malignant hemangioendothelioma of the cervical spine. J Bone Joint Surg [Am] 52:805–808, 1970
223. Jaffe JW, Mesgarzadeh M et al: Case report 519. Skeletal Radiol 18:50, 1989
224. Lye DJ, Wepfer JF, Haskell DS: Case report 458. Skeletal Radiol 17:57, 1988
225. Martinez-Tello FJ, Marcos-Robles J, Blanco-Lorenzo F: Case report 520. Skeletal Radiol 18:55, 1989
226. Abrahams TG, Bula W, Jones M: Epithelioid hemangioendothelioma of bone. Skeletal Radiol 21:509–513, 1992
227. Carmody E, Loftus B et al: Case report 759. Skeletal Radiol 21:538–541, 1992
228. Addison AK, Payne SR: Primary liposarcoma of bone. J Bone Joint Surg [Am] 64:301–304, 1982
229. Retz LD: Primary liposarcoma of bones: Report of a case and review of the literature. J Bone Joint Surg [Am] 43:123–129, 1961
230. Schwartz A, Shuster M, Becker SM: Liposarcoma of bone: Report of a case and review of the literature. J Bone Joint Surg [Am] 52:171–177, 1970
231. Downey EF, Worsham GF, Brower AC: Liposarcoma of bone with osteosarcomatous foci. Skeletal Radiol 8:47–50, 1982
232. Milgram JW: Malignant transformation in bone lipomas. Skeletal Radiol 19:347–352, 1990
233. Berlin O, Angervall B et al: Primary leiomyosarcoma of bone. Skeletal Radiol 16:364–376, 1987

Imaging of Bone Tumors: A Multimodality Approach,
edited by George B. Greenfield and John A. Arrington.
J. B. Lippincott Company, Philadelphia © 1995.

c h a p t e r

THREE

BENIGN BONE TUMORS

Differential Diagnosis of Benign Conditions of Bone
Imaging of Specific Benign Tumors and Related Conditions
Osteoma
Osteoid Osteoma
Osteoblastoma
Osteochondroma
Enchondroma
Juxtacortical Chondroma
Chondroblastoma
Chondromyxoid Fibroma
Nonossifying Fibroma
Fibrous Cortical Defect
Desmoplastic Fibroma
Periosteal Desmoid
Unicameral Bone Cyst
Aneurysmal Bone Cyst
Hemangioma
Massive Osteolysis
Stress Fractures
Rare Lesions

DIFFERENTIAL DIAGNOSIS OF BENIGN CONDITIONS OF BONE

Many imaging features that we associate with malignancy may be found in a benign lesion on conventional radiographs, computed tomography (CT), and magnetic resonance imaging (MRI). Equally dense bone production may be found in osteosarcoma, osteoid osteoma, Garré osteomyelitis, or a Charcot joint. Spiculated and laminated periosteal reaction atypically may be found in benign tumors, osteomyelitis, and healing fractures (Fig. 3-1). Malignant tumor spicules tend to be long, thin, and filiform, but benign spicules are short and squat (Fig. 3-2). A soft-tissue reaction and marrow edema may be associated with benign lesions such as osteoid osteoma, chondroblastoma, and eosinophilic granuloma.

Benign bone tumors most frequently occur in late childhood and adolescence. Exceptions are giant cell tumor, most often seen in patients between 20 and 40 years of age; enchondroma, which is almost evenly distributed in the 10- to 50-year range; and unicameral bone cyst, which has its greatest frequency in patients between 3 and 14 years of age. Benign bone tumors rarely occur in the elderly.

The most frequent site of involvement of these lesions is in the long bones, particularly in the metaphyses about the knee. A unicameral bone cyst does not tend to involve the knee, but instead affects the proximal humerus and proximal femur. Enchondroma has a predilection for the short tubular bones of the hands. The vertebrae are most frequently involved by an aneurysmal bone cyst or osteoblastoma. Osteoblastoma tends to involve the neural arch. Giant cell tumor of the spine is uncommon.

In the long bones, most lesions occur in the metaphysis, except giant cell tumor and benign chondroblastoma, which almost always involve the epiphysis. Giant cell tumor extends to the articular cortex, but chondroblastoma abuts or straddles the epiphyseal cartilage plate. Before epiphyseal fusion, a giant cell tumor involves the metaphysis in the rare instances in which it affects a younger-aged patient. An aneurysmal bone cyst also involves the epiphysis after fusion of the growth plate. A nonossifying fibroma typically is in the diametaphyseal region.

The lesion most characterized by a location off the central axis is aneurysmal bone cyst. Nonossifying fibroma, chondromyxoid fibroma, giant cell tumor, and osteoid osteoma usually have off-axis locations. A centrally located lesion is typically a unicameral bone cyst.

The benign lesions that often attain a larger size are aneurysmal bone cyst, unicameral bone cyst, fibrous dysplasia, and chondromyxoid fibroma. The lesions that are typically small are fibrous cortical defect, the nidus of osteoid osteoma, and enchondroma in the short tubular bones. Malignant bone tumors are usually larger than 6 cm when first seen by a physician.

Most of the these lesions are ovoid. The long axis of the tumor is parallel to the long axis of the bone. Giant cell tumor is typically round. A unicameral bone cyst has the shape of a truncated pyramid with its wide base abutting the physis. It usually does not expand the cortex beyond the width of the epiphyseal cartilage plate. The greatest expansion is produced by an aneurysmal bone cyst.

The margin of a benign tumor is usually well defined. Cartilaginous tumors are likely to have dense marginal sclerosis, which may extend some distance from the lesion. The most pronounced reactive sclerosis is caused by intracortical osteoid osteoma. The sclerosis may be severe enough to obscure the nidus, which itself shows various degrees of calcification. Sclerotic residuals occur in healed fibrous cortical defects and brown tumor of hyperparathyroidism.

The matrix in enchondroma and in about half of the cases of benign chondroblastoma shows a characteristic stippled, punctate, or streaky linear calcification, typifying cartilage. Most other benign tumors are radiolucent. Some may show light trabeculation, such as brown tumor of hyperparathyroidism. Lesions that may show heavier trabeculation are desmoplastic fibroma and chondromyxoid fibroma.

Periosteal reaction is sparse in benign neoplasms. Aneurysmal bone cyst may show solid periosteal elevation near the margin of the lesion, with a periosteal buttress. Chondroblastoma, eosinophilic granuloma, and osteoid osteoma may also show periosteal new

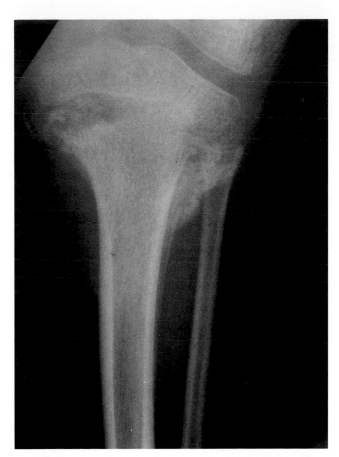

FIGURE 3-1. The anteroposterior view of the proximal tibia shows a healing metaphyseal fracture with laminated periosteal new bone formation laterally. No tumor is present.

bone. Thick, solid periosteal new bone in an untreated lesion suggests benignity, but this finding should be regarded with caution.

Some malignant tumors, such as a solitary myeloma, blow-out metastasis from kidney or thyroid carcinoma, and secondary chondrosarcoma within an enchondroma, may simulate a benign, expansile lesion and be misleading in making the differential diagnosis. MRI of some benign lesions may have a misleading aggressive appearance.[1] The greater sensitivity of MRI demonstrates features that are not seen on plain films or CT scans. These include inflammatory reactions caused by the lesion in adjacent bone marrow and soft tissues. Bone marrow edema and a soft-tissue mass showing low signal intensity on T1-weighted images with an increase in signal intensity on T2-weighted images, but without defined margins, may be seen, most often in children. These lesions include osteoid osteoma, chondroblastoma, eosinophilic granuloma, and stress fractures. Lesions containing dense fibrous tissue show low signal intensity on T1-weighted and T2-weighted spin echo images.

IMAGING OF SPECIFIC BENIGN TUMORS AND RELATED CONDITIONS

Osteoma

An osteoma is a benign tumor of bone tissue origin. It contains only dense compact bone, and a solitary osteoma develops in intramembranous bone. The most

FIGURE 3-2. Thyroid acropachy of the hands. Spiculated periosteal new bone formation is present bilaterally and symmetrically. The first and second radials show the most pronounced changes at the radial side, and the fifth radial shows the most pronounced changes at the ulnar side. Soft-tissue masses are associated with the periosteal new bone formation. The spicules are short and squat, characteristic of a benign spiculative process. (From Greenfield GB, Escamilla CH, Schorsch HA: The hand as an indicator of generalized disease. AJR Am J Roentgenol 99:736–745, 1967)

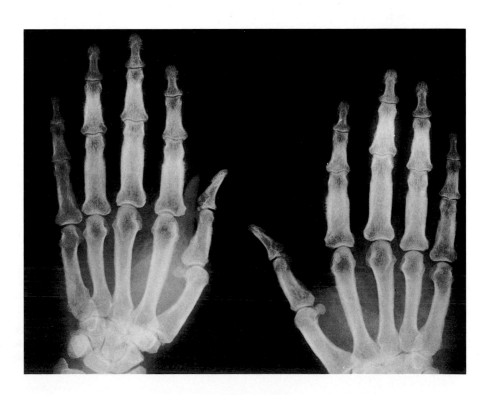

common sites of origin are the inner and outer tables of the skull, the paranasal sinuses, and the mandible, and rarely the nasal bones. The lesions are asymptomatic unless they block the ostia of the paranasal sinuses. They may cause mucoceles or involve the orbit or cranium.[2] Other reported complications include proptosis, reversible blindness,[3] and recurrent pyogenic meningitis due to frontal sinus osteomas.[4] Osteomas are often discovered in adulthood and show neither progression nor malignant change. Osteomas of the temporal bone, located in the internal acoustic meatus, middle ear, and on the posterior surface of the petrous ridge, have also been reported.[5]

Radiologically, the tumors are characterized by a dense radiopaque and structureless appearance. Round or ovoid and well-circumscribed, they rarely attain a size larger than 2 cm in diameter (Fig. 3-3), although a greater size is possible. If situated in a paranasal sinus, usually the frontal or ethmoid sinuses (Fig. 3-4) are involved. The tumor may cause expansion of the sinus walls. An osteoma-like bone response to tropical ulcer has been reported.[6] Osteomas of long and flat bones may rarely occur, in which case, they may be intraosseous, surface, or parosteal lesions. Some investigators postulate that these may represent hamartomas.

Gardner Syndrome

Gardner syndrome is a rare syndrome consisting of osteomas, soft-tissue tumors, and intestinal polyposis, chiefly of the colon.[7] It is transmitted in an autosomal dominant manner. The colonic polyps are premalignant, and a colonic carcinoma may be present at the time of diagnosis. Polyposis of the gastrointestinal tract may be present outside the colon, and adenocarcinoma

of the duodenum has been reported. The bone lesions may precede the intestinal polyposis. Multiple dense osteomas of various sizes, from slight focal cortical thickening to large masses, are distributed throughout the skeleton. The skull and mandible are characteristically show osteomas. The maxilla and hard palate may also be involved (Fig. 3-5). In the mandible, dense, protuberant, lobulated osteomas arise from the mandibular angle. Osteomas at the roots of the teeth and other dental abnormalities are seen. The tubular bones show localized or wavy cortical thickening and possibly exostoses or pedunculated osteoma-like lesions. The ribs and the pelvis may also have cortical thickening. Small, dense osteomas of the scaphoid may also occur.

Osteoid Osteoma

Osteoid osteoma is a common benign lesion of bone.[8–10] The lesion is 1 cm or smaller in diameter and is called the nidus. This nidus, initially uncalcified, later may develop calcification, which can range from minimal to complete. If located in the cortex, the lesion evokes a great deal of reactive sclerosis with cortical thickening, periosteal new bone, and a possible reactive soft-tissue mass. The degree of reactive new bone formation varies according to the location of the nidus. The nidus consists of osteoid within a highly vascular stroma with giant cells, and it is sharply demarcated from the surrounding reactive sclerosis.

The clinical hallmark of this lesion is local pain, which is worse at night and relieved by activity and aspirin. It has been shown that prostaglandins, which have been recovered in large amounts in this tumor,

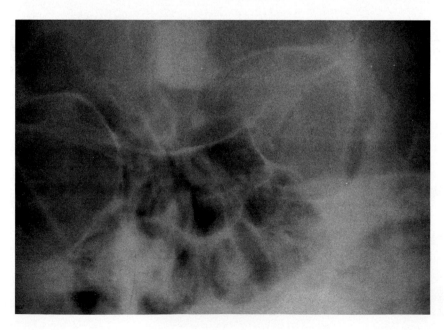

FIGURE 3-3. Osteoma of the frontal sinus. A dense, structureless, ossific mass is seen within the frontal sinus.

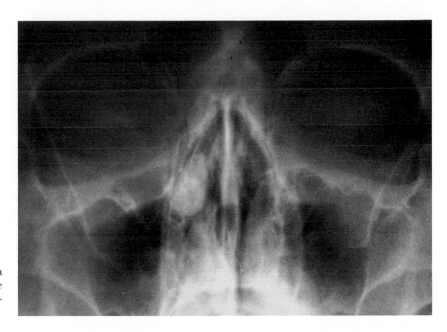

FIGURE 3-4. The Water view shows a dense, ovoid, structureless mass in the right ethmoid sinuses, indicating an osteoma.

are probably responsible for the pain. Prostaglandin inhibitors provide some relief.[11] The duration of symptoms before presentation usually ranges from 6 months to 2 years. The pain may be referred to a nearby joint, and it later increases in severity. Focal soft-tissue swelling, point tenderness, and limitation of motion also occur. Heat and erythema do not occur. If in the lower extremities, limp, weakness, muscle atrophy, and depressed deep tendon reflexes are seen. With spinal involvement, osteoid osteoma produces a painful, rigid scoliosis causing nerve irritation simulating a neurologic lesion.[12] Scoliosis and back pain may result from

osteoid osteoma of a rib.[13] Radicular pain and torticollis may occur in a cervical spinal location.[14] There are no systemic symptoms. Rarely, a lesion may not be painful.[15] In the capitate bone, the tumor has presented with symptoms of carpal tunnel syndrome.[16] In the elbow, it may present with osteosclerosis, joint effusion, and a periosteal reaction.[17] Leg-length discrepancy with tibial osteoid osteoma has been reported.[18] Joint pain occurs with a juxtaarticular lesion.[19–21] Osteoarthritis has developed in half of the patients with intraarticular hip lesions.[22]

Ninety percent of patients are seen before the age

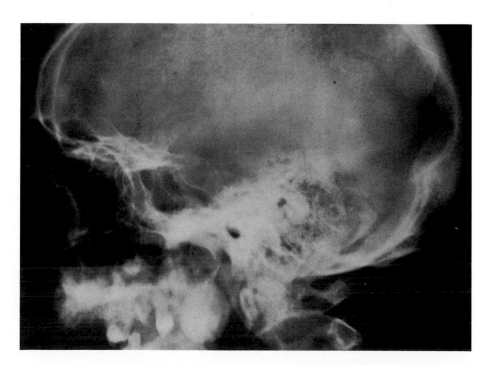

FIGURE 3-5. Gardner syndrome of the skull. There are multiple osteomas of the calvarium, maxilla, and hard palate. The patient had colonic polyposis, carcinoma of the sigmoid colon, and subcutaneous nodules.

of 25 years. The lesion is rare in patients younger than 2 years of age or older than 50 years of age, but it has been reported in the tibia of an 8-month-old boy.[23] The ratio of males to females is 2 to 1. One half of the lesions are in the femur and tibia. Other common sites are the fibula, humerus, and vertebral arch, but any bone may be involved, including the tarsals, metatarsals,[24] and skull.[25,26] The nidus may be intracortical, intramedullary, subperiosteal, or within a joint capsule. Double and triple nidi have been reported,[27–29] as have osteoid osteomas in adjacent bones.[30]

The typical imaging appearance is that of a small, radiolucent intracortical nidus less than 1 cm in diameter, surrounded by a large, dense, sclerotic zone of cortical thickening (Fig. 3-6), and there may be a solid or, rarely, a laminated or spiculated periosteal reaction. The dense sclerotic reaction may obscure the nidus on conventional films, and CT may be necessary for its demonstration. The nidus may be uncalcified, partially calcified, or have its center calcified, which presents

radiologically as a radiolucent halo within the sclerotic zone. The nidus is not always centrally located within the area of sclerosis but may be eccentrically placed or even at the edge. Synovitis may occur in an adjacent joint not involved by an intracapsular lesion.[31,32] An intramedullary nidus causes little bone sclerosis and may cause endosteal thickening.

A subperiosteal nidus is less common (Fig. 3-7). It presents as a small, radiolucent bulge of the contour of the bone. A thin margin and variable cortical thickening are seen.

A common location for an intramedullary osteoid osteoma is in the femoral neck, where it results in local osteoporosis and possible growth disturbances. Lymphofollicular synovitis and soft-tissue inflammation has been reported for intraarticular osteoid osteoma.[31,32] The findings include uniform narrowing of the joint space and subperiosteal bone formation involving the affected bone and adjacent bones.[20]

In the spine, it is the neural arch that is usually affected by osteoid osteoma. With lamina involvement, there may be enlargement of the adjacent transverse process. The appearance is similar to that seen in other bones involved with osteoid osteoma. In one series of spinal osteoid osteomas, conventional radiographs

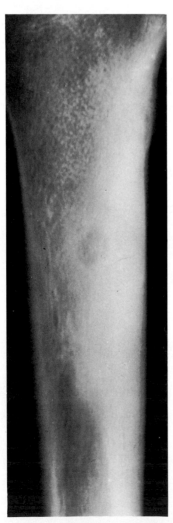

FIGURE 3-6. Osteoid osteoma of the femur. There is dense cortical thickening with a radiolucent nidus.

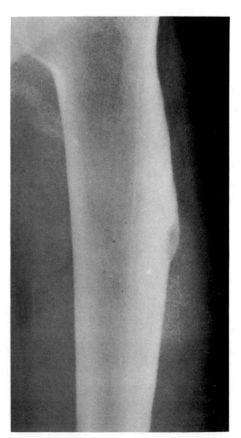

FIGURE 3-7. Subperiosteal osteoid osteoma. There is bulging of the periosteum by the nidus and cortical thickening.

were normal for all patients. Bone scans were positive and useful in localizing the lesion and directing CT to the appropriate level. In all cases, CT accurately demonstrated the location, nidus, and other diagnostic radiographic features of osteoid osteoma.[33]

The lesion may often be seen well only on CT scans, which are particularly valuable in diagnosing osteoid osteoma of the femoral neck (Fig. 3-8). The nidus

is usually readily identified unless it is completely calcified. Rarely, a spiculated periosteal pattern may be seen on CT. Deformity of the femoral neck with widening and shortening and with flattening of the femoral capital epiphysis may occur if the diagnosis of an intracapsular lesion is delayed.[34]

Radioscintigraphy is of particular value for osteoid osteomas in the spine, joints, and small bones of the

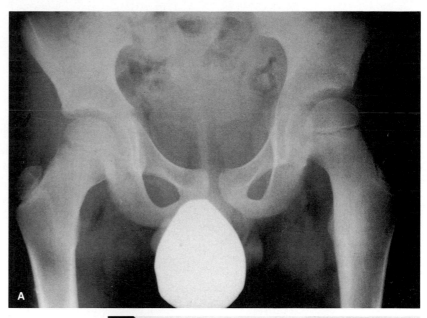

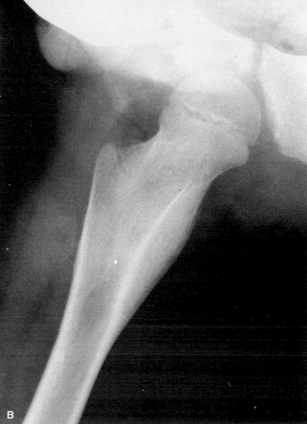

FIGURE 3-8. Osteoid osteoma involving the left proximal femur in an 8-year-old girl.
(**A**) The anteroposterior view of the pelvis shows marked cortical thickening medially. This is centered at the level of the lesser trochanter. (**B**) A lateral view of the left proximal femur shows marked cortical thickening and layered periosteal new bone formation blending with the cortex. (**C**) The CT examination shows the nidus within an area of cortical thickening medially. The CT scan at a higher level shows cortical thickening with spiculated periosteal new bone formation anteriorly. (**D**) The radionuclide bone scan shows increased activity in the left hip and proximal femur to the subtrochanteric region.   *continued*

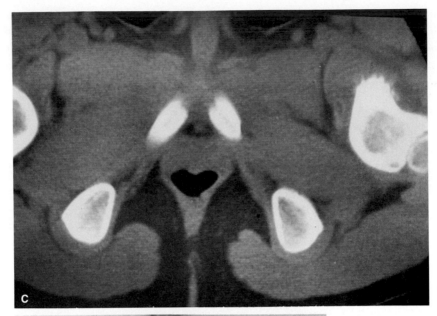

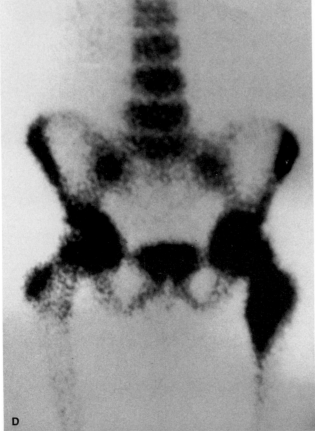

FIGURE 3-8. *(Continued)*

foot. On the triple-phase flow scan, an osteoid osteoma produces a discretely localized blush.[35] A characteristic pattern of uptake of this lesion is called the "double-density" sign.[36] A smaller, more intense focus of activity is superimposed on a lesser increase in activity of a larger area of bone (Fig. 3-9). A bone scan is particularly helpful in assessing intracapsular osteoid osteomas of the femoral neck, because it can provide guidance for CT planning.

The radionuclide scan is also useful in the operative management of the patient. The specimen can be evaluated by autoradiography to determine whether the nidus has been removed.[11,37]

MRI demonstrates abnormalities in all cases of osteoid osteoma. The nidus may not be identified[38] or may show signal intensity characteristics from low to intermediate on all pulse sequences. Mild to inhomogenous enhancement after gadolinium infusion may oc-

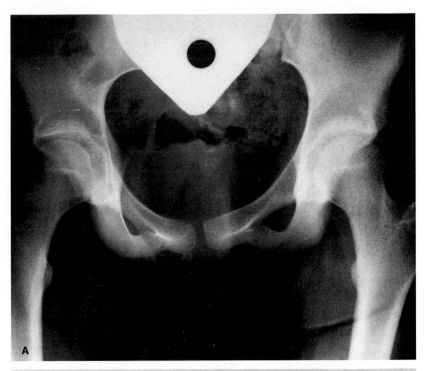

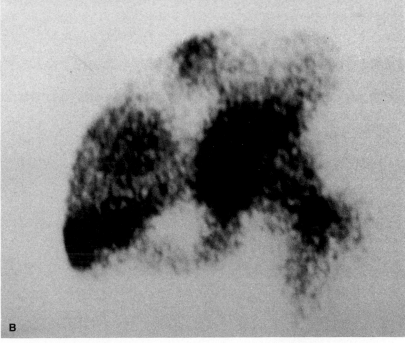

FIGURE 3-9. Osteoid osteoma of the left proximal femur in a 14-year-old girl. (**A**) The anteroposterior view of the pelvis shows local osteoporosis of the left femoral head, neck, and trochanters. (**B**) A radionuclide bone scan shows increased activity in the left hip, femoral neck, and intertrochanteric region. Superimposed on this diffuse increased activity is a small focus of greater activity at the base of the femoral neck. (**C**) The tomogram shows the nidus of the osteoid osteoma at the base of the femoral neck. *continued*

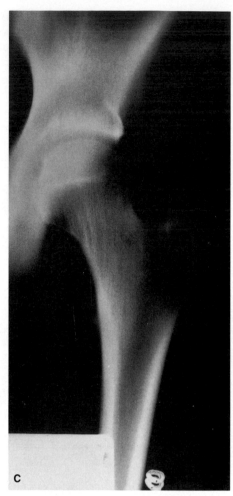

FIGURE 3-9. *(Continued)*

cur in the nidus, and the adjacent bone marrow may be enhanced. This area also shows low signal intensity on T1-weighted images, which increases on T2-weighted images. A thickened cortex is seen as a signal void. Peritumoral edema and a reactive soft-tissue mass adjacent to the nidus also occurs. This is fairly well defined but varies in size. It may have inhomogeneous low to high signal intensity on T1-weighted images and increased signal intensity on T2-weighted images (Fig. 3-10).[39,40]

Angiographically, osteoid osteomas are hypervascular, with an intense, uniform vascular stain located only in the nidus. The feeding vessels to the nidus arise from surrounding soft tissues and completely opacify it. They are best seen on subtraction films. Tumor stain usually persists late into the venous phase.[41]

The differential diagnosis includes an intracortical abscess, which may present a similar imaging appearance. Enhancement on postinfusion CT of the nidus correlating with the histologic vascular stroma in osteoid osteoma can aid in the differentiation. A necrotic abscess cavity demonstrates no such finding. If the ni-

dus is not seen, differentiation from osteosarcoma must be made.

If an osteoid osteoma is incompletely excised, it may recur as an osteoblastoma.[42]

Osteoblastoma

Osteoblastoma (i.e., benign osteoblastoma, giant osteoid osteoma) is a rare benign bone tumor.[12,43–48] It is similar to osteoid osteoma in microscopic appearance, characterized by osteoblasts and giant cells in a vascular connective tissue stroma. The peak incidence is among patients between 7 and 20 years of age, with a range of 3 to 78 years. Males are more frequently affected. Pain, not as severe as in osteoid osteoma, and a palpable mass may develop along with local tenderness. With spinal involvement, neurologic symptoms and scoliosis may occur.[49] Some tumors may be quite aggressive.

Approximately half of the patients with osteoblastoma have vertebral involvement, most commonly in the the transverse and spinous processes (Fig. 3-11), but the vertebral bodies may also be affected. Atlas involvement has been reported.[50] Two adjacent vertebrae may be involved. The tubular bones of the hands and feet,[51,52] the femur and tibia, and the calvarium are other possible sites. The calvarium may have an appearance of button sequestra. The other long bones, scapula, ribs, sacrum, carpals, tarsals,[53] patella, maxilla, mandible, and pelvis may occasionally be involved. In the tubular bones, the lesions are located in the metaphysis or shaft, without epiphyseal involvement. An expansile, well-circumscribed lesion is typical (Fig. 3-12). The lesion may be surrounded by thick periosteal reaction or a thin, fine margin. There may be cortical breakthrough with a soft-tissue component. The matrix may be radiolucent, contain spotty calcific areas, or be radiopaque because of extensive calcification. The tumor is usually 2 to 12 cm in diameter. Rapid growth and pathologic fracture may occur. The margin is usually well defined but can be poorly defined. There may be dense, reactive bone sclerosis, almost the same as that seen in osteoid osteoma. Periosteal new bone formation may be present. A small bone may be involved, with reactive sclerosis and periosteal new bone formation which, is difficult to differentiate from an osteosarcoma.

MRI may reveal a diffuse, reactive, inflammatory infiltrate in vertebrae adjacent to the lesion, nearby ribs, or paraspinal soft tissues. This pattern is called the flare phenomenon.[54]

Malignant change occurs in very few cases.[46] Unusual cases of osteoblastoma with aggressive features

(text continues on page 180)

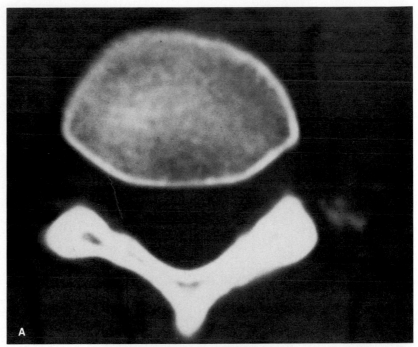

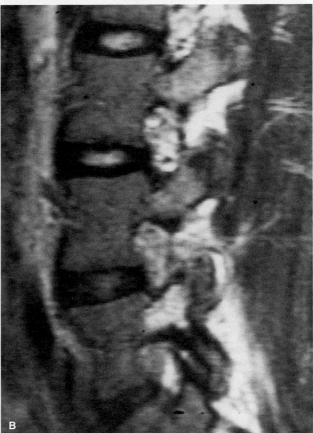

FIGURE 3-10.   Osteoid osteoma in an 18-year-old man involving the left side of the neural arch of L5. (**A**) A CT scan shows cortical thickening and sclerosis of the left pedicle. (**B**) The sagittal MR (SE 4000/96) image shows high signal intensity in the left pedicle of L5. (**C**) MRI (SE 800/15). The axial section shows cortical thickening corresponding to that seen on the CT scan of the left lamina. The soft-tissue fat planes are obliterated on the left side but not on the right. (**D**) MRI (SE 2000/80). The soft tissues adjacent to the left lamina show an increase in signal intensity. The well-circumscribed appearance somewhat suggests a mass. This represents soft-tissue reaction. No tumor or organism was found in the soft tissues on biopsy. (**E**) The CT scan shows a nidus at the junction of the left lamina and pedicle.   *continued*

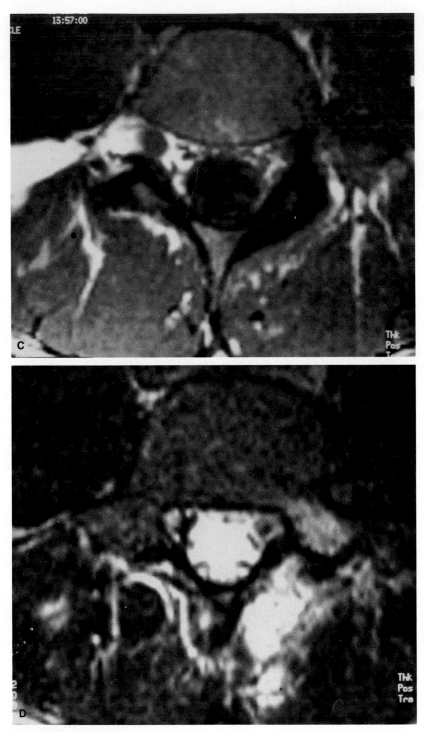

FIGURE 3-10. *(Continued)*

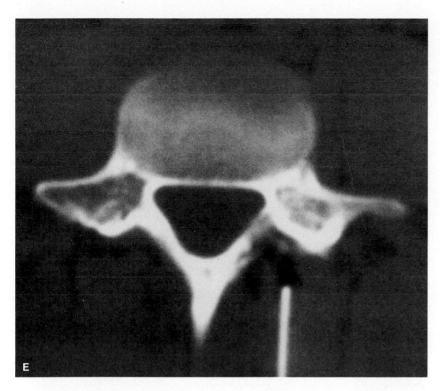

FIGURE 3-10. *(Continued)*

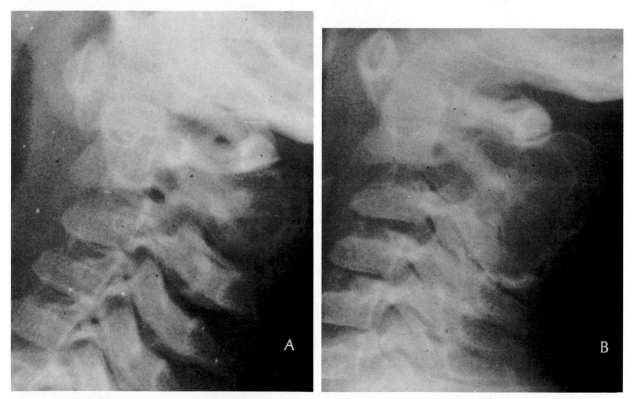

FIGURE 3-11. Benign osteoblastoma of the cervical spine. (**A**) Well-circumscribed, expansile lesion situated between the spinous processes of the second and third cervical vertebrae. The bony margin is intact. Some calcification of the matrix is present. (**B**) Nine months after **A**, there has been progressive growth of the lesion, with involvement of the spinous processes of C2 and C3. The cortical shell of the lesion remains intact. (Courtesy of Dr. Harvey White, Children's Memorial Hospital, Chicago, IL.)

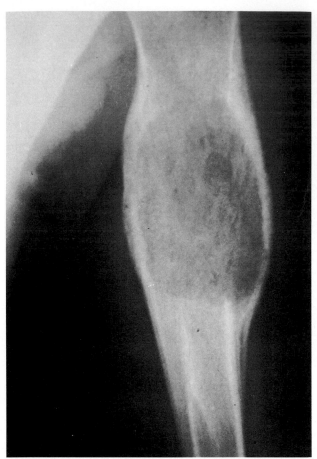

FIGURE 3-12. Benign osteoblastoma of the humerus. Notice the expansile lesion with a thick cortical shell in the proximal humeral diaphysis. Extensive ossification of the matrix is evident. A minimal amount of periosteal new bone formation, which has a laminated appearance, can be seen at the distal aspect of the lesion, forming a buttress. There is no periosteal new bone formation around the periphery of the lesion. (Courtesy of Dr. Harvey White, Children's Memorial Hospital, Chicago, IL.)

Osteochondroma

Solitary osteochondroma (i.e., solitary osteochondroma, osteocartilaginous exostosis) is a bony projection with a cartilaginous cap. It usually forms at the metaphysis of a tubular bone. This is the most common benign skeletal growth. The mechanism of formation is similar to that in hereditary multiple exostoses.

Not all exostoses are osteochondromas. Several different entities may have a similar appearance. A supracondylar process is a small bony spur projected mediodistally at the distal humerus 5 to 7 cm above the medial epicondyle and joined to it by a band of fibrous tissue forming an arch (Fig. 3-13).[57] It is an atavism to the lemur, and has been erroneously termed a "seal

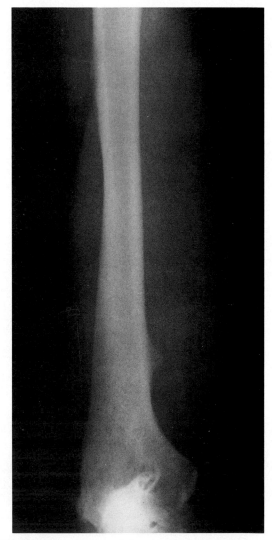

FIGURE 3-13. Supracondylar process. A bony spur projects medially 6 cm above the medial epicondyle of the humerus. It has a triangular configuration, and the cortex is distinct from the spur.

have been reported.[55] Aggressive osteoblastoma is characterized by pain, rapid growth, and a high recurrence rate. Distant metastases occurred in one patient after curettage, radiation therapy, and chemotherapy. A malignant variant has been documented.[56] Angiographically, the lesion is moderately vascular, with no evidence of invasion of vessels nor of large obstructed veins.

In the differential diagnosis, the chief problem is identifying the ossifying character of the lesion. Differentiation from cartilaginous tumors can be made by the lack of cartilage calcification patterns. Differentiation from giant cell tumor can be made by the nonepiphyseal location and matrix calcification of osteoblastoma.

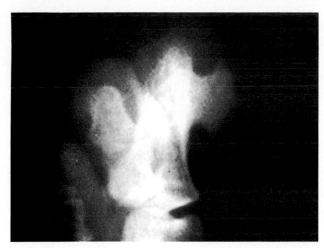

FIGURE 3-14.   Subungual exostosis of the distal phalanx of the great toe. Notice the bony protrusion at the dorsal aspect of the distal phalanx. The cortex of the toe does not blend with the lesion.

bone." The median nerve and the brachial artery pass through the formed arch, and a fracture of this spur may result in compression of the median nerve.[58]

A subungual exostosis is a painful bony spur under a fingernail or toenail (Fig. 3-14).[59] Some bone protrusions originate as myositis ossificans or as ossification within a soft tissue lipoma, and they subsequently

blend with bone (Fig. 3-15). An exostosis may follow irradiation[60] or trauma (Fig. 3-16). Enchondroma protuberans of a rib may resemble an osteochondroma.[61] A transitory exostosis at the medial tibial metaphysis may rarely be seen in children which later regresses.[62] Advanced Blount disease may simulate an osteochondroma (Fig. 3-17). An intracapsular osteochondroma arising from the epiphyseal articular surface represents Trevor disease, also called dysplasia epiphysialis hemimelica (Fig. 3-18).

A true osteochondroma has a cartilaginous cap. The cortex is continuous with the cortex of the parent bone, as is the periosteum. Growth of the osteochondroma continues during the active growth period and stops at maturity. The lesion may attain a very large size. Most patients are 10 to 20 years of age at the time of discovery of the lesion. The most frequent finding is a painless mass, but symptoms may be produced by pressure on contiguous vessels and nerves. Complications include pain[63] and unilateral leg edema.[64] A pseudoaneurysm of the popliteal artery resulting from transection by an osteochondroma has been reported.[65] Trauma may result in a fracture of the pedicle.

Malignant change to chondrosarcoma probably occurs in fewer than 1% of patients with osteochondroma, and this usually occurs in later life. Cases of development of osteosarcoma and fibrosarcoma have also been

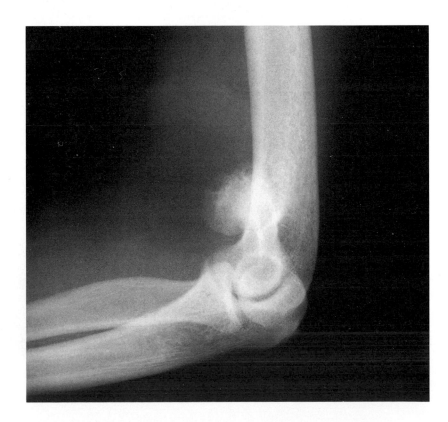

FIGURE 3-15.   Lipoma of the antecubital region, showing an ossific mass in the soft tissues that has blended with the distal humerus. The cortex of the humerus is distinct from the bony mass.

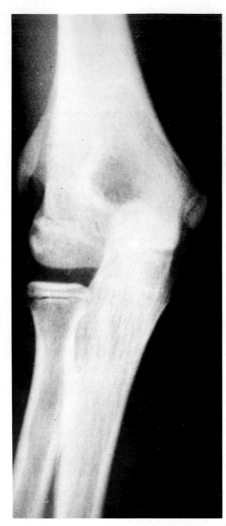

FIGURE 3-16. Posttraumatic exostosis of the distal humerus.

row base (Fig. 3-19). The direction of this type is away from the adjacent joint because of muscle pull, inspiring the common term "coat-hanger exostosis." If visualized en face, a dense ring of cortex surrounding the base is seen superimposed on the cartilage cap. This should be differentiated from an enchondroma. The sessile form is broad-based without an elongated projection, forming a local widening of the shaft of the bone (Fig. 3-20). The radiologic hallmark of both types is the continuity of the cortex of the osteochondroma with the cortex of normal bone. The cap shows irregularity, and the cartilage may calcify extensively, with an amorphous spotty appearance. Undertubulation of the metaphysis may occur. A giant osteochondroma may occasionally be seen.

The most common appearance in flat bones is a dense, localized area of amorphous calcification. The attachment to bone may not be apparent. On plain films, in the pelvis this form may be confused with a

reported.[66] The rapid growth of a prior stable lesion indicates malignant change. A case of spontaneous resolution of a sessile osteochondroma in the midhumeral shaft has been reported.[67] An osteochondroma can regress if the lesion becomes incorporated into the growing bony metaphysis.[68]

The common sites for osteochondroma are the lower femur and the upper tibia, at or near the metaphyses. Rarely, the lesions may be situated away from the metaphysis. Most solitary osteochondromas occur in the long bones, with more than half in the lower extremities. Bone preformed in cartilage also may be involved. The scapula, pelvis, ribs, vertebrae,[69] and sacrum are less common sites.

There are four distinct forms of osteochondroma: pedunculated, sessile, calcific, and giant. The pedunculated form is an osteocartilaginous cap on a long, nar-

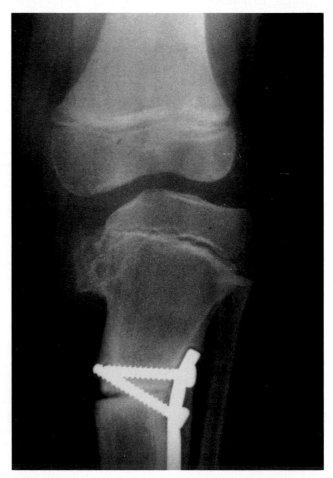

FIGURE 3-17. Blount disease produces widening and irregularity of the medial tibial metaphysis, simulating an osteochondroma. An osteotomy is apparent in this radiograph.

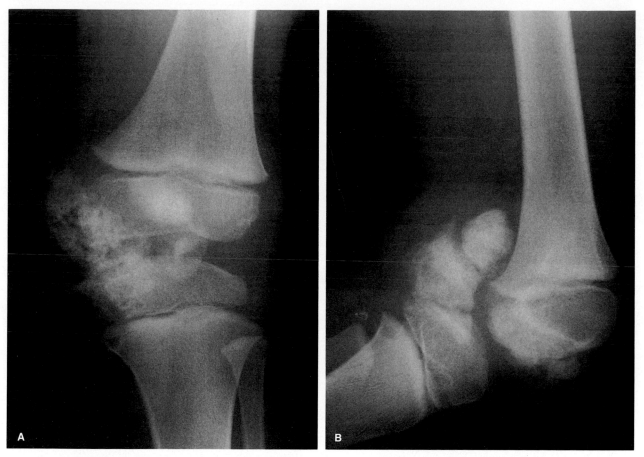

FIGURE 3-18. Dysplasia epiphysealis hemimelica, or Trevor disease, in a 4-year-old boy. (**A**) The anteroposterior view of the knee shows a calcific mass originating from the proximal tibial epiphysis and extending medially. (**B**) The lateral view of the left knee shows the mass situated posteriorly, originating from the posterior aspect of the proximal tibial epiphysis. A second calcification originates from the distal femoral epiphysis.

calcified uterine fibroid (Fig. 3-21). Conversely, a mesenteric calcification may simulate an osteochondroma on frontal view (Fig. 3-22). This form may also resemble thyroid calcification when situated at the thoracic inlet (Fig. 3-23).

MRI can demonstrate anatomic relations and assess the thickness of the cartilaginous cap.[70] The cap shows a high signal intensity on T2-weighted images and is best evaluated with GRE techniques. A band of low signal intensity covers the cap and represents the perichondrium (Fig. 3-24). The cortex of the osteochondroma is continuous with the cortex of the parent bone. The marrow signal within the osteochondroma is the same as that of of the parent bone (Fig. 3-25). A radionuclide bone scan shows increased uptake of isotope in a benign osteochondroma (Fig. 3-26). An osteochondroma may develop in children after radiation therapy with a dosage in a range starting at 1300 cGy to an epiphyseal growth zone.[71]

Malignant transformation may be suspected if growth takes place in a previously stable lesion. Extensive calcification may be present in a benign lesion, but a large associated soft-tissue mass that contains streaky calcification should be suspected of being malignant. A soft-tissue mass with a thickness greater than 2 cm on CT or MRI scans should arouse suspicion of a malignancy, but a thickened bursal sac may form around the osteochondroma, simulating malignant change.[72]

Invasion and destruction of the base of the osteochondroma are definitive signs of chondrosarcomatous change.

Hereditary Multiple Exostoses

Hereditary multiple exostoses (i.e., diaphyseal aclasia) is a disorder characterized by multiple osteochondromas, principally at the metaphyses.[73] There are

(text continues on page 186)

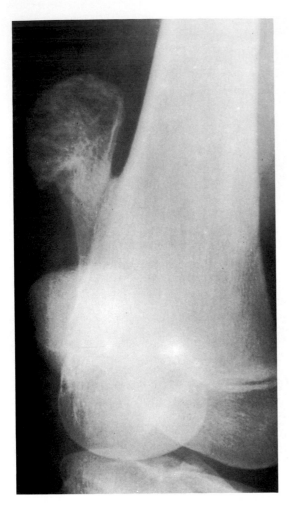

FIGURE 3-19. Pedunculated form of solitary osteochondroma of the distal femur. There is a narrow base, with blending of the cortex of the parent bone with the lesion. A calcified cartilaginous cap containing several streaks of calcification is visible. The orientation of the lesion is away from the joint because of muscle pull—hence the term "coat-hanger exostosis."

FIGURE 3-20. Osteochondroma of the humerus involving the metaphysis and proximal shaft. This is the broad-based sessile type and is quite large; it is called a giant osteochondroma. The bone is widened, and the cortex of bone is continuous with the osteochondroma. A densely calcified cartilaginous cap is seen, but there is no evidence of malignant change.

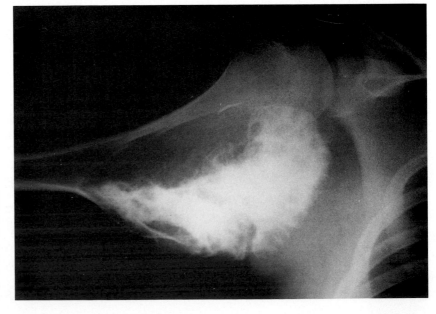

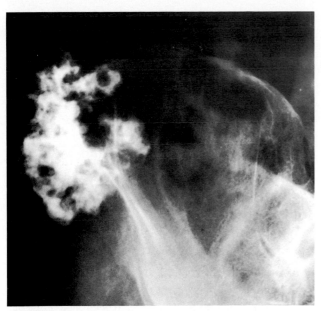

FIGURE 3-21. Calcified-type osteochondroma of the iliac crest. An amorphous area of spotty calcification can be seen at the iliac crest. The precise site of attachment to the iliac bone cannot be discerned.

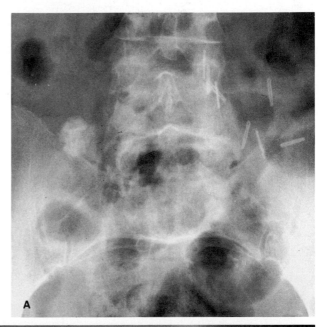

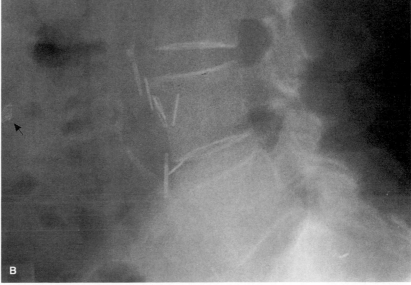

FIGURE 3-22. Mesenteric calcification simulating an osteochondroma. (**A**) The anteroposterior view of the sacroiliac region shows an amorphous, calcific density projected at the right sacral wing. This closely resembles the cartilaginous cap of an osteochondroma. (**B**) The lateral view shows that calcification is in the mid-abdomen.

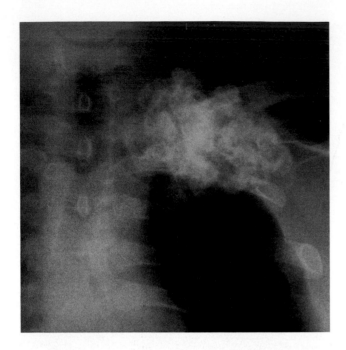

FIGURE 3-23. An amorphous, lobulated, calcific mass originating from the scapula is projected over the left thoracic inlet. This represents the calcific type of osteochondroma.

defects found in the juxtaepiphyseal regions of the periosteal ring along with disturbed function of the periosteum in forming small islets of cartilage. These factors allow enchondral bone growth perpendicular to the shaft. These exostoses are similar to solitary osteochondroma. Physial dysplasia has also been implicated.[73a]

This is a relatively common condition, which is most often discovered in patients between the ages of 2 and 10 years. Males are affected twice as often as females. The mode of inheritance may be a mendelian dominant pattern. Hard, painless masses near joints, which form and enlarge only during the growth period, and deformities with bone shortening and curvature occur. The distribution is usually bilateral and symmetric, but there may be a unilateral predilection in some cases. About one third of patients show a characteristic "bayonet hand" deformity due to shortening of the ulna and an ulnar tilt of the radius (Fig. 3-27).[74] Asymmetric shortening of the lower extremities results in compensatory scoliosis. The exostoses interfere with joint function. Symptoms from pressure on vessels, nerves, and the spinal cord may develop.[75] Bursae form at the cartilaginous margins and may lead to inflammatory changes. Perforation of the popliteal artery with false aneurysm formation in the popliteal fossa has been reported.[76] Perforation of the lung has also been reported.[77]

The lesions range in number from a few to a thousand, which in the long bones are clustered around the metaphyseal region. There is interference with bone remodeling leading to undertubulation, which gives the alternate name for this condition of diaphyseal aclasia. Epiphyseal exostoses do not represent this entity, but instead are signs of Trevor disease (i.e., dysplasia epiphysealis hemimelica; see Fig. 3-18).

The long bones are the most common sites of involvement, particularly in the lower extremities, where the knees are most severely affected (Fig. 3-28). In the lower extremities, all ends of bones show lesions, but in the upper extremities, the elbow tends to be spared of exostoses but may show dislocation of the radial head. There is shortening of the ulna and of the fibula. Ulnar shortening causes curvature of the radius and a false articulation between the two. There may be ulnar deviation of the carpus and subluxation of the radius resulting in bayonet-hand deformity (see Fig. 3-27).

A large exostosis causes pressure erosion or deformity of the adjacent bone (Fig. 3-29). There may be interlocking exostoses or synostoses in these bones. Shortening or deformity of the metacarpals and phalanges occurs. The base of the skull may be involved, but the calvarium and mandible are spared. The scapula is frequently involved at the vertebral margin and inferior angle (Fig. 3-30). Pelvic lesions occur at the iliac crest and the ischiopubic synchondroses. The ribs are involved most frequently at the costochondral junctions. The sternum and clavicles also may show lesions. The vertebrae are rarely involved but may have lesions of the spinous processes. The os calcis may be in-

(*text continues on page 191*)

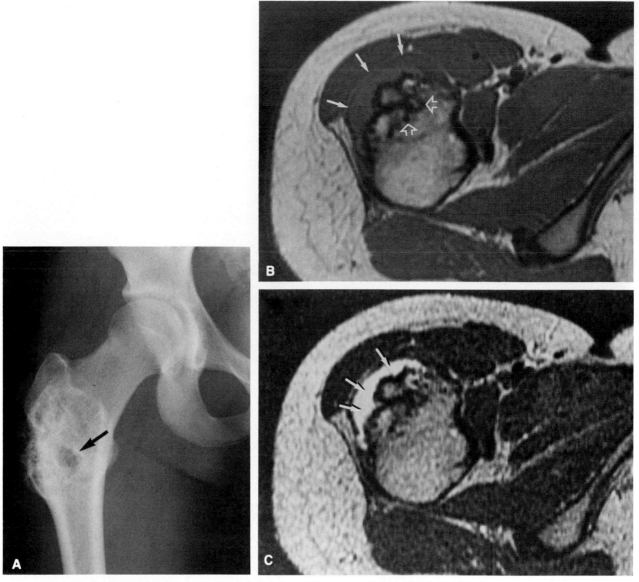

FIGURE 3-24. Osteochondroma in a 19-year-old woman. (**A**) Radiograph of right proximal femur shows anteriorly protruding osteochondroma containing irregular areas of mineralization and a poorly defined external margin. Radiolucency is seen in the subtrochanteric region of the proximal femur (*arrow*), suggesting malignant degeneration. Subsequent histologic examination showed this to represent an area of nonossified cartilage. (**B**) In a transaxial MR image (TR = 1200 msec, TE = 20 msec), the intact perichondrium is seen as a low-signal-intensity area (*arrows*). Irregular areas of signal absence in the base of the lesion are consistent with extensive matrix mineralization (*open arrows*). (**C**) T2-weighted transaxial MR image (TR = 1200 msec, TE = 75 msec). Exostotic cartilage cap is seen as an area of high signal intensity (*arrows*). (From Lee JK, Yao L, Wirth CR: MR imaging of solitary osteochondromas: Report of eight cases. AJR Am J Roentgenol 149:557–560, 1987)

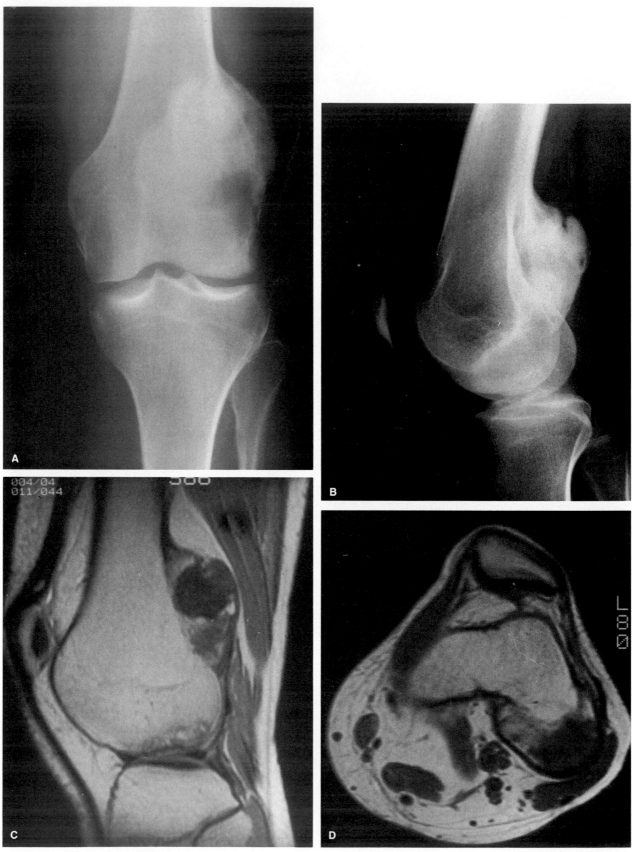

FIGURE 3-25.

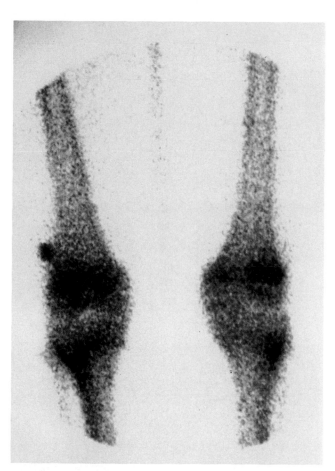

FIGURE 3-26. A radionuclide bone scan of a 16-year-old girl with an osteochondroma of the right distal femoral metaphysis. A focus of increased uptake is adjacent to the bone.

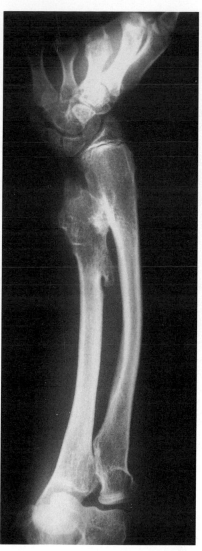

FIGURE 3-27. Multiple osteochondromatosis. The anteroposterior view of the forearm reveals shortening of the ulna with osteochondromas at the distal aspect and a coat-hanger exostosis. There is curvature of the radius. A false articulation between the radius and the distal ulna is seen, and there is an ulnar shift of the carpus. The radial epiphyseal ossification center is deficient at its ulnar aspect.

◀ **FIGURE 3-25.** Densely calcified sessile-type osteochondroma involves the posterior distal femoral metaphysis. (**A**) The anteroposterior view of the knee reveals a densely calcified mass projecting over the lateral aspect of the distal femoral metaphysis. (**B**) The lateral view of the knee reveals a densely calcified mass at the posterior distal tibial metaphysis. (**C**) The sagittal MR (SE 2700/20) section reveals a lesion posteriorly. The cortex of bone is continuous with the cortex of the lesion. The marrow signal surrounding the calcific signal void is the same as that of normal marrow in the shaft. (**D**) The axial MR (SE 2700/20) section shows the cortex of bone to be continuous with the cortex of the lesion. The densely calcified cartilaginous portion is seen as a signal void. The marrow signal within the lesion is the same as the marrow signal within the bone. These findings prove that this represents an osteochondroma rather than a parosteal sarcoma.

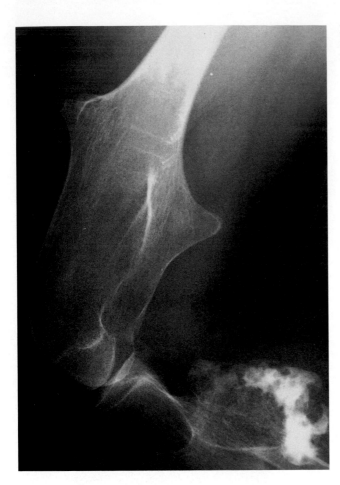

FIGURE 3-28. The lateral view of the knee shows sites of multiple osteochondromatosis. A partially calcified cartilaginous cap at the osteochondroma of the fibula is seen.

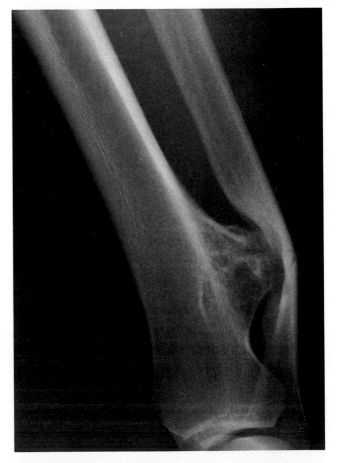

FIGURE 3-29. Osteochondroma of the distal tibia, which has deformed and eroded the fibula. The fracture line in the fibula is traumatic.

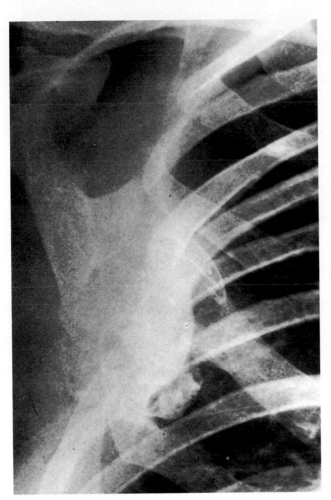

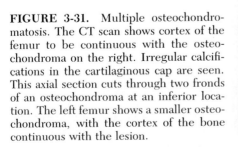

FIGURE 3-30. Multiple exostoses. There are deformities of several ribs due to a large osteochondroma with an area of calcification and an osteochondroma involving the axillary margin of the scapula.

volved, but other small bones are usually spared. A bursa occasionally forms around an exostosis, and this may rarely contain calcific loose bodies or may be inflamed.[78]

CT shows the cortex of the parent bone to be continuous with the lesion and shows a cartilaginous cap with punctate and linear calcifications (Fig. 3-31). MRI shows the same changes as in a solitary osteochondroma (Fig. 3-32), with the cortex of the lesion being continuous with the cortex of bone and the marrow signal of the lesion appearing the same as the marrow signal of the parent bone. Various degrees of signal void and low signal intensity reflect cartilage calcification and bony sclerosis. The radionuclide bone scan shows increased uptake in the cartilage (Fig. 3-33). In the event of sarcomatous change, the imaging appearance is the same as that of a secondary chondrosarcoma in a solitary exostosis, with rapid enlargement, destruction of the bony base, and wildly irregular calcification. Osteochondromatosis and enchondromatosis rarely coexist.

Dysplasia Epiphysealis Hemimelica

Dysplasia epiphysealis hemimelica (i.e., Trevor disease) is a rare, unilateral, asymmetric growth of the epiphyses resulting in swelling, deformities, and functional impairment of the involved joints. The knees and ankles are most commonly involved. The findings are limitation of motion, knock knees, bowed legs, and flat feet.

Radiologically, the lesion is limited to one half of the epiphysis. There may be irregular cartilage overgrowth or an epiphyseal osteocartilaginous exostosis

FIGURE 3-31. Multiple osteochondromatosis. The CT scan shows cortex of the femur to be continuous with the osteochondroma on the right. Irregular calcifications in the cartilaginous cap are seen. This axial section cuts through two fronds of an osteochondroma at an inferior location. The left femur shows a smaller osteochondroma, with the cortex of the bone continuous with the lesion.

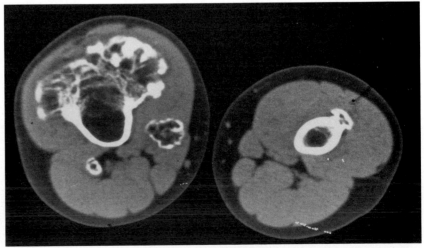

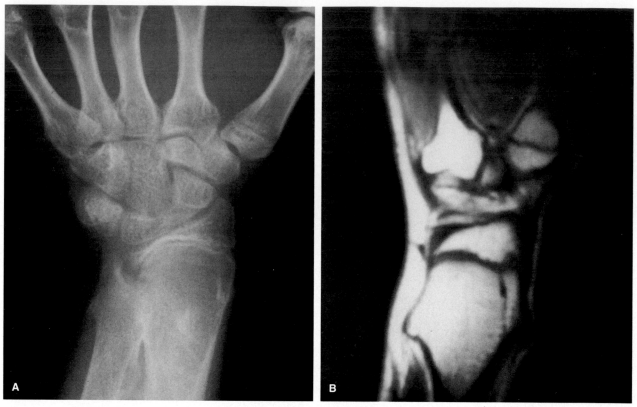

FIGURE 3-32. Multiple osteochondromatosis. (**A**) An anteroposterior view of the right wrist shows multiple osteochondromas involving the distal radius and ulna. (**B**) The coronal MR (SE 800/20) section of the right radius shows an osteochondroma with the cortex of bone continuous with the cortex of the lesion and the marrow signal within the lesion the same as the marrow signal within the bone.

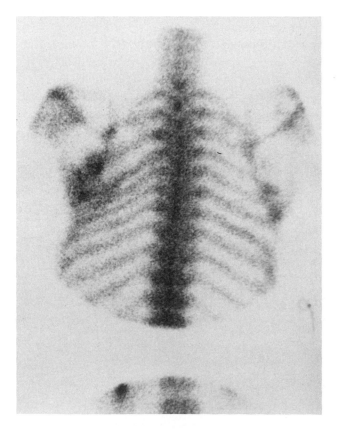

FIGURE 3-33. The radionuclide scan shows osteochondromas of both scapulae and bilateral increased activity in both scapular regions.

(see Fig. 3-18). The affected limb may be longer or shorter than normal and have a varus or valgus deformity. The most frequent sites of involvement are the talus, the distal femur, and the distal tibia. This condition rarely may be associated with various cartilaginous tumors, including intracapsular chondroma, extraskeletal osteochondroma, and typical osteochondroma.

Enchondroma

Solitary Enchondroma

A solitary enchondroma is a benign tumor of cartilage located within the medullary cavity.[8] It originates from a cartilage rest displaced from the epiphyseal plate.

Microscopically, the cellularity varies but does not approach that of a chondrosarcoma, although differentiation can be difficult at times. The cartilage cells are regularly small and uninuclear. The major tissue is mature hyaline cartilage. Lesions centrally located in the skeleton have more malignant potential than those in the periphery.

Enchondroma is a common tumor. The incidence is greatest between the second and fifth decades of life. Men and women are equally affected. The lesions are usually asymptomatic in the short tubular bones and are discovered as incidental findings or after a pathologic fracture occurs. If a long bone is involved, pain or pathologic fracture may be the presenting complaint.

The short tubular bones of the hand are affected in half of these patients; solitary enchondroma is the most common tumor of the bones of the hand. The humerus, femur, toes, metatarsals, tibia, fibula, and ulna are not uncommon sites, and any bone preformed in cartilage may be involved. Rarely, the ribs, sternum, pelvis, patella,[79] carpal bones,[80] and vertebrae may be affected.

The origin of the tumor in a tubular bone is usually the metaphysis, with apparent migration down the shaft. It may extend into the epiphysis after fusion of the growth plate. The epiphysis is not involved before epiphyseal closure. The lesion usually involves the middle and distal aspects of the metacarpals and the proximal aspects of the phalanges (Fig. 3-34). Initially, it is located off axis, but it grows toward a central location. The size varies from small to extensive involvement of a long bone. These lesions may attain enormous size (Fig. 3-35); one as large as 11.5 kg has been reported.[81] Such tumors are called giant enchondromas.

The lesion may appear as a well-marginated radiolucency or as an expansile, well-demarcated lesion with a thin cortical margin or with a thickened cortex with endosteal scalloping. A subperiosteal enchondroma shows external cortical erosion and an expanded shell of periosteal new bone surrounding its outer margin. There is no cortical breakthrough. The appearance of the matrix may be radiolucent, contain a few flecks of calcification, or have extensively amorphous, linear, ring-like, or spotty calcification. Occasionally, an enchondroma may be seen as a dense intramedullary collection of stippled calcifications without expansion and

(text continues on page 196)

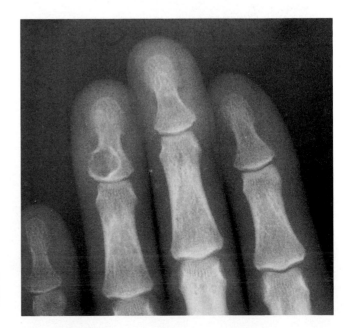

FIGURE 3-34. Enchondroma of the distal phalanx of the ring finger. A well-circumscribed radiolucent lesion involving the base of the distal phalanx is seen with a small area of calcification within the lesion.

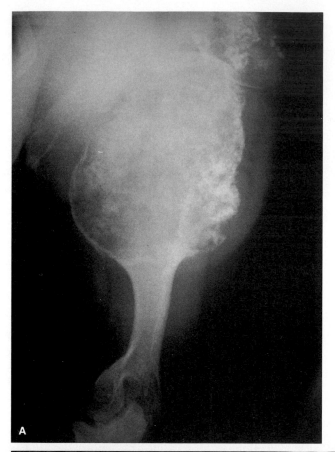

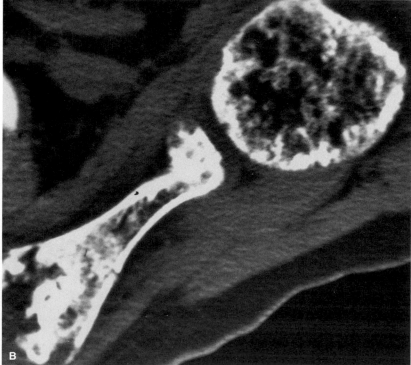

FIGURE 3-35. Giant enchondroma involving the left proximal humerus with enchondromas also involving the scapula. (**A**) The anteroposterior view of the humerus shows a markedly expansile lesion originating centrally within the proximal humerus. Amorphous calcification of the cartilage is evident. Similar changes are seen in the scapula, including the body and acromial process. (**B**) The CT scan shows a markedly expanded humeral shaft with a large amount of amorphous calcification within the enchondroma. Similar changes are seen in the scapula. (**C**) MR (SE 800/20) coronal image. The enchondroma is seen as an inhomogeneous, expansile mass in the proximal left humerus. (**D**) MR (SE 3000/20) axial section. The enchondromas in the proximal humerus and in the scapula are seen as heterogeneous, intermediate-signal-intensity, expansile lesions. (**E**) MR image (SE 3000/80). The enchondromas are increased in signal intensity and heterogeneous.

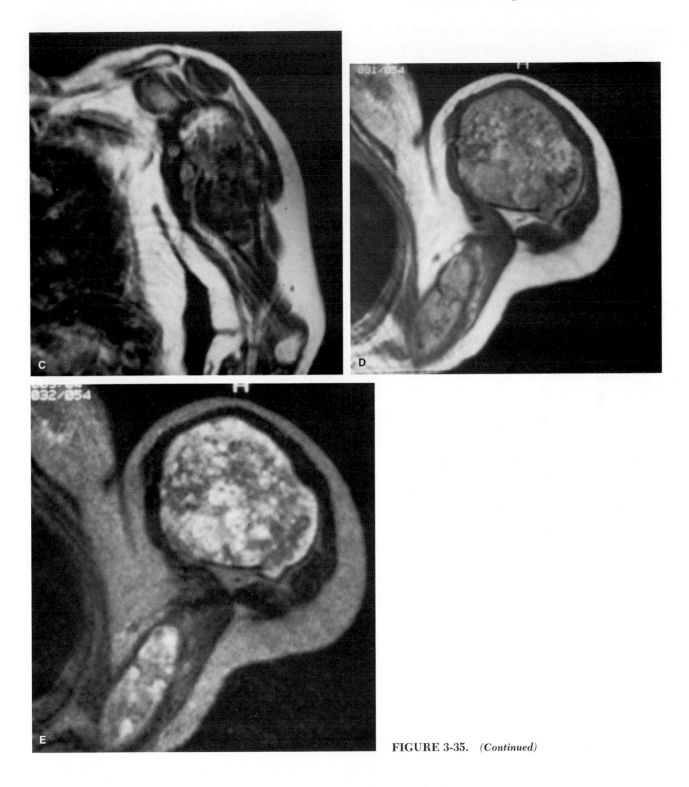

FIGURE 3-35. *(Continued)*

without a radiolucent component (Fig. 3-36). The adjacent cortex may be normal or thickened. This lesion must then be differentiated from a medullary bone infarct, which has a characteristic dense limiting margin and a serpiginous pattern of calcification (Fig. 3-37), neither of which occur in enchondroma.

On CT scans, a medullary bone infarct is seen as a calcified shell within the bone, an appearance not shared by enchondroma. Rarely, an uncalcified, completely radiolucent appearance is seen. For a large tumor, it is not possible to radiologically differentiate a benign enchondroma from a chondrosarcoma unless invasion has occurred. Histologic differentiation may also be difficult. Malignant transformation to a secondary chondrosarcoma may occur.[82] It is more likely to occur in a tumor that is more centrally located in the skeleton. Radionuclide bone scan shows increased isotope uptake within an enchondroma.

MRI shows replacement of marrow fat on T1-weighted images by the low signal intensity of the tumor. Increased signal intensity of the cartilaginous portion of the tumor is seen on T2-weighted images (Fig. 3-38), and the calcifications, if dense enough, are seen as a signal void (Fig. 3-39). Gadolinium-enhanced T1-weighted images show rings and arcs of enhancement reflecting the lobuated growth pattern of the tumor.[83]

An epidermoid inclusion cyst of a distal phalanx may simulate an enchondroma. The lack of calcification, loss of cortical definition, and a history of penetrating trauma can clarify the diagnosis (Fig. 3-40).

Multiple Enchondromatosis

Multiple enchondromatosis is an osseous dysplasia characterized by hypertrophic cartilage that has not been resorbed and ossified normally at the metaphyses.[84] This condition is probably sporadic and is usually discovered before the patient is 10 years of age, but it has been seen as early as 6 months of age.

(text continues on page 201)

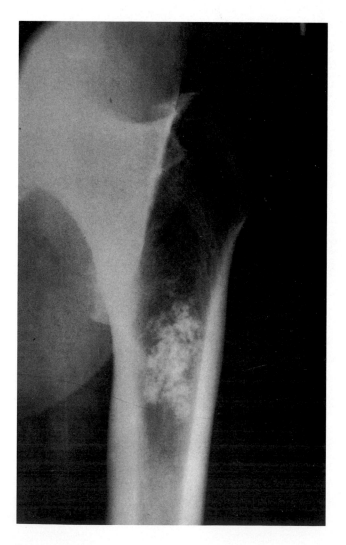

FIGURE 3-36. Enchondroma of the proximal femur. Amorphous, stippled calcification is seen without an outer limiting margin. Very lucent areas at the superior and inferior aspects of the calcification and endosteal scalloping at the upper medial margin are evident in the radiograph.

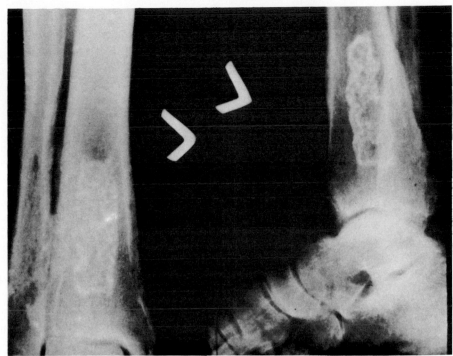

FIGURE 3-37. Mature metaphyseal infarct of the distal tibia. There is a well-circumscribed, dense area of calcification that is sharply delimited from normal bone. Notice the serpiginous anterior contour of infarct and the periosteal reaction caused by chronic stasis.

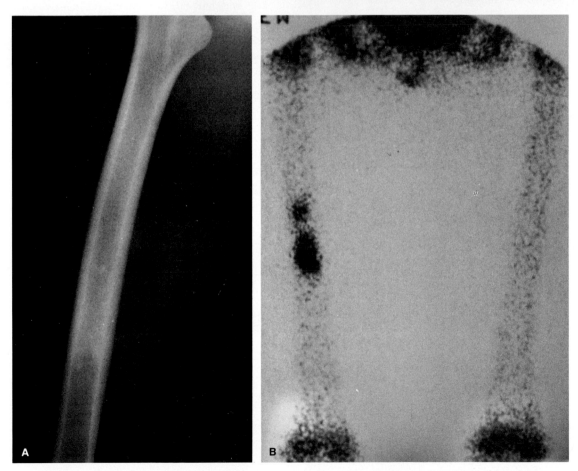

FIGURE 3-38. A 17-year-old girl with an enchondroma of the right femoral shaft. (**A**) The lateral view of the right femur shows amorphous calcification within the midfemoral shaft and slight cortical thickening. (**B**) The radionuclide bone scan shows increased activity within the enchondroma. Two distinct areas correspond to the distribution of calcifications. (**C**) MR image (SE 650/20). An area of marrow replacement can be seen in the midfemoral shaft, with residual marrow within the lesion corresponding to the area between the two foci of increased uptake in **B**. (**D**) MR image (SE 3000/80). The enchondroma shows high signal intensity within the medullary cavity. There is no surrounding reaction. *continued*

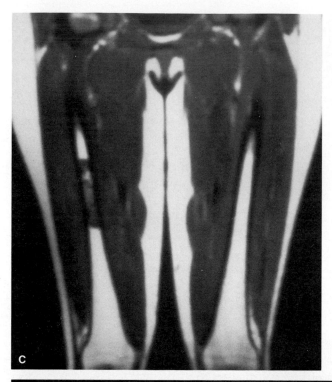

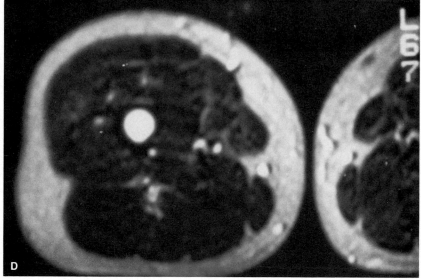

FIGURE 3-38. *(Continued)*

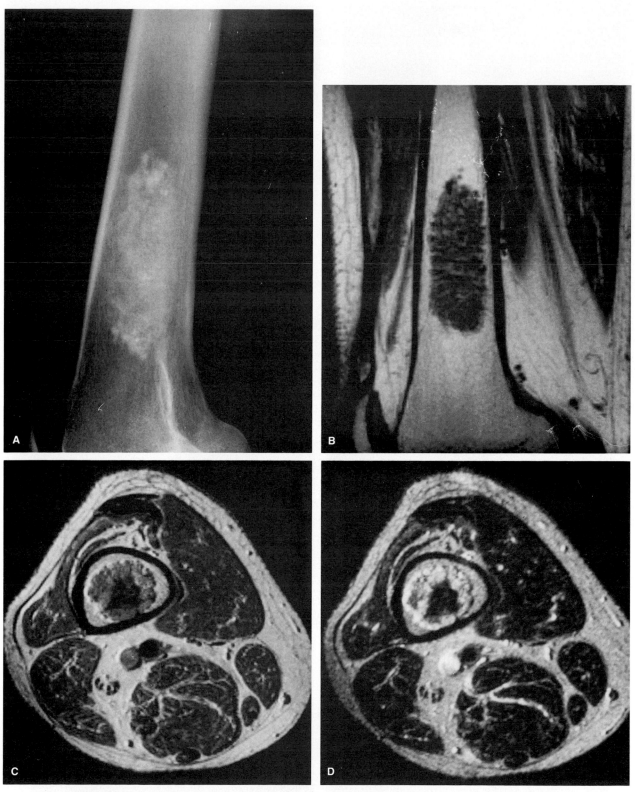

FIGURE 3-39.   A 66-year-old man with an enchondroma of the distal right femur. (**A**) The lateral view of the femur shows dense calcifications within the medulla without an outer limiting margin. (**B**) MR image (SE 800/15). The enchondroma is seen as a dense, irregular, low-signal-intensity area within the medullary cavity. The cortex is not involved. (**C**) MR image (SE 2000/22). The enchondroma is seen as irregular marrow replacement, with the central low-signal-intensity area representing calcification. (**D**) MR image (SE 2000/85). The enchondroma is seen as a central low-signal-intensity area representing calcification. The periphery is of high signal intensity, indicating the cartilaginous component. The cortex is intact, and there is no reaction.

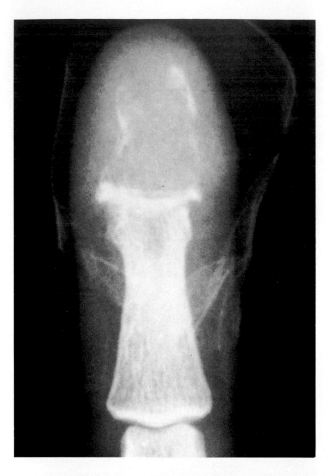

FIGURE 3-40. Epidermoid inclusion cyst of the distal phalanx. An expansile lesion involving the entire distal phalanx demonstrates loss of cortex at the terminal tuft and along the margins. There is no calcification within the lesion. In considering the differential diagnosis, the loss of cortical definition would be an unusual finding for an enchondroma.

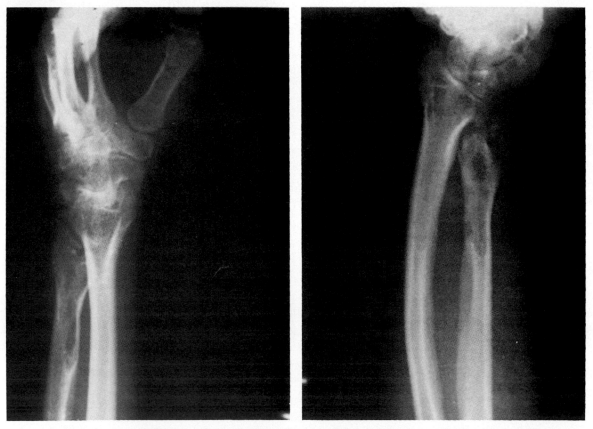

FIGURE 3-41. Maffucci syndrome. Enchondromas of the distal radius and ulna are present with shortening of the ulna and bowing of the radius, soft-tissue irregularities, and calcifications indicating phleboliths in hemangiomas.

Marked shortening of an extremity, severe deformity, deforming masses, and facial asymmetry may be present. Laboratory values are within normal limits. If associated with hemangiomatosis, it is called Maffucci syndrome, which is associated with a higher incidence of malignant change. Soft-tissue irregularity and calcifications, which are called phleboliths, are then seen (Fig. 3-41).

Radiologically, rounded or linear radiolucencies in the metaphyses and shafts of tubular bones are characteristic (Fig. 3-42). The lesions may be expansile, and they may or may not show stippled central calcifications. Shortening of the bone and deformities due to eccentric growth and undertubulation are common (Fig. 3-43). Rarely, the flat bones are involved. The iliac crest may have a scalloped appearance, with radiating bands of cartilage. This may result in severe iliac bone deformity (Fig. 3-44). The disease may show generalized distribution or be unilateral. It is then called Ollier disease. It may only involve the hands and feet. Malignant change occurs, but precise figures are not available.

CT shows an expansile mass containing stippled calcifications (Fig. 3-45). MRI shows replacement of marrow fat by low-signal-intensity enchondromas on T1-weighted images and high-signal-intensity lesions on T2-weighted images (Fig. 3-46). MRI can help to identify malignancy. Chondrosarcomas may show higher signal intensity than enchondromas on T2-weighted images.[85] Radionuclide bone scan shows increased uptake of isotope within the multiple enchondromas.

Astrocytomas in the brain and abdominal tumors rarely occur as associated findings.[86] Enchondroma protuberans is an eccentrically located lesion simulating an osteochondroma and has been reported in the humerus and rib.[87]

Juxtacortical Chondroma

Juxtacortical chondroma or periosteal chondroma is a rare, benign, cartilaginous tumor.[88,89] It develops in association with the periosteum or parosteal connective tissue.[90] It is usually solitary, but rarely may be multiple. The age-related and sex-related incidence is the same as for enchondroma. The patient complains of a small, firm, painless mass.

Radiologically, a soft-tissue mass adjacent to the cortex of a tubular bone is seen. It may also be at the tibial tuberosity.[91] It is rarely larger than 4 cm in diameter and usually contains amorphous, spotty calcifications (Fig. 3-47). It may be outlined by a thin, calcific rim. The cortex adjacent to the mass shows some de-

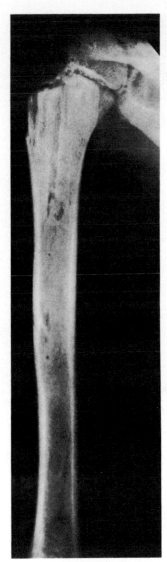

FIGURE 3-42. Enchondromatosis of the humerus. Linear radiolucencies occur at the proximal humeral metaphysis; the epiphysis is spared. Notice the radiolucencies at the midshaft of the humerus and a rounded radiolucency with a well-defined margin in the scapula.

gree of pressure erosion. Reactive cortical sclerosis can be seen. A periosteal chondroma may show cortical scalloping with overhanging margins.[92,93]

Chondroblastoma

Chondroblastoma is an uncommon bone tumor originating from chondroblasts in the epiphyseal cartilage plate.[94–97] It is generally considered to be benign.

Microscopically, the cells are moderate-sized polyhedral cells with little intercellular connective tissue.

(text continues on page 204)

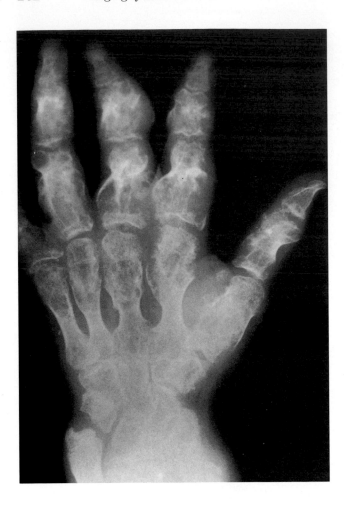

FIGURE 3-43. Enchondromatosis in a 12-year-old girl. The anteroposterior view of the hand shows multiple, expansile enchondromas involving all of the phalanges and metacarpals. There is also a large enchondroma of the distal radius, which has caused shortening.

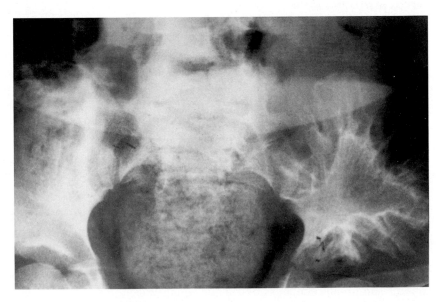

FIGURE 3-44. A 4-year-old boy with Ollier disease. The anteroposterior view of the pelvis shows marked irregularity of the left iliac bone, caused by multiple enchondromas.

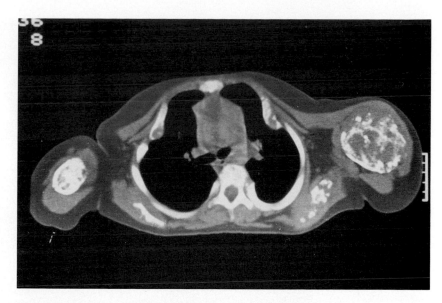

FIGURE 3-45. Enchondromatosis in a 12-year-old girl. The CT scan shows a markedly expansile lesion with calcific stippling in the left upper humerus and similar changes to a lesser extent in the right upper humerus and in the left scapula, ribs, and right scapula.

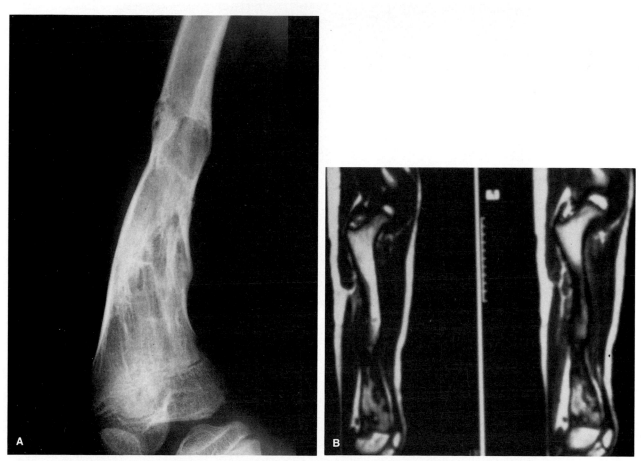

FIGURE 3-46. Multiple enchondromatosis in a 10-year-old boy. (**A**) An oblique view of the femur shows expansion and deformity of the distal femur. The enchondromas assume linear and rounded configurations. (**B**) MR image (SE 705/15). The deformity of the femur is evident. Circular areas of low signal intensity indicate marrow replacement by cartilage. (**C**) MR image (SE 2700/80). Lobulated, high-signal-intensity areas correspond to cartilage. The cortex is not evident on this frame. There is no high-signal-intensity area within the soft tissues. (**D**) The CT scan shows irregularity of the cortex with a lack of cortex medially. MR confirmed there was no soft tissue invasion. This image shows benign enchondromatosis. *continued*

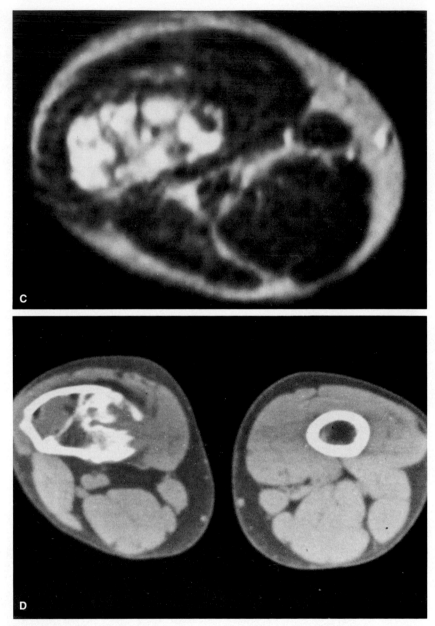

FIGURE 3-46.   *(Continued)*

Focal areas of calcification, necrosis, and giant cells may be seen. Differentiation from clear cell chondrosarcoma may be difficult.[98]

The age distribution peaks between 10 and 25 years of age, with a range of 8 to 59 years. The symptoms are joint pain, tenderness, heat, swelling, limitation of motion, weakness, numbness, and muscle atrophy.

The tumor arises in the epiphyseal cartilage plate and extends into the epiphysis (Fig. 3-48), sometimes involving the adjacent metaphysis, but to a lesser extent. Rarely, it may be confined to the metaphysis, abutting the epiphyseal cartilage plate.[99] The sites of most frequent involvement[90] are the lower femur, upper tibia, upper humerus, lower tibia, femoral head and greater trochanter, calcaneus,[100] astragalus, ilium, and ischium. It has also been reported in the patella,[101,102] finger,[103] rib, scapula, proximal fibula, and distal radius and more rarely in the manubrium, capitate, metatarsal, vertebra, mandibular condyle, calvarium, and mastoid. The hands, feet, and tarsals may also be involved, with a predilection for the calcaneus and talus. Tumors in the pelvis tend to arise from the triradiate cartilage. Extensive osteolysis with an intrapelvic soft-tissue mass has been reported.[104]

This tumor typically presents as a well-demar-

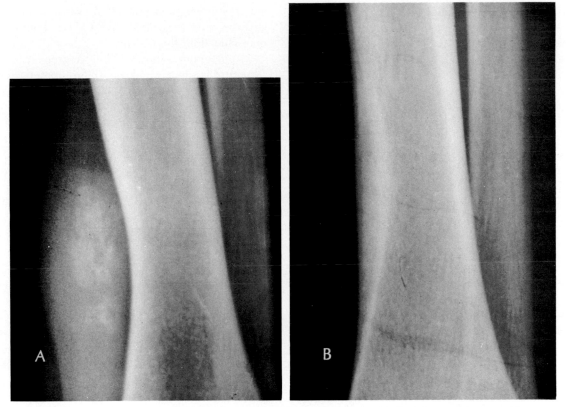

FIGURE 3-47. Juxtacortical chondroma. (**A**) There is a 2-cm, ovoid, soft-tissue mass at the anterior aspect of the tibia that contains amorphous spotty calcifications. Pressure erosion of the anterior tibial cortex has occurred. (**B**) Nine-months after surgery for removal of juxtacortical chondroma, cortical thickening at the site of erosion has occurred and is progressing toward a normal contour.

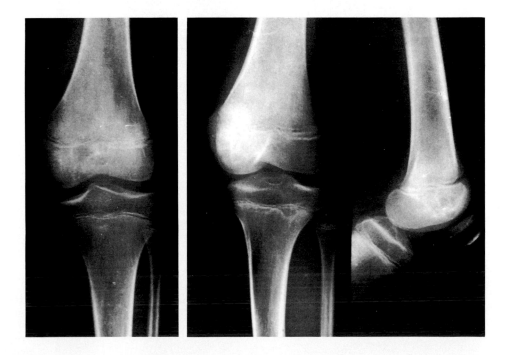

FIGURE 3-48. Benign chondroblastoma of the distal femoral epiphysis. There are radiolucent areas in the epiphyseal ossification center with a fine sclerotic margin and several stippled calcifications. (Courtesy of Dr. Heriberto Garcia, Chicago, IL.)

cated, oval or round radiolucency (Fig. 3-49) that is usually between 3 and 6 cm in diameter. It may eccentrically expand the cortex.[105] A thin, sharply demarcated sclerotic bony margin is usually part of the picture and is occasionally scalloped. The metaphyseal portion of the tumor may not show this sclerotic rim. The outer cortex may be eroded (Fig. 3-50). Surrounding nonuniform reactive bone sclerosis may be seen at a slight distance from the tumor. A thick, solid periosteal reaction that extends distally along the shaft has been reported in about half of all chondroblastomas.[106] In a minority of cases, there is amorphous, spotty calcification reflecting its cartilaginous origin. Pathologic fracture is rare, but synovitis of the adjacent joint may occur.

Radionuclide bone scan shows increased activity but is not useful in differentiating benign from malignant forms.[98] CT is most useful for defining the bony extent and location of the tumor. It can also demonstrate matrix calcification.

MRI can identify the tumor, which shows low to intermediate signal intensity on T1-weighted images with variable to high signal intensity on T2-weighted images. Extensive bone marrow edema may be seen with low signal intensity on T1-weighted images, which increases on T2-weighted images. This area may enhance after gadolinium infusion. The adjacent soft tissue may show edematous changes with low signal intensity on T1-weighted images and high signal intensity on T2-weighted images. An effusion may affect an adjacent joint (Fig. 3-51).[1,106] Cystic chondroblastoma may show fluid-fluid levels.

Angiography shows a low degree of vascularity. Chondroblastoma must be differentiated from giant cell tumor and, in the femoral head, from ischemic necrosis.[107] Complications include the formation of a secondary aneurysmal bone cyst, development of a malignant chondroblastoma, and fibrosarcoma after radiation therapy.[108] Malignant chondroblastomas of bone have been reported.[109] These may represent a variant of chondrosarcoma or clear cell chondrosarcoma.

Chondromyxoid Fibroma

Chondromyxoid fibroma is a rare benign bone tumor.[110-115] It originates from cartilage-forming connective tissue and is characterized by chondroid tissue and an intercellular mucin-like substance. Histologically, the lesion may be mistaken for a chondrosarcoma.

It most commonly occurs in the second and third decades of life, with a range of between 3 and 79 years. Males are affected more often than females. Pain of several months' duration and swelling may be present. Pathologic fracture is rare.

One half of the patients with chondromyxoid fibroma have tibial involvement, including the tuberosity.[116] Other sites of involvement are the femur, pelvis,

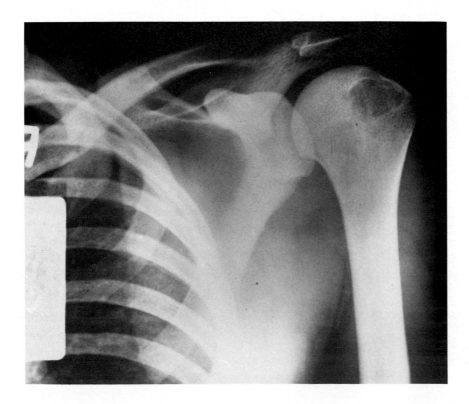

FIGURE 3-49. Benign chondroblastoma. The radiolucent area in the outer aspect of the proximal humeral epiphysis has a thin, sharp, sclerotic margin and contains light trabeculae.

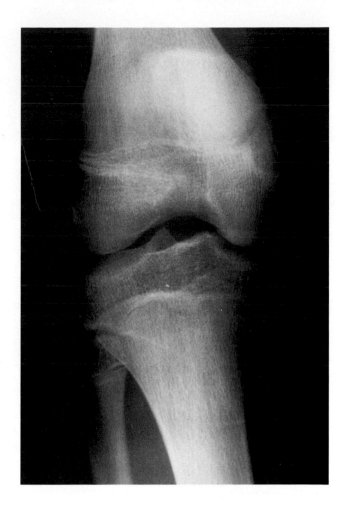

FIGURE 3-50. Chondroblastoma. The anteroposterior view of the knee. A radiolucent lesion is seen in the medial aspect of the distal femoral epiphysis. The major portion lies in the epiphysis, and a smaller portion lies in the metaphysis. The outer cortex is eroded. A sclerotic margin is seen only in the epiphyseal portion of the tumor.

humerus, fibula, calcaneus, metatarsals and tarsals, ribs, and phalanges. Vertebral, radial, ulnar, mastoid, and scapular involvement have also been reported, as have a sesamoid bone[117] and the temporomandibular joint.[118] In the tubular bones, the site is most often metaphyseal. It may extend into the epiphysis, but it does not involve the epiphysis alone.

The characteristic appearance is an ovoid, eccentric, radiolucent lesion that causes asymmetric cortical expansion (i.e., bone blister). The lesion is usually about 3 cm in its longest diameter, but it may be as large as 10 cm in its long axis. In a small bone, the lesion may involve the full width of the shaft. A cortical origin may rarely be seen without medullary involvement (Fig. 3-52). The limiting periosteal shell may be thick, thin, or not visible. No periosteal new bone formation is visible. The inner margin of the lesion may be a thin, dense line or thickened, sclerotic bone. Cortical thickening may be seen at a short distance beyond the lesion. In the flat and cuboid bones (Fig. 3-53), an expansile lesion is seen. Stippled calcification, common in chondroblastoma, is very rarely seen in this lesion.

Periosteal elevation in an aggressive form of this

tumor has been described. Rare cases of recurrence of this tumor as chondrosarcoma have been reported.

Nonossifying Fibroma

Nonossifying fibroma (i.e., fibroxanthoma) is a common benign bone tumor arising from fibrous tissue. It bears a relation to fibrous cortical defect, which is smaller and may ossify. Some researchers consider these to be the same entity.

Histologically, whorled bundles of spindle-shaped connective tissue cells contain cytoplasmic hemosiderin granules. Large nests of lipid-containing foam cells may be present. New bone formation is usually lacking.

The peak age-related incidence is in the second decade of life, in contrast to fibrous cortical defect, which has usually spontaneously regressed at this age. Many lesions are asymptomatic and are discovered as incidental findings. Malignant change has not been reported. Pathologic fracture may occur.

The most common sites of involvement are the

(text continues on page 210)

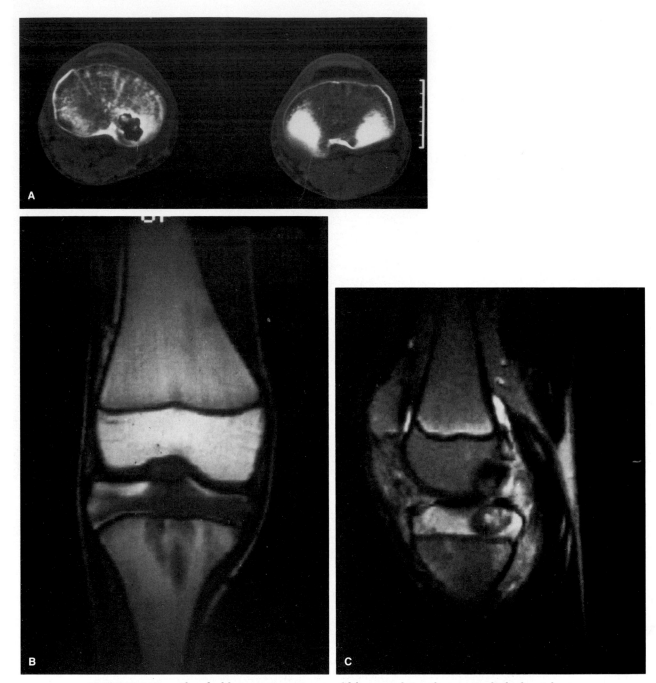

FIGURE 3-51. Chondroblastoma in a 16-year-old boy involving the proximal tibial epiphysis. (**A**) The CT scan shows a well-defined, low-density lesion with sclerotic margins that contains several calcifications in the epiphysis. (**B**) MR image (SE 700/17). The low signal intensity of the proximal tibial epiphysis extends down to the metaphysis in a streaky fashion. This represents bone marrow edema. (**C**) The sagittal MR (SE 2500/90) section shows the low-signal-intensity chondroblastoma within the epiphysis containing high-signal-intensity cartilage. The high signal intensity of the remainder of the epiphysis indicates edema. Soft-tissue edema and joint effusion are of high signal intensity.

FIGURE 3-53. Chondromyxoid fibroma of the talus. An expansile, lightly trabeculated lesion with a sharp sclerotic margin is seen. (**A**) Lateral view. (**B**) Oblique view. ▶

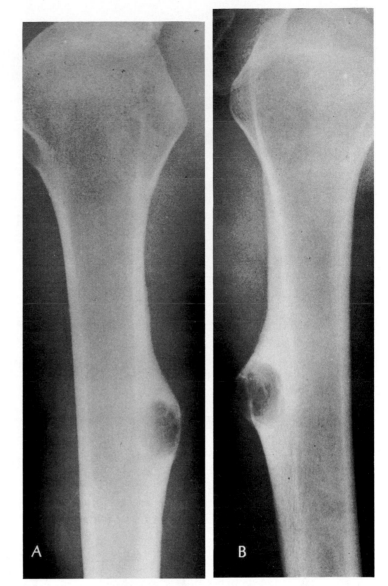

FIGURE 3-52. Chondromyxoid fibroma of the proximal humeral shaft. (**A**) An ovoid, radiolucent, expansile lesion that originated in the cortex has ballooned out of the outer cortical margin without involving the endosteum. Cortical thickening, extending a small distance on either side of the lesion, is also visible. The lesion is very lightly trabeculated but contains no calcific stippling. There is no periosteal new bone formation. (**B**) The same lesion shows loss of cortical definition of the outer margin of the lesion; this is caused by lack of visibility rather than destruction and breakthrough. Light trabeculation without stippled amorphous calcification can be seen.

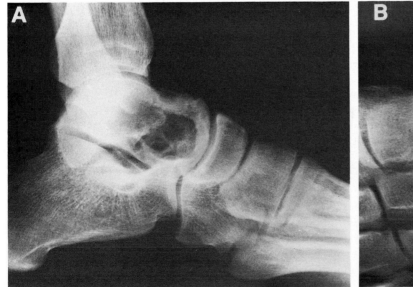

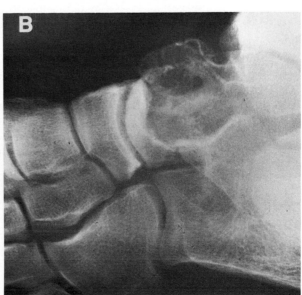

FIGURE 3-53.

long bones of the lower extremities. The upper extremities and small bones are not spared. The lesion is usually situated in the diametaphyseal area and may extend to the diaphysis. The epiphysis is not involved.

The characteristic appearance is an off-axis, ovoid radiolucency between 2 and 7 cm in its largest diameter. The margins are scalloped, and it may appear multilocular. The cortex is thin and expanded, and the inner margin has a sclerotic appearance. The long axis of the lesion is parallel to the axis of the bone. Periosteal new bone formation is not seen. A large tumor may extend across the entire diameter of the bone (Fig. 3-54). Pathologic fracture may occur. These tumors may rarely be multiple.

CT is useful in defining the extent of the lesion (Fig. 3-55). A radionuclide bone scan may or may not show some increase in activity. MRI can differentiate this lesion from a unicameral bone cyst. In nonossifying fibroma, both T1-weighted and T2-weighted images show low signal intensity, whereas a cyst shows high signal intensity on T2-weighted images (Fig. 3-56).

Fibrous Cortical Defect

A fibrous cortical defect is an asymptomatic small focus of cellular fibrous tissue in the cortex, originating from the periosteum in the metaphysis.[119,120] With increasing bone growth, it apparently migrates toward the diaphysis. As the lesion increases in size, it shows increasing marginal sclerosis, followed by progressive ossification, which starts on the diaphyseal side. This results in sclerosis and its subsequent disappearance.[121] The peak incidence is between 4 and 8 years of age, and it is rarely seen in patients younger than 2 years of age. Males are affected more often than females. Some investigators consider this to be the same entity as a nonossifying fibroma. However, a nonossifying fibroma can enlarge and lead to pathologic fracture, but a fibrous cortical defect scleroses and eventually disappears.

The most frequent sites for the lesion are the posterior medial aspect of the distal femoral metaphysis, the proximal tibia, and the fibula. The lesions rarely extend into the epiphysis and only rarely occur in the upper extremity.[122]

The characteristic appearance is a small, ovoid, cortical radiolucency (Figs. 3-57 and 3-58). The average size is from 1 to 2 cm in the longest diameter. The long axis of the lesion parallels the long axis of the bone. The margins are well defined. Lobulation or slight bulging of the cortex may be seen. Local weakening may be produced by this lesion, increasing susceptibility to an avulsion fracture if at an enthesis. An irregular periosteal reaction may follow, which should not be mistaken

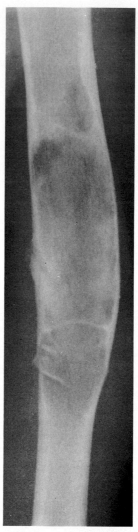

FIGURE 3-54. Large, nonossifying fibroma of the midshaft of the humerus with a pathologic fracture. Thinning and expansion of the cortex to a mild degree can be seen. There is no calcification of the matrix. The differential diagnosis from a unicameral bone cyst would be difficult.

for a malignant tumor.[123] The lesion may remodel to a normal appearance or persist as a sclerotic focus.

Desmoplastic Fibroma

Desmoplastic fibroma of bone is a rare, locally aggressive, fibrous tumor characterized by the presence of fibroblasts in a dense collagenous matrix with no atypia or new bone formation.[124–128] The age distribution peaks in the second decade, with a range of 8 to 40 years of age or rarely older. Complaints include local pain and swelling.

The mandible, tibia, humerus, femur, and other long bones and the scapula, vertebra, os calcis, innominate, and pubis[126] may be involved. The desmoplastic

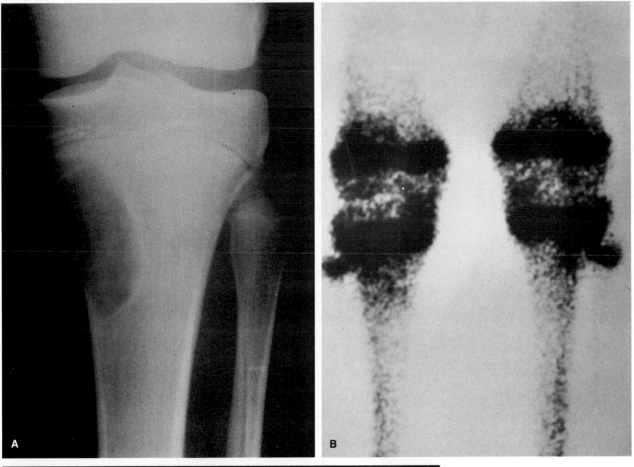

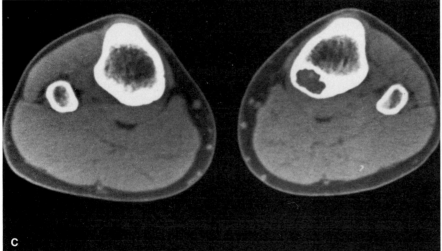

FIGURE 3-55. Nonossifying fibroma in a 14-year-old boy. (**A**) An anteroposterior view of the tibia shows an ovoid radiolucency in the medial tibial metaphysis with a sclerotic margin. There is no periosteal new bone formation. (**B**) The radionuclide bone scan shows that there is no increased activity within this nonossifying fibroma. (**C**) The CT scan shows a low-density focus in the medial tibial cortex that contains a slight amount of calcification. The lesion is well circumscribed.

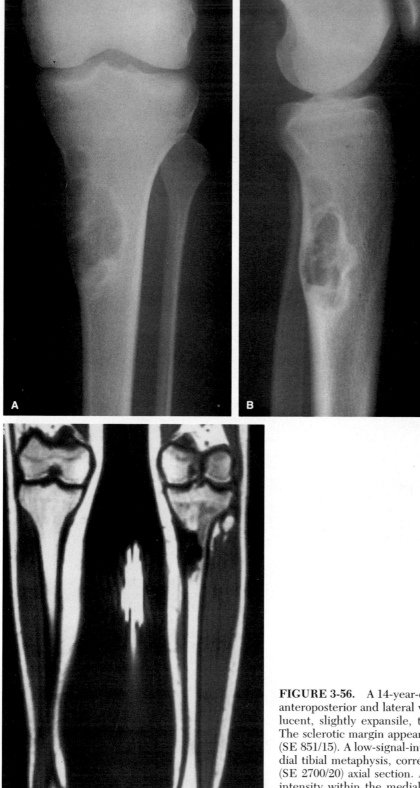

FIGURE 3-56. A 14-year-old girl with nonossifying fibroma. (**A,B**) The anteroposterior and lateral views of the left proximal tibia show a radiolucent, slightly expansile, trabeculated lesion with a sclerotic margin. The sclerotic margin appears thicker on the lateral view. (**C**) MR image (SE 851/15). A low-signal-intensity lesion replaces marrow fat in the medial tibial metaphysis, corresponding to that seen on **A** and **B**. (**D**) MR (SE 2700/20) axial section. A nonossifying fibroma is seen as low signal intensity within the medial tibial cortex. (**E**) MR image (SE 2700/80). The nonossifying fibroma is still seen as a signal void on this T2-weighted image. (**F**) The CT scan shows the nonossifying fibroma within the medial tibial cortex. A bony ridge is also apparent. The bony structure is evident on CT, but it could not be differentiated on the MR examination.

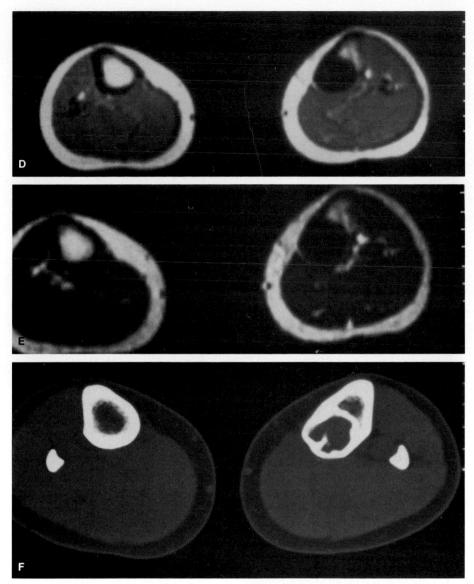

FIGURE 3-56.   *(Continued)*

fibroma is most likely to be located near the metaphysis, although it may extend into the epiphysis (Fig. 3-59). Most lesions are centrally located.

Characteristically, a large geographic radiolucency, usually well demarcated with nonsclerotic margins, is seen. The lesion may have a honeycomb appearance, be heavily trabeculated, or rarely present as a radiolucency with a sclerotic margin. Cortical destruction or thickening may be seen. Scant periosteal or reactive bone is present. A permeative destructive appearance in the diaphysis of the radius has been reported.[129] CT reveals an expansile lesion with well-defined bony margins. Cortical breakthrough with soft-tissue extension may occur.[130] MRI shows intermediate signal intensity

on T1-weighted images. T2-weighted images show predominantly intermediate signal intensity with inhomogeneous increased-signal-intensity foci representing areas of cystic necrosis.[128]

Periosteal Desmoid

Periosteal desmoid is a rare fibrous lesion arising in the periosteum.[131–134] Microscopically, adult fibroblasts and intercellular collagen are seen. Bone erosion due to osteoclastic activity can also be seen.

The usual age range of patients is 8 to 20 years. The site is not uncommonly the metaphysis of distal femur.

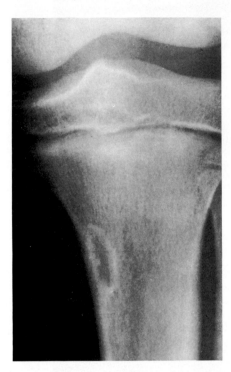

FIGURE 3-57. Fibrous cortical defect of the proximal tibia. There is a small, ovoid radiolucency involving the medial cortex, with a thin, dense margin. There is no calcification of the matrix.

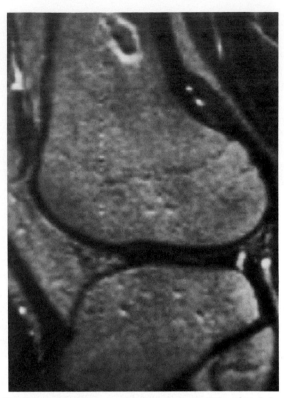

FIGURE 3-58. Fibrous cortical defect of the distal femur seen on a T2-weighted MR image. An ovoid, high-signal-intensity focus in the distal femoral diamet region is seen with a central low signal intensity. The marrow fat signal intensity is low in this T2-weighted image.

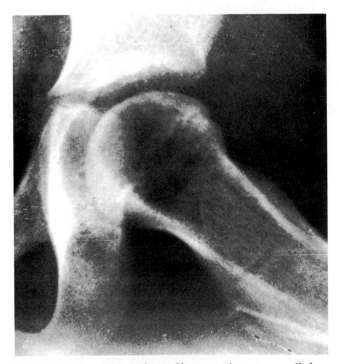

FIGURE 3-59. Desmoplastic fibroma. There is a well-defined area of radiolucency in the femoral head and neck, crossing the epiphyseal cartilage plate. There is no calcification of the matrix or expansion of bone. (Courtesy of Dr. Harvey White, Children's Memorial Hospital, Chicago, IL.)

It originates subperiosteally, resulting in destruction of the outer margin of the cortex. The endosteal margin of the cortex remains sharply defined. A slight amount of periosteal new bone formation usually occurs. An small soft-tissue mass may also be seen. Normal irregularities on the surface of the distal tibial metaphysis occur and should be taken into account in the differential diagnosis.[135] CT may be helpful in the diagnosis.[136] A periosteal ganglion may also cause cortical erosion and spiculated periosteal new bone formation. A periosteal osteosarcoma may give rise to a somewhat similar picture (Fig. 3-60). A negative radionuclide bone scan is helpful in the differentiation.

Unicameral Bone Cyst

A unicameral bone cyst (i.e., simple bone cyst) is a true cyst and a common lesion.[137] It has a wall of fibrous tissue and is fluid filled. Classically, two types are described; active and latent.[90] Active cysts are located immediately adjacent to the epiphyseal cartilage plate and are in the process of formation, and latent cysts are displaced away from the growth plate by normal bone formation and usually remain static. However, the term latent should not be taken literally, because enlargement of bone cysts in the shaft (Fig. 3-61) and pathologic fractures may occur.[138]

The cyst wall comprises fibrous and vascular tissue. Osteoid, osteoclasts and multinuclear giant cells may also be present. The fluid is clear and yellowish unless there has been a recent fracture, in which case, it may be bloody.

The peak age-related incidence is between 3 and 14 years, with a reported range of 2 months to more than 50 years. The male to female ratio is 2 to 1. Cysts behave more aggressively in childhood, and the recurrence rate is four times greater than in adolescents.[138] The highest incidence of pathologic fractures is among patients younger than 10 years of age. An active cyst grows until the time of epiphyseal fusion. It is asymptomatic unless pathologic fracture occurs.

The proximal metaphyses of the humerus and femur are the most common sites. The tibia, fibula, ribs, ilium, radius, ulna, phalanges,[139] and rarely, the calcaneus (Fig. 3-62)[140] and sacrum[141] are other locations.

Two cysts occurring simultaneously have been reported.[142]

An active lesion lies immediately adjacent to the epiphyseal cartilage plate. Rarely, it may extend into the base of the epiphyseal ossification center (Fig. 3-63).[143] A latent cyst may migrate down the shaft because of normal bone growth at the physis (Fig. 3-64). Growth retardation and deformity of the proximal humerus has been reported.[144] A cyst is most often centrally located, although it may rarely be in an off-axis position.

Characteristically, the lesion is seen as a moderate to large radiolucency that is broader at the metaphysis than at the diaphysis, resulting in a truncated cone appearance. The expanded cortex rarely exceeds the diameter of the epiphyseal plate. A latent cyst may be located far along the midshaft. A true cyst never penetrates the cortex to extend into the soft tissues and is sharply demarcated from normal bone. Trabeculations may be seen. No periosteal new bone formation occurs except after a pathologic fracture. In the event of a pathologic fracture with a free fragment, the fluid con-

(*text continues on page 219*)

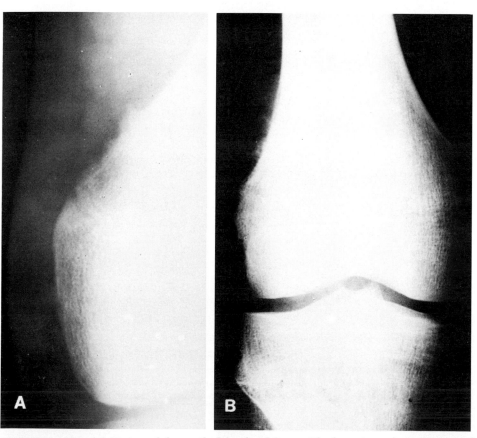

FIGURE 3-60. (**A**) Periosteal desmoid of the distal femur. The bony irregularity has a thick, squat appearance. (**B**) Osteosarcoma in similar location for comparison. Filiform spiculated periosteal new bone formation is seen.

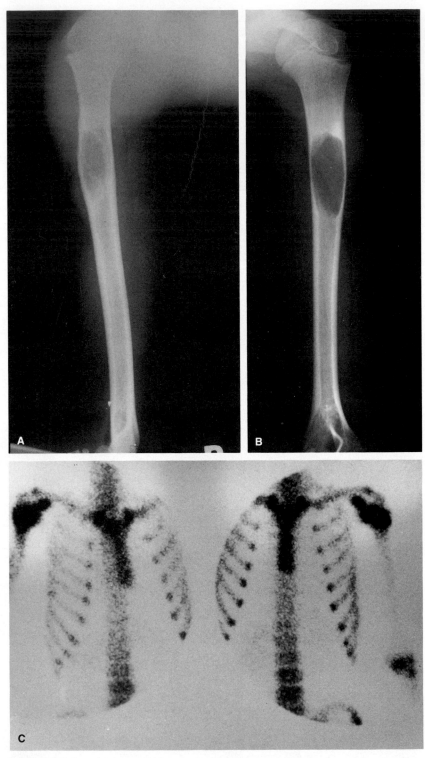

FIGURE 3-61. Unicameral bone cyst that enlarged in a diaphyseal location in a 10-year-old boy. (**A**) A radiolucent, slightly expansile cyst in the proximal humeral diaphysis. (**B**) A radiograph taken 6 months after **A** shows enlargement of the cyst. (**C**) A radionuclide bone scan shows increased activity in the right proximal humeral shaft.

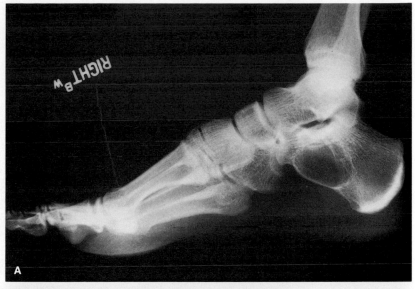

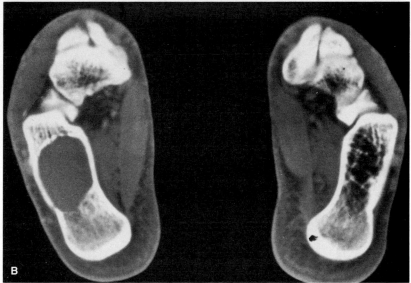

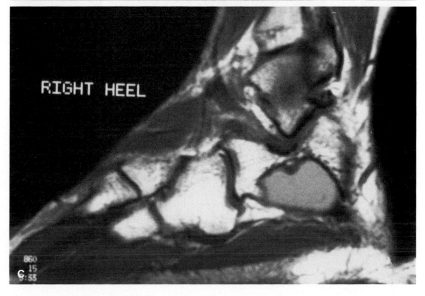

FIGURE 3-62. An 18-year-old man with a cyst in the calcaneus. (**A**) The lateral view of the right foot shows a radiolucent cyst in the calcaneus with a thin, sharp margin. (**B**) The CT scan shows a well-defined, thinly marginated cyst. The contents are of uniform density. (**C**) MR image (SE 850/15). The cyst is seen within the calcaneus as an intermediate-signal-intensity, homogeneous lesion with a thin low-signal-intensity margin. (**D**) MR STIR image. The cyst has increased in signal intensity and remains homogeneous. *continued*

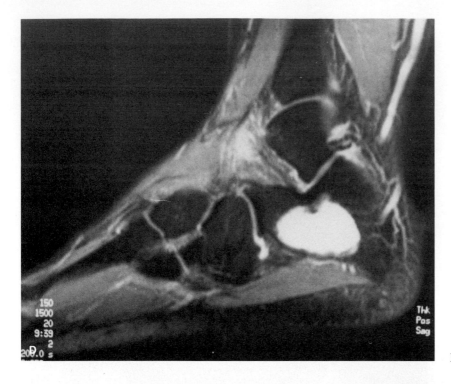

FIGURE 3-62. *(Continued)*

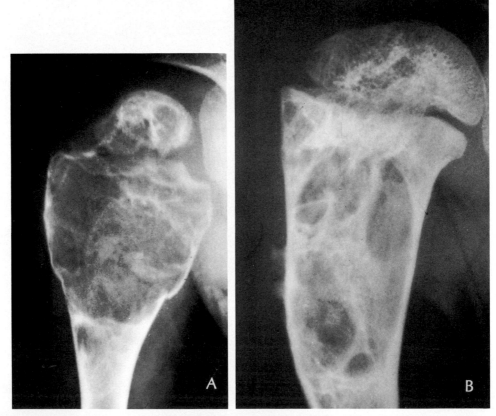

FIGURE 3-63. Unicameral bone cyst. (A) An expansile lesion at the proximal humeral metaphysis can be seen, with light trabeculation and thinning of the cortex. The lesion has crossed the unfused epiphyseal cartilage plate and involves the epiphyseal ossification center, an unusual finding in a unicameral bone cyst. (B) Fourteen-months after surgery, the typical roentgen appearance of postsurgical bone cyst in the proximal humerus can be seen, separated about 1 cm from the cartilage plate. There is a truncated appearance with a lack of tubulation of the proximal humeral shaft. The epiphyseal ossification center is residually involved.

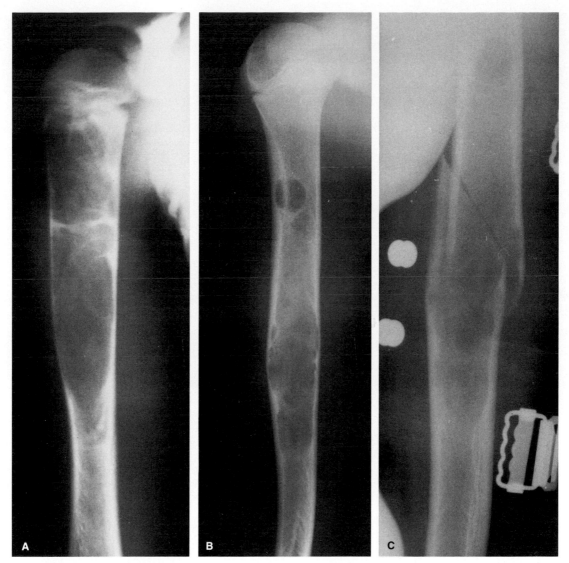

FIGURE 3-64. (A) The anteroposterior view of the humerus in an 8-year-old boy shows a unicameral bone cyst originating at the metaphysis and extending down the shaft. The lesion is thinly marginated and lightly trabeculated but does not expand beyond the width of the metaphysis. (B) Six years after A, the cyst is located in the diaphysis as a result of normal bone growth. Expansion of the humeral shaft is seen. (C) One year after B, a pathologic fracture has occurred through the cyst.

tent of the cyst allows the bony fragment to fall to a dependent portion, differentiating a cyst from a solid tumor. This is known as the "fallen fragment" sign (Fig. 3-65).[145] The radiolucent cystic area usually shows no calcification, but calcification or ossification within the cyst rarely may occur because of changes in old fibrin coagula.[146]

The differential diagnosis includes giant cell tumor and benign chondroblastoma, which have an epiphyseal location; aneurysmal bone cyst, which usually is eccentric and very expansile; enchondroma, which sometimes contains calcifications; and chondromyxoid

fibroma, which is more eccentric in location and causes more cortical expansion. A nonossifying fibroma may cause difficulty. Intrasacral defects due to meningocele also occur, as does a Tarlov cyst (i.e., perineural cyst), which may cause bone erosion and loculated erosion or expansion of the sacrum (Fig. 3-66). The original description defined a perineural cyst as not communicating with the dural sac, but common usage does not make this distinction. MRI shows the same signal characteristics as cerebrospinal fluid (Fig. 3-67).

A true cyst may be mimicked by other conditions. A triangular radiolucency between trabeculae in the

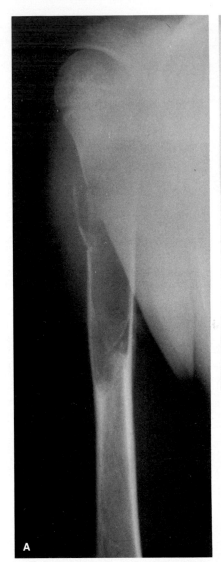

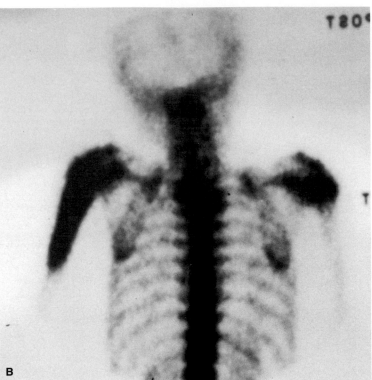

FIGURE 3-65. A 7-year-old girl with a pathologic fracture of a cyst in the right humerus. (**A**) The anteroposterior view of the humerus shows a pathologic fracture at the proximal aspect of the cyst. A sharply defined fragment is seen at the inferior aspect of the cyst, not at the fracture site. This is the "fallen-fragment" sign. (**B**) The radionuclide bone scan shows a large amount of increased activity of the proximal humerus after a pathologic fracture.

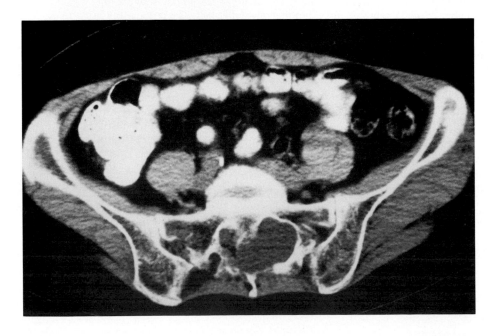

FIGURE 3-66. Tarlov cyst in a 65-year-old woman. The CT scan shows an expansile, well-marginated lesion in the body of the sacrum with uniform attenuation of the contents.

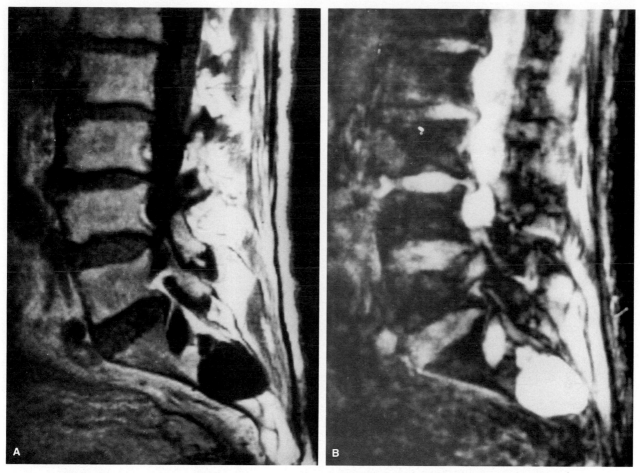

FIGURE 3-67. A 65-year-old man with a Tarlov cyst. (**A**) MR image (SE 600/15). For the multilocular Tarlov cyst in the sacrum, the signal intensity is the same as that of cerebrospinal fluid. (**B**) MR image (SE 2000/40). The Tarlov cyst increases in signal intensity to match that of the cerebrospinal fluid.

calcaneus can simulate a cyst.[147] Cyst-like rarefactions in the proximal humerus, particularly in older patients, should not be confused with a tumor.[148] Subchondral cysts associated with arthritis may be large and expansile.[149] Posttraumatic cysts may form.[150–152] Areas of apparent rarefaction in the region of the greater tuberosity, called "pseudocysts of the humerus," which contain normal bone, have been described.[153]

When cysts are located in the pelvic bones, CT can help in the differential diagnosis.[154] The expansile and intact appearance of the cortex can be demonstrated and the water density of the cystic fluid measured. Similar findings are seen in the long bones.

One method of treatment is direct steroid injection. Postinjection healing changes include reduced size, increased internal density, cortical thickening, and bone remodeling. Recurrence is delineated by renewed rarefaction and bone expansion.[155]

The radionuclide bone scan may be normal or show slightly increased activity. The center of the cyst may show decreased activity (Fig. 3-68). Increased activity occurs in the event of a pathologic fracture.

MRI shows a sharply marginated lesion with trabeculations in the cyst wall. The cyst fluid has the same signal characteristics as water or cellular tumors: a low signal intensity on T1-weighted images and a high signal intensity on T2-weighted images (Fig. 3-69).[156]

Aneurysmal Bone Cyst

Aneurysmal bone cyst is a lesion characterized by a highly expansile appearance.[157–161] There are two types: a primary cyst occurs without an associated lesion, and a secondary cyst occurs in association with a bone tumor. The radiologic appearance of a secondary aneurysmal bone cyst is most often that of the associated

(*text continues on page 225*)

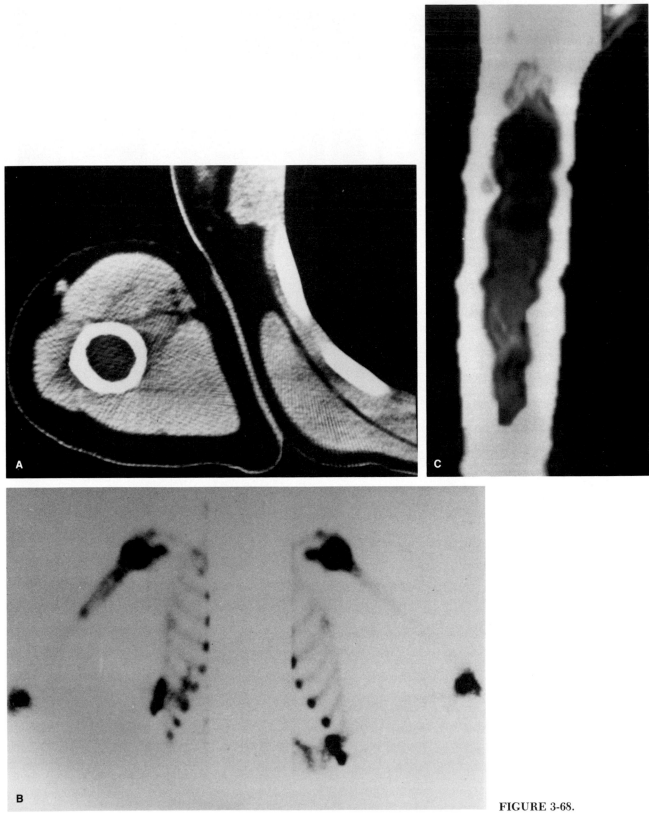

FIGURE 3-68.

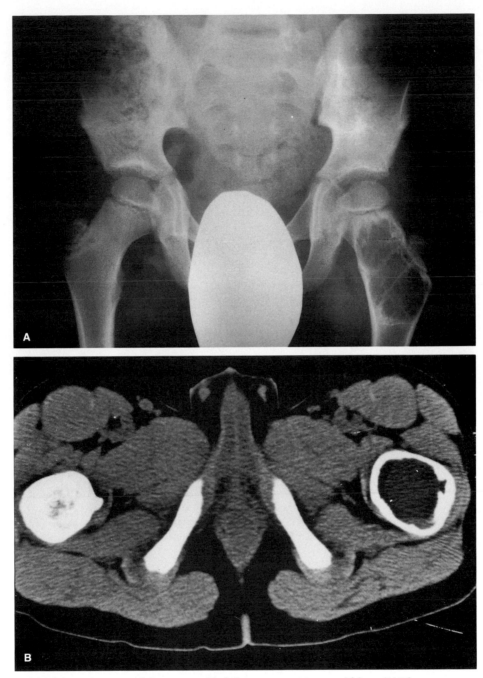

FIGURE 3-69.   Cyst of the proximal left femur in an 11-year-old boy. (**A**) The anteroposterior view of the pelvis shows a lightly trabeculated, expansile lesion in the proximal femoral metaphysis that is well circumscribed. There is a healing fracture of the medial femoral cortex. (**B**) The CT scan shows cortical expansion with a uniform low attenuation of the cyst fluid. (**C**) MR image (SE 600/16). The cyst is expanding the left femoral cortex, producing a homogeneous intermediate signal intensity. (**D**) MR image (SE 4000/36). The cyst fluid shows a homogeneous increase in signal intensity. There is no surrounding reaction.

continued

◀ **FIGURE 3-68.**   Simple bone cyst in an 11-year-old girl. (**A**) The CT scan through the midsection of the cyst shows expanded bone with a low-attenuation center. (**B**) The radionuclide bone scan shows increased activity in the cyst of the right proximal humerus, with an increase at the periphery and small foci at the superior and inferior aspects of the cyst. (**C**) Three-dimensional reconstruction shows bone formation at the superior and inferior aspects of the cyst that correspond with the foci of increased activity in **B**.

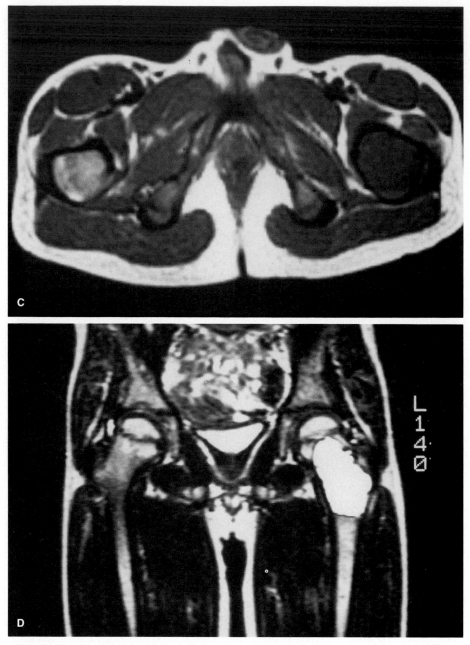

FIGURE 3-69. *(Continued)*

bone lesion. The ratio of primary to secondary lesions is 2 to 1.

The bone lesions that occur with an aneurysmal bone cyst are presented in order of frequency[157]:

- giant cell tumor
- osteosarcoma
- solitary bone cyst
- nonossifying fibroma
- fibrous dysplasia[162]
- metastatic carcinoma
- chondromyxoid fibroma
- hemangioendothelioma
- osteoblastoma
- chondroblastoma
- fibromyxohemangioma[163]
- fracture.[163]

The histologic appearance is of interconnecting cavernous spaces separated by fibrous septa filled with unclotted blood that may show thin bone formation. An endothelial lining of the blood spaces and numerous multinuclear giant cells may be seen. A solid portion of fibroblastic, fibrohistiocytic, and osteoblastic proliferation with osteoid production is also evident. Rarely, the latter portion predominates, and the tumor is devoid of cavernous spaces. This has been called a solid aneurysmal bone cyst. Its radiologic appearance may include an osteolytic lesion with a wide zone of transition, cortical expansion, and destruction with soft-tissue invasion.[164,165]

Older children and young adults are most often affected, with complaints of mild, local pain, swelling, and impairment of function of a contiguous joint of several months' duration. If a vertebral body is involved, pathologic fracture often ensues, sometimes with neurologic symptoms. Females are affected more often than males.

The femur (Fig. 3-70) is the most common site of involvement. In most cases, the lesion is found in a segment of the long bones or spine, including the bodies and neural arch.[166] Any bone may be involved, including the flat bones (Fig. 3-71), ribs, calvarium,[167] orbits,[168] small bones, calcaneus, pubis, and zygoma. Multiple aneurysmal bone cysts in a 3-month-old infant have been reported.[169]

In the tubular bones, the origin is usually in the metaphysis, but it may later involve the entire epiphysis (Fig. 3-72). The lesion has been reported to extend into an unfused epiphyseal ossification center.[170]

The typical appearance is a radiolucency off of the central axis with marked ballooning of a thinned cortex. Light trabeculation within the lesion is usually seen. It may be in a subperiosteal location, in which case it presents as a bone blister (Fig. 3-73). Periosteal new bone

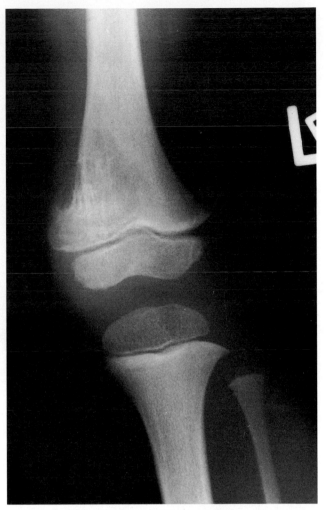

FIGURE 3-70. Aneurysmal bone cyst. The anteroposterior view of the knee reveals an expansile lesion in the distal femoral metaphysis with a thin outer margin located off of the central axis. The lesion is well defined but has no sclerotic margin with the bone. The epiphyseal ossification center has not yet fused, and there is no involvement of the epiphysis.

is usually limited to the margins, where a periosteal buttress is sometimes seen. The long axis of the lesion is parallel to the long axis of the bone, and it may be as long as 8 cm. The thin outer cortical shell may not be seen on conventional radiographs. There may be a thin sclerotic zone of transition, and pathologic fracture may occur.

Vertebral involvement is seen as an expansile, lightly trabeculated lesion that may attain large size. The body, arch, transverse, and spinous processes (Fig. 3-74) are affected alone or in combination. The vertebral body may collapse.

In flat bones, an expansile lesion with thin or thick margins may be seen (Fig. 3-75). In the ribs, it may

(text continues on page 230)

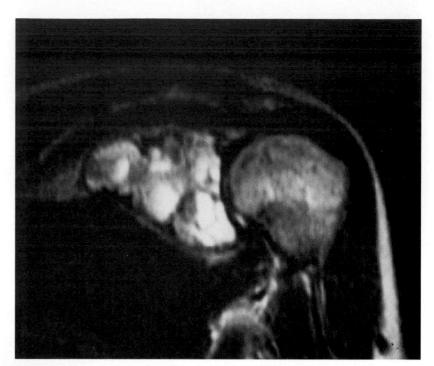

FIGURE 3-71. Aneurysmal bone cyst involving the scapula. The T2-weighted MR image shows an area of lobulated high signal intensity extending to the articular surface of the glenoid fossa.

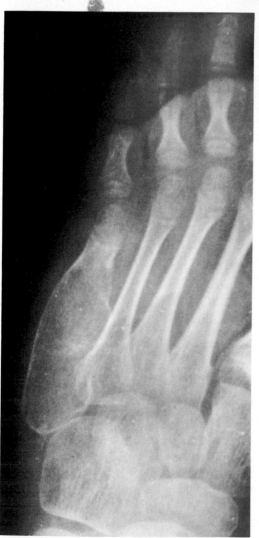

FIGURE 3-72. Aneurysmal bone cyst of the foot. There is an expansile lesion in the fifth metatarsal with involvement of the proximal end and the major portion of the shaft. There is considerable ballooning of the cortex, but the cortical shell is intact. No periosteal new bone formation is seen. This represents the intraosseous type of aneurysmal bone cyst. (Courtesy of Dr. Harvey White, Children's Memorial Hospital, Chicago, IL.)

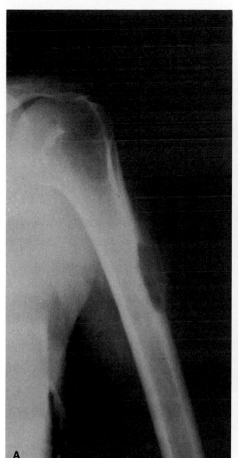

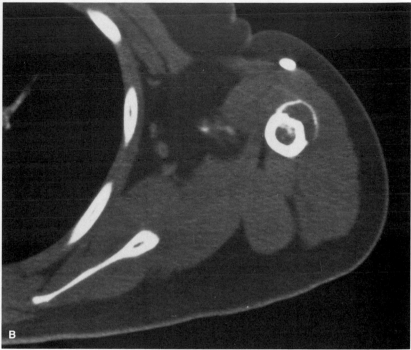

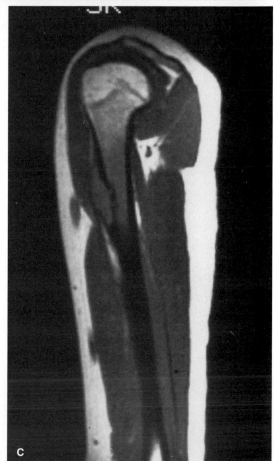

FIGURE 3-73. Subperiosteal aneurysmal bone cyst of the proximal humerus. (**A**) The anteroposterior view of the humerus shows an expansile lesion involving the outer cortex with a thin outer margin and sharp inner definition. Periosteal buttressing is seen at its superior aspect. (**B**) The CT scan shows the lesion with a thin outer calcific margin. Cortical irregularity and calcification are seen within the medullary cavity. (**C**) A T1-weighted sagittal MR image shows the subperiosteal location of the lesion and cortical irregularity. The signal intensity is intermediate and homogeneous. (**D**) A proton density axial MR image shows the homogeneous, slightly increased signal intensity of the lesion. The signal intensity of the marrow cavity matches that of the subperiosteal location indicating involvement there as well. (**E**) The T2-weighted MR image shows the high signal intensity of the lesion in the subperiosteal and medullary components. There is a suggestion of lobulation within the subperiosteal portion. The cortex is intact. *continued*

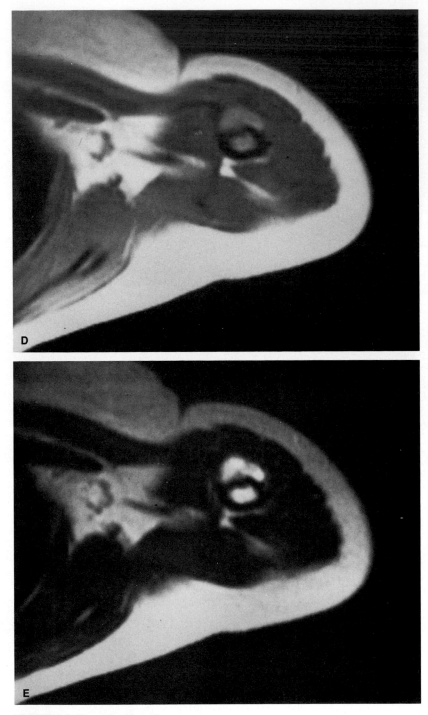

FIGURE 3-73. *(Continued)*

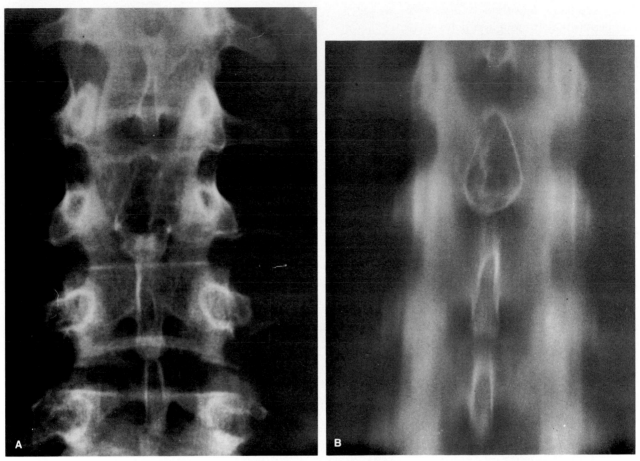

FIGURE 3-74.   Aneurysmal bone cyst of the spinous process in a 17-year-old girl. (**A**) The anteroposterior view of the lumbar spine reveals expansion of the spinous process of the third lumbar vertebra. (**B**) A conventional tomogram shows an expanded spinous process with a thin and intact outer shell containing light trabeculation.

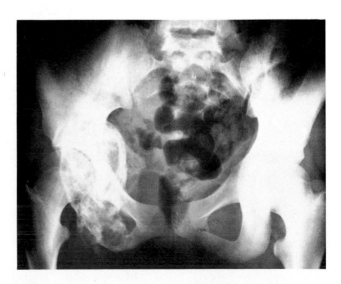

FIGURE 3-75.   Aneurysmal bone cyst of the pelvis. An expansile trabeculated lesion involves the ilium, ischium, and pubis. (Courtesy of Dr. Harold Rosenbaum, Lexington, KY.)

present as a large, intrathoracic mass.[171] In the pelvis, these lesions may present as a pelvic mass. In the calvarium, the occipital bone is most frequently involved. Aneurysmal bone cysts have been described in the sacrum,[172] where it had radiographic appearances similar to a simple bone cyst, both with significant exophytic components (Fig. 3-76).[141]

CT may show fluid-fluid levels with the proper window and level settings if the patient is immobilized long enough.[173,174] This is the result of blood layering in blood-filled spaces of various sizes.

A radionuclide bone scan shows increased uptake of isotope.[175] Some patients show an extended uptake beyond the margins of the lesion. Angiographically, the lesion is hypervascular, with large vascular spaces (Fig. 3-77).[41]

MRI findings are characteristic.[176] Internal septa-

tions; cystic loculations, occasionally with fluid-fluid levels of various signal intensities; and an expanded low-signal-intensity rim surrounding the lesion are seen (Figs. 3-78 and 3-79). Portions of the lesion have high signal intensity on T1-weighted and T2-weighted images. Fluid-fluid levels may also be seen in telangiectatic osteosarcoma, giant cell tumor, cystic chondroblastoma, and tumoral calcinosis.

Hemangioma

Hemangioma of bone is a benign condition and falls into two histologic types, cavernous and capillary, depending on the size of the involved vessels.[177,178] Cavernous hemangioma is composed of of large thin-walled vessels and sinuses lined by a single layer of endothelial

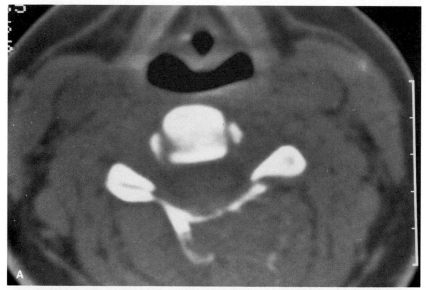

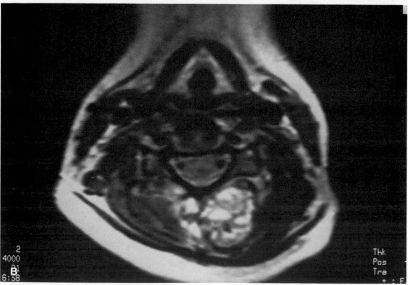

FIGURE 3-76. Aneurysmal bone cyst. (**A**) The CT scan shows an expanded neural arch. (**B**) Gradient echo MR image. Fluid-fluid levels are seen within the lesion.

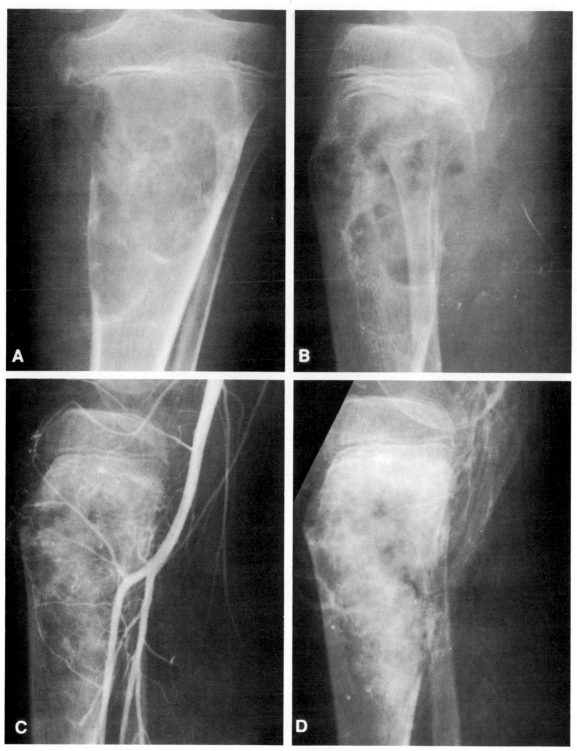

FIGURE 3-77.   Aneurysmal bone cyst in a 13-year-old boy with a 12-month history of limping and pain in the right knee. Conventional (**A**) anteroposterior and (**B**) lateral radiographs of the knee reveal a multiloculated radiolucent bone lesion involving the metaphysis of the proximal end of the tibia. Radiographically, due to age of the patient and location of the lesion, the lesion was diagnosed as aneurysmal bone cyst. Arteriographic findings in early (**C**) arterial and (**D**) capillary phases reveal numerous, small arteries arising from the soft tissues that supply the lesion. There is close attachment of the arteries without evidence of the soft-tissue extension typical for these tumors. Uneven tumor stain is seen with numerous cavity-like spaces full of contrast media. Notice the absence of vascularity in some parts of the lesion. Biopsy and postsurgical curettage specimens proved the diagnosis of aneurysmal bone cyst. (Courtesy of Dr. Issa Yaghmai, Medical College of Virginia, Richmond, VA.)

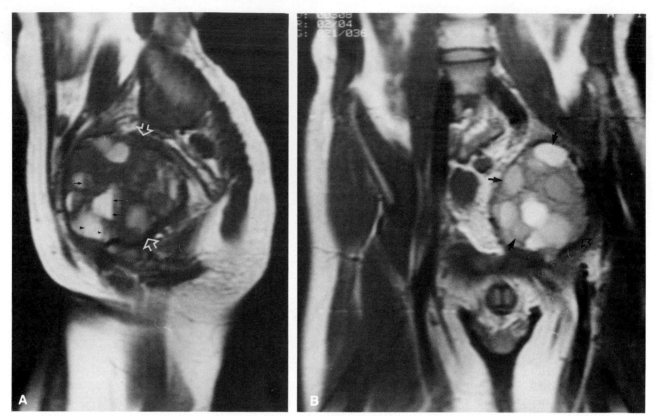

FIGURE 3-78. Aneurysmal bone cyst. (**A**) The sagittal MR image (PS 500/25) shows multiple cysts with fluid levels (*arrows*). The largest cyst has more than one fluid level (*arrowheads*). There is a rim of decreased signal intensity surrounding the lesion (*open arrows*). (**B**) Coronal MR image (SE 2000/25 × 4) shows multiple cysts with different signal characteristics (*arrows*) and a dark rim (*open arrow*). (From Beltran J, Simon DC, Levy M et al: Aneurysmal bone cysts: MR imaging at 1.5 T. Radiology 158:689–690, 1986)

cells in intimate relation with the bone trabeculae. This results in their resorption. Capillary hemangiomas consist of fine, peripherally radiating capillary loops.

Cavernous hemangiomas of the vertebrae are usually small and asymptomatic. Their incidence in the spine at autopsy is estimated to be greater than 10%. It is usually a single lesion, but occasionally, two or more vertebrae may be involved. The site is usually in the body, but the neural arch may also be affected. Hemangioma of the spine has been reported in patients as young as 10 years of age. The patient may complain of vague and intermittent pain. Compression fractures can occur, which may be complicated by spinal cord or cauda equina compression. Resultant neurologic symptoms ensue, which may include paraplegia. Cord compression can also result from hematoma, epidural extension (Fig. 3-80), or bony expansion.[179] Spinal stenosis or block may occasionally occur because of chronic hemorrhage and fibrous reaction, and at surgery, only dense fibrosis is seen (Fig. 3-81).

Radiologically, a vertically striped orientation of the bone trabeculae gives a corduroy-cloth appearance, or a reticular texture may be seen. CT may show the entire vertebral body or only a portion of it involved with a cross section of the coarsened trabeculae, yielding a stippled appearance (Fig. 3-82). These changes may also involve the pedicle, transverse and spinous processes, and the adjoining ribs (Fig. 3-83).[177] The cortex is usually intact, but there may be posterior bulging or a paraspinal mass.

MRI shows increased signal intensities on T1-weighted and T2-weighted images that may be focal or involve the entire vertebral body (Fig. 3-84). A mottled increase in signal intensity is seen on T1-weighted images in the intraosseous portion because of fat tissue within the hemangioma.[180] It has been suggested that a large amount of fat represents the inactive cases and that those with low degrees of fat signal are more prone to cord compression and fractures.[181] Extraosseous components lack fat and have low signal intensity on

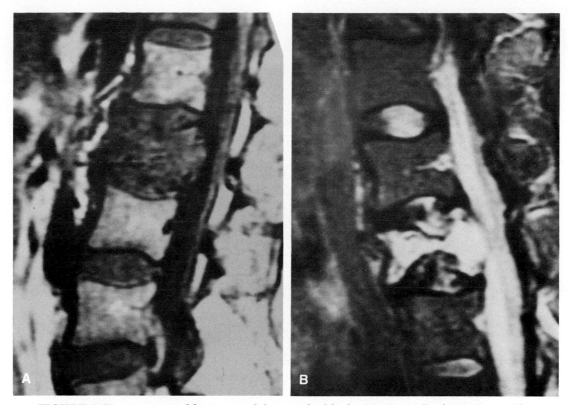

FIGURE 3-79. Aneurysmal bone cyst of the vertebral body. (**A**) T1-weighted MR image. The second lumbar vertebral body has lost signal intensity because of replacement of marrow fat by the aneurysmal bone cyst. Collapse of the vertebral body is seen. (**B**) T2-weighted MR image. The lesion shows increased signal intensity. The marrow fat has decreased signal intensity. Compression of the dural sac is seen on both images. (Courtesy of Dr. Harold Posniak, Loyola University, Maywood, IL.)

T1-weighted images, which increases with T2 weighting.[182]

Hemangiomas rarely occur in the long bones.[183–185] When they do occur, the ends of the bone are most often involved with an expansile, loculated, radiolucent lesion. Rarely, sclerosis may occur (Fig. 3-85). Typically in the flat bones, particularly in the calvarium, a stippled or sunburst appearance may be seen (Fig. 3-86). A capillary hemangioma of the sphenoid bone producing unilateral optic atrophy has been reported.[186] Lymphangioma of bone has also been well described.[187,188]

Massive Osteolysis

Massive osteolysis (i.e., vanishing bone disease, Gorham disease) is a rare condition of unknown etiology characterized by the progressive resorption of large segments of bone.[189–195] It does not involve malignant cells and is associated with hemangioma or lymphangioma. It usually affects patients younger than 30 years of age, with a reported range of 14 months to 58 years. There is no evidence of heredity, metabolic, or endocrine disturbances. Pain and progressive weakness occurs, followed by deformity and sometimes followed by pathologic fracture. The progress of the disease is unpredictable. It may spontaneously arrest[196] or may progress to death, particularly with rib cage involvement. Laboratory studies show no characteristic changes. At surgery, bone is absent at the involved site. Bone grafts also may be resorbed. Cases have been reported with spontaneous reossification.[197]

Large areas of bone resorption are seen. Any bone may be affected, but involvement is most frequent in the shoulders, hips, pelvis, ribs (Fig. 3-87), spine, and long bones. Joints and intervertebral disks are not a barrier to spread, allowing massive areas of bone loss. The characteristic appearance in a tubular bone is a tapered margin. There is no osteosclerosis, periosteal reaction, coarsening of the trabecular pattern, soft-tissue debris, nor phleboliths. Skip areas are not usually seen.

(text continues on page 238)

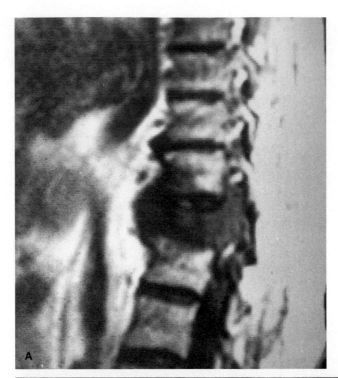

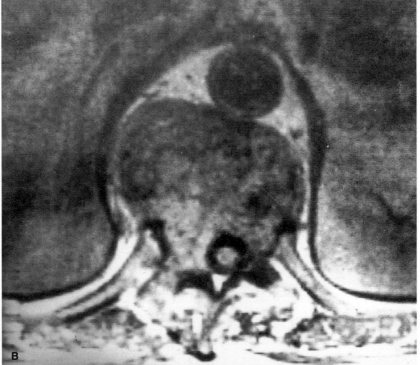

FIGURE 3-80. Hemangioma of a thoracic vertebra. (**A**) A sagittal MR (SE 300/ 17) image of the thoracic spine reveals low siganl intensity and a partially col- lapsed vertebral body with an extension anteriorly and posteriorly impacting on the spinal canal. (**B**) MR image (SE 1000/28). Inhomogeneous signal intensity in the vertebral body and posterior extension of the hemangioma into the spinal canal are seen. The patient is a 51-year-old man.

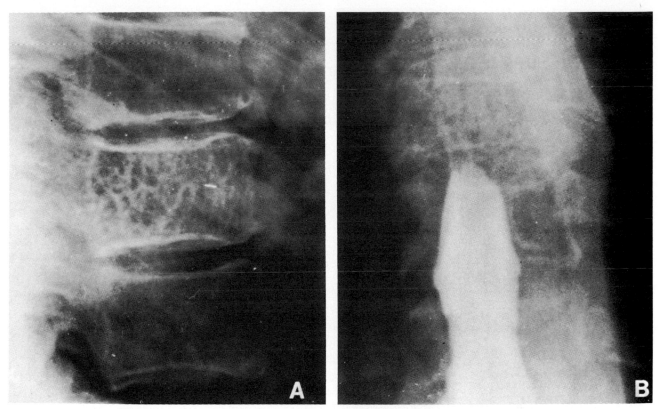

FIGURE 3-81.   Hemangioma of the vertebrae in a paraplegic patient. (**A**) A lateral view of the spine shows the typical striated appearance of a vertebral body hemangioma. (**B**) The myelogram shows a complete block at the level of the hemangioma. An associated soft-tissue mass in the paraspinal region is also seen. At surgery, this patient had meningeal thickening caused by small, chronic hemorrhages without evidence of a large, recent hemorrhage.

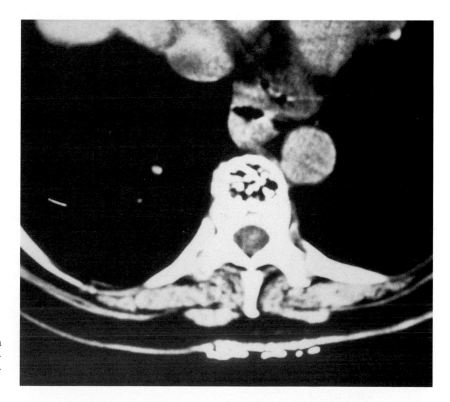

FIGURE 3-82.   The CT scan shows a hemangioma of the vertebra in a 72-year-old woman. The vertebral body has a stippled appearance.

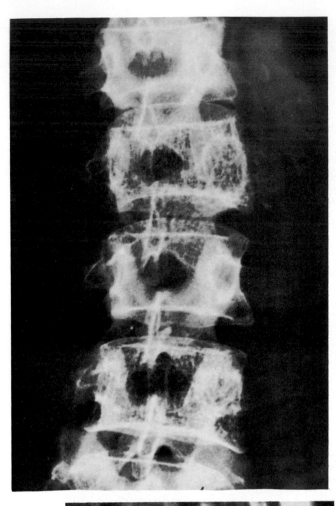

FIGURE 3-83. Hemangiomas of the spine involving the second and fourth lumbar vertebrae are seen in this antero-posterior view. Notice the loss of bone density and accentuation of the trabecular pattern, with predominantly vertical stripes. The pedicles are involved, and there is expansion of the left transverse process of L2. The vertebral end-plates are intact.

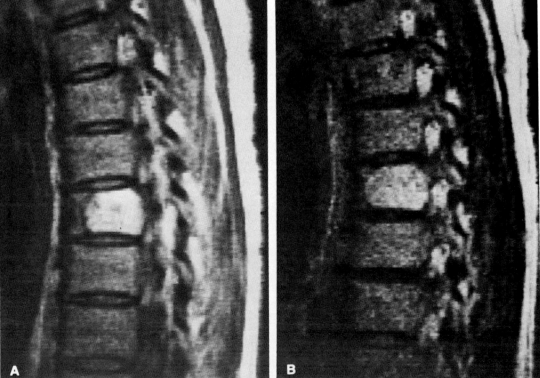

FIGURE 3-84.

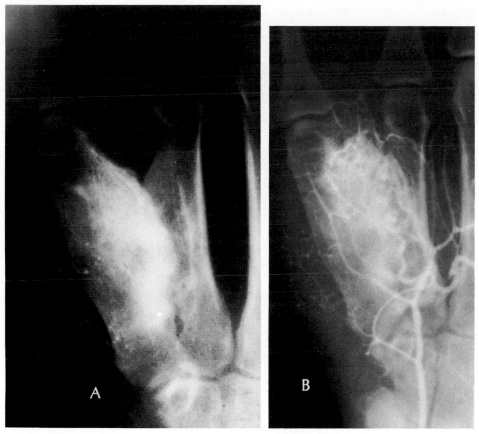

FIGURE 3-85. Hemangioma of the fifth metacarpal. (**A**) Unusual, dense, sclerotic cortical thickening is seen. (**B**) An arteriogram of the hemangioma shows hypervascularity.

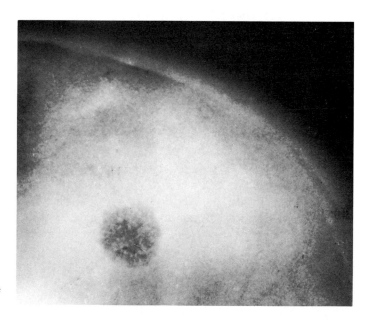

FIGURE 3-86. Hemangioma of the skull. Notice the area of radiolucency showing small, punctate stippling.

◀ **FIGURE 3-84.** Hemangiomas of the spine. (**A**) T1-weighted MR image. A high signal intensity is seen in the posterior two thirds of the body of the seventh thoracic vertebra. A low signal margin surrounds the lesion. (**B**) The T2-weighted image shows a persistent high signal. High signal intensity of the T1-weighted and T2-weighted images is characteristic of a hemangioma, reflecting a hemorrhagic component.

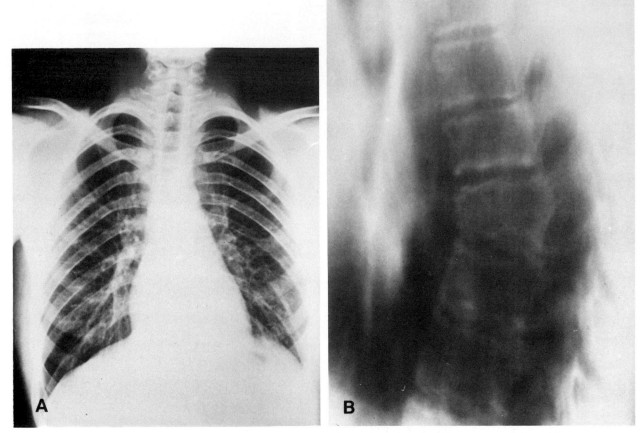

FIGURE 3-87. Massive osteolysis or vanishing bone disease. (**A**) Posteroanterior chest film. Destruction of the left eighth and ninth ribs is seen. (**B**) Tomogram of dorsal spine. Partial collapse of the middorsal vertebrae occurred with sharp gibbus formation. (Courtesy of Dr. Tom Hinckle, Beaumont, TX.)

Stress Fractures

Fractures without a single notable traumatic event may occur in normal or weakened bone. If repeated unusual stress occurs in normal bone, a fracture is called a *stress fracture* (e.g., fracture occurring while marching). If it occurs in structurally weakened bone with deficient elastic resistance, as in osteoporosis or irradiated bone (Fig. 3-88), it is called an *insufficiency fracture*. These fractures occur at all ages and are specific in location. The most frequent sites are metatarsals, calcaneus, navicular, tibia,[198] fibula, femoral neck,[199] pelvis, humerus, and ulna.[200] Stress fractures of the ribs and insufficiency fractures of the tibial condyles,[201] sacrum,[202] and the sternum may occur.[203] Calcaneal fractures may be associated with diabetes mellitus, in which case they are extraarticular and confined to the posterior aspect.[204] Multiple insufficiency fractures have been occurred in patients with rheumatoid arthritis.[205] Stress fractures may not be initially visible on plain films, or they may first present radiologically as only periosteal

new bone formation and later as callus formation (Fig. 3-89).[206] Care must be taken not to interpret early callus as tumor osteoid histologically. Light, irregular linear sclerosis may traverse the diameter of the bone at the fracture site.

CT can demonstrate a stress fracture line earlier than conventional films.[207] CT findings, in addition to a fracture line, are increased medullary density, endosteal sclerosis, callus formation, and soft-tissue swelling.[208] Radionuclide bone scans are helpful in early diagnosis, showing focal increased uptake when plain films may be negative.[209,210] Radiation-induced insufficiency fractures of the pelvis show often symmetric areas of increased activity in the radiation field.[211]

MRI shows a fracture as a line or band of low signal intensity on T1-weighted images. Extensive decreased signal intensity in the marrow cavity on T1-weighted images with high signal intensity on T2-weighted images is caused by marrow edema. Early changes may not include a low-signal-intensity line.[212,213] Soft-tissue reactive changes surrounding the bone, sometimes

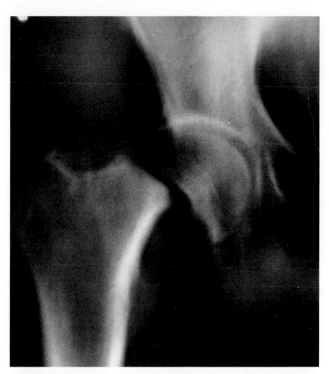

FIGURE 3-88. Insufficiency fracture after radiation therapy. The conventional tomogram shows a smooth, linear fracture traversing the subcapital region of the right femur with displacement of the fragments.

simulating a mass, may be seen in acute cases. A chronic stress fracture shows surrounding callus formation that produces a low signal intensity on all pulse sequences (Fig. 3-90).

Rare Lesions

Glomus Tumor

Glomus tumor may involve the distal aspect of a terminal phalanx.[214] A small, central, circumscribed radiolucency is seen in an intraosseous or subungual lesion that resembles an enchondroma. It is painful, however. Ultrasound has been used in the diagnosis.[215] Glomus tumors of the coccygeal body may cause coccydynia.[216]

Arteriovenous Malformation

Arteriovenous malformation may cause erosion of bone and local bone overgrowth. Extensive arteriovenous malformations occur in Klippel-Weber-Trenaunay disease with marked bony deformities (Fig. 3-91).

Ossifying Fibroma

Ossifying fibroma of the skull, face, and mandible is a distinct lesion presenting as a smooth round expan-

sile mass.[217] A paranasal sinus may be expanded. Reactive bone sclerosis or calcification of the tumor matrix (Fig. 3-92) may occur. There are no differences in this tumor based on location, and there is a range of histologic maturation.[218]

Intraosseous Lipoma

Intraosseous lipoma is a rare tumor that can affect the elderly.[219] It may occur in the metaphyses of the long bones, skull, ribs, spine, sacrum,[220] extremities, and the calcaneus. Radiologically, there is an expansile lesion with a thin cortex, which may progress to cortical breakthrough with a soft-tissue component. Involution with tissue necrosis and internal foci of calcification or ossification may be present.[221] Multiple lipomas may be seen in patient with hyperlipoproteinemia.[222] On CT images, the low attenuation of fat may be seen, which can be simulated by necrosis in chronic osteomyelitis.[223] On MRI, the high signal intensity of fat, which is brighter than that of fatty marrow, is seen in T1-weighted images (Fig. 3-93). Malignant transformation to liposarcoma or malignant fibrous histiocytoma very rarely occurs, followed by rapid bone destruction.[224] (text continues on page 242)

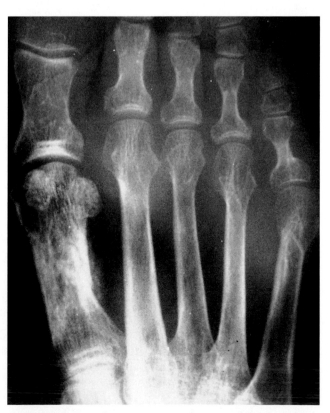

FIGURE 3-89. The anteroposterior view of the foot shows a stress fracture of the first metatarsal with callus formation and reactive bony sclerosis.

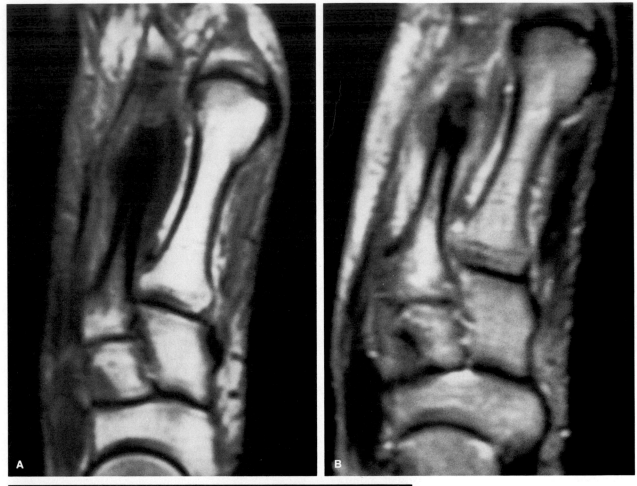

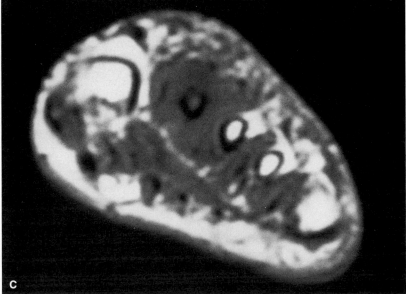

FIGURE 3-90. Stress fracture of the second metatarsal in a 28-year-old man. (**A**) MR image (SE 500/18). The low signal intensity of the second metatarsal involves the marrow cavity and extends into the soft tissues. (**B**) MR image (SE 4000/35). The low signal intensity of the fracture line of the second metatarsal is seen with the intermediate signal intensity in the surrounding soft tissue. There is no increase in signal intensity. (**C**) The axial MR (SE 700/18) section through the tarsus reveals a soft-tissue prominence surrounding the second metatarsal. The signal intensity of its medullary cavity does not match the fat intensity of the other bones.

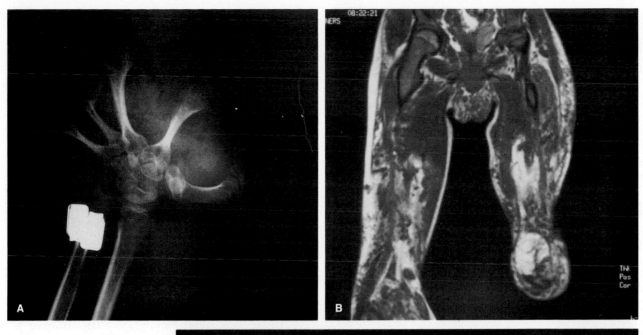

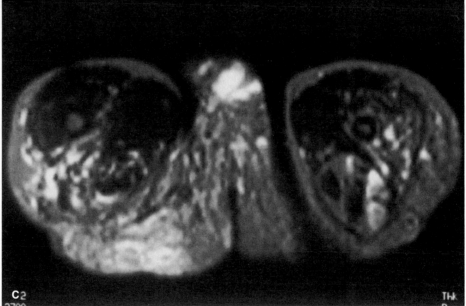

FIGURE 3-91. Klippel-Weber-Trenaunay disease. **(A)** The anteroposterior view of the hand shows a marked bony deformity and lobulated soft-tissue masses. **(B)** MRI (SE 650/15). Multiple arteriovenous malformations are of low signal intensity in the subcutaneous fat and other tissues. The left foot had been amputated. **(C)** MR image (2700/80). The arteriovenous malformations have increased in signal intensity and are widely distributed in a serpiginous pattern.

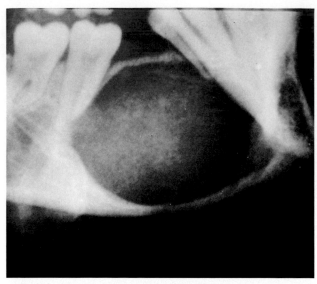

FIGURE 3-92. Ossifying fibroma of the mandible. Notice the smooth, well-marginated, expansile lesion in the body of the mandible. Several small flecks of calcification are within the tumor, and there is a fine, diffuse, calcific distribution.

Neurilemoma

Neurilemoma (i.e., schwannoma) may rarely be situated in the medullary cavity of a bone.[225] Radiologically, it is seen as a circumscribed or multilocular radiolucency with a thin sclerotic margin. It may be sub-periosteal with erosion of the outer aspect of the cortex.

Fibromyxoma

Fibromyxoma is a rare, benign, fibrous tumor of bone.[226-228] It may involve the tibia, iliac bone, and other sites. The radiologic appearance is not characteristic, although a well-marginated osteolytic lesion, possibly containing some calcifications, may be seen.

Plasma Cell Granuloma

Plasma cell granuloma is a rare condition of bone. Histologically, it is a granuloma with large masses of plasma cells and a mingling of other cells. Widespread sclerotic lesions may be present.[229] Growth is slow, and the laboratory findings are normal.

Anterior Sacral Meningocele

An anterior sacral meningocele may present as a pelvic mass with marked erosion of the sacrum (Fig. 3-94). MRI is useful in the diagnosis, showing signal characteristics within the mass similar to that of cerebrospinal fluid (Fig. 3-95).[230]

Arachnoid Cyst

An arachnoid cyst may also cause a destructive lesion in the sacrum, which can be diagnosed by char-

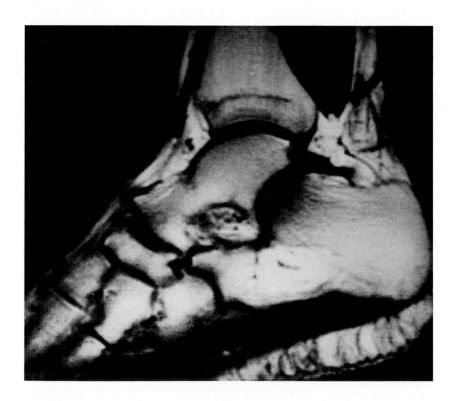

FIGURE 3-93. The MR (SE 600/20) image shows a lipoma within the calcaneus with the high signal intensity of fat. A low-signal-intensity streak within the mass represents a fibrotic strand.

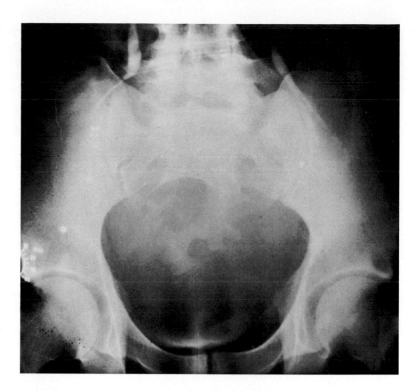

FIGURE 3-94. Anterior meningocele. Notice the large pelvic mass and deformity and erosion of the sacrum. (Courtesy of Dr. D. Christou, Athens, Greece.)

acteristic MR signal intensities.[231] A perineural or Tarlov cyst may also cause destructive or expansile sacral changes (see Figs. 3-66 and 3-67).

Epidermoid Inclusion Cyst

Epidermoid inclusion cyst develops as a result of penetrating trauma with implantation of an epidermoid rest.[232,233] It frequently involves the terminal phalanx, with a well-circumscribed radiolucency showing a thin cortical margin that may not be visible in its entirety

(see Fig. 3-40). The cyst has also been reported in the ulna.[234]

Thorn- and Twig-induced Granulomas

Thorn- and twig-induced granulomas produce lytic, sclerotic, or mixed lesions.[235] An area of bone destruction with cortical thickening and periosteal reaction, sometimes laminated, may be seen. A wood splinter-induced pseudotumor of bone has been described.[236] A wood sliver can also cause the formation

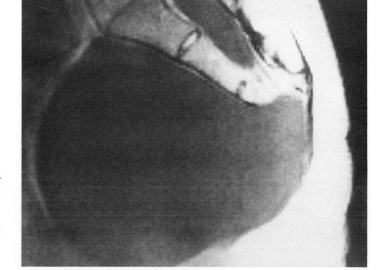

FIGURE 3-95. The sagittal MR image (SE 450/26) shows anterior sacral meningocele as a large mass of low signal intensity, similar to cerebrospinal fluid within the thecal sac. Notice the sacral abnormality and the presence of fibrofatty connective tissue with a mixed signal intensity. (From Martin B, de Latour FB: MR imaging of anterior sacral meningocele. J Comput Assist Tomogr 12:166–167, 1988)

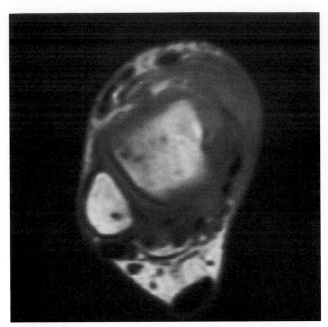

FIGURE 3-96. Granuloma secondary to a wood sliver from a palm tree. The T1-weighted MR image shows a soft-tissue mass medially adjacent to the bone.

of a soft-tissue granuloma. MRI may then show a low-signal-intensity area on T1-weighted and T2-weighted images (Fig. 3-96).

Intraosseous Ganglion

Intraosseous ganglion is a rare osteolytic lesion of bone.[237–240] A well-defined radiolucency with a sclerotic margin is seen, usually near an articular surface (Fig. 3-97), but possibly in other locations. The tibia and femoral head and neck are often involved. The lesions may be any size up to 7 cm in diameter. A periosteal ganglion may cause various degrees of cortical erosion and periosteal new bone formation, which may be spiculated. CT shows a well-defined tissue mass sharply eroding the cortex. MRI shows the signal intensity to be homogenous and isointense with muscle on T1-weighted images and to markedly increase on T2-weighted images, reflecting the fluid contents of the ganglion.[241]

Echinococcus Cyst

Echinococcus cyst presents as a radiolucency within a bone, which may be large.[242–244] It causes endosteal scalloping and expansion, and daughter cysts may be present. Cortical breakthrough and soft-tissue masses may occur. It is usually monostotic. The pelvis (Fig. 3-98), spine, and long bones are common sites. The ribs may rarely be involved.

Alveolar Echinococcosis

Alveolar echinococcosis, caused by *Echinococcus multilocularis*, is different from the unilocular disease caused by *E. granulosus*. Alveolar echinococcosis may secondarily involve bone. Spinal involvement with bone destruction, spondylitis, and spread to ribs and soft tissues has been reported.[245] CT demonstrates the extent of the disease in bone and soft tissues.

Actinomycosis

Actinomycosis usually involves the mandible and may extend to the facial bones. It often presents with a mixed destructive and sclerotic appearance. The ribs

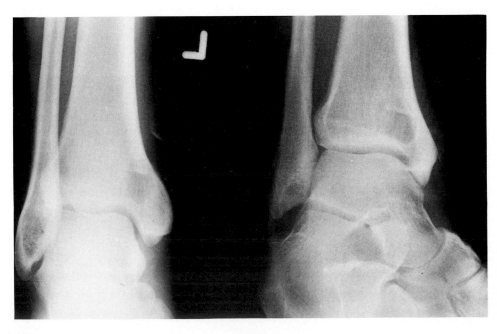

FIGURE 3-97. Intraosseous ganglion of the distal tibia is seen as a small, well-margin-ated radiolucency. (Courtesy of Dr. Harold Rosenbaum, Lexington, KY.)

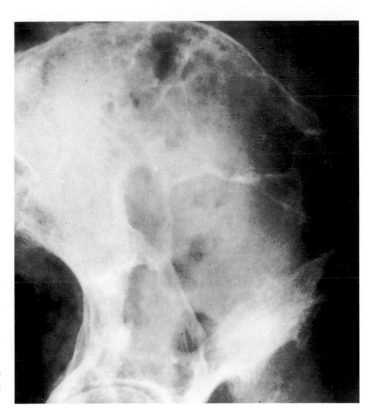

FIGURE 3-98. Echinococcus cyst of the ilium. Notice the large area of radiolucency involving almost the entire bone and the extensive light trabeculation.

(Fig. 3-99), vertebrae (Fig. 3-100), and peripheral skeleton may also be involved.

Blastomycosis

Blastomycosis affects the skeleton as part of a generalized disease.[246,247] Osteolysis initially is seen (Figs. 3-101 and 3-102), followed by sclerosis. The vertebrae, skull, ribs, tibia, tarsus, and knees are most frequently involved.

Coccidioidomycosis

Coccidioidomycosis involves bone by hematogenous spread. A solitary osteolytic lesion is usually first seen without periosteal reaction (Fig. 3-103), and multiple lesions often occur. The lumbar vertebrae are frequently involved (Fig. 3-104). Rib lesions are often associated with an extrapleural mass. Chronic disease may produce some degree of sclerosis.

(*text continues on page 249*)

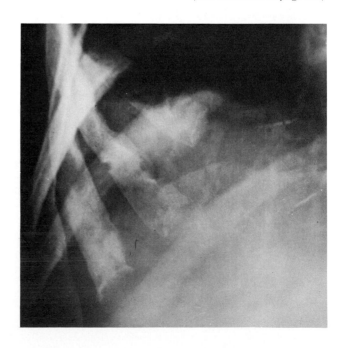

FIGURE 3-99. Actinomycosis of the ribs. Sclerosis and destruction of multiple lower ribs are seen. (Courtesy of Dr. Dharmashi V. Bhate, VA Hospital, Hines, IL.)

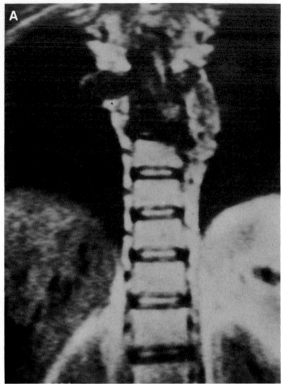

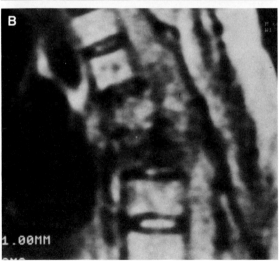

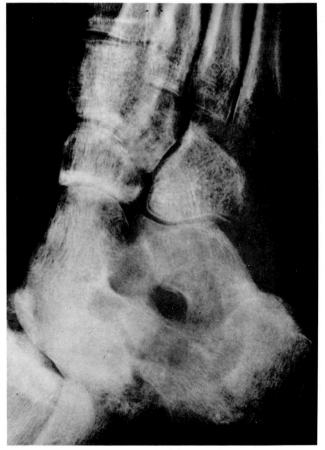

FIGURE 3-100. Actinomycosis of the upper thoracic spine. (**A**) The MR coronal image shows a destructive, low-signal-intensity lesion involving the sixth and seventh thoracic vertebral bodies and their intervertebral space. Paraspinal extension is also evident. (**B**) The sagittal MR image shows destruction as low signal intensity replacing normal marrow fat in the bodies of T6 and T7. Patchy low signal intensity in the bodies of T5 and T8 indicates involvement. Posterior extension of the process into the spinal canal is seen on the T1-weighted images. (Courtesy of Dr. Bong Yoon, Chicago, IL.)

FIGURE 3-101. Blastomycosis of the tarsus. Lytic lesions in the calcaneus and local osteoporosis can be seen.

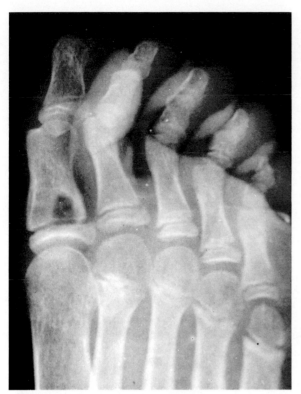

FIGURE 3-102. Blastomycosis. There are radiolucent lesions in the metaphysis of the proximal phalanx of the great toe. No reactive sclerosis is present. There is a minimal amount of periosteal new bone formation at the medial aspect of the shaft. (Courtesy of Dr. Harvey White, Children's Memorial Hospital, Chicago, IL.)

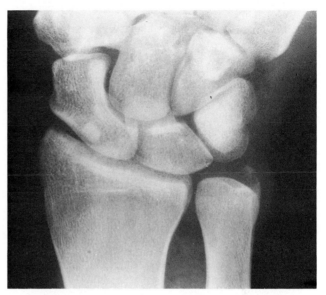

FIGURE 3-103. Coccidioidomycosis of the wrist. Destruction of the ulnar styloid process is associated with soft-tissue swelling. (Courtesy of Dr. Dharmashi V. Bhate, VA Hospital, Hines, IL.)

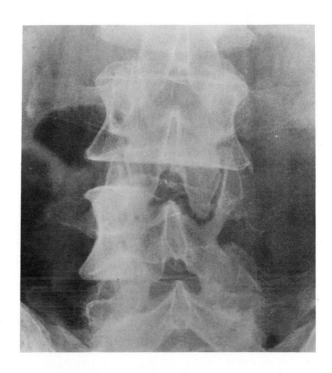

FIGURE 3-104. Coccidioidomycosis. The anteroposterior view reveals destruction of the left half of the body of the fifth lumbar vertebra. (Courtesy of Dr. Dharmashi V. Bhate, VA Hospital, Hines, IL.)

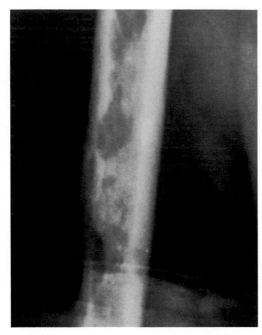

FIGURE 3-105. Sporotrichosis of the humerus. There are osteolytic lesions with cortical destruction and endosteal scalloping. There is no periosteal new bone formation in this patient.

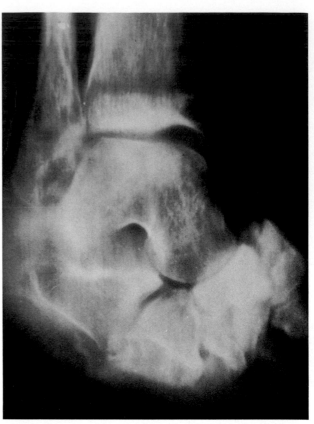

FIGURE 3-106. Sporotrichosis is revealed in a tomogram of the tarsal bones. This is the same patient as in Figure 3-105. Notice the destructive changes and reactive sclerosis.

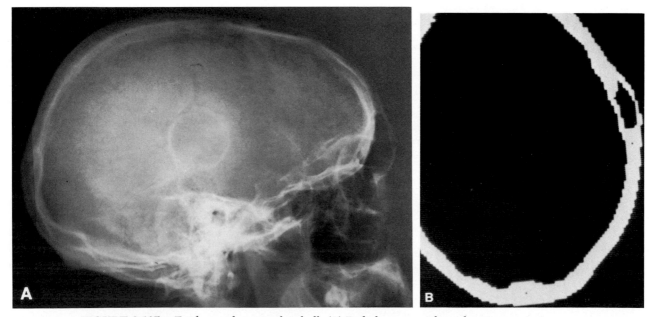

FIGURE 3-107. Epidermoid rest in the skull. (**A**) Radiolucency with a sclerotic margin is seen in the calvarium. (**B**) Computed tomography shows the lesion to be intradiploic and expanding the outer table.

Sporotrichosis and Aspergillosis

Sporotrichosis is caused by the fungus *Sporothrix schenkii*.[248–250] It may involve the bones or joints. In the osseous type, osteoporosis and destructive lesions can be seen (Fig. 3-105). Synovial involvement may resemble pigmented villonodular synovitis, and a destructive arthritis may occur (Fig. 3-106). The knees, elbows, wrists, and small joints of the hands are most often involved. Aspergillosis is another fungus that may involve bone and the paranasal sinuses.[251,252]

Epidermoid Rest

An epidermoid rest in the skull presents as an intradiploic expansile radiolucency with a sclerotic margin en face due to elevation of the edges. CT can demonstrate its location in the calvarium (Fig. 3-107).

Primary Amyloidoma

Primary amyloidoma may affect bones and rarely involve the spine. Destruction of a vertebral body with a paraspinal soft-tissue mass can be seen.[253] Secondary amyloidomas of bone may occur with multiple myeloma and in patients on long-term hemodialysis. Multiple, well-defined, juxtaarticular osteolytic lesions without calcification are seen.[254]

Cementoma

Cementoma of the tubular bones is a rare tumor that resembles tooth cementum histologically. It occurs in patients younger than 20 years of age and may occur in the metaphyses of the femur or humerus. It appears as a multiloculated cyst involving the entire diameter of the bone.[255–256]

Focal Hematopoietic Hyperplasia

Focal hematopoietic hyperplasia of a rib has been reported without underlying hematologic disease. A solitary, expansile rib lesion with focal hyperplasia of all hematopoietic elements was described.[257]

References

1. Hayes CW, Conway WF, Sundaram M: Misleading aggressive MR imaging appearance of some benign musculoskeletal lesions. Radiographics 12:111–134, 1992
2. Sadry F, Hessler C et al: The potential aggressiveness of sinus osteomas. Skeletal Radiol 17:427–430, 1988
3. Güttich H, Müller ES: Brosses stirnhöhlenosteom und reversible blindheit. HNO 15:155–158, 1967
4. Siegler J: Recurrent pyogenic meningitis due to an osteoma of the frontal sinus. J Laryngol Otol 78:226–228, 1964
5. Beale DJ, Phelps PD: Osteomas of the temporal bone: A report of three cases. Clin Radiol 38:67–69, 1987
6. Kolawole TM, Bohrer SP: Ulcer osteoma: Bone response to tropical ulcer. AJR Am J Roentgenol 109:611–618, 1970
7. Chang CH, Piatt ED, Thomas KE, Watne AL: Bone abnormalities in Gardner's syndrome. AJR Am J Roentgenol 103:645–652, 1968
8. Dahlin DC, Unni KK: Bone Tumors. 4th ed. Springfield, IL, Charles C Thomas, 1986
9. Lechner G, Knahr K, Riedl P: Das osteoid-osteom (osteoid osteoma). Fortschr Geb Rontgenstr 128:511–520, 1978
10. Swee RG, McLeod RA, Beabout JW: Osteoid osteoma. Radiology 130:117–123, 1979
11. Bilchik T, Heyman S, Siegel A et al: Osteoid osteoma: The role of radionuclide bone imaging, conventional radiograpy and computed tomography in its management. J Nucl Med 33:269–271, 1992
12. Pettine KA, Klassen RA: Osteoid-osteoma and osteoblastoma of the spine. J Bone Joint Surg [Am] 68:354–361, 1986
13. Kehl DK, Alonso JE, Lovell WW: Scoliosis secondary to an osteoid-osteoma of the rib. J Bone Joint Surg [Am] 65:701–703, 1983
14. Scott M, Lignelli GJ, Shea FJ: Cervical radicular pain secondary to osteoid osteoma of spine. JAMA 217:964–965, 1971
15. Lawrie TR, Aterman K, Path FC, Sinclair AM: Painless osteoid osteoma: A report of 2 cases. J Bone Joint Surg [Am] 52:1357–1363, 1970
16. Herndon JH, Eaton RG, Littler JW: Carpal-tunnel syndrome: An unusual presentation of osteoid-osteoma of the capitate. J Bone Joint Surg [Am] 56:1715–1718, 1974
17. Moser RP, Kransdorf MJ, Brower AC et al: Osteoid osteoma of the elbow. Skeletal Radiol 19:181–186, 1990
18. Greenfield GB: Radiology of Bone Diseases. 5th ed. Philadelphia, JB Lippincott, 1990
19. Brabants K, Geens S et al: Subperiosteal juxta-articular osteoid osteoma. J Bone Joint Surg 68:320–324, 1986
20. Cronemeyer RL, Kirchmer NA, DeSmet AA et al: Intraarticular osteoid-osteoma of the humerus simulating synovitis of the elbow. J Bone Joint Surg [Am] 63:1172–1174, 1981
21. Kattapuram SV, Kushner DC, Phillips WC et al: Osteoid osteoma: An unusual cause of articular pain. Radiology 147:383–387, 1983
22. Norman A, Abdelwahab IF et al: Osteoid osteoma of the hip stimulating an early onset of osteoarthritis. Radiology 158:417–420, 1986
23. Habermann ET, Stern RE: Osteoid osteoma of the tibia in an 8-month-old boy: A case report. J Bone Joint Surg [Am] 56:633–636, 1974
24. Shereff MJ, Cullivan WT, Johnson KA: Osteoid osteoma of the foot. J Bone Joint Surg [Am] 65:638–641, 1983
25. Daly JG: Case report: Osteoid osteoma of the skull. Br J Radiol 46:392–393, 1973
26. Prabhakar B, Reddy DR, Dayananda B, Rao GR: Osteoid osteoma of the skull. J Bone Joint Surg [Br] 54:146–148, 1972
27. Alcalay M, Clarac JP, Bontoux D: Double osteoid-osteoma in adjacent carpal bones. J Bone Joint Surg [Am] 64:779–780, 1982
28. Glynn JL, Lichtestein L: Osteoid osteoma with multicentric nidus. J Bone Joint Surg [Am] 55:855–858, 1973
29. Rand JA, Sim FH, Unni KK: Two osteoid-osteomas in one patient. J Bone Joint Surg [Am] 64:1243–1245, 1982
30. O'Dell CW et al: Osteoid osteomas arising in adjacent bones: Report of a case. J Can Assoc Radiol 27:298–300, 1976
31. Sherman FS: Osteoid osteoma associated with changes in the adjacent joint: Report of 2 cases. J Bone Joint Surg 29:483–490, 1947
32. Snarr JW, Abell MR, Martel W: Lymphofollicular synovitis with osteoid osteoma. Radiology 106:557–560, 1973
33. Gamba JL, Martinez S, Apple J et al: Computed tomography of axial skeletal osteoid osteomas. AJR Am J Roentgenol 142:769–772, 1984

34. Schlesinger AE, Hernandez RJ: Intracapsular osteoid osteoma of the proximal femur: Findings on plain film and CT. AJR Am J Roentgenol 154:1241–1244, 1990
35. Bassett LW, Gold RH, Webber MM: Radionuclide bone imaging. Radiol Clin North Am 19:675–702, 1981
36. Helms CA, Hattner RS, Vogler JB: Osteoid osteoma: Radionuclide diagnosis. Radiology 151:779–784, 1984
37. Ghelman B, Vigorita VJ: Postoperative radionuclide evaluation of osteoid osteomas. Radiology 146:509–512, 1983
38. Goldman AB, Schneider R, Pavlov H: Osteoid osteomas of the femoral neck: Report of four cases evaluated with isotopic bone scanning, CT, and MR imaging. Radiology 186:227–232, 1993
39. Woods ER, Martel W, Mandell SH et al: Reactive soft-tissue mass associated with osteoid osteoma: Correlation of MR imaging features with pathologic findings. Radiology 186:221–225, 1993
40. Biebuyck JC, Katz LD, McCauley T: Soft tissue edema in osteoid osteoma. Skeletal Radiol 22:37–41, 1993
41. Yaghamai I: Angiography of Bone and Soft Tissue Lesions. New York, Springer-Verlag, 1979
42. Bettelli G, Tigani D, Picci P: Recurring osteoblastoma initially presenting as a typical osteoid osteoma. Report of two cases. Skeletal Radiol 20:1–4, 1991
43. Kopp WK: Benign osteoblastoma of the coronoid process of the mandible: Report of a case. J Oral Maxillofac Surg 27:653–655, 1969
44. Lichtenstein L, Sawyer WR: Benign osteoblastoma: Further observations and report of 20 additional cases. J Bone Joint Surg [Am] 46:755–765, 1964
45. McLeod RA, Dahlin DC, Beabout JW: The spectrum of osteoblastoma. AJR Am J Roentgenol 126:321–335, 1976
46. Schajowicz F, Lemos C: Osteoid osteoma and osteoblastoma. Acta Orthop Scand 41:272–291, 1970
47. Tulloh HP, Harry D: Osteoblastoma in a rib in childhood. Clin Radiol 20:337–338, 1969
48. Kroon HM, Schurmans J: Osteoblastoma: Clinical and radiologic findings in 98 new cases. Radiology 175:783–790, 1990
49. Akbarnia BA, Rooholamini SA: Scoliosis caused by benign osteoblastoma of the thoracic or lumbar spine. J Bone Joint Surg [Am] 63:1146–1155, 1981
50. Gelberman RH, Olson CO: Benign osteoblastoma of the atlas: A case report. J Bone Joint Surg [Am] 56:808–810, 1974
51. Segal P, Hoeffel JC et al: Osteoblastome du premier metatarsien. J Radiol 68:533–535, 1987
52. Hoeffel JC, Segal P, Abadou H et al: Osteoblastoma of the first metatarsal bone. Fortschr.Rontgenstr 151:506–507, 1989
53. Capanna R, Van Horn JR et al: Osteoid osteoma and osteoblastoma of the talus: A report of 40 cases. Skeletal Radiol 15:360–364, 1986
54. Crim JR, Mirra JM, Edkardt JJ et al: Widespread inflammatory response to osteoblastoma: The flare phenomenon. Radiology 177:835–836, 1990
55. Mitchell ML, Ackerman LV: Metastatic and pseudomalignant osteoblastoma: A report of two unusual cases. Skeletal Radiol 15:213–218, 1986
56. Lingg VG, Roessner A et al: Zur roentgenmorphologie und pathologischen anatomie des osteoblastoms. Fortschr Geb Rontgenstr 145:49–56, 1986
57. Delahaye RP, Metges PJ, Lomazzi R, Capeau F: About 3 cases of sus epitrochlear process of the humerus: Radioclinical approach and review of the literature. J Radiol 57:341–345, 1976
58. Newman A: The supracondylar process and its fracture. AJR Am J Roentgenol 105:844–849, 1969
59. Evison G, Price CHG: Subungual exostosis. Br J Radiol 39:451–455, 1966
60. Murphy FD, Blount WB: Cartilaginous exostosis following irradiation. J Bone Joint Surg [Am] 44:662–668, 1962
61. Keating RB, Wright PW et al: Enchondroma protuberans of the rib. Skeletal Radiol 13:55–58, 1985
62. Caffey J, Silverman FN: Pediatric X-ray Diagnosis. 5th ed. Chicago, Year Medical Book Publishers, 1967
63. Vallance R, Hamblen DL et al: Vascular complications of osteochondroma. Clin Radiol 36:639–642, 1985
64. Matthews MG: Unilateral oedema of the lower limb caused by osteochondroma. J Bone Joint Surg [Br] 69:339–340, 1987
65. Gomez-Reino JJ, Radin A, Gorevic PD: Pseudoaneurysm of the popliteal artery as a complication of an osteochondroma. Skeletal Radiol 4:26–28, 1979
66. Anderson RL, Popowitz L, Li JKH: An unusual sarcoma rising in a solitary osteochondroma. J Bone Joint Surg [Am] 51:1199–1204, 1969
67. Callan JE, Wood VE: Spontaneous resolution of an osteochondroma. J Bone Joint Surg [Am] 57:723, 1975
68. Paling MR: The "disappearing" osteochondroma. Skeletal Radiol 10:40–42, 1983
69. Novick GS, Pavlov H, Bullough PG: Osteochondroma of the cervical spine: Report of two cases in preadolescent males. Skeletal Radiol 8:13–15, 1982
70. Lee JK, Yao L et al: MR imaging of solitary osteochondromas: Report of eight cases. AJR Am J Roentgenol 149:557–560, 1987
71. DeSimone DP, Abdelwahab IF, Kenan S et al: Case report 785. Skeletal Radiol 22:289–291, 1993
72. Griffiths HJ, Thompson RC, Galloway HR et al: Bursitis in association with solitary osteochondromas presenting as mass lesions. Skeletal Radiol 20:513–516, 1991
73. Stark JD, Adler NN, Robinson WH: Hereditary multiple exostoses. Radiology 59:212–215, 1952
73a. Ogden JA: Multiple hereditary osteochondromata. Report of an early case. Clin Orthop 116:48–60, 1976
74. Bock GW, Reed MH: Forearm deformities in multiple cartilaginous exostoses. Skeletal Radiol 20:483–486, 1991
75. Twersky J, Kassner EG, Tenner MS, Camera A: Vertebral and costal osteochondromas causing spinal cord compression. AJR Am J Roentgenol 124:124–128, 1975
76. Hershey SL, Lansden FT: Osteochondromas as a cause of false popliteal aneurysms: Review of the literature and report of 2 cases. J Bone Joint Surg [Am] 54:1765–1768, 1972
77. Schmoller H, Suwandschieff N: Eine aussergewöhnliche komplikation bei multiplen kartilaginären exostosen. Fortschr Geb Rontgenstr 123:273–275, 1975
78. Resnik CS, Levine AM, Aisner SC et al: Case report 522. Skeletal Radiol 18:66–69, 1989
79. Lammot TR: Enchondroma of the patella: A case report. J Bone Joint Surg [Am] 50:1230–1232, 1968
80. Takigawa K: Chondroma of the bones of the hand: A review of 110 cases. J Bone Joint Surg [Am] 53:1591–1600, 1971
81. Pandey S: Giant chondromas arising from the ribs. J Bone Joint Surg [Br] 57:519–522, 1975
82. Hamlin JA, Adler L, Greenbaum EI: Central enchondroma: A precursor to chondrosarcoma. J Can Assoc Radiol 22:206–209, 1971
83. Aoki JA, Sone S, Fujioka F et al: MR of enchondroma and chondrosarcoma: Rings and arcs of Gd-DDPTA enhancement. J Comp Asst Tomogr 15:1011–1016, 1991
84. Rubin R: Dynamic Classification of Bone Dysplasias. Chicago, Year Book Medical Publishers, 1964
85. Unger EC, Kessler HB et al: MR imaging of Maffucci syndrome. AJR Am J Roentgenol 150:351–353, 1988
86. Schwartz HS, Zimmerman NB et al: The malignant potential of enchondromatosis. J Bone Joint Surg 69:269–274, 1987
87. Keating RB, Wright PW et al: Enchondroma protuberans of the rib. Skeletal Radiol 13:55–58, 1985
88. Cary GR: Juxtacortical chondroma: A case report. J Bone Joint Surg [Am] 47:1405–1407, 1965
89. Rockwell MA, Saiter ET, Enneking WF: Periosteal chondroma. J Bone Joint Surg [Am] 54:102–108, 1972

90. Jaffe HL: Tumors and Tumorous Conditions of the Bones and Joints. Philadelphia, Lea & Febiger, 1958
91. McLeod RA, Beabout JW: The roentgenographic features of chondroblastoma. AJR Am J Roentgenol 118:464–471, 1973
92. Boriani S, Bacchini P, Bertoni F: Periosteal chondroma. J Bone Joint Surg [Am] 65:205–212, 1983
93. deSantos LA, Spjut HJ: Periosteal chondroma: A radiographic spectrum. Skeletal Radiol 6:15–20, 1981
94. Nolan DJ, Middlemiss H: Chondroblastoma of bone. Clin Radiol 26:343–350, 1975
95. Plum GE, Pugh DG: Roentgenologic aspects of benign chondroblastoma of bone. AJR Am J Roentgenol 79:584–591, 1958
96. Schajowicz F, Gallardo H: Epiphyseal chondroblastoma of bone. J Bone Joint Surg [Br] 52:205–226, 1970
97. Sundaram TKS: Benign chondroblastoma. J Bone Joint Surg [Br] 48:92–104, 1966
98. Hudson TM, Hawkings IF: Radiological evaluation of chondroblastoma. Radiology 139:1–10, 1981
99. Fechner RE, Wilde HD: Chondroblastoma in the metaphysis of the femoral neck. J Bone Joint Surg [Am] 56:413–415, 1974
100. Kricun ME, Kricun R, Haskin ME: Chondroblastoma of the calcaneus: Radiographic features with emphasis on location. AJR Am J Roentgenol 128:613–616, 1977
101. Cohen J, Cahen I: Benign chondroblastoma of the patella: A case report. J Bone Joint Surg [Am] 45:824–826, 1963
102. Moser RP Jr, Brockmole DM et al: Chondroblastoma of the patella. Skeletal Radiol 17:413–419, 1988
103. Neviaser RJ, Wilson JN: Benign chondroblastoma of the finger. J Bone Joint Surg [Am] 54:389–392, 1972
104. Matsuno T, Hasegawa I et al: Chondroblastoma arising in the triradiate cartilage. Skeletal Radiol 16:216–22, 1987
105. Braunstein E, Martel W, Weatherbee L: Periosteal bone apposition in chondroblastoma. Skeletal Radiol 4:34–36, 1979
106. Brower AC, Moser RP, Kransdorf MJ: The frequency and diagnostic significance of periostitis in chondroblastoma. AJR Am J Roentgenol 154:309–314, 1990
107. Gohel VK, Dalinka MK, Edeiken J: Ischemic necrosis of the femoral head simulating chondroblastoma. Radiology 107:545–546, 1973
108. Bloem JL, Mulder JD: Chondroblastoma: A clinical and radiological study of 104 cases. Skeletal Radiol 14:1–9, 1985.
109. McLaughlin RE, Sweet DE, Webster T, Merritt WM: Chondroblastoma of the pelvis suggestive of malignancy: Report of an unusual case treated by wide pelvic excision. J Bone Joint Surg [Am] 57:549–550, 1975
110. Beggs IG, Stoker DJ: Chondromyxoid fibroma of bone. Clin Radiol 33:671–679, 1982
111. Dahlin DC, Wells AH: Chondromyxoid fibroma of bone: Report of 2 cases. J Bone Joint Surg [Am] 35:831–834, 1953
112. Feldman F, Hecht HL, Johnston AD: Chondromyxoid fibroma of bone. Radiology 94:249–260, 1970
113. Murphy NB, Price CHG: The radiological aspects of chondromyxoid fibroma of bone. Clin Radiol 22:261–269, 1971
114. Vix VA: Unusual appearance of a chondromyxoid fibroma. Radiology 92:365–366, 1969
115. Wilson AJ, Kyriakos M, Ackerman LV: Chondromyxoid fibroma: Radiographic appearance in 38 cases and in a review of the literature. Radiology 179:513–518, 1991
116. Gherlinzoni F, Rock M, Picci P: Chondromyxoid fibroma. J Bone Joint Surg [Am] 65:198–204, 1983
117. Ribalta T, Ro JY, Carrasco CH et al: Case report 638. Skeletal Radiol 19:549–551, 1990
118. Sellami M, Doyon D, Deboise A et al: Fibrome chondromyxoide de l'articulation temporo-mandibulaire. J Radiol 65:97–100, 1984
119. Prentice AID: Variations on the fibrous cortical defect. Clin Radiol 25:531–533, 1974
120. Schmidt M, Thiel HJ, Spitz J: Der fibroese kortikalisdefekt. Fortschr Geb Rontgenstr 128:521–524, 1978
121. Ritschl P, Karnel F et al: Fibrous metaphyseal defects: Determination of their origin and natural history using a radiomorphological study. Skeletal Radiol 17:8–15, 1988
122. Freyschmidt VJ, Ostertag H, Saure D: Der fibrose metaphysare defekt (fibroser kortikalisdefekt nicht-ossifizierendes knochenfibrom). Fortschr Geb Rontgenstr 134:392–400, 1981
123. Kumar R, Swischuk LE, et al: Benign cortical defect: Site for an avulsion fracture. Skeletal Radiol 15:553–555, 1986
124. Bertoni F, Calderoni P, Bacchini P et al: Desmoplastic fibroma of bone. J Bone Joint Surg [Br] 66:265–268, 1984
125. Cohen P, Goldenberg RR: Desmoplastic fibroma of bone: Report of 2 cases. J Bone Joint Surg [Am] 47:1620–1625, 1965
126. Sugiura I: Desmoplastic fibroma: A case report and review of the literature. J Bone Joint Surg [Am] 58:126–129, 1976
127. Crim JR, Gold RH, Mirra JM et al: Desmoplastic fibroma of bone: Radiographic analysis. Radiology 172:827–832, 1989
128. Greenspan A, Unni KK. Case report 787. Skeletal Radiol 22:296–299, 1993
129. Omojola MF, Cockshott WP, Beatty EG: Desmoplastic fibroma. J Can Assoc Radiol 31:273–275, 1980
130. Young WR, Aisner SC et al: Computed tomography of desmoid tumors of bone: Desmoplastic fibroma. Skeletal Radiol 17:333–337, 1988
131. Brower AC, Culver JE, Keats TE: Histological nature of the cortical irregularity of the medial posterior distal femoral metaphysis in children. Radiology 99:389–392, 1971
132. Castleman B, McNeill MJ: Bone and Joint Clinicopathological Conferences of the Massachusettes General Hospital. Boston, Little, Brown & Co, 1966
133. Feine VU, Ahlemann LM: Das periostal desmoid im metaphysenbereich und seine differentialdiagnostiche abgrenzung von bosartigen knochentumoren durch das knochenszintigramm. Fortschr Geb Rontgenstr 135:193–196, 1981
134. Kimmelstiel P, Rapp IH: Cortical defect due to periosteal desmoids. Bull Hosp Joint Dis Orthop Inst 12:286–297, 1951
135. Barnes GR, Gwinn JL: Distal irregularities of the femur simulating malignancy. AJR Am J Roentgenol 122:180–185, 1974
136. Pennes DR, Braunstein EM, Glazer GM: Computed tomography of cortical desmoid. Skeletal Radiol 12:40–42, 1984
137. Cohen J: Etiology of simple bone cyst. J Bone Joint Surg [Am] 52:1493–1497, 1970
138. Norman A, Schiffman M: Simple bone cysts: Factors of age dependency. Radiology 124:779–782, 1977
139. Ewald FC: Bone cyst in a phalanx of a 2 -year-old child. J Bone Joint Surg [Am] 54:399–401, 1972
140. Smith RW, Smith CF: Solitary unicameral bone cyst of the calcaneus: A review of 20 cases. J Bone Joint Surg [Am] 56:49–56, 1974
141. Ehara S, Rosenberg AE, El-Khoury GY: Sacral cysts with exophytic components. A report of two cases. Skeletal Radiol 19:117–119, 1990
142. Sadler AH, Rosenhain F: Occurrence of 2 unicameral bone cysts in the same patient. J Bone Joint Surg [Am] 46:1557–1560, 1964
143. Hutter CG: Unicameral bone cyst: A report of an unusual case. J Bone Joint Surg [Am] 32:430–432, 1950
144. Moed BR, LaMont RL: Unicameral bone cyst complicated by growth retardation. J Bone Joint Surg [Am] 64:1379–1381, 1982
145. Reynolds J: The "fallen fragment sign" in the diagnosis of unicameral bone cysts. Radiology 92:949–953, 1969
146. Sanerkin NG: Old fibrin coagula and their ossification in simple bone cysts. J Bone Joint Surg [Br] 61:194–199, 1979

147. Keats TK, Harrison RB: The calcaneal nutrient foramen: A useful sign of the differentiation of true from simulated cysts. Skeletal Radiol 3:239–240, 1979

148. Resnick D, Conne RO: The nature of humeral pseudocysts. Radiology 150:27–28, 1984

149. Glass TA, Dyer R, Fisher L et al: Expansile subchondral bone cyst. AJR Am J Roentgenol 139:1210–1211, 1982

150. Phillips CD, Keats TE: The development of post-traumatic cyst-like lesions in bone. Skeletal Radiol 15:631–634, 1986

151. Taxin RN, Feldman F: The tumbling bullet sign in a post-traumatic bone cyst. AJR Am J Roentgenol 123:140–143, 1975

152. Moore TE, King AR, Travis RC et al: Post-traumatic cysts and cyst-like lesions of bone. Skeletal Radiol 18:93–97, 1989

153. Helms CA: Pseudocysts of the humerus. AJR Am J Roentgenol 131:287–288, 1978

154. Blumberg ML: CT of iliac unicameral bone cysts. AJR Am J Roentgenol 136:1231–1232, 1981

155. Fernbach SK, Blumenthal DH, Poznanski AK et al: Radiographic changes in unicameral bone cysts following direct injection of sterioids: A report on 14 cases. Radiology 140:689–695, 1981

156. Lemmens JAM, Huynen CHJN et al: MR imaging of cystic lesion of the bone. Fortschr Geb Rontgenstr 143:362–364, 1985

157. Bonakdarpour A, Levy WM, Aegerter E: Primary and secondary aneurysmal bone cyst: A radiological study of 75 cases. Radiology 126:75–83, 1978

158. Carlson DH, Wilkinson RH, Bhakkaviziam A: Aneurysmal bone cysts in children. AJR Am J Roentgenol 116:644–650, 1972

159. Dahlin DC, Besse BE, Pugh DG, Ghormley RK: Aneurysmal bone cysts. Radiology 64:56–65, 1955

160. Dahlin DC, McLeod RA: Aneurysmal bone cyst and other nonneoplastic conditions. Skeletal Radiol 8:243–250, 1982

161. Slowick FA, Campbell CJ, Kettlekamp DB: Aneurysmal bone cyst: An analysis of 13 cases. J Bone Joint Surg [Am] 50:1142–1151, 1968

162. Diercks RL, Sauter AJM et al: Aneurysmal bone cyst in association with fibrous dysplasia: A case report. J Bone Joint Surg [Br] 68:144–146, 1986

163. Dabezies EJ, D'Ambrosia RD, Chuinard RG et al: Aneurysmal bone cyst after fracture. J Bone Joint Surg [Am] 64:617, 1982

164. Buirski G, Watt I: The radiological features of "solid" aneurysmal bone cysts. Br J Radiol 57:1057–1065, 1984

165. Chateil JF, Coindre JM et al: Localisation rachidienne d'un kyste aneurysmal solide: Aspects cliniques, radiographiques et histopathologiques. J Radiol 68:805–808, 1987

166. Hay MC, Paterson D, Taylor TKF: Aneurysmal bone cysts of the spine. J Bone Joint Surg [Br] 60:406, 1978

167. Burns-Cox CJ, Higgins AT: Aneurysmal bone cyst of the frontal bone. J Bone Joint Surg [Br] 51:344–345, 1969

168. O'Gorman AM, Kirkham TH: Aneurysmal bone cyst of the orbit with unusual angiographic features. AJR Am J Roentgenol 126:896–899, 1976

169. Huettig G, Rittmeyer K: Multiple aneurysmatische knochenzysten bei 3 monate altem saeugling. Fortschritte a/d Gebiet Röntgenstrahlen 129:796, 1978

170. Dyer R, Stelling CB, Fechner RE: Epiphyseal extension of an aneurysmal bone cyst. AJR Am J Roentgenol 137:172–173, 1981

171. Henley FT, Richetts GL: Aneurysmal bone cyst presenting as a chest mass: A case report. Radiology 92:1103–1104, 1969

172. Capanna R, Van Horn JR, Biagini R et al: Aneurysmal bone cyst of the sacrum. Skeletal Radiol 18:109–113, 1989

173. Hertzanu Y, Mendelsohn DB, Gottschalk F: Aneurysmal bone cyst of the calcaneus. Radiology 151:51–52, 1984

174. Hudson TM: Fluid levels in aneurysmal bone cysts. AJR Am J Roentgenol 142:1001–1004, 1984

175. Hudson TM: Scintigraphy of aneurysmal bone cysts. AJR Am J Roentgenol 142:761–765, 1984

176. Beltran J, Simon DC et al: Aneurysmal bone cysts: MR imaging at 1.5 T. Radiology 158:689–690, 1986

177. Mohan V, Gupta SK, Tuli SM, Sanyal B: Symptomatic vertebral haemangiomas. Clin Radiol 31:575–579, 1980

178. Sherman RS, Wilner D: Roentgen diagnosis of hemangioma of bone. AJR Am J Roentgenol 66:587–594, 1951

179. Baker ND, Greenspan A et al: Symptomatic vertebral hemangiomas: A report of four cases. Skeletal Radiol 15:458–463, 1986

180. Ross JS, Masaryk TJ et al: Vertebral hemangiomas: MR imaging. Radiology 165:165–169, 1987

181. Laredo JD, Assouline E, Gelbert F et al: Vertebral hemangiomas: Fat content as a sign of aggressiveness. Radiology 177:467–472, 1990

182. Braitinger VS, Weigert F, Held P et al: CT und MRI von Wirbelhamangiomen. Fortschr Geb Roentgenstr 151,4: 399–407, 1989

183. Karlin CA, Brower AC: Multiple primary hemangiomas of bone. AJR Am J Roentgenol 129:162–164, 1977

184. Sherman RS, Wilner D: Roentgen diagnosis of hemangioma of bone. AJR Am J Roentgenol 86:1146–1159, 1961

185. Singh R, Grewal DS, Bannerjee AK, Bênsal VP: Haemangiomatosis of the skeleton. J Bone Joint Surg [Br] 56:136–138, 1974

186. Suss RA, Kumar AJ, Dorfman HD et al: Capillary hemangioma of the sphenoid bone. Skeletal Radiol 11:102–107, 1984

187. Bullough PG, Goodfellow JW: Solitary lymphangioma of bone: A case report. J Bone Joint Surg [Am] 58:418–419, 1976

188. Kopperman M, Antoine JE: Primary lymphangioma of the calvarium. AJR Am J Roentgenol 121:118–120, 1974

189. Abrahams J, Ganick D, Gilbert E et al: Massive osteolysis in an infant. AJR Am J Roentgenol 135:1084–1086, 1980

190. Blundell G, Midgley RL, Smith GS: Massive osteolysis: Disappearing bones. J Bone Joint Surg [Br] 40:494–501, 1958

191. Cadenat H, Combelles R, Fabert G, Clovet M: Ostéolyse cryptogénétique de la mandibule. J Radiol 59:509–512, 1978

192. Kery L, Wouters HW: Massive osteolysis: A report of 2 cases. J Bone Joint Surg [Br] 52:452–459, 1970

193. Patrick JH: Massive osteolysis complicated by chylothorax successfully treated by pleurodesis. J Bone Joint Surg [Br] 58:347–349, 1976

194. Sacristan HD, Portal LF, Castresana FG, Pena DR: Massive osteolysis of the scapula and ribs: A case report. J Bone Joint Surg [Am] 59:405–406, 1977

195. Sage MR, Allen PW: Massive osteolysis. J Bone Joint Surg [Br] 56:130–135, 1974

196. Kolar J, Zidková H, Vohralik M et al: Langristige teilremission des Gorhamschen syndroms. Fortschr Geb Rontgenstr 134:214–215, 1981

197. Campbell J, Almond HGA, Johnson R: Massive osteolysis of the humerus with spontaneous recovery. J Bone Joint Surg [Br] 57:238–240, 1975

198. Daffner RH, Martinez S, Gehweller JA et al: Stress fractures of the proximal tibia in runners. Radiology 142:63–65, 1982

199. Kaltsas DS: Stress fractures of the femoral neck in young adults. J Bone Joint Surg [Br] 63:33–37, 1981

200. Daffner RH, Pavlov H: Stress fractures: Current concepts. AJR Am J Roentgenol 159:245–252, 1992

201. Bauer G, Gustafsson K, Mortensson W et al: Insufficiency fractures in the tibial condyles in elderly individuals. Acta Radiol [Diagn] 22:619–622, 1981

202. Gaucher A, Regent D et al: Les fractures par insuffisance osseouse du sacrum. J Radiol 68:433–440, 1987

203. Aymard A, Chevrot A et al: Fracture spontanee du sternum. J Radiol 68:593–595, 1987

204. Kathol MH, El-Khoury GY, Moore TE et al: Calcaneal insufficiency avulsion fractures in patients with diabetes mellitis. Radiology 180:725–729, 1991
205. Miller B, Markheim HR, Towbin MN: Multiple stress fractures in rheumatoid arthritis: A case report. J Bone Joint Surg [Am] 49:1408–1414, 1967
206. Levin DC, Blazina ME, Levine E: Fatigue fractures of the shaft of the femur: Simulation of malignant tumor. Radiology 89:883–885, 1967
207. Murcia M, Brennan RE, Edeiken J: Computed tomography of stress fracture. Skeletal Radiol 8:193–195, 1982
208. Yousem D, Magid D et al: Computed tomography of stress fractures. J Comput Assist Tomogr 10:92–95, 1986
209. Nussbaum AR, Treves ST et al: Bone stress lesions in ballet dancers: Scintigraphic assessment. AJR Am J Roentgenol 150:851–855, 1988
210. Greaney RB, Gerber FH, Laughlin RL et al: Distribution and natural history of stress fractures in U.S. Marine recruits. Radiology 146:339–346, 1983
211. Abe H, Nakamura M, Takahashi S et al: Radiation-induced insufficiency fractures of the pelvis: Evaluation with ^{99m}Tc-methylene diphosphonate scintigraphy. AJR Am J Roentgenol 158:599–602, 1992
212. Lee JK, Yao L: Stress fractures: MR imaging. Radiology 169:217–220, 1988
213. Brahme SK, Cervilla V, Vint V et al: Magnetic resonance appearance of sacral insufficiency fractures. Skeletal Radiol 19:489–493, 1990
214. Tang TT et al: Angioglomoid tumor of bone. J Bone Joint Surg [Am] 58:873–876, 1976
215. Fornage BD: Glomus tumors in the fingers: Diagnosis with US. Radiology 167:183–185, 1988
216. Pambakian H, Smith MA: Glomus tumours of the coccygeal body associated with coccydynia. J Bone Joint Surg [Br] 63:424–426, 1981
217. Schwarz E: Ossifying fibroma of the face and skull. AJR Am J Roentgenol 91:1012–1015, 1964
218. Majewski VA, Freyschmidt J, Steinmeyer R et al: Das ossifizierende knochenfibrom (OF). Fortschr Geb Rontgenstr 140:179–187, 1984
219. Hanelin LG, Sclamberg EL, Bardsley JL: Intraosseous lipoma of the coccyx: Report of a case. Radiology 114:343–344, 1975
220. Ehara S, Kattapuram SV, Rosenberg AE: Case report 619. Skeletal Radiol 19:375–376, 1990
221. Milgram JW: Intraosseous lipomas with reactive ossification in the proximal femur. Skeletal Radiol 7:1–13, 1981
222. Freiberg RA, Air GW, Glueck J et al: Multiple intraosseous lipomas with type IV hyperlipoproteinemia: A case report. J Bone Joint Surg [Am] 56:1729–1732, 1974
223. Ramos A, Castello J et al: Osseous lipoma: CT appearance. Radiology 157:615–619, 1985
224. Milgram JW: Malignant transformation in bone lipomas. Skeletal Radiol 19:347–352, 1990
225. Agha FP, Lilienfeld RM: Roentgen features of osseous neurilemmoma. Radiology 102:325–326, 1972
226. Caballes RL: Fibromyxoma of bone. Radiology 130:97–99, 1979
227. Hill JA et al: Myxoma of the toes: A case report. J Bone Joint Surg [Am] 60:128–130, 1978
228. Abdelwahab IF, Hermann G, Klein MJ et al: Fibromyxoma of bone. Skeletal Radiol 20:95–98, 1991
229. Sartoris DJ, Pate D et al: Plasma cell sclerosis of bone: A spectrum of disease. J Can Assoc Radiol 37:25–34, 1986
230. Martin B, deLatour FB: MR imaging of anterior sacral meningocele: Case report. J Comput Assist Tomogr 12:166–167, 1988
231. Sundaram M, Awwad EE: Magnetic resonance imaging of arachnoid cysts destroying the sacrum. AJR Am J Roentgenol 146:359–360, 1986
232. Hensley CD: Epidermoid cyst of the distal phalanx occurring in an 8-year-old child: A case report. J Bone Joint Surg [Am] 48:946–948, 1966
233. Lerner MR, Southwick WO: Keratin cysts in phalangeal bones: Report of an unusual case. J Bone Joint Surg [Am] 50:365–372, 1968
234. Mollan RAB, Wray AR, Hayes D: Traumatic epidermoid cyst of the ulna. J Bone Joint Surg [Br] 64:456–457, 1982
235. Weston WJ: Thorn and twig-induced pseudotumours of bone and soft tissues. Br J Radiol 36:323–326, 1963
236. Swischuk LE, Jorgenson F, Caden D: Wooden splinter induced "pseudotumors" and "osteomyelitis-like" lesions of bone and soft tissue. AJR Am J Roentgenol 122:176–179, 1974
237. Crabbe WA: Intraosseous ganglions in bone. Br J Surg 53:15–17, 1966
238. Feldman F, Johnston A: Intraosseous ganglion. AJR Am J Roentgenol 118:328–343, 1973
239. Prager PJ, Menges V, DiBiase M: The intraosseous ganglion. Fortschr Geb Rontgenstr 123:458–461, 1975
240. Seymour N: Intraosseous ganglia: Report of 2 cases. J Bone Joint Surg [Br] 50:134–137, 1968
241. Abdelwahab IF, Kenan S, Hermann G et al: Periosteal ganglia: CT and MR imaging features. Radiology 188:245–248, 1993
242. Hsieh CK: Echinococcus involvement of bone with x-ray examination. Radiology 14:562–575, 1930
243. Pintilie DC, Panoza GH, Hatman VD, Fahrer M: Echinococcosis of the humerus: Treatment by resection and bone grafting. J Bone Joint Surg [Am] 48:957–962, 1966
244. Torricelli P, Martinelli C, Biagini R et al: Radiographic and computed tomographic findings in hydatid disease of bone. Skeletal Radiol 19:435–439, 1990
245. Claudon M, Bracard S et al: Spinal involvement in alveolar echinococcosis: Assessment of two cases. Radiology 162:571–572, 1987
246. Joyce PF et al: A rare clinical presentation of blastomycosis. Skeletal Radiol 2:239–242, 1977
247. Moore RM, Green NE: Blastomycosis of bone. J Bone Joint Surg [Am] 64:1097–1101, 1982
248. Comstock C, Wolson AH: Roentgenology of spoirotrichosis. AJR 125:651–655, 1975
249. Winter TQ, Pearson KD: Systemic sporothrixosis. Radiology 104:579–584, 1972
250. Chang AC, Destouet JM, Murphy WA: Muscuoskeletal sporotrichosis. Skeletal Radiol 12:23–28, 1984
251. Grossman M: Aspergillosis of bone. Br J Radiol 48:57–59, 1975
252. Rudwan MA, Sheikh NA: Aspergilloma of paranasal sinuses: A common cause of unilateral proptosis in Sudan. Clin Radiol 27:497–502, 1976
253. Pawar S, Kay CJ, Anderson HH et al: Primary amyloidoma of the spine. J Comput Assist Tomogr 6:1175–1177, 1982
254. Ross LV, Ross GJ, Mesgarzadeh M et al: Hemodialysis-related amyloidomas of bone. Radiology 178:263–265, 1991
255. Adler CP: Tumour-like lesions in the femur with cementum-like material: Does a "cementoma" of long bone exist? Skeletal Radiol 14:26–37, 1985
256. Kolar JJ, Horn V, Zidkova H et al: Cementifying fibroma (so-called "cementoma") of tibia. Br J Radiol 54:989–992, 1981
257. Edelstein G, Kyriakos M: Focal hematopoietic hyperplasia of the rib: A form of pseudotumor. Skeletal Radiol 11:108–118, 1984

Imaging of Bone Tumors: A Multimodality Approach,
edited by George B. Greenfield and John A. Arrington,
J. B. Lippincott Company, Philadelphia © 1995.

chapter

FOUR

SOFT-TISSUE TUMORS

Imaging Modalities for Evaluating Soft-Tissue Tumors
> Conventional Radiography
> Ultrasonography
> Computed Tomography
> Radionuclide Bone Scanning
> Arteriography
> Magnetic Resonance Imaging
> Arthrography

Staging of Soft-Tissue Tumors
Classification of Soft-Tissue Tumors
Differential Diagnosis of Soft-Tissue Tumors
> Fibrohistiocytic and Fibrous Tumors
> Fatty Tumors
> Vascular Soft-Tissue Tumors
> Muscle Tumors
> Synovial Tumors
> Tumors of Peripheral Nerves and Nerve Sheaths
> Calcified Soft-Tissue Masses
> Soft-Tissue Infections
> Soft-Tissue Edema

IMAGING MODALITIES FOR EVALUATING SOFT-TISSUE TUMORS

Conventional Radiography

All soft-tissue tumors are seen as equal to water density on conventional radiographs except those containing fat, hemosiderin, or calcium,[1,2] and a definitive diagnosis based on the plain film appearance is only rarely possible. There are no soft-tissue tumor diagnostic features, as there are in the assessment of bone tumors (e.g., patterns of cortical and periosteal response) to give us a clue to the diagnosis on plain films. However, the fat, hemosiderin, and calcium content can be seen. The behavior of the tumor with respect to bone (e.g., saucerization, erosion or invasion, sclerotic reaction) can be better seen in the extremities with conventional radiographs than with other modalities. Infiltration of a fatty tumor along muscle planes may be determined, and specific characteristics, such as phleboliths and patterns of calcification and bone formation, are important clues to the identity of a tumor and best seen on conventional films.

Ultrasonography

Sonography is useful in the evaluation of soft-tissue masses, especially in the distal extremities, where fat is sparse. It can define solid, cystic, or mixed lesions and evaluate the size of a lesion. Discrete echo patterns, with reduced echoes and a clearly defined lesion margin, are likely to be malignant.[3] Ultrasonography is particularly useful for determining the relation of a soft-tissue tumor to a major nerve or vessel. Color flow Doppler is useful in demonstrating the vascularity of a mass and in determining whether a mass represents a vascular malformation. Ultrasonography is useful in routine follow-up and in localization for needle biopsies.

Magnetic resonance imaging (MRI) and sonography have been reported to be equally useful in detecting local recurrences of soft-tissue sarcomas, except in the early postoperative period, during which MRI is more conclusive.[4]

Computed Tomography

Computed tomography (CT) is second only to MRI as a modality in the work-up of a patient with a soft-tissue mass.[5,6] It can demonstrate a lesion based on differences in tissue attenuation, anatomic changes, and vascular enhancement. One advantage is its ability to define fatty tumors. It is not possible to correlate attenuation values with the histologic type or grade of malignancy.[5] An isodense lesion is very difficult to detect. The size of a lesion can usually be determined, and bony changes can be well seen, better than with MRI.

A contrast-enhanced examination is of value, although most soft-tissue lesions show little enhancement.[6] Anatomic detail and the relations to the neurovascular bundle can be demonstrated, but not as well as on MR images. CT can be used to diagnose aneurysms and show relations to major blood vessels. It is invaluable as a guide for needle biopsy.

CT is useful in detecting skeletal muscle metastases. Muscle enlargement with low-density masses and loss of normal fat planes and tumor invasion of adjacent bone may be seen.[7]

Radionuclide Bone Scanning

Radionuclide scanning with bone-seeking agents and with gallium is of value in diagnosing soft-tissue masses. Many types of soft-tissue masses may reveal increased uptake of technetium diphosphonate on the scans. If the results are positive, it is important to correlate the scan with a radiograph, because soft-tissue calcification or ossification may be present. The absence of soft-tissue densities does not rule out microscopic foci of calcification or heterotopic bone formation below the limits of resolution of the radiograph. Bone-forming and calcifying tumors, such as osteosarcoma, neuroblastoma, and colonic carcinoma metastases, may yield positive pictures on bone scans. Lesions that do not typically show calcification may also concentrate the bone-seeking agents, including various benign or malignant soft-tissue tumors.

Bone scintigraphy often reveals periosteal invasion that is not detected by conventional radiography. Blood pool scintigraphy with bone agents is quite sensitive for malignant disease. Gallium scintigraphy is reported to be a reliable preoperative indicator of malignant disease of soft-tissue. Combined gallium and bone scintigraphy with blood pool imaging allows a reliable prediction of the presence of a malignant lesion in patients with a soft-tissue mass in an extremity.[8]

Arteriography

The angiographic features of malignant tumors of soft-tissue are the same as those in other locations, including tumor stain, vessel encasement, and early venous filling. Although these angiographic features are diagnostic, arteriography is rarely used in the diagnostic workup of a soft-tissue mass. Diagnostic angiography is reserved for suspected vascular malformations and if CT or MRI does not adequately assess vascular encasement or displacement. Because intraarterial chemotherapy is in use, arteriography and the vascular pattern is important in follow-up evaluation after chemotherapy. The decrease in tumor vascularity is a good indicator of tumor response.

Magnetic Resonance Imaging

MRI is the method of choice for the evaluation of soft-tissue masses because of superior tissue contrast. Muscles, fat, tendons, ligaments, and blood vessels are clearly defined and are reliably differentiated. Soft-tissue tumors are readily demonstrated on MR images and usually have higher signal intensity than muscle on proton density PD-weighted and T2-weighted images. MRI is of particular value in the diagnosis of soft-tissue masses of the hand, wrist,[9] and foot.[10] The advantages of MRI compared with CT are higher contrast resolution and multiplanar imaging. The anatomic site of a soft-tissue tumor can be defined with respect to compartments. The tumor's relation to major vessels, nerves, and bone can be accurately assessed. Early reports indicated that periosteal reaction, cortical erosion, and bone destruction are better seen on CT and plain films,[11-14] but it has been well demonstrated that cortical and periosteal changes can be defined on MR images.[15] The extent and pattern of soft-tissue calcification cannot be reliably conveyed with current spin echo techniques. Gradient echo imaging is much more

sensitive in detecting calcium but does not reliably demonstrate the pattern of calcifications. Although MRI cannot reliably differentiate between malignant and benign soft-tissue tumors,[16] the degree of aggressiveness can be assessed by evaluating the margination, size, extent, and signal homogeneity.[17]

Lesions within or abutting the muscles or in the intramuscular septa are best seen on T2-weighted images. Those located next to or within the subcutaneous fat are best seen on T1-weighted images. Both images are necessary for a complete evaluation.[18] On T1-weighted images, soft-tissue masses with cellular or water content are of low signal intensity and show a high signal intensity with T2 weighting. Edema shows high signal intensity on T2-weighted images, and differentiation from tumor extension or invasion is difficult. Many edematous areas are found to contain tumor cells. Cysts containing fluid show low signal intensity with T1 weighting and high signal intensity with T2 weighting, but cysts containing highly proteinaceous fluid may show high signal intensity on both images. Masses that contain fat or blood may have a high signal intensity on T1-weighted images.[19] Hematomas have a complex pattern, depending on the time of evolution of the various breakdown products of hemoglobin. Soft-tissue hemorrhage is usually detected as irregular areas of high signal intensity on T1-weighted images because the hemorrhage is usually subacute or chronic when imaged. A hemorrhagic component also has irregular signal characteristics on T1-weighted and T2-weighted images. A large soft-tissue hematoma can mimic a hemorrhagic soft-tissue neoplasm in signal characteristics and appearance.

Increased MR signal intensity on T2-weighted images in skeletal muscle adjacent to malignant tumors may represent tumor invasion or edema. Infections, hematomas, and myositis may show similar signal intensities to neoplasms.

It is not possible to reliably diagnose the cell of origin of most soft-tissue neoplasms. Many pathologists consider all soft-tissue sarcomas to be mesenchymal tumors, with the cells differentiating to resemble various mature tissues, after which they are named and classified. Conflicting reports appear in the radiologic literature about the ability to differentiate benign from malignant neoplasms.[16,20-22] The following parameters should be considered:

- size
- margination
- broaching of compartments
- invasion of muscle, subcutaneous tissue, and skin
- involvement of bone, vessels, or nerves
- signal homogeneity
- signal intensity.

A small size appears to be a good indicator of benignity, at least in adults. In one series, there were no malignant tumors smaller than 3 cm.[20] However, a smaller size for malignant tumors is possible in infants (Fig. 4-1). Compartmental and subcutaneous invasion (Fig. 4-2) and involvement of major vessels and nerves indicate malignancy. Cortical bone involvement may be invasive or erosive. MR images may not be able to differentiate the two, and conventional x-ray films or CT may be necessary if no focal marrow changes are seen (Fig. 4-3).

Margination is not a reliable criterion. Malignant

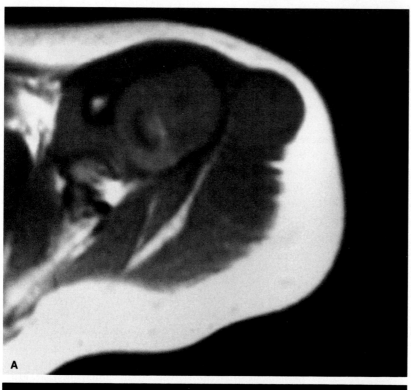

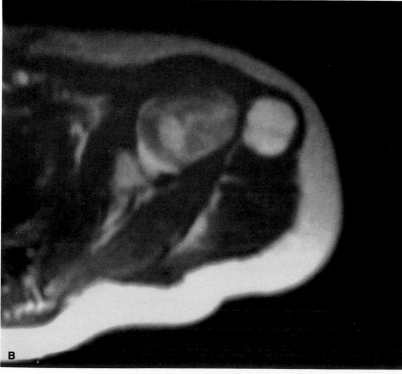

FIGURE 4-1. A 15-month-old boy. (**A**) MR image (SE 650/20). A 1.5-cm well-encapsulated mass is seen within the deltoid muscle. (**B**) MRI (SE 2000/80). The mass increases in signal intensity and is homogeneous. Biopsy showed an embryonal rhabdomyosarcoma. (From Greenfield GB, Arrington JA, Kudryk BT: MRI of soft tissue tumors. Skeletal Radiol 22:77–84, 1993)

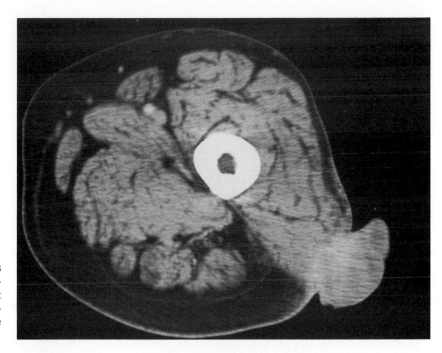

FIGURE 4-2.   A pleomorphic sarcoma is seen using enhanced CT. A large soft-tissue mass extends out of the lateral aspect of the thigh. (From Greenfield GB, Arrington JA, Kudryk BT: MRI of soft tissue tumors. Skeletal Radiol 22:77–84, 1993)

tumors may also have a smooth margin (see Fig. 4-1) and muscle infiltration is a characteristic of benign intramuscular lipoma. The visible margination also varies with pulse sequence and section level (Fig. 4-4). Signal inhomogeneity may reflect necrosis, hemorrhage, or calcification. The same tumor may be inhomogeneous on one pulse sequence and show homogeneity on another (Fig. 4-5). Although a large, inhomogeneous tumor should be highly suspect of being malignant, a benign tumor may also be inhomogeneous (Fig. 4-6). In one series, most benign and malignant tumors had inhomogenous signal intensities and at least partially irregular margins.[21] Signal intensities on T1-weighted and T2-weighted images characterize the type of tissue that is present. Several benign and malignant tumors

(text continues on page 263)

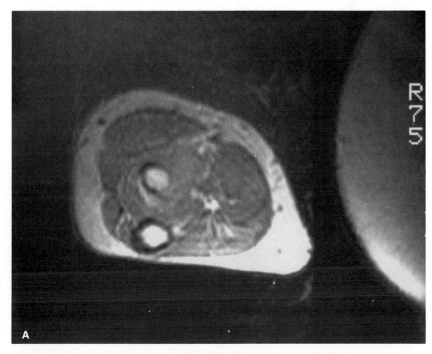

FIGURE 4-3.   (**A**) MR image (SE 3000/ 20). A soft-tissue mass involves the medial aspect of the bony cortex. The marrow signal appears normal. (**B**) MR image (SE 3000/80). The soft-tissue mass increases in signal intensity. The cortex is involved, and the marrow cavity is spared. (**C**) Example of a destroyed cortex. A large soft-tissue fibrosarcoma has invaded and destroyed the cortex with a saucerized appearance. (**D**) Example of an eroded cortex. A slow-growing soft-tissue mass has eroded the cortices of the tibia and fibula. MR images may not show enough bony detail to differentiate between erosion and destruction. (From Greenfield GB, Arrington JA, Kudryk BT: MRI of soft tissue tumors. Skeletal Radiol 22:77–84, 1993)   *continued*

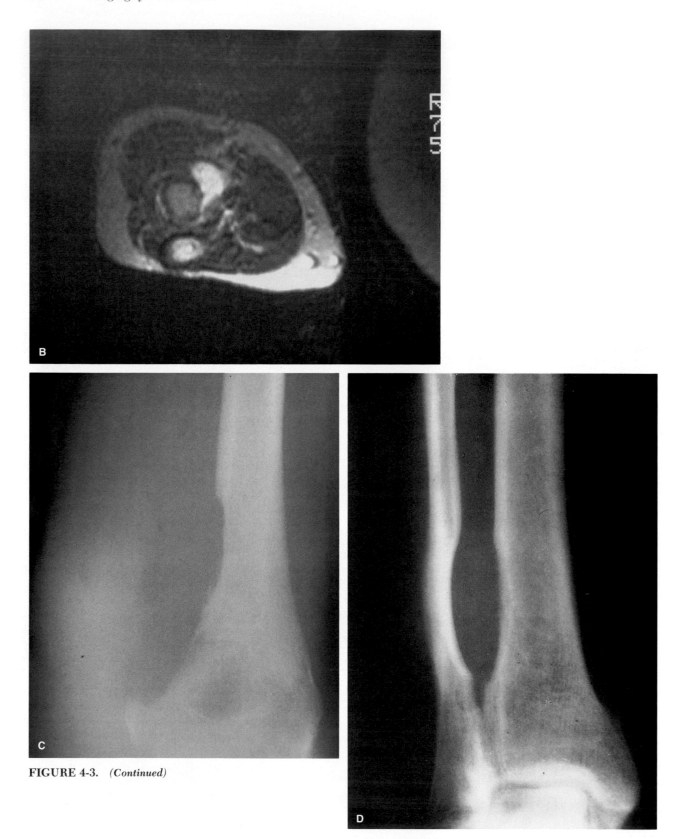

FIGURE 4-3. *(Continued)*

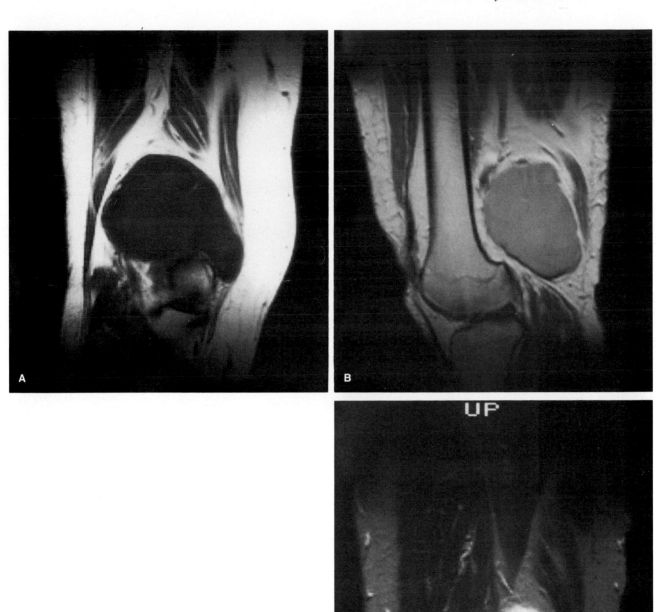

FIGURE 4-4. Myxoid liposarcoma. (**A**) MR image (SE 500/
17). A smoothly marginated low-signal-intensity mass is detected in the popliteal fossa. (**B**) A sagittal MR (SE 2300/25)
section shows the mass of intermediate signal intensity with
smooth inferior and posterior margins, but with slight shad-
ing-off of its superior margins. (**C**) A sagittal MR (SE 2300/90)
section shows the mass to be of high signal intensity with
invasion through the musculature at its anterior surface. The
superior and inferior aspects of the lesion also show irregular
margination. (From Greenfield GB, Arrington JA, Kudryk
BT: MRI of soft tissue tumors. Skeletal Radiol 22:77–84,
1993)

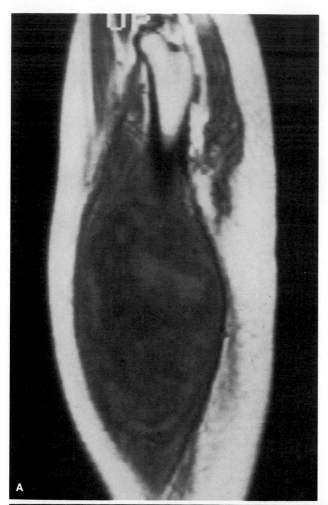

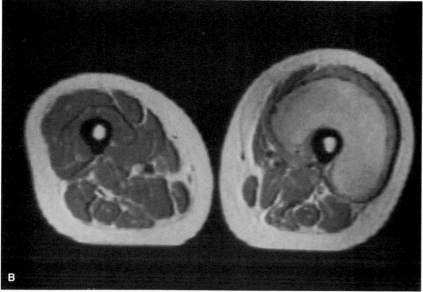

FIGURE 4-5. Malignant fibrous histiocytoma. (**A**) MR image (SE 800/20). A large, ovoid, inhomogeneous tumor mass is seen in the thigh. (**B**) MR (SE 2500/25) axial section. The tumor mass produces a homogeneous appearance in this image. (**C**) MR (SE 2500/80) axial section. The tumor mass has increased in signal intensity and shows signal inhomogeneity. (From Greenfield GB, Arrington JA, Kudryk BT: MRI of soft tissue tumors. Skeletal Radiol 22:77–84, 1993)

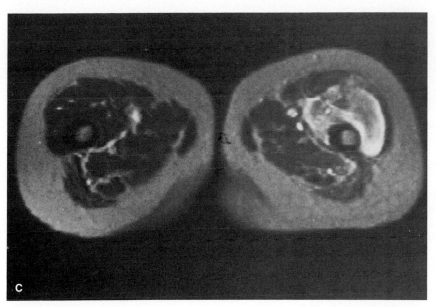

FIGURE 4-5.   *(Continued)*

may have similar appearances with respect to margination and homogeneity (Figs. 4-7 and 4-8). A biopsy should be done after the MRI examination, not before. MRI shows a change in the tumor volume after therapy, but it is not reliable in predicting the percentage of tumor necrosis.[22]

Gadolinium-DPTA enhancement of soft-tissue tumors has been reported to give better delineation in richly vascularized parts of tumors and in compressed tissue and atrophic muscle.[23] This benefit may be only minimal. Enhanced MRI more clearly delineates cystic areas, which is of little benefit in diagnosis, but it may be helpful in evaluating the response to chemotherapy.

Arthrography

Arthrography is the gold standard for diagnosing and demonstrating popliteal cysts and bursal extensions. Synovial tumors and intraarticular masses can be satisfactorily demonstrated using this modality, and ruptured synovial and bursal cysts can be shown (Fig. 4-9).

STAGING OF SOFT-TISSUE TUMORS

The staging of soft tissue sarcomas is a most important function of imaging, and the modality best suited to this task is MRI. The TNM (i.e., tumor, node, metastasis) classification of the American Joint Committee Task Force on Soft Tissue Sarcomas is presented in Table 4-1). The basis of this staging is the histologic grade.

All grade 1 tumors are stage 1, grade 2 tumors are stage 2, and grade 3 tumors are stage 3. Tumors are further subclassified according to size. Masses smaller than 5 cm in diameter are placed in subclass A, and those larger than 5 cm in diameter are placed in subclass B. If regional nodes are present in any grade tumor, it is staged as 3C. If major structures are involved, it is 4A, and if distant metastases are present, it is classified as 4B.[24]

Survival statistics for 1215 cases of lower extremity sarcomas were reviewed by the American Joint Committee Task Force on Soft Tissue Sarcomas and cited by Arlen and Marcove.[24] The findings based on tissue type and staging show that prognosis depends more on the stage of the disease than the cell of origin of the tumor (Table 4-2). The type of tumor is important with respect to radiosensitivity and propensity to lymphatic metastasis. The overall 5-year survival rate for all tumors in all stages was 41%. The range for all tumors was from 75% for stage 1 to 7% for stage 4. The lowest 5-year survival rate for all stages was for rhabdomyosarcoma (23%), and the highest was for liposarcoma (55%). Most were in the 30% and 40% range.

The inability of MRI to allow a specific diagnosis for most soft-tissue tumors does not make this examination less important. A biopsy of a suspected malignant tumor is always necessary because the stage is the histologic grade, relegating a prediction of histology based on imaging to academic interest. MRI provides vital information about the size of the lesion and its aggressiveness.

(text continues on page 268)

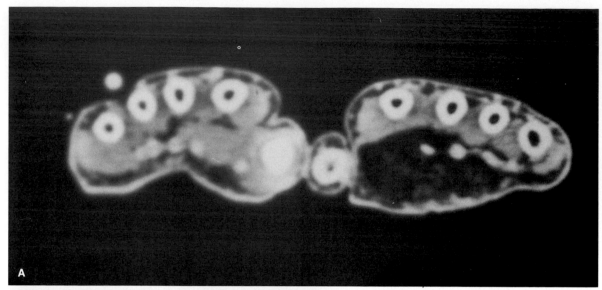

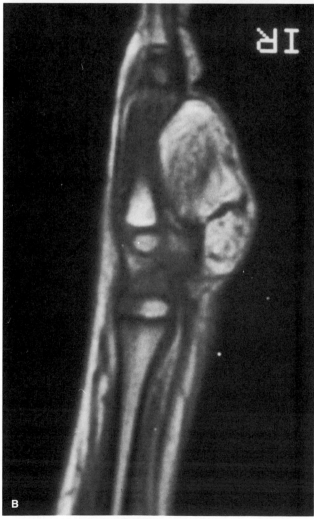

FIGURE 4-6. Twelve-year-old girl with a benign lipoma of the hand. (**A**) A low-density mass is seen on the CT scan at the palmar aspect of the left hand. (**B**) MR image (IR 600/20). The mass produces a high-intensity signal, similar to that of subcutaneous fat. Low-density streaks traverse the mass. (From Greenfield GB, Arrington JA, Kudryk BT: MRI of soft tissue tumors. Skeletal Radiol 22:77–84, 1993)

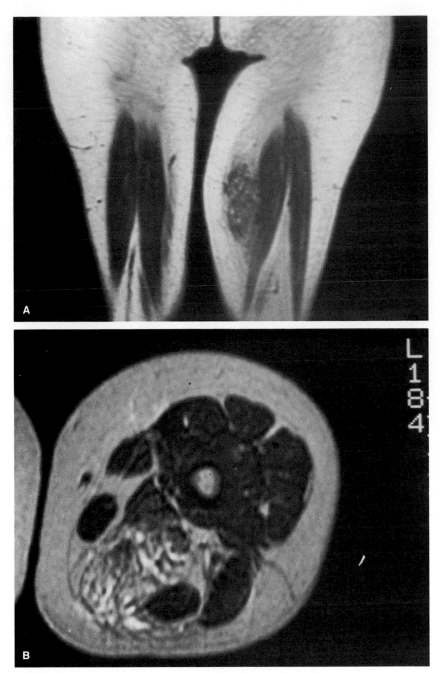

FIGURE 4-7.   Hemangioma of the thigh. (**A**) MR (SE 650/20) coronal image. An irregular mass of mixed signal intensity is seen medially. The high-signal-intensity areas within the tumor are caused by fat contained within it. (**B**) MR image (SE 3000/80). The hemangioma involves the semimembranosus, semitendinosus, and gracilis muscles and infiltrates adjacent fascial planes. There is marked signal in-homogeneity. (From Greenfield GB, Arrington JA, Kudryk BT: MRI of soft tissue tumors. Skeletal Radiol 22:77–84, 1993)

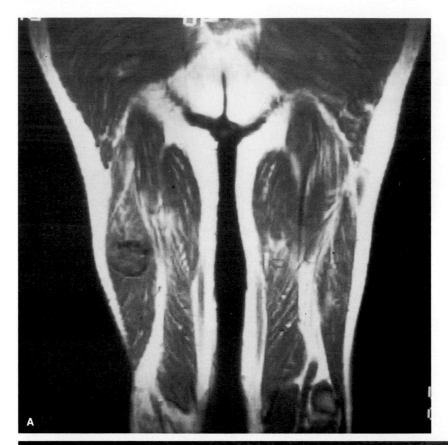

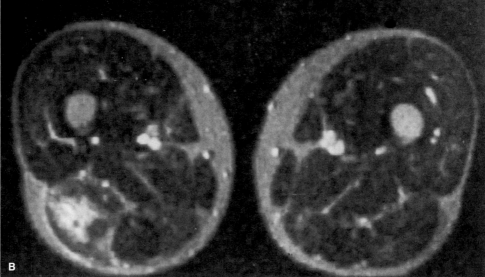

FIGURE 4-8. Seventy-year-old man with a mass in the right thigh.
(**A**) MR image (SE 600/20). A low-signal-intensity mass with somewhat irregular margination is seen in the lateral aspect of the right thigh. (**B**) MR image (SE 2500/90). The mass increases in signal intensity but remains inhomogeneous and irregularly marginated. The mass is in the biceps femoris muscle. Biopsy revealed a malignant fibrous histiocytoma. (From Greenfield GB, Arrington JA, Kudryk BT: MRI of soft tissue tumors. Skeletal Radiol 22:77–84, 1993)

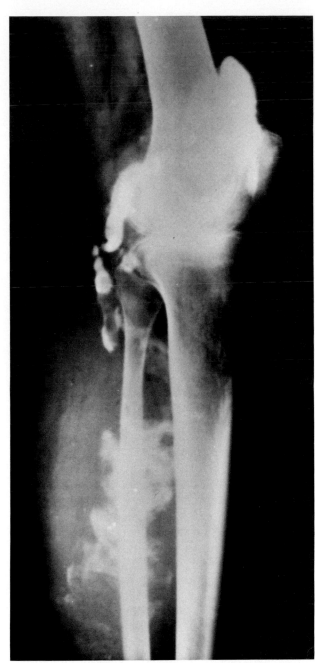

FIGURE 4-9. The arthrogram shows a giant ruptured bursa of the knee of a patient with rheumatoid arthritis. Contrast material has dissected down the calf. (Courtesy of Dr. Dharmashi V. Bhate, Veterans Administration Hospital, Hines, IL.)

TABLE 4-1.
Tumor Staging System

PRIMARY TUMOR (T)

Tx	Minimum requirements cannot be met
T0	No demonstrable tumor
T1	Tumor <5 cm in diameter
T2	Tumor ≥5 cm in diameter
T3	Tumor that grossly invades bone, major vessel, or major nerve

NODAL INVOLVEMENT (N)

Nx	Minimum requirements cannot be met
N0	No histologically verified metastases to lymph nodes
N1	Histologically verified regional lymph node metastases

DISTANT METASTASIS (M)

Mx	Not assessed
M0	No (known) distant metastasis
M1	Distant metastasis present

STAGE

Stage I

IA	G1 T1 N0 M0
	Grade 1 tumor, <5 cm in diameter, no regional lymph node or distant metastases
IB	G1 G2 N0 M0
	Grade 1 tumor, ≥5 cm in diameter, no regional lymph node or distant metastases

Stage II

IIA	G2 T1 N0 M0
	Grade 2 tumor, <5 cm in diameter, no regional lymph node or distant metastases
IIB	G2 T2 N0 M0
	Grade 2 tumor, ≥5 cm in diameter, no regional lymph node or distant metastases

Stage III

IIIA	G3 T1 N0 M0
	Grade 3 tumor, <5 cm in diameter, no regional lymph node or distant metastases
IIIB	G3 T2 N0 M0
	Grade 3 tumor, ≥5 cm in diameter, no regional lymph node or distant metastases
IIIC	Any G T1,2 N1 M0
	Tumor of any histologic grade or size, (no invasion) with regional lymph node metastases but without distant metastases

Stage IV

IVA	Any G T3 Any N M0
	Tumor of any histologic grade of malignancy that grossly invades bone, major vessels, or major nerves, with or without regional lymph node metastases, but without distant metastases
IVB	Any G Any T Any N M1
	Tumor with distant metastases

TABLE 4-2.
Survival Rates for the Histologic Types of Lower Extremity Sarcomas

Tumor Type	All Stages	Stage I	Stage II	Stage III	Stage IV
All types	41*	75	(55)	29	7
Fibrosarcoma	48	(73)	5/15	(43)	1/12
Malignant fibrohistiocytoma	46	11/13	(72)	(22)	1/7
Liposarcoma	55	(78)	10/17	(35)	0/12
Angiosarcoma	24	2/2	1/2	0/9	1/4
Synovial sarcoma	(43)	4/5	4/6	(16)	2/5
Rhabdomyosarcoma	23	0/1	0/0	(30)	0
Leiomyosarcoma	(32)	8/14	1/5	3/11	1/11
Malignant schwannoma	(45)	8/10	1/6		0/1

Rates in parentheses have standard errors between 5% and 10%.

CLASSIFICATION OF SOFT-TISSUE TUMORS

The World Health Organization histologic classification of soft-tissue tumors is presented in Table 4-3.[25]

The usual age range in years of common soft tissue sarcomas is presented below:

Malignant fibrous histiocytoma: 45 to 70 or older
Malignant schwannoma: 30 to 60
Liposarcoma: 25 to 55
Fibrosarcoma: 15 to 40
Synovial sarcoma: 15 to 30
Rhabdomyosarcoma: birth to 15.

DIFFERENTIAL DIAGNOSIS OF SOFT-TISSUE TUMORS

A wide spectrum of soft-tissue tumors and conditions should be considered in an imaging differential diagnosis.[26] These are discussed in the following sections.

Fibrohistiocytic and Fibrous Tumors

The spectrum of fibrohistiocytic and fibrous tumors and conditions of the extremities includes the following types.

MALIGNANT	BENIGN
Malignant fibrous histiocytoma	Fibroma
Fibrosarcoma	Fibromatosis
Postirradiation fibrosarcoma	Fasciitis
Fibrosarcoma in burn scars	

MALIGNANT *(continued)*
Congenital fibrosarcoma
Myxofibrosarcoma
Dermatofibrosarcoma
protuberans

Malignant Fibrous Histiocytoma

Malignant fibrous histiocytoma (MFH) is the most common sarcoma of soft-tissue in the extremities, and it typically presents in the fifth, sixth, and seventh decades of life.[27–30] The tumor is of fibrous and histiocytic origin with a variety of histologic patterns, the subtypes of which are storiform-pleomorphic, myxoid (i.e., myxofibrosarcoma), giant cell, inflammatory, and angiomatoid.[25] Most tumors are in the storiform group. Angiomatoid MFH occurs most frequently in the first and second decades of life, and it most often involves the dermis and subcutaneous tissues of the extremities.

Men are more frequently affected than women. The lower extremity is most often involved, followed by the upper extremity, but the tumor can occur almost anywhere. Most cases occur in the thigh, buttock, and groin regions. The tumor is most often located within skeletal muscle or adjacent to deep fascia, with only a small percentage in the subcutaneous tissues. The patient typically presents with a painless soft-tissue mass in a limb of several months' duration or accelerated growth with recent rapid increase in size, associated with pain.

On conventional radiographs, an ill-defined soft-tissue mass with possible punctate calcifications is seen. Adjacent bone may be destroyed in advanced lesions. CT is useful in assessing the size and extent of the tumor in soft tissues.[31] MR images show an intermediate or low signal intensity on T1-weighted images and high signal intensity on T2-weighted images of the tumor. There may be irregularity of the margin and sig-

TABLE 4-3.
Classification of Soft-Tissue Tumors

I. Tumors and tumor-like lesions of fibrous tissue
   A. Benign
      1. Fibroma
      2. Nodular fasciitis, including intravascular and cranial types
      3. Proliferative fasciitis
      4. Proliferative myositis
      5. Fibroma of tendon sheath
      6. Elastofibroma
      7. Nuchal fibroma
      8. Nasopharyngeal fibroma
      9. Keloid
   B. Fibrous tumors of infancy and childhood
      1. Fibrous hamartoma of infancy
      2. Myofibromatosis (solitary, multicentric)
      3. Fibromatosis colli
      4. Infantile digital fibromatosis
      5. Infantile fibromatosis, desmoid type
      6. Giant cell fibroblastoma
      7. Gingival fibromatosis
      8. Calcifying aponeurotic fibroma
      9. Hyalin fibromatosis
   C. Fibromatoses
      1. Superficial fibromatoses
         a. Palmar and plantar fibromatosis
         b. Penile (i.e., Peyronie) fibromatosis
         c. Knuckle pads
      2. Deep fibromatoses
         a. Abdominal fibromatosis
         b. Extraabdominal fibromatosis
         c. Intraabdominal fibromatosis
         d. Mesenteric fibromatosis (i.e., Gardner syndrome)
         e. Postradiation fibromatosis
         f. Cicatricial fibromatosis
   D. Malignant
      1. Adult fibrosarcoma
      2. Congenital and infantile fibrosarcoma
      3. Inflammatory fibrosarcoma
      4. Postradiation fibrosarcoma
      5. Cicatricial fibrosarcoma
II. Fibrohistiocytic tumors
   A. Benign
      1. Fibrous histiocytoma
         a. Cutaneous (i.e., dermatofibroma)
         b. Deep
      2. Atypical fibroxanthoma
      3. Juvenile xanthogranuloma
      4. Reticulohistiocytoma
      5. Xanthoma
   B. Intermediate
      1. Dermatofibrosarcoma protuberans
      2. Bednar tumor
   C. Malignant
      1. Malignant fibrous histiocytoma
         a. Storiform-pleomorphic
         b. Myxoid (i.e., myxofibrosarcoma)
         c. Giant cell (i.e., malignant giant cell tumor of soft parts)
         d. Inflammatory (i.e., malignant xanthogranuloma, xanthosarcoma)
         e. Angiomatoid

III. Tumors and tumor-like lesions of adipose tissue
   A. Benign
      1. Lipoma (cutaneous, deep, and multiple)
      2. Angiolipoma
      3. Spindle cell and pleomorphic lipoma
      4. Lipoblastoma and lipoblastomatosis
      5. Angiomyolipoma
      6. Myelolipoma
      7. Intramuscular and intermuscular lipoma
      8. Lipoma of tendon sheath
      9. Lumbosacral lipoma
      10. Interneural and perineural fibrolipoma
      11. Diffuse lipomatosis
      12. Cervical symmetrical lipomatosis (i.e., Madelung disease)
      13. Pelvic lipomatosis
      14. Hibernoma
   B. Malignant
      1. Liposarcoma, predominantly
         a. Well-differentiated
            (1) Lipoma-like
            (2) Sclerosing
            (3) Inflammatory
         b. Myxoid
         c. Round cell (i.e., poorly differentiated myxoid)
         d. Pleomorphic
         e. Dedifferentiated
IV. Tumors of muscle tissue
   A. Smooth muscle
      1. Benign
         a. Leiomyoma (cutaneous and deep)
         b. Angiomyoma (i.e., vascular leiomyoma)
         c. Epitheliod leiomyoma (i.e., benign leiomyoblastoma)
         d. Intravenous leiomyomatosis
         e. Leiomyomatosis peritonealis disseminata
      2. Malignant
         a. Leiomyosarcoma
         b. Epitheliod leiomyosarcoma (i.e., malignant leiomyoblastoma)
   B. Striated muscle
      1. Benign
         a. Adult rhabdomyoma
         b. Genital rhabdomyoma
         c. Fetal rhabdomyoma
      2. Malignant
         a. Rhabdomyosarcoma, predominantly
            (1) Embryonal, including botryoid
            (2) Alveolar
            (3) Pleomorphic
            (4) Mixed
         b. Ectomesenchymoma (i.e., rhabdomyosarcoma with ganglion cell differentiation)

(continued)

TABLE 4-3.
(Continued)

V. Tumors and tumor-like lesions of blood vessels
  A. Benign
      1. Hemangioma
          a. Capillary, including juvenile
          b. Cavernous
          c. Arteriovenous
          d. Venous
          e. Epitheliod (i.e., angiolymphoid hyperplasia, Kimura disease)
          f. Granulation tissue type (i.e., pyogenic, granuloma)
      2. Deep hemangioma (intramuscular, synovial, perineural)
      3. Hemangiomatosis
      4. Glomus tumor
      5. Hemangiopericytoma
      6. Papillary endothelial hyperplasia (i.e., intravascular vegetant hemangioendothelioma of Masson)
  B. Intermediate
      1. Hemangioendothelioma
          a. Epitheliod
          b. Spindle cell
          c. Malignant endovascular papillary angioendothelioma
  C. Malignant
      1. Angiosarcoma
      2. Kaposi sarcoma
      3. Malignant glomus tumor
      4. Malignant hemangiopericytoma
VI. Tumors of lymph vessels
  A. Benign
      1. Lymphangioma
          a. Cavernous
          b. Cystic (i.e., cystic hygroma)
      2. Lymphangiomatosis
      3. Lymphangiomyoma and lymphangiomyomatosis
  B. Malignant
      1. Angiosarcoma
VII. Tumors and tumor-like lesions of synovial tissue
  A. Benign
      1. Giant cell tumor of tendon sheath
          a. Localized (i.e., nodular tenosynovitis)
          b. Diffuse (i.e., florid synovitis)
  B. Malignant
      1. Synovial sarcoma (i.e., malignant synovioma), predominantly
          a. Biphasic (fibrous and epithelial)
          b. Monophasic (fibrous or epithelial)
      2. Malignant giant cell tumor of tendon sheath
VIII. Tumors of mesothelial tissue
  A. Benign
      1. Localized fibrous mesothelioma (i.e., subserosal fibroma)
      2. Multicystic peritoneal mesothelioma
      3. Mesothelioma of the genital tract (i.e., adenomatoid tumor)

  B. Malignant
      1. Diffuse and localized mesothelioma, predominantly
          a. Epithelial
          b. Fibrous
          c. Biphasic
IX. Tumors and tumor-like lesions of peripheral nerves
  A. Benign
      1. Traumatic neuroma
      2. Morton neuroma
      3. Neuromuscular hamartoma
      4. Nerve sheath ganglion
      5. Neurilemonma (i.e., benign schwannoma)
      6. Neurofibroma, solitary
          a. Localized
          b. Diffuse
          c. Pacinian
          d. Pigmented
      7. Granular cell tumor
      8. Neurofibromatosis (i.e., von Recklinghausen disease)
          a. Localized
          b. Plexiform
          c. Diffuse
      9. Pigmented neuroectodermal tumor of infancy (i.e., retinal anlage tumor)
      10. Ectopic meningioma
      11. Nasal glioma
      12. Neurothekeoma
  B. Malignant
      1. Malignant schwannoma, including malignant schwannoma with rhabdomyoblastic differentiation (i.e., malignant Triton tumor), glandular malignant schwannoma, and epithelioid malignant schwannoma
      2. Peripheral tumors of primitive neuroectodermal tissues (i.e., neuroepithelioma)
      3. Malignant pigmented neuroectodermal tumor of infancy (i.e., retinal anlage tumor)
      4. Malignant granular cell tumor
X. Tumors of autonomic ganglia
  A. Benign
      1. Ganglioneuroma
      2. Melanocytic schwannoma
  B. Malignant
      1. Neuroblastoma
      2. Ganglioneuroblastoma
      3. Malignant melanocytic schwannoma
XI. Tumors of paraganglionic structures
  A. Benign
      1. Paraganglioma (solitary, multiple, familial)
  B. Malignant
      1. Malignant paraganglioma

continued

TABLE 4-3.
(Continued)

XII. Tumors and tumor-like lesions of cartilage and bone-forming tissues
    A. Benign
        1. Panniculitis ossificans
        2. Myositis ossificans
        3. Fibrodysplasia (i.e., myositis) ossificans progressiva
        4. Extraskeletal chondroma or osteochondroma
        5. Extraskeletal osteoma
    B. Malignant
        1. Extraskeletal chondrosarcoma
           a. Well-differentiated
           b. Myxoid (i.e., chordoid sarcoma)
           c. Mesenchymal
        2. Extraskeletal osteosarcoma
XIII. Tumors and tumor-like lesions of pluripotential mesenchyme
    A. Benign
        1. Mesenchymoma
    B. Malignant
        1. Malignant mesenchymoma

XIV. Tumors and tumor-like lesions of disputed or uncertain histogenesis
    A. Benign
        1. Congenital granular cell tumor
        2. Tumoral calcinosis
        3. Myxoma (cutaneous and intramuscular)
        4. Aggressive angiomyxoma
        5. Amyloid tumor
        6. Parachordoma
    B. Malignant
        1. Alveolar soft part sarcoma
        2. Epithelioid sarcoma
        3. Clear cell sarcoma of tendons and aponeuroses (i.e., malignant melanoma, soft parts)
        4. Extraskeletal Ewing sarcoma
XV. Unclassified soft-tissue tumors and tumor-like lesions

---

nal inhomogeneity (Fig. 4-10; see Figs. 4-5 and 4-8). There may be invasion across compartments and in subcutaneous tissues. Major vessels and nerves may show involvement with encasement or invasion. MR images can best differentiate recurrent or residual tumor from postoperative changes if performed more than 3 months after surgery.[27] Preoperative chemotherapy may result in hemorrhage within the tumor, resulting in considerable enlargement. MR images can differentiate this hemorrhage from tumor growth, particularly on T1-weighted images.[32] Angiography shows increased vascularity, tumor stain, vessel encasement, and early venous filling. Rare cases have been reported with metaplastic bone and cartilage formation visible on the radiograph. The reactive ossification tends to be peripheral in location, involving the pseudocapsule of the sarcoma or its fibrous septa. There may be a zoning pattern with peripheral or polar orientation, simulating myositis ossificans.[33]

MYXOFIBROSARCOMA. Myxofibrosarcoma is a subtype of MFH with a peak incidence in the seventh decade of life. It is highly malignant. It is characterized histologically by myxoid areas associated with cellular areas of ordinary MFH. On MR images, low signal intensity is seen on T1-weighted images, with a high signal on T2-weighted images. Gadolinium-enhanced T1-weighted images show irregular enhancement. The myxomatous components do not enhance (Fig. 4-11).

Fibrosarcoma

Fibrosarcoma is defined as a malignant spindle cell tumor of fibroblasts that shows no evidence of differ-

entiation into other types of cells. Many earlier reported cases now meet the criteria of malignant fibrous histiocytoma, and this entity is no longer considered a common tumor. Clinically, it usually presents as a relatively painless mass between 3 and 8 cm in diameter. The average duration of symptoms is 3 to 4 years, and it is most commonly diagnosed in patients between the ages of 30 and 55,[25] although it also occurs in older persons. An ill-defined soft-tissue mass is seen on conventional x-ray films. Small, calcific flecks may be present, and the adjacent bone may be invaded with a typical saucerized appearance (see Fig. 4-3C). MR images show an intermediate- to low-signal-intensity mass on T1-weighted images with some heterogeneity. On T2-weighted images, the signal intensity does not generally increase (Fig. 4-12). The subcutaneous tissues may show involvement and lymphedema. The margination varies.

Postradiation fibrosarcomas and those occurring in burn scars have been reported. Congenital and infantile fibrosarcomas have also been reported,[34] but these lesions are rare, tend to be well differentiated, and have a favorable course.

Benign Fibromas

Benign fibromas of the soft tissues are a heterogenous group and are given various names according to anatomic location, age of the patient, and shape of the lesion: fibroma of a tendon sheath, elastofibroma, pedunculated fibroma, and juvenile aponeurotic fibroma. Keloids are also classified in this group. Cutaneous and

(text continues on page 274)

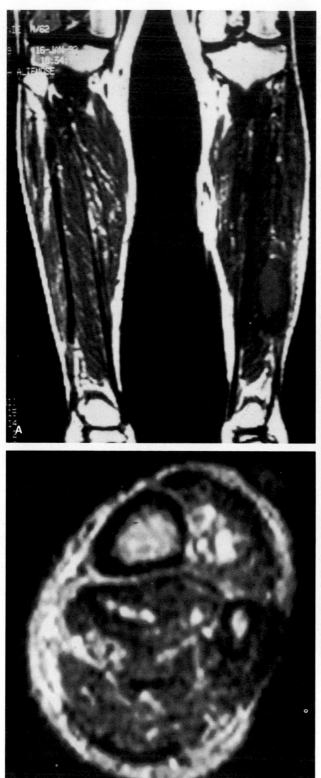

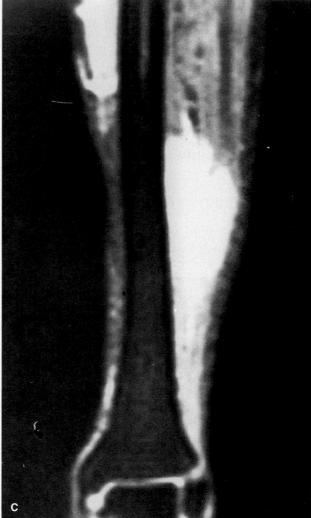

FIGURE 4-10. Malignant fibrous histiocytoma in a 62-year-old man. (**A**) MR image (SE 810/15). A 5-cm, ovoid, low-signal-intensity soft tissue mass is adjacent to the left tibia. (**B**) MR (SE 3000/80) axial section. The mass yields an inhomogeneous increase in signal intensity. (**C**) Inversion recovery MR image (IRM 150, TR 1500, TE 20). The mass is better seen on this pulse sequence with high signal intensity.

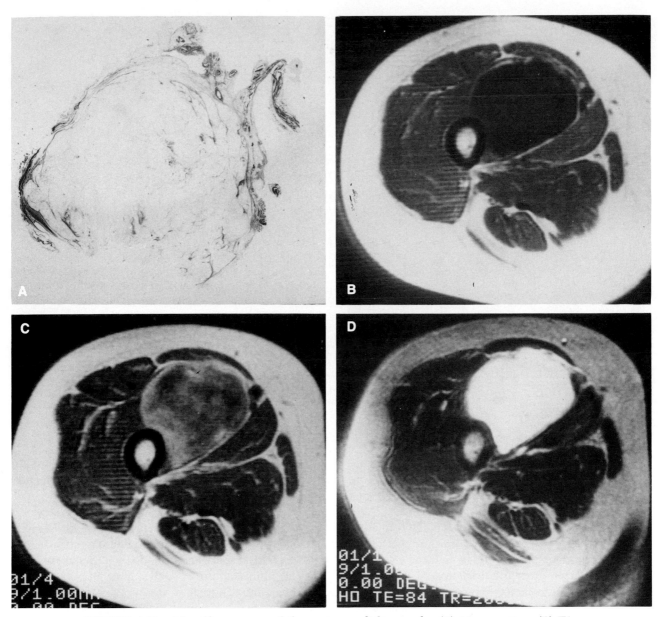

FIGURE 4-11. Myxofibrosarcoma of the vastus medialis muscle. (**A**) Macrosection, (**B**) T1-weighted plain, (**C**) T1-weighted, gadolinium-enhanced, and (**D**) T2-weighted plain sections through the tumor. The whole tumor has a low signal intensity in T1-weighted plain image and a high signal intensity in the T2-weighted plain image. The T1-weighted gadolinium-enhanced image reveals an irregular enhancement, corresponding to the vascularized strands of fibrous tissue within the tumor. The myxomatous parts of the tumor are not enhanced. There is also enhancement of the pseudocapsule, which is composed of compressed, richly vascularized atophic muscle. (From Pettersson H, Eliasson J, Egund N et al: Gadolinium-DPTA enhancement of soft tissue tumors in magnetic resonance imaging—preliminary clinical experience in five patients. Skeletal Radiol 17:319–323, 1988)

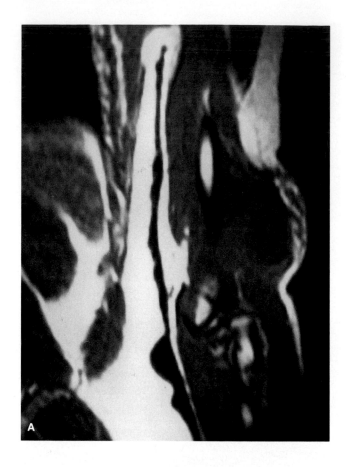

FIGURE 4-12. Grade II fibrosarcoma in a 73-year-old man. (**A**) The coronal MR (FSE 650/10 Ef) view shows a low-intensity-signal, heterogeneous mass in the musculature of the left arm. Dilated lymphatic channels in the subcutaneous tissues are also seen. The mass is heterogeneous. (**B**) MR image (FSE 4000/17 Ef). The subcutaneous fat signal intensity decreases to match the signal intensity of the tumor. The tumor abuts the cortex of the humerus but has not caused bone marrow changes. Dilated subcutaneous lymphatic channels are seen. The brachial artery is seen within the tumor. (**C**) The tumor does not increase in signal intensity in this T2-weighted MR (FSE 4000/85 Ef) image and matches the intensity of subcutaneous fat. The brachial artery is contained within the tumor.

deep benign fibrous histiocytomas occur. Fibrous tumors of infancy have a different histologic picture and behavior than those of older children and adults.[25]

Fibromatoses are a category of diverse soft-tissue fibrous lesions.[35–37] MR images show variable signal characteristics, depending on the amount of cellularity and dense collagen present in each area. They may be hyperintense, isointense, or hypointense with respect to skeletal muscle. The margination in most cases is well defined, but it may be poorly defined. On T2-weighted images, linear areas of decreased signal within the lesion or heterogeneity may be present.

Aggressive Fibromatosis

Aggressive fibromatosis is a term synonymous with musculoaponeurotic fibromatosis, extraabdominal desmoid, and periosteal desmoid.[38,37] It is also applied to some cases of desmoplastic fibroma involving the skeleton.[39] Aggressive fibromatosis is a benign proliferation of fibrous tissue that, when located around the shoulder, exhibits a characteristic behavior. It presents as a soft-tissue mass in the shoulder or upper portion of the back, displacing the scapula (Fig. 4-13). It is seen without calcification. The mean age of these patients at diagnosis is 23 years. The tumor may be tender and painful. Bone may be involved. It is highly aggressive and tends to invade adjacent soft tissues. Involvement of

the posterior mediastinum has been reported with fatal hemorrhage[40] and enlargement of the vertebral pedicles.[41] It has a high recurrence rate but typically does not metastasize. CT can show the extent of disease.

These tumors are typically isodense or slightly hypodense with respect to muscle without the use of contrast medium, and they enhance after infusion of contrast material. They may rarely be hyperdense on preinfusion scans, although this is not related to their histologic appearance.[42] They may appear echopenic on ultrasonography.[43] Arteriograms may show hypervascularity and help to delineate the extent of involvement and vessels that are poorly seen on CT. Radionuclide bone scans may show involvement of adjacent bones,[44] although they are less useful in this respect than CT.[45] MR images show a heterogeneous mass with a well-defined low-signal-intensity periphery. Cellular areas show moderate enhancement on T1-weighted images after infusion of gadolinium.[37] Multicentric, aggressive fibromatosis of the extremities has been demonstrated by MRI.[46]

Desmoid Fibromatosis

Desmoid fibromatosis (i.e., fibrosarcoma, grade I desmoid type) in the extremities demonstrates bone erosion and a frond-like periosteal reaction. There may be local recurrence after excision.[47]

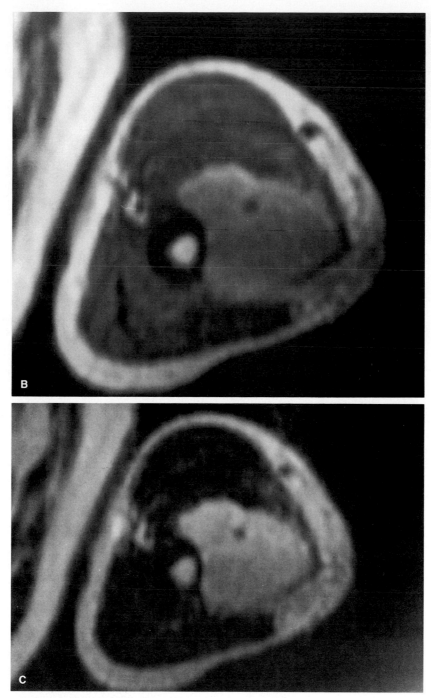

FIGURE 4-12. *(Continued)*

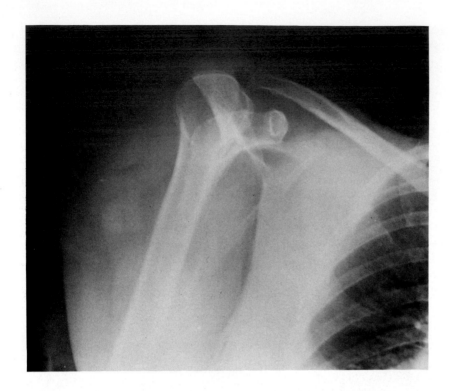

FIGURE 4-13. Aggressive fibromatosis. A large, lobulated, soft-tissue mass is seen in the right shoulder region. It has markedly displaced the scapula away from the chest wall.

Nodular Fasciitis

Nodular fasciitis (i.e., pseudosarcomas) are "quasi-neoplastic benign proliferations of connective tissue" that, because of their cellularity and frequently rapid growth, are readily mistaken for sarcoma.[1,48,49] These entities represent reactive cellular proliferations. They usually present as small, rapidly growing, tender masses that may or may not be well circumscribed. They may be subcutaneous, intramuscular, or fascial, and they usually occur in young adults but may occur in children. Histologic differentiation from angiomatoid malignant fibrous histioma is difficult.

Fatty Tumors

A spectrum of fatty tumors can arise in the extremities.[25,50]

MALIGNANT	BENIGN
Liposarcoma	Lipoma
Atypical lipoma	Intramuscular lipoma
Well-differentiated liposarcoma	Lipoma of a joint or tendon sheath
Round cell liposarcoma	Lipoma arborescens
Pleomorphic liposarcoma	Neural fibrolipoma
Myxoid liposarcoma	Lipoblastoma
Dedifferentiated liposarcoma	Cutaneous angiolipoma
	Infiltrating angiolipoma
	Lipomatosis
	Hibernoma

Liposarcoma

Liposarcoma is the second most frequently occurring soft-tissue malignant neoplasm of the extremities in adults, exceeded only by MFH.[1,50] It is usually encountered in the fourth to sixth decades of life. It is rare in children, in whom lipoblastomas are the most common of fatty tumors. It is rare in subcutaneous fat and distal extremities, and it is most often seen in deep structures.[25] The most common type is the myxoid liposarcoma, which accounts for about half of all of these tumors and commonly contains less than 10% mature fat. In the extremities, this tumor has a predilection for the medial thigh and popliteal area (Fig. 4-14; see Fig. 4-4). Other histologic types are the well-differentiated, round cell, and pleomorphic tumors. The well-differentiated tumors include a lipoma-like lesion called the atypical lipoma. Liposarcoma arises from primitive mesenchyme, not mature fat cells. Malignant transformation, such as lipoma to liposarcoma, is rare in bone, and it has been reported in the soft tissues,[51] although this change is not generally accepted.

Clinically, a slow-growing, deep-seated mass is usually large when first seen. Pain and tenderness are experienced by a minority of patients.

On CT, an inhomogeneous or a nonspecific soft-tissue mass, possibly enhancing after intravenous contrast administration, may be seen. A low-density area is usually not apparent.

On MRI, the signal characteristics depend on the amount of differentiation and correlate with the histo-

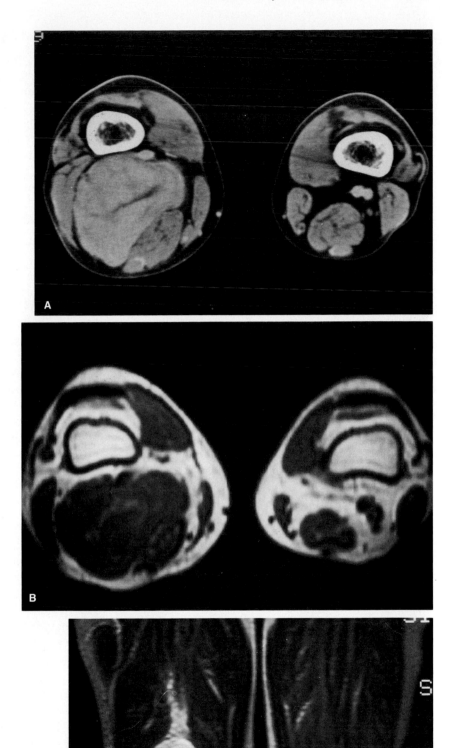

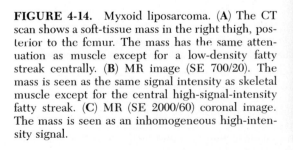

FIGURE 4-14. Myxoid liposarcoma. (**A**) The CT scan shows a soft-tissue mass in the right thigh, posterior to the femur. The mass has the same attenuation as muscle except for a low-density fatty streak centrally. (**B**) MR image (SE 700/20). The mass is seen as the same signal intensity as skeletal muscle except for the central high-signal-intensity fatty streak. (**C**) MR (SE 2000/60) coronal image. The mass is seen as an inhomogeneous high-intensity signal.

logic subtypes with regard to the amount of mature fat present.[52] In subtypes that are not well differentiated, the major portion of the tumor shows heterogenous low signal intensity on T1-weighted images and high signal intensity on T2-weighted images. Myxoid liposarcoma is encapsulated and usually septated. A lacy high signal may be seen within a mildly heterogeneous, low-signal-intensity mass on T1-weighted images.[53] Round cell and pleomorphic subtypes tend to be more heterogenous than the myxoid. In well-differentiated types with a considerable amount of fatty tissue, T1-weighted images show a moderately high signal intensity, usually reflecting a lobulated, inhomogeneous mass (Fig. 4-15), which decreases in signal intensity on T2-weighted images. The nonfatty cellular components increase in signal intensity. Some fatty liposarcomas show an atypical appearance on short tau inversion recovery (STIR) sequence in that they do not have the signal characteristics of subcutaneous fat but show a high signal intensity on these fat-suppression images. One lipoma was also reported in this series.[54] Dedifferentiated liposarcoma is a tumor in which a well-differentiated liposarcoma is associated with a high-grade nonfatty sarcoma. It occurs most often in the trunk but has been reported as a rare event in the lower extremities, with a patient age range of 33 to 79 years. MR images and CT scans show fatty and nonfatty components juxtaposed within a large neoplasm, and calcification and ossification were seen on plain x-ray films.[55]

Atypical Lipomas

Atypical lipomas differ histologically from simple lipomas, consisting of mature fat cells interspersed with multinucleated cells, collagen bundles, and adipocytes with large hyperchromic nuclei, similar to well-differentiated liposarcomas.[56] They differ from liposarcoma, because they have no tendency for distant metastases, but they may locally recur. They may simulate a well-differentiated liposarcoma histologically and appear as a liposarcoma on CT scans and MR images.

Lipomas

Lipomas are soft, well-encapsulated, benign, fatty tumors. They occur most commonly in the fifth and sixth decades of life. They may be demonstrated on conventional films by their radiolucency (Fig. 4-16) or readily seen on CT (Fig. 4-17) by their low-attenuation fat content. They do not enhance after injecting intravenous contrast material. In MR images, these tumors show high signal intensity on T1-weighted images,[19] with a decrease of intensity on T2-weighted images (Fig. 4-18), similar to that of subcutaneous fat. Strands of low signal intensity due to fibrous tissue may be present in some tumors (see Fig. 4-6). An intramuscular lipoma may be poorly marginated and infiltrate muscle planes. If phleboliths are seen within the tumor, the diagnosis of infiltrating angiolipoma is suggested.[57] Ossification may occur within a benign lipoma

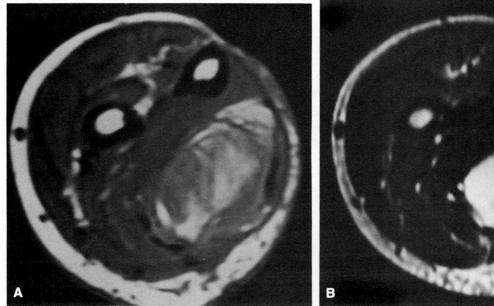
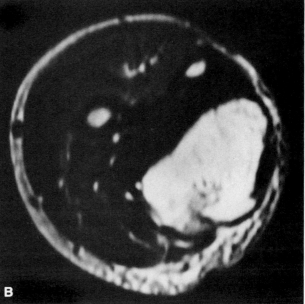

FIGURE 4-15. Liposarcoma of the forearm. (**A**) T1-weighted MR image. A well-circumscribed tumor displays mixed signal intensity. The high signal intensity is caused by fatty components. Low-signal areas within the subcutaneous fat are also seen. (**B**) T2-weighted MR image. The tumor is predominantly of high signal intensity. The cellular components of the tumor have increased in signal intensity with T2-weighting. Fatty components have decreased in signal intensity, particularly at the margins. Cellular infiltration of the subcutaneous fat is also seen as high signal intensity. (Courtesy of Dr. Harold Posniak, Loyola University, Maywood, IL.)

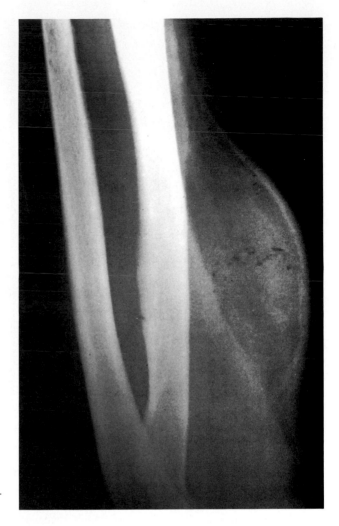

FIGURE 4-16. Lipoma of the forearm. There is a radiolucent, ovoid mass between the soft-tissue planes.

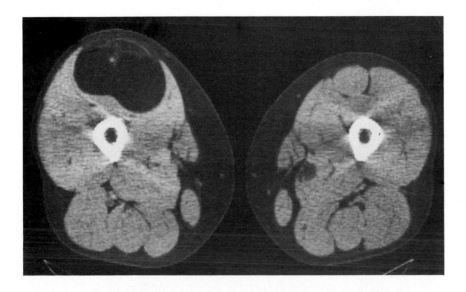

FIGURE 4-17. CT scan of a lipoma of the left thigh. A well-circumscribed, low-density region anterior to the right femur, principally in the vastus intermedius muscle, is seen. This area has the same density as the subcutaneous fat and represents a lipoma. A smaller lipoma exists medially on the left side.

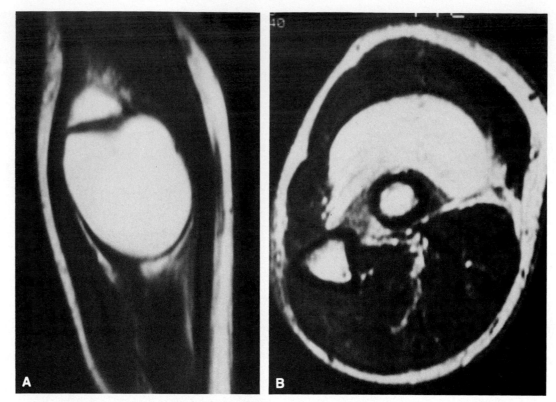

FIGURE 4-18. Lipoma. (**A**) T1-weighted MR sagittal image. The lipoma is seen as a high-signal-intensity, well-encapsulated lesion displacing the musculature. (**B**) T2-weighted MR axial image. The fat intensity has diminished somewhat, but the lipoma retains its high signal intensity, contrasted with the musculature. The lipoma has the same signal intensity as that of the subcutaneous fat. (Courtesy of Dr. H. Posniak, Loyola University, Maywood, IL.)

(Fig. 4-19). Overgrowth of bone may be seen in cases of neural fibrolipoma, an example of which is macrodactyly (Fig. 4-20). Lipomas may arise in a tendon sheath or within a joint, where the form may be discrete or more often composed of hypertrophic synovial villi containing fat. This type is called lipoma arborescens and most commonly occurs in the knee. Angiolipomas are cutaneous lesions containing fatty and vascular tissue. The infiltrating form is deeper and has a tendency to recur.

Congenital Lipomatosis

Congenital lipomatosis is a rare malformation of adipose tissue occurring early in life in which the fat cells, in addition to forming a mass, appear to infiltrate adjacent tissues. Bone changes due to increased vascularity that involve the underlying ribs have been reported.[58]

Lipoblastomatosis

Lipoblastomatosis, an unusual benign neoplastic condition of embryonal fat, occurs most frequently in the first year of life and should not be confused with myxoid liposarcoma.[59] Myxoid liposarcoma is the most common soft tissue sarcoma in adults but rarely occurs in children. The lower extremity is involved most frequently. The soft-tissue mass with relative radiolucency may evoke a bone reaction.

Hibernoma

Hibernoma is an encapsulated lesion similar to the natural brown fatty tissue of hibernating animals, such as bears. It is a rare tumor that usually occurs about the scapula, presenting as a slowly growing, painless mass. It is a vascular tumor that on CT shows a density somewhat higher than fat and that enhances on postinfusion studies.

Vascular Soft-Tissue Tumors

A spectrum of vascular soft-tissue tumors can be considered in the differential diagnosis.[25]

MALIGNANT	BENIGN
Angiosarcoma	Hemangioma
Stewart-Treves syndrome	Angiomatosis
Kaposi sarcoma	Hematoma

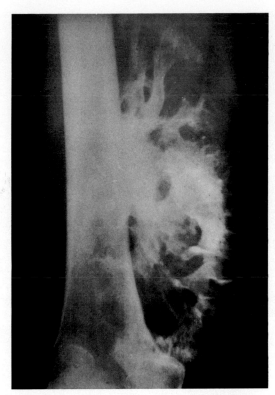

FIGURE 4-19. Lipoma of the thigh contains extensive ossification. The radiolucent character of the fatty tissue is apparent.

Angiosarcomas

Angiosarcomas are rare, highly malignant tumors with a wide spectrum of histologic forms, varying from hemangioma-like lesions to anaplastic tumors. This category includes a variety of terms for describing microscopic appearance, and there is a lack of standardization. Hemangiosarcoma and lymphangiosarcoma are in this category, as is hemangioendothelioma, which is considered by some pathologists to be the same as angiosarcoma. The tumors tend to be cutaneous or superficial and rarely arise from major vessels, with a smaller percentage arising in deep tissues and organs (Fig. 4-21).[25] Radiation, carcinogens, and chronic lymphedema have been implicated as etiologic factors.

Stewart-Treves Syndrome

Stewart-Treves syndrome is the rare development of angiosarcoma in a patient with chronic lymphedema. This event was originally described after radical mastectomy and axillary lymph node dissection; the tumors occurred an average of 10 years after mastectomy. Although radiation therapy could contribute to this development, many patients with this condition never received radiation treatment. This setting accounts for about 90% of cases, with the remainder arising in

chronic lymphedema from other causes, including idiopathic,[60] congenital, traumatic, and filarial cases and after lymph node dissection for carcinoma of the penis.[25] The tumor manifests itself by mottling, erythema, pain, nodulation, and ulceration with a serosanguineous discharge and progression of edema. CT shows skin thickening, nodulation, septal thickening, and tumor infiltration (Fig. 4-22), unlike the reticular and dilated lymphatic channel pattern of uncomplicated lymphedema.

Kaposi Sarcoma

Kaposi sarcoma is a neoplasm with angiomatous and fibrosarcoma-like components and a complex pathogenesis, usually affecting the lower extremities. The non-AIDS (acquired immunodeficiency syndrome)-related chronic form occurs in the sixth or seventh decade of life, and is rare outside of Africa. Bluish red nodules are seen, usually in the distal lower extremity, and they increase in size and number to coalesce and ulcerate. The most frequent occurrence of this tumor is among AIDS patients. Most patients with Kaposi sarcoma are young adult men, and many are homosexuals. There is also an increased incidence

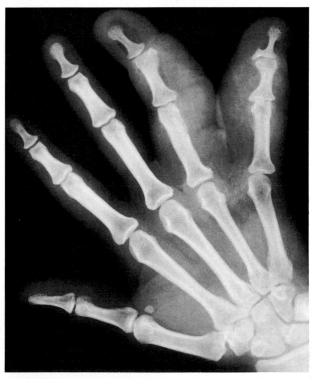

FIGURE 4-20. Macrodactyly of the hand. Enlargement of the fourth and fifth fingers. There is soft-tissue swelling, predominantly at the ulnar side of the fourth finger and at the radial side of the fifth finger. The biopsy revealed fatty tissue. This condition was not present at birth and represents the noncongenital type of idiopathic macrodactyly often complicated by fatty tissue.

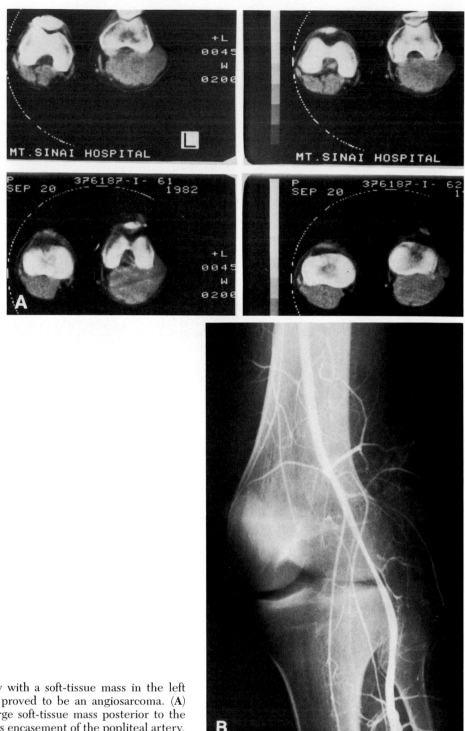

FIGURE 4-21. A 19-year-old boy with a soft-tissue mass in the left popliteal region, which on biopsy proved to be an angiosarcoma. (**A**) Computed tomography shows a large soft-tissue mass posterior to the left knee. (**B**) The arteriogram shows encasement of the popliteal artery, displacement of vessels around the soft-tissue mass, and tumor stain.

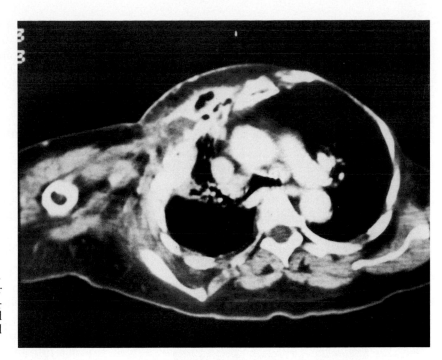

FIGURE 4-22. Stewart-Treves syndrome. A 69-year-old woman had breast cancer and bilateral mastectomies. Tumor infiltrated the right axilla and chest wall and involved the rib. Pulmonary changes and chest wall emphysema are also depicted.

among organ transplantation patients. Although Kaposi sarcoma is usually superficial, it may involve bone.[61] The bone changes include multiple osteolytic lesions in the central skeleton and proximal joints. A radionuclide bone scan may not detect early lesions.[62] MR images may demonstrate skin thickening, a subcutaneous honeycomb appearance with lymphedema and fluid collections, and variable muscle involvement.[63]

Cavernous Hemangioma

Cavernous hemangioma is a relatively common soft-tissue tumor of the extremities, with a predilection for sites distal to the elbow and knee. Fewer than 1% of all hemangiomas occur in muscle or deep soft tissue.[64] On conventional x-ray films, lobulated soft-tissue masses that may contain phleboliths are seen (Fig. 4-23).[65] CT can define the extent of the lesion,[65] but the exact timing of contrast infusion is critical. MRI is the preferred method,[66] showing these tumors as high-signal-intensity areas on T1-weighted images because of their fat content and also as high signal intensities on T2-weighted images due to their soft-tissue content (Fig. 4-24).[19] They may have a serpiginous, lobulated (see Fig. 4-7), or striated-septated pattern on T2-weighted images. Fluid-fluid levels may be seen.[66a] Radiographic examination followed by MRI has been recommended for initial staging.[67] The lesions may be associated with muscle atrophy.[68–71] The regional bone may be deformed and overgrown. If associated with enchondromatosis, it is called the Maffucci syndrome.

Capillary Hemangioma

Capillary hemangioma is a superficial lesion with smaller-diameter vessels than found in a cavernous hemangioma. Other vascular abnormalities, detectable on MR images, include arteriovenous malformations, which show high flow with flow voids; venous malformations, which show slow flow; lymphatic malformations, which show slow flow and may be cystic; and lymphaticovenous malformations, which show slow flow and may have a fibrofatty matrix. The findings for lymphangioma are similar to those for hemangioma on plain films, except that there are no phleboliths (Fig. 4-25).[72] Ossification of skeletal muscle hemangiomas with a radiographic Swiss-cheese appearance has been reported.[73]

Angiomatosis

Angiomatosis is a rare condition of widespread involvement with vascular malformation and proliferation.[25] Klippel-Trenaunay-Weber syndrome is an example of an extreme form, producing bone overgrowth, deformities, and erosions.

Hematoma

On plain films and CT scans, a hematoma appears as a smooth, uniform mass (Fig. 4-26). On ultrasonography, a sonolucent area is seen (Fig. 4-27). In MR images, a complex pattern develops, depending on time and hemoglobin breakdown products. The appearance

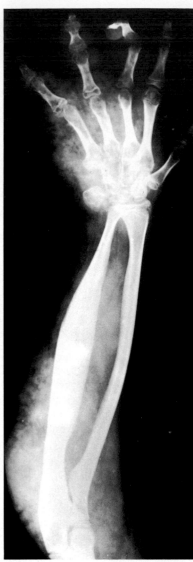

FIGURE 4-23. Hemangioma of the forearm and hand. Notice the soft-tissue swelling, with small, irregular lobulations. The bones are deformed, and the ulna has a fusiform contour. Several phleboliths are present.

in the brain is well documented. Acute hematomas initially show isointense signal intensity for as long as 12 hours because of the presence of oxyhemoglobin. From 1 day to 1 week, the presence of deoxyhemoglobin produces low-signal-intensity T2-weighted images and no signal intensity changes on T1-weighted images. After several days to possibly months, the signal increases on both T1-weighted and T2-weighted images (Fig. 4-28). The hematoma may infiltrate muscle planes (Fig. 4-29) or be bounded by a low-signal-intensity rim of hemosiderin (Fig. 4-30). This picture helps in differentiating a hematoma from most tumors. Muscle tears[74] presenting with pain or a palpable mass may be confused with

a tumor. MR images show signal intensity changes according to the age of the hematoma. Changes in muscle bulk depend on the site and extent of the tear, and there need not be high signal intensity on T1-weighted images (Fig. 4-31).

Muscle Tumors

The common malignant tumors of muscle are rhabdomyosarcoma and leiomyosarcoma. The benign tumors, rhabdomyoma and leiomyoma of deep soft tissue, are rare, as is an intramuscular myxoma.

Rhabdomyosarcoma

Rhabdomyosarcoma[25] is a common soft-tissue malignancy. One half are the embryonal type that affect infants and young children (see Fig. 4-1). These tumors are usually found in the head, neck, genitourinary tract, and retroperitoneum. Only 5% have been found in the extremities (Fig. 4-32). The second subgroup is the alveolar type, which involves the extremities more frequently and affects older children and young adults. The least common is the pleomorphic type, which involves skeletal muscle in adults, usually the thigh in patients older than 45 years of age. Mixed forms may also occur.

Clinically, a deep-seated mass with rapid or slow growth is found. Although initially painless, pain may later develop in patients with large masses. The MRI characteristics are the same as for other nonfatty soft tissue sarcomas. Bone involvement is rare, but it may occur.

Leiomyosarcomas

Leiomyosarcomas are rare tumors occurring outside the retroperitoneum and abdomen. They are rare in children. The tumors are of vascular wall origin and usually arise from the iliac, femoral, or saphenous veins in the lower extremity.[25] They present as deep-seated intramuscular or intermuscular tumors of the extremities. Leg edema may ensue. Hypervascularity, vascular compression, and intravenous tumor growth may be demonstrated on angiography.[75] Heterogenous signal intensity may be seen on MR images, with signal characteristics indistinguishable from other cellular nonfatty soft-tissue malignancies (Fig. 4-33).

Deep-seated leiomyomas of vascular origin[76] may mimic sarcomas because of their vascularity, size, and location. They are richly vascular, may attain large size, and may contain scattered calcifications. CT can demonstrate these features.

(text continues on page 293)

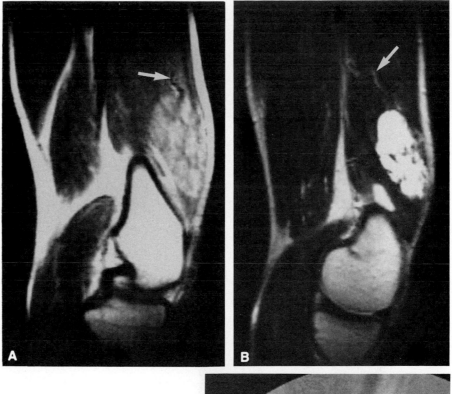

FIGURE 4-24.   Hemangioma of the vastus medialis muscle in an 18-year-old man. Sagittal MR scans show high signal intensity. (**A**) Relatively T1-weighted MR image (TR = 683 msec, TE = 26 msec). Signal-voided vessels may represent the feeding artery (*arrow*). (**B**) T2-weighted MR image (TR = 2000 msec, TE = 80 msec). Enhanced vessels may represent slow-flowing draining veins (*arrow*). Contrast between skeletal muscle hemangioma and normal muscle is much greater in **B** than in **A**. (**C**) Digital subtraction angiography. Contrast material puddles within the tumor and superiorly in the vasculature. (**A,B**: From Yuh WTC, Kathol MH, Sein MA, et al: Hemangiomas of skeletal muscle: MR findings in five patients. AJR Am J Roentgenol 149:765–768, 1987)

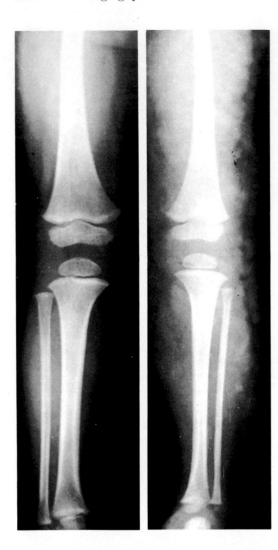

FIGURE 4-25. Lymphangioma. Lobular soft-tissue masses and soft-tissue enlargement in the left leg have resulted in a lack of bone development, both in length and in caliber. (Courtesy of Dr. Harvey White, Children's Hospital, Chicago, IL.)

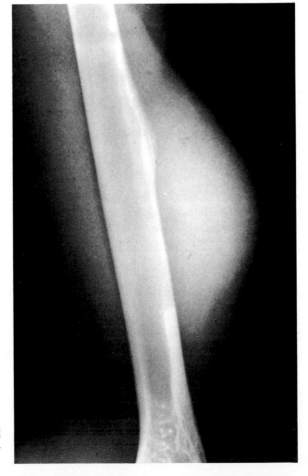

FIGURE 4-26. Chronic hematoma was confirmed by two biopsies. There is a smooth soft-tissue mass at the outer aspect of the arm and a small amount of laminated periosteal new bone formation. The laminations appear to be thick.

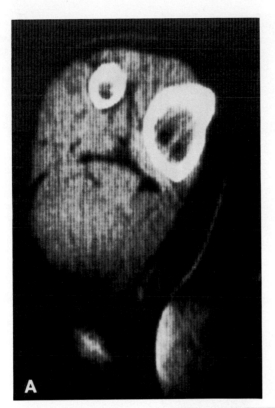

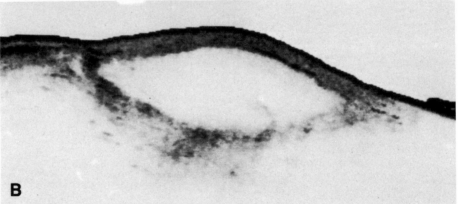

FIGURE 4-27.   Hematoma. A 65-year-old woman taking anticoagulants developed a mass posterior to the left knee. **(A)** Computed tomography shows a mass of soft-tissue density located posteriorly in the proximal leg. **(B)** Ultrasound demonstrates a clear, sonolucent region with a moderate backwall echo.

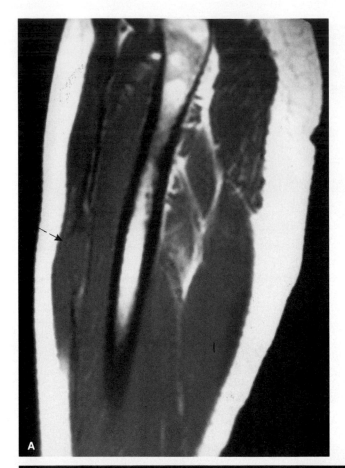

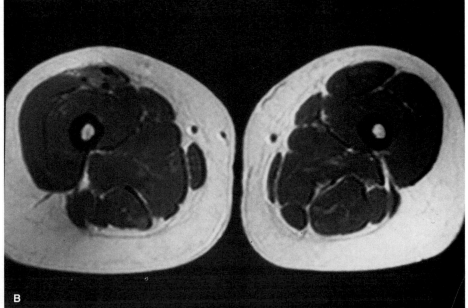

FIGURE 4-28. Hematoma of the rectus femoris muscle. (**A**) MR image (SE 500/20). A 3-cm hematoma, seen anteriorly, is isointense with muscle. (**B**) MR image (SE 2000/20). The major portion of the hematoma increases in signal intensity. Several foci are seen as signal voids. (**C**) MR image (SE 2000/80). A small area of the hematoma markedly increases in signal intensity, whereas other areas are signal voids or isointense with muscle.

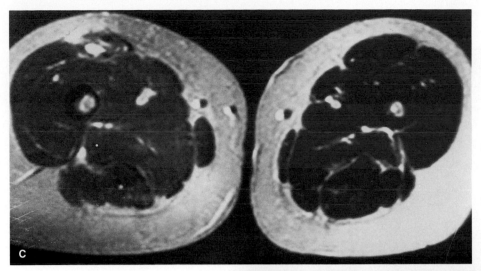

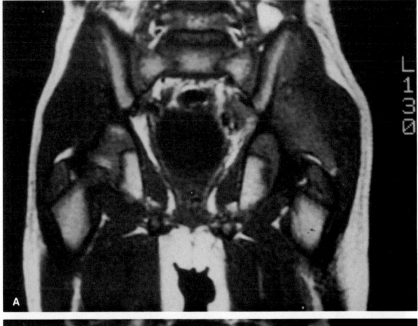

FIGURE 4-28. *(Continued)*

FIGURE 4-29. Gluteal hematoma in a hemophiliac. (**A**) A bulge in the contour of the left gluteus musculature was palpated and determined clinically to be a mass. High signal intensity medially in the muscle is seen. (**B**) MR image (SE 2200/80). The hemorrhagic area has increased in signal intensity and is infiltrating the outer portion of the muscle. (From Greenfield GB, Arrington JA, Kudryk BT: MRI of soft tissue tumors. Skeletal Radiol 22:77–84, 1993)

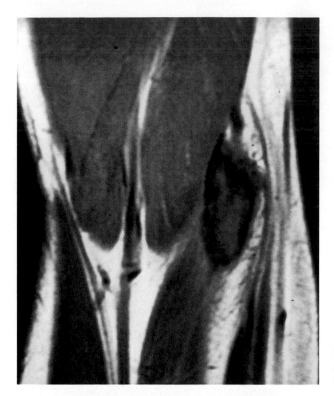

FIGURE 4-30. Chronic hematoma in an 11-year-old boy. MR image (SE 600/19). A low-signal-intensity rim surrounds the hematoma, which is situated medially in the soft tissues.

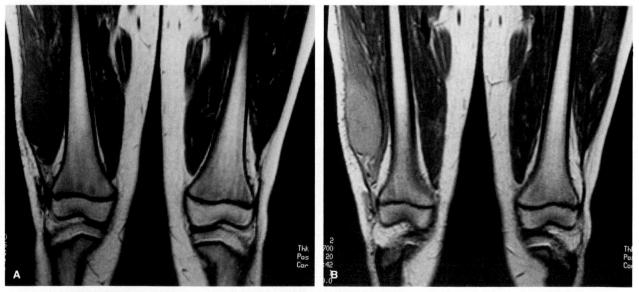

FIGURE 4-31. Muscle tear in a 16-year-old girl. (**A**) MR (SE 810/15) coronal image. Enlargement of the vastus lateralus compartment was secondary to a muscle tear. The lesion is isodense compared with muscle, but the textural pattern is effaced. (**B**) MRI (SE 2700/20). The region of the tear is increased in signal intensity. The pattern is homogeneous. (**C**) MR image (SE 2700/80). The muscle compartment is seen as a heterogeneous, high-intensity signal with high-signal-intensity linear and reticular changes in the subcutaneous tissues.

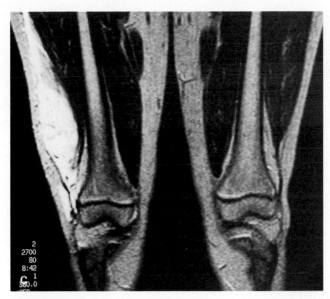

FIGURE 4-31. *(Continued)*

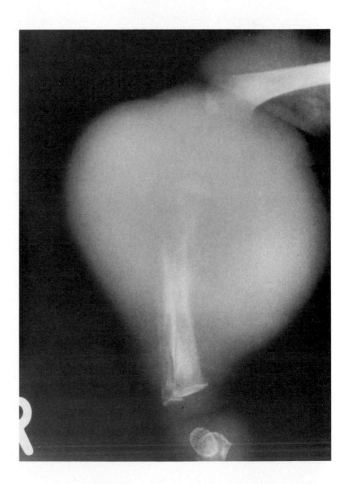

FIGURE 4-32. Rhabdomyosarcoma in a 3-day-old boy. A large soft-tissue mass has produced marked destruction of the tibia and fibula.

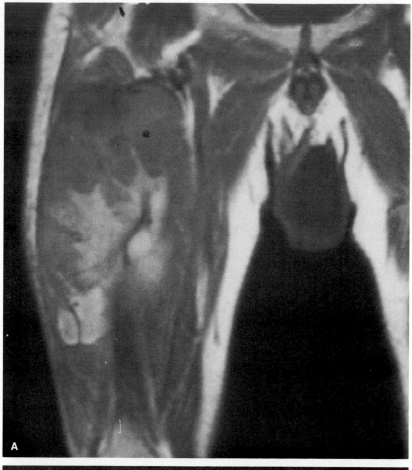

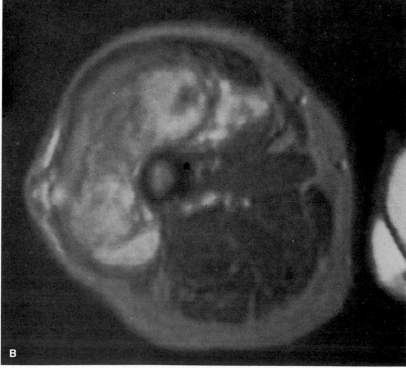

FIGURE 4-33. Leiomyosarcoma. (**A**) MR image (SE 800/20). A large, inhomogeneous, soft-tissue mass is seen in the thigh. The subcutaneous tissue laterally shows a reticular low-signal-intensity pattern. (**B**) MR image (SE 2500/80). The tumor is of mixed signal intensity and invades the subcutaneous tissue laterally. (From Greenfield GB, Arrington JA, Kudryk BT: MRI of soft tissue tumors. Skeletal Radiol 22:77–84, 1993)

Intramuscular Myxoma

Intramuscular myxoma is a rare benign tumor that most often occurs in patients between 40 and 70 years of age. It presents as a firm, painless, palpable mass. It most frequently arises in the muscles of the thigh, buttocks, shoulder, and upper arm. It is not to be confused with other tumors containing myxoid tissue, most notably myxoid liposarcoma. MR images show a well-circumscribed mass arising from muscle with uniform decreased intensity on T1-weighted images, inhomogeneous contrast enhancement, and uniform increased signal intensity on T2-weighted images.[77] Angiography shows poor vascularization.

Synovial Tumors

The synovium may be involved with malignant tumors, most often with synovial sarcoma, also called synovioma, and very rarely with synovial chondrosarcoma. Benign conditions include pigmented villonodular synovitis (PVNS), synovial osteochondromatosis, lipoma arborescens, hemangioma, and cysts.

Synovioma

Synovioma, or synovial sarcoma, is a common, highly malignant fibroblastic neoplasm. The lower extremities are most often involved, especially the knees. Only 10% of these tumors are located primarily within a joint capsule, arising instead near a joint or from a tendon sheath anywhere along a limb. The buttocks, back, neck, chest, hands, feet, hips, abdominal wall, and orbits are other reported sites. The sarcomas may occur in unusual locations and have even been reported in the oropharynx.[78] The peak age incidence is between 18 and 35 years. In one series, 69% of the tumors occurred in the lower extremity; 25% occurred in the upper extremity; and 6% occurred in the trunk. The histologic characteristics include a predominantly bimorphic pattern, with epithelial and spindle cell components in 33% of the tumors, a monomorphic pattern in 31%, and a mixed pattern in 36%.[79] The patients usually present with a mass associated with pain and tenderness.

On plain films, a soft-tissue mass is seen, which may be lobulated and quite large. Calcification occurs in about 30% of cases,[25] which may be the only definitive finding on conventional x-ray films. This contrasts with PVNS, which rarely calcifies. Locally, the bone shows osteoporosis or invasion with irregular destructive changes with possibly more than one bone involved (Fig. 4-34). CT may demonstrate calcification within a mass.[80] MR images show the tumor as a low-signal-intensity area on T1-weighted images and higher-signal-intensity area on T2-weighted images, usually as an inhomogeneous, septated mass with infiltrative margins, possibly with hemorrhage near a joint (Fig. 4-35).[81] Fluid-fluid levels may be seen. It may cause destruction or erosion of several adjacent bones (Fig. 4-36). The tumor may involve the carpal or tarsal tunnel (Fig. 4-37). The pattern and extent of the calcification cannot be accurately depicted on MR images with current techniques. Angiography shows marked vascularity (Fig. 4-38).

Synovial Chondrosarcoma

Synovial chondrosarcoma[82-84] is a rare tumor that may arise de novo or develop in a joint from malignant change in synovial osteochondromatosis.[85,86] A large mass and bony invasion may be seen. If synovial chondromatosis is present, the calcifications may be displaced away from the joint. Calcifications may also appear displaced posterior to the knee joint if they are in a Baker cyst.

(text continues on page 298)

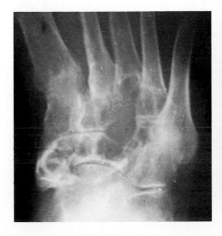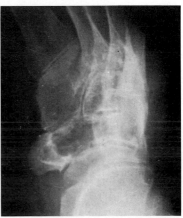

FIGURE 4-34. Synovioma of the tarsus. Extensive tarsal destruction and destruction of the metatarsal bases are seen. (Courtesy of Dr. Antonio Pizarro, Hines Veterans Administration Hospital, Hines, IL.)

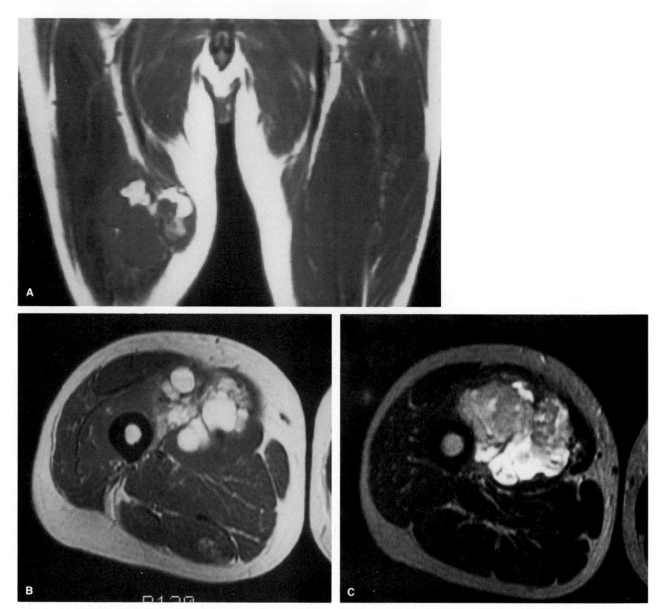

FIGURE 4-35. Synovial sarcoma of a thigh that contains hemorrhage. (**A**) MR (SE 600/20) coronal section. A large, irregular, lobulated, inhomogeneous mass of mixed signal is depicted medially in the right thigh. (**B**) MR (SE 3000/20) axial section. A large, lobulated mass of mixed signal intensity involves principally the vastus medialis muscle and extends into adjacent musculature. A fluid-fluid level is seen in the uppermost lobulation. (**C**) MR image (SE 3000/80). The low-signal-intensity portions of the tumor that were seen on previous images have increased in signal intensity. Irregularity of margination is evident. (From Greenfield GB, Arrington JA, Kudryk BT: MRI of soft tissue tumors. Skeletal Radiol 22:77–84, 1993)

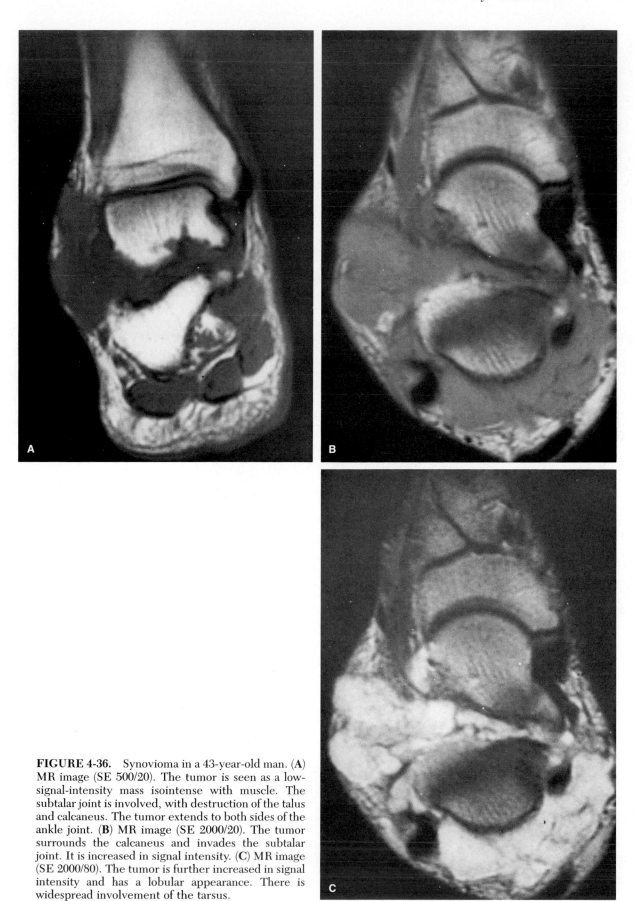

FIGURE 4-36. Synovioma in a 43-year-old man. (**A**) MR image (SE 500/20). The tumor is seen as a low-signal-intensity mass isointense with muscle. The subtalar joint is involved, with destruction of the talus and calcaneus. The tumor extends to both sides of the ankle joint. (**B**) MR image (SE 2000/20). The tumor surrounds the calcaneus and invades the subtalar joint. It is increased in signal intensity. (**C**) MR image (SE 2000/80). The tumor is further increased in signal intensity and has a lobular appearance. There is widespread involvement of the tarsus.

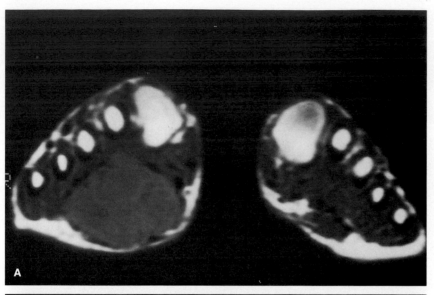

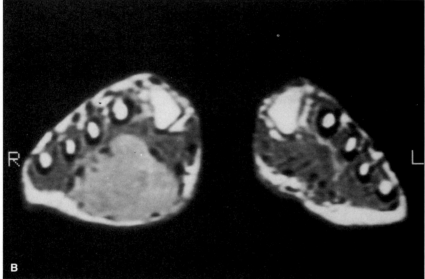

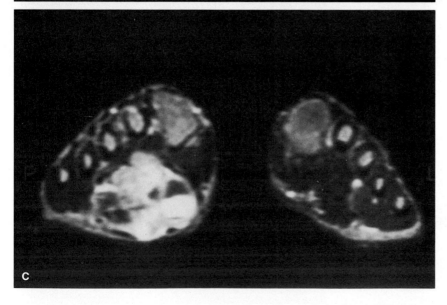

FIGURE 4-37. Synovial sarcoma. (**A**) MR image (SE 750/20). A large, low-signal-intensity soft-tissue mass is seen at the plantar aspect of the right foot, which appears fairly homogeneous. (**B**) MR image (SE 2000/20). The mass is increased in signal intensity and retains its fairly homogeneous appearance. (**C**) MR image (SE 2000/80). The mass shows high signal intensity. The various tendons are of low signal intensity. (From Greenfield GB, Arrington JA, Kudryk BT: MRI of soft tissue tumors. Skeletal Radiol 22:77–84, 1993)

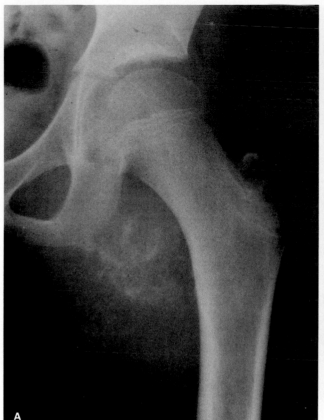

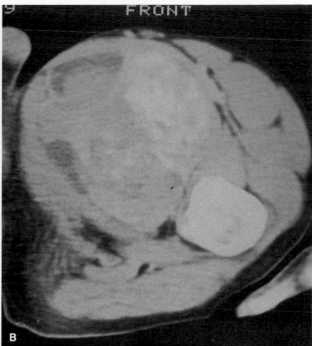

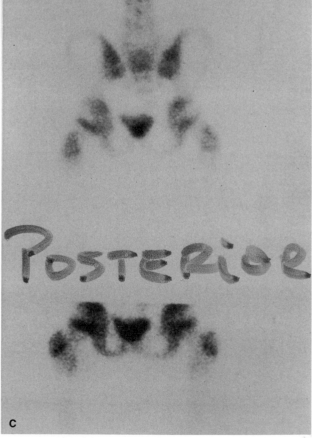

FIGURE 4-38.   Synovial sarcoma of the hip in a 10-year-old boy. (**A**) An anteroposterior view of the left hip shows a large soft-tissue mass containing multiple, small calcifications. These calcifications do not have the linear or circular pattern of cartilage calcifications. (**B**) The CT scan shows a large soft-tissue mass with calcifications and necrotic areas. The posterior aspect of the bony cortex is minimally involved. (**C**) The radionuclide bone scan shows minimally increased activity in the left subtrochanteric region. (**D**) MR image (SE 600/20). A large, inhomogeneous mass in the soft tissues adjacent to the hip extends down the medial thigh. (**E**) MR image (SE 2500/80). The mass is of high signal intensity and has irregular margins and internal septations. (**F**) Digital subtraction angiography shows the mass to be markedly hypervascular, displacing the major vessels. Early venous filling is also depicted.   *continued*

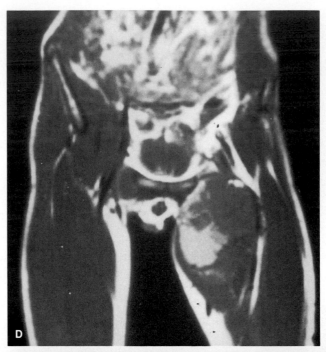

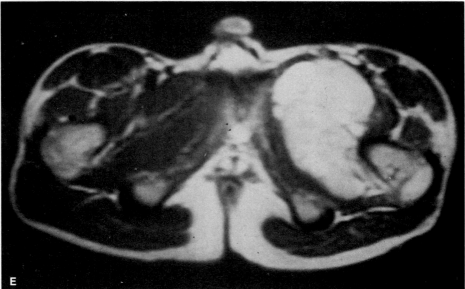

FIGURE 4-38. *(Continued)*

Pigmented Villonodular Synovytis and Villonodular Tenosynovitis

PVNS and villonodular tenosynovitis[87–90] are chronic proliferations, probably caused by inflammatory reactions that occur in the synovia of the joints, tendons, and bursae. They are also called giant cell tumors and xanthomas. The disease most commonly affects young adults with intermittent pain and swelling of a joint. PVNS is classified as a diffuse form that affects the entire synovial membrane and as a localized form that affects tendon sheaths or a small portion of the synov-

ium.[91] There may be a solitary lesion. The lesions are usually monarticular, but biarticular involvement has been reported.[92–94] The disease most commonly occurs in the knee joint, but temporomandibular joint involvement has been reported.[95] Polyarticular disease has also been reported in six joints.[96]

Erosion or invasion of bone involves subchondral areas and the articular margin (Figs. 4-39 and 4-40). Various sizes of cyst-like defects have sharp and sclerotic margins, which rarely may progress to joint destruction. Characteristically, joint space narrowing and osteoporosis are absent. An intracapsular location and

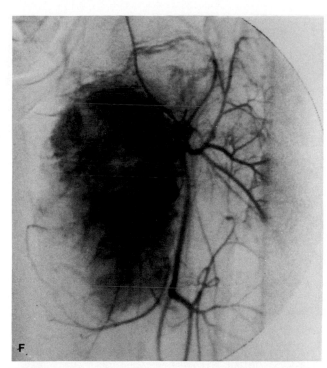

FIGURE 4-38. *(Continued)*

lack of calcification help differentiate this lesion from synovial sarcoma.

Lobular soft-tissue masses do not calcify but may appear denser on conventional films because of hemosiderin deposition. Ultrasound can demonstrate synovial thickening, joint effusion, and echogenic villous projections.[97] CT can determine the nature and extent of this disorder. It can show the entire area of involvement. The lesions enhance with intravenous contrast administration.[98]

MR images show inflamed and thickened synovium as intermediate in signal intensity on T1-weighted images and as increased in signal intensity on T2-weighted images. The synovium is interspersed in the hemosiderin deposits, which are seen as foci of decreased signal intensity. The hemosiderin deposition can be greatly accentuated with the GRE technique.[99,100] The masses themselves do not increase in signal intensity on T2-weighted images because of their hemosiderin content (Fig. 4-41).

Arthrography demonstrates capsular distention and multiple nodular filling defects in the diffuse form, which may be of various sizes and may be sessile or pedunculated. This pattern is referred to as a cobble-

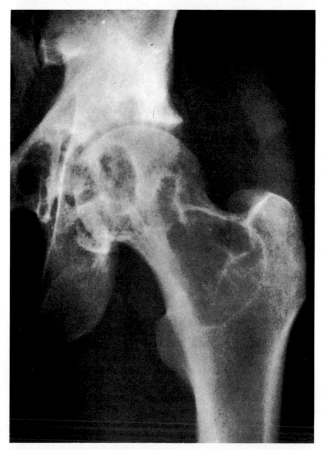

FIGURE 4-39. Endosteal-type pigmented villonodular synovitis of the hip. There are multiple large and small erosions of the femoral head and neck in the acetabular region. The joint space is maintained. Bulging of the soft-tissue fascial planes at the superior aspect of the hip joint can be seen.

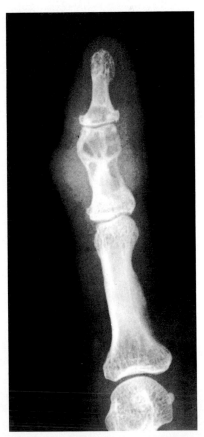

FIGURE 4-40. Pigmented villonodular tenosynovitis of the finger. There is soft-tissue swelling in the middle phalanx of the fifth finger that is associated with multiple bone erosions.

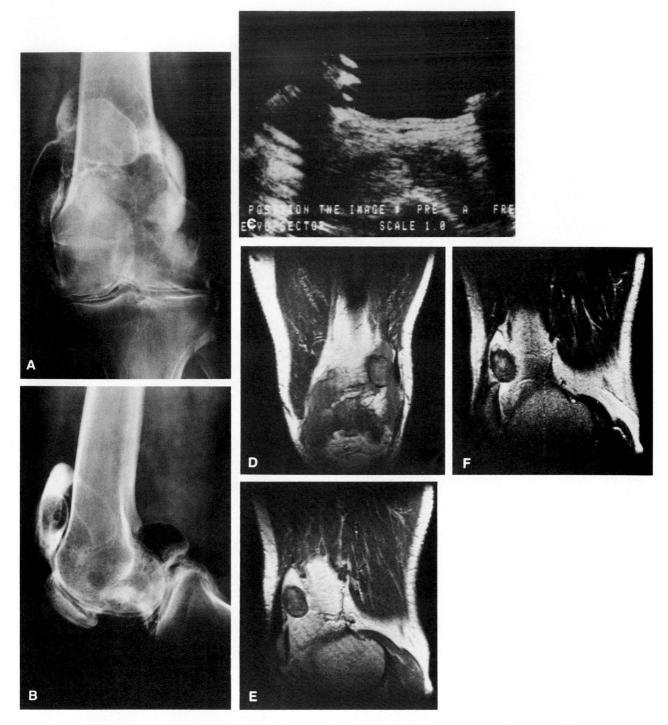

FIGURE 4-41. Benign tenosynovial giant cell tumor. (**A**) Double-contrast arthrogram of the knee shows a large, well-circumscribed mass in the suprapatellar bursa attached to the synovium on its medial side. (**B**) Lateral arthrogram shows the mass as a well-circumscribed filling defect in the contrast-filled suprapatellar bursa. (**C**) Ultrasound examination shows this lesion as a solid, well-circumscribed, echogenic mass. (**D**) A T1-weighted coronal MR image shows a well-circumscribed, intermediate-intensity mass surrounded by a low-signal-intensity capsule. (**E**) T1-weighted sagittal MR image shows an intermediate-signal-intensity mass that is inhomogeneous, surrounded by a low-signal-intensity capsule. (**F**) A T2-weighted MR image shows a patchy area of high signal intensity within the lesion.

stone synovium.[91] In the focal form, a solitary intracapsular filling defect is seen.

Involvement of a lumbar vertebral facet joint has been reported. An extradural mass behind the vertebral body was seen displacing the dural sac on a myelogram, and the tumor was associated with destructive changes of the facet joint.[101] Another site of possible involvement in the knee is the infrapatellar region associated with the fat pad, which can be demonstrated by arthrography.[102] Rare cases of metastases have been observed, which raise questions about this lesion's inflammatory nature.[103]

Synovial Osteochondromatosis

Synovial osteochondromatosis is not a neoplasm but a proliferative condition of chondrometaplasia in which foci of cartilage develop in the synovia and eventually become calcified and ossified.[104–106] The areas later become detached and become free within the joint cavity. The size of the foci increase, nourished by the synovial fluid. They may coalesce into large masses.

Usually monarticular, the condition occurs in adults and is rare in children.[107,108] Males are affected more often than females. It is mildly painful. The most frequent joint involved is the knee,[109] followed by the hip, elbow, and shoulder. Hip involvement has been associated with an intrapelvic mass.[110] Involvement of the ankle,[111,112] and temporomandibular joint[113,114] have been reported. A mass in the temporomandibular joint may have an extension into the middle cranial fossa.[115,116] Bursae[117] and tendons may be involved.

Multiple calcified or ossified densities as large as several centimeters in diameter are seen within the joint capsule. Rarely, it may be solitary. Osteoporosis is rare. There may be osteoarthritis with joint space narrowing, osteophytes, and joint effusion. Extensive erosions of bone, particularly in the hip, may occur.[118] Pathologic fracture of the hip may occur as a presenting feature.[119] These lesions can be well demonstrated by CT and MRI (Fig. 4-42). Ultrasound is useful in the diagnosis. Arthrography is also useful, particularly in demonstrating noncalcified masses.

The calcifications are smaller in younger patients

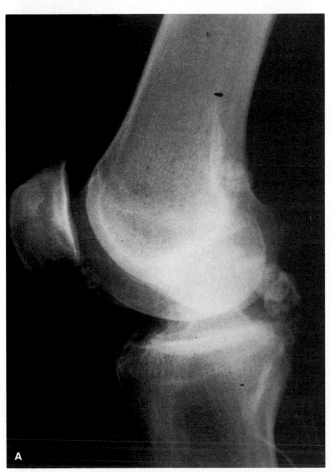
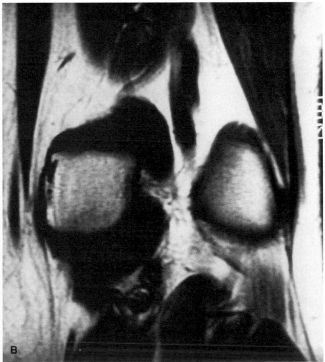

FIGURE 4-42. Synovial osteochondromatosis in a 40-year-old man. (**A**) A lateral view of the knee reveals moderate-sized, rounded calcifications located posteriorly within the joint capsule. (**B**) MR image (SE 600/14). The synovial osteochondromas are moderate-sized areas with a signal-void rim corresponding to the calcification and mixed-signal-intensity interiors.

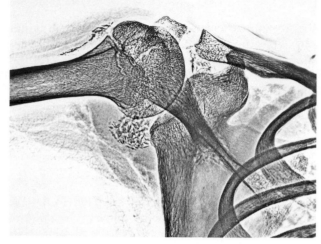

FIGURE 4-43. Idiopathic-type synovial osteochondromatosis of the shoulder, is shown in a xeroradiograph of an asymptomatic 13-year-old girl. The lesion was not biopsied. Multiple, small, intracapsular calcifications are revealed.

(Fig. 4-43). Fewer but larger intraarticular calcifications and ossifications are more likely to result from trauma, neuropathic arthropathy, or osteochondrosis dissecans (Fig. 4-44). Rarely, some calcifications may be extraarticular, occurring in combination with PVNS and synovial hemangioma. Malignant transformation of extraarticular synovial chondromatosis to a chondrosarcoma has been reported.[85,83]

Synovial Hemangioma

Synovial hemangioma is a rare benign tumor that most often involves the knee.[120,121] Other joints, including the elbow and temporomandibular joint, may also be involved. Adolescents and young adults are most often affected, exhibiting joint enlargement, pain, muscle atrophy, and limitation of motion. Joint aspiration may yield hemorrhagic fluid. The adjacent bone and soft tissues may have concomitant angiomas. There are two types: circumscribed and diffuse.

This condition is often not seen on conventional x-ray films, but phleboliths and a soft-tissue mass about the joint may be present. There may be limb-length discrepancy, accelerated maturation of the epiphyses, and destructive regional bone changes. Osteoporosis, osteoarthritis, periosteal new bone formation, joint ankylosis, and hemophilia-like changes have been described. Arthrography may demonstrate a lobulated synovial mass. Arteriography may show a network of tortuous and irregular small vessels.

Lipoma Arborescens

Lipoma arborescens is a polypoid, fatty synovial proliferation most often associated with degenerative joint disease.[122] Soft-tissue swelling that need not be

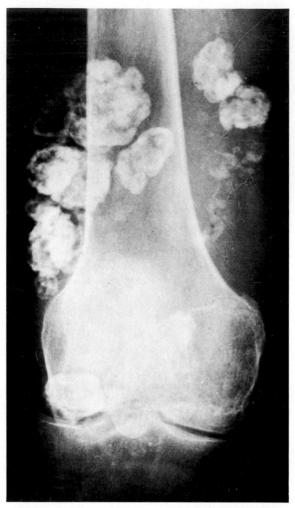

FIGURE 4-44. Large-sized synovial osteochondromas are associated with degenerative disease of the knee.

radiolucent is evident radiologically. Arthrography may demonstrate a lobulated, radiolucent defect.

Popliteal Cyst

A popliteal cyst, or Baker cyst, results from posterior herniation of the synovium of the knee, usually between the medial head of the gastrocnemius and semimembranosus muscles. On CT, a thin, well-defined cyst wall with fluid-density contents, central septa, and medial popliteal location with mediocaudal extension are seen. This picture may be changed because of gelatinous cyst contents, rupture of the synovial membrane, or metaplasia of the cyst wall.[123] On MR images, an uncomplicated cyst or well-circumscribed homogeneous mass, with or without communication to the knee joint, may be seen. The signal intensity is the same as that of synovial fluid on all pulse sequences. One complication of popliteal cysts is occlusion of the popliteal artery.[124] Extension and rupture with dissection along the calf musculature may occur, particularly in association with rheumatoid arthritis (Fig. 4-45). The cyst may also extend superiorly, and then magnetic resonance angiography (MRA) is employed to rule out an aneurysm or tumor (Fig. 4-46). A malignant tumor of the popliteal region may simulate a Baker cyst.[125] A hemorrhagic Baker cyst may simulate a solid mass on ultrasound and show signal characteristics of blood on MR images. It should be differentiated from a clotted popliteal artery aneurysm.[126] Synovial osteochondromatosis may rarely be found in a Baker cyst (Fig. 4-47).

Tumors of Peripheral Nerves and Nerve Sheaths

Malignant tumors arising from the peripheral nerves and nerve sheaths include malignant schwannoma and, rarely, neuroepithelioma. Benign tumors include neurofibroma, neurofibromatosis, neurilemoma, and neuroma.

Malignant Schwannoma

Malignant schwannoma,[25] also called malignant peripheral nerve sheath tumor, may arise from a peripheral nerve or a neurofibroma. There is a 4% chance for late sarcomatous change of neurofibromatosis, and about half of these tumors occur with neurofibromatosis. Most tumors occur in patients between the ages of 20 and 50 years and arise along major nerve trunks.

CT demonstrates low-attenuation areas that histopathologically correlate with necrosis, hemorrhage, or cystic degeneration. The density differences may be enhanced by intravenous contrast administration.[127] Angiography demonstrates the extent and vascularity of these sarcomas and can guide selection of the biopsy site and help in planning surgical resection.[128] Low to intermediate signal intensities are seen on T1-weighted images, with an increase in signal intensity with T2 weighting. The lesions may be fairly well circumscribed and may show some internal inhomogeneities (Fig. 4-48).

Neuroepithelioma

Neuroepithelioma is a primitive neuroectodermal tumor (PNET) arising in the periphery that histologically resembles Ewing tumor and neuroblastoma.

(*text continues on page 306*)

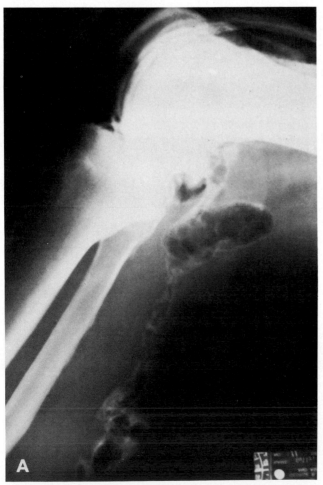

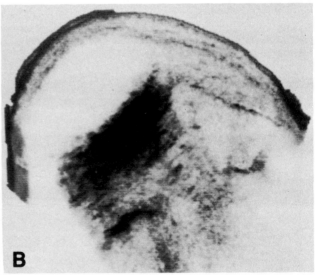

FIGURE 4-45. Baker cyst that has extended down the calf. (**A**) Pneumoarthrogram. A double-contrast outline of the cyst shows its downward extension. The cyst has ruptured and dissected down to the calf. (**B**) Ultrasound examination shows a sonolucent area posterior to the knee that has a strong backwall echo.

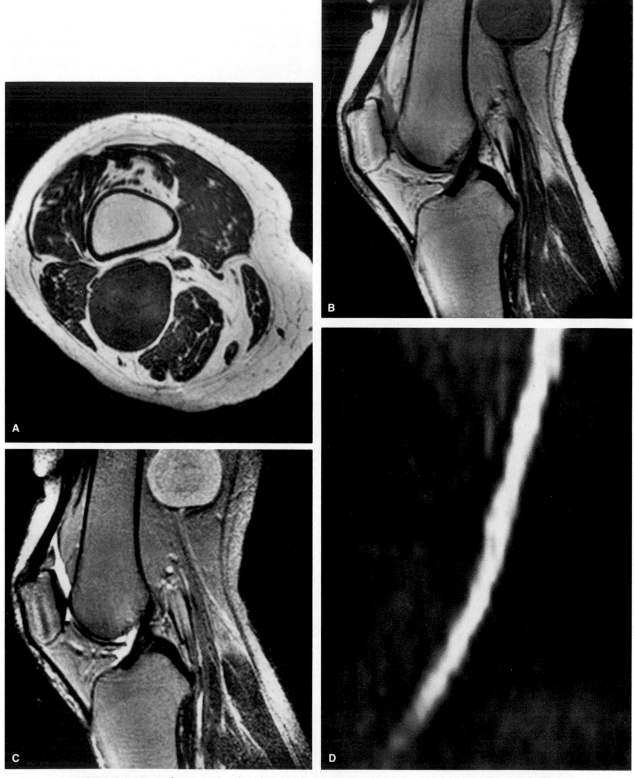

FIGURE 4-46. Baker cyst that has dissected superiorly. (**A**) MR image (SE 600/20). A rounded, well-circumscribed collection resides posteriorly between the biceps femoris muscle and the semimembranosus. The signal intensity is isointense with muscle. (**B**) MR image (SE 2200/20). The collection lies superiorly to the knee joint with a thin stalk extending from the knee region. The signal intensity is slightly greater than muscle. (**C**) MR image (SE 2200/80). The signal intensity of the collection is increased and shows heterogeneity. The stalk is still seen. The synovial fluid appears much brighter than the cyst. (**D**) Magnetic resonance angiography shows the popliteal artery is intact.

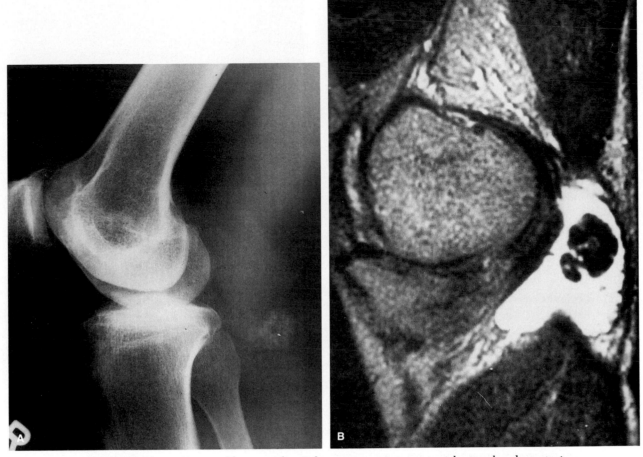

FIGURE 4-47. A 41-year-old man with a Baker cyst containing synovial osteochondromatosis. (**A**) A lateral view of the knee shows irregular calcification in the soft tissues posterior to the knee joint. The calcific bodies contain a dense, calcified outer margin. (**B**) MRI (SE 2700/80). A Baker cyst posterior to the knee joint contains calcification, seen with a low-signal-intensity periphery.

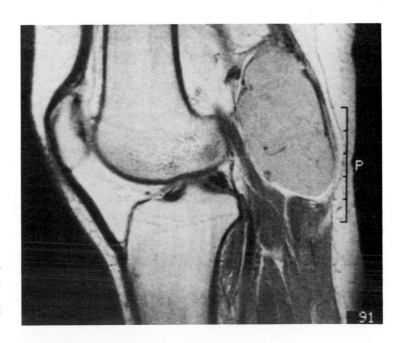

FIGURE 4-48. T1-weighted MR image. A 6-cm, ovoid mass is in the popliteal fossa. A curvilinear small blood vessel and light marginal septations are seen within the mass, which is displacing muscle. On biopsy, this lesion proved to be a malignant schwannoma.

These are small, round cell tumors. It is a rare tumor that may occur at any age and may be confused with metastatic neuroblastoma.

Neurofibromatosis

Neurofibromatosis, classified a phakomatosis (i.e., neurocutaneous syndrome), is a hereditary dysplasia of mesodermal and neuroectodermal tissues.[129-134] It occurs in approximately 1 of 3000 live births, and expression of the disease ranges from minimal to extensive involvement. It is transmitted as an autosomal dominant trait with a high degree of penetrance. Males are more frequently affected. The basic lesions are neurofibromas of the peripheral and cranial nerves. Café au lait spots with smooth margins or coast-of-California type, skin and subcutaneous neurofibromas, plexiform neurofibromas, bone deformities (including severe angular kyphoscoliosis that may lead to paraplegia and localized gigantism), elephantoid skin hypertrophy, intrathoracic meningocele, glial tumors, hypertrophied sebaceous glands, and lipomas are frequently associated features. Skeletal deformities are caused by the basic mesodermal dysplasia in this condition and erosions from the neurofibromas.

Solitary neurofibromas outnumber cases of neurofibromatosis.[25] They show the same characteristics as the lesions of the multiple variety. Malignant change rarely occurs in solitary lesions.

Subcutaneous and skin neurofibromas can be seen as multiple, soft-tissue densities, particularly on CT.[135] The peripheral nerves may develop enlarged diameters or fusiform focal enlargement.[136] Approximately half of these patients develop bone abnormalities. The spine may show a sharp angular kyphoscoliosis with dysplasia of the vertebral bodies, and dislocation of the spine has also been reported.[137] Erosions, particularly in the intervertebral foramina, may occur from dumbbell neurofibromas (Fig. 4-49). Posterior scalloping of the vertebral bodies may occur (Fig. 4-50).[138] Intrathoracic meningocele may simulate a paravertebral neurofibroma. Anterior and lateral scalloping of the vertebral bodies and vertebral body collapse may occur.

The skull shows a characteristic defect involving the posterosuperior wall of the orbit that is caused by a developmental defect of the wings of the sphenoid and the orbital plate of the frontal bone. The ribs show erosions at their superior and inferior margins from intercostal neurofibromas, or there may be a twisted-ribbon appearance.

The long bones may show localized enlargement in areas of plexiform neurofibromas.[139] There may also be overtubulation with a long, slender, bowed appearance. The bones rarely may be smaller than normal.

Pseudarthroses are common,[140] usually without neurofibromatous tissue at the pseudarthrotic site.

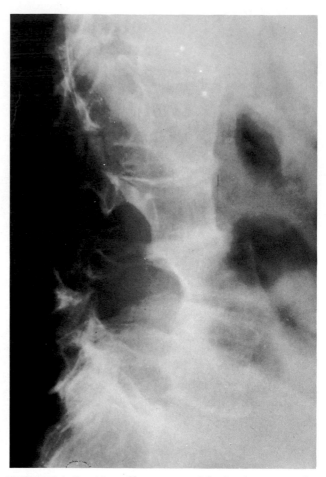

FIGURE 4-49. Neurofibromatosis of the lumbar spine. The lateral view shows marked erosions of the intervertebral foramina due to dumbbell neurofibromas and posterior scalloping of the upper lumbar vertebral bodies.

Plexiform neurofibromas may be demonstrated on CT (Fig. 4-51) and MR images (Fig. 4-52).

Osteomalacia may rarely be associated with neurofibromatosis, resulting from renal failure due to stenosis of the renal artery. There is a high incidence of associated congenital anomalies that are not specific for this disease.[141] Technetium 99m diethylenetriamine pentaacetic acid is taken up by benign soft-tissue neurofibromas. This may be seen on conventional scintigraphy[142] or single photon emission computed tomography (SPECT).[143] MR images show each neurofibroma as having homogeneous low signal intensity on T1-weighted images and high signal intensity on T2-weighted images (Fig. 4-53). Clusters of neurofibromas may be irregularly marginated (Fig. 4-54).

Other benign tumors of peripheral nerves or their sheaths include neurilemoma (i.e., benign schwannoma) and neurinoma. On MR images, these tumors exhibit an intermediate signal intensity on T1-weighted images, and they brighten on T2-weighted images, with some inhomogeneity. The diagnosis is suggested

FIGURE 4-50. Neurofibromatosis of the lumbar vertebrae. The myelogram shows posterior scalloping of the lumbar vertebrae and dural ectasia.

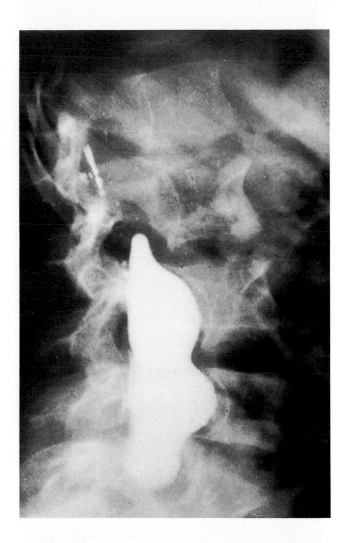

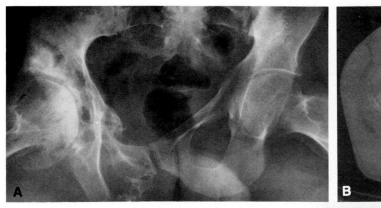

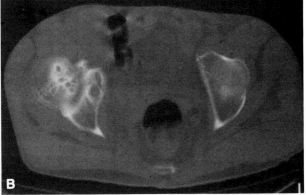

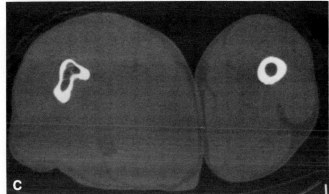

FIGURE 4-51. Neurofibromatosis of the pelvis. (**A**) The deformity of the pelvis is principally on the right side, with multiple cysts, particularly about the acetabulum. (**B**) CT. Cysts of the acetabulum and the femoral head are seen on the patient's right. (**C**) CT. A plexiform neurofibroma has enlarged the right thigh and deformed the femur.

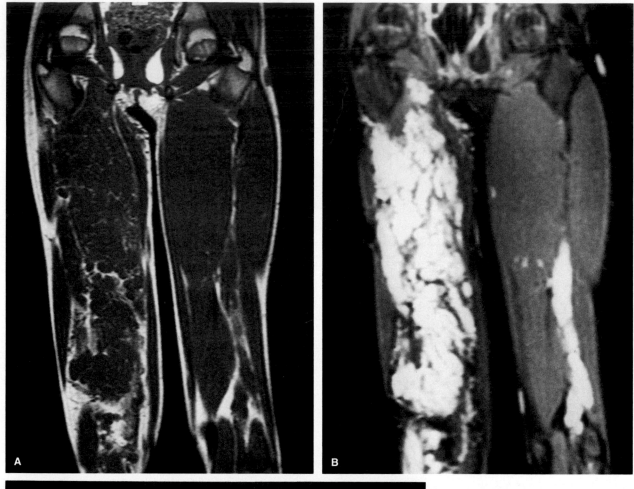

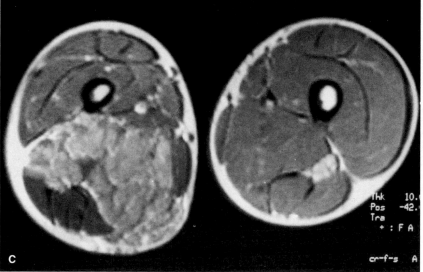

FIGURE 4-52. Plexiform neurofibromatosis in a 10-year-old girl. (**A**) MR image (SE 800/17) of the lower extremities shows marked soft-tissue irregularities of the entire thigh. These represent a plexiform neurofibroma, which is isointense with muscle. Similar changes occur to a much lesser extent on the patient's left side. (**B**) MRI (SE 3000/20). The signal intensity is markedly increased, and the signal area is heterogeneous and lobular. Similar changes occur to a lesser extent on the left side. (**C**) MR image (SE 2700/20) shows that the subcutaneous tissue is also involved. It has a lobular appearance, and the signal intensity is higher than that of muscle.

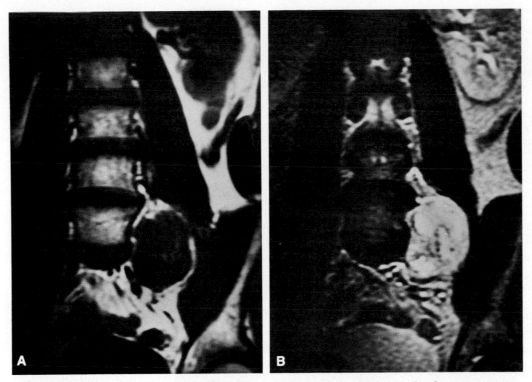

FIGURE 4-53. Neurofibroma lateral to the lumbosacral spine. (**A**) T1-weighted MR image. A well-encapsulated lesion of low signal intensity is adjacent to the lumbosacral region. (**B**) T2-weighted MR image. The tumor has high signal intensity and is nonhomogenous. A high-intensity vascular pattern surrounds the tumor. (Courtesy of Dr. Harold Posniak, Loyola University, Maywood, IL.)

by the presence of the tumor near a large nerve trunk that is associated with atrophy of its innervated muscles.[144]

Morton neuroma is a mass of perineural fibrosis of a plantar digital nerve resulting in pain in the sole of the foot between the metatarsals. Edema and fibrosis occur within the nerve. Ultrasound reveals an ovoid hypoechoic mass parallel to the long axis of the metatarsals.[145]

Extraosseous Ewing Sarcoma

Extraosseous Ewing sarcoma is a rare, highly malignant, soft-tissue tumor with a predilection for persons between 15 and 30 years of age.[25,146,147] The tumor ranges from 2 to 20 cm in diameter. Males are more often affected than females. This tumor rarely develops in patients of African descent. The areas chiefly involved are the paravertebral region, the chest wall, and the extremities. It presents as a rapidly growing, deep-seated mass. Histologically, this is a round cell tumor identical to that originating within bone. Hemorrhage frequently occurs within the tumor, and pulmonary metastases are common.

CT shows a mass with attenuation lower than muscle, without calcification, and with some enhancement after contrast material infusion. MRI is the only method that can demonstrate the full extent of the tumor. T1-weighted images show intermediate to low signal intensity, and T2-weighted images show increased signal intensity. The lesion margins may be relatively smooth, although careful inspection is warranted. MRI can demonstrate noninvolvement of the bone marrow cavity (Fig. 4-55).

Calcified Soft-Tissue Masses

Tumoral Calcinosis

Tumoral calcinosis is a rare, possibly autosomal dominant, hereditary disorder of phosphorus metabolism in which focal collections of calcium hydroxyapatite are deposited in the soft tissues, often in the vicinity of joints.[148–157] Calcium pyrophosphate may also be deposited in the soft-tissue masses. Other abnormalities include angioid streaks of the retina and hyperphosphatemia. The cause is considered to be a defect in phosphate excretion in the proximal renal tubules,[158] with hyperphosphatemia and elevated 1,25-dihydroxy-vitamin D_3 levels in some cases. Calcium levels are

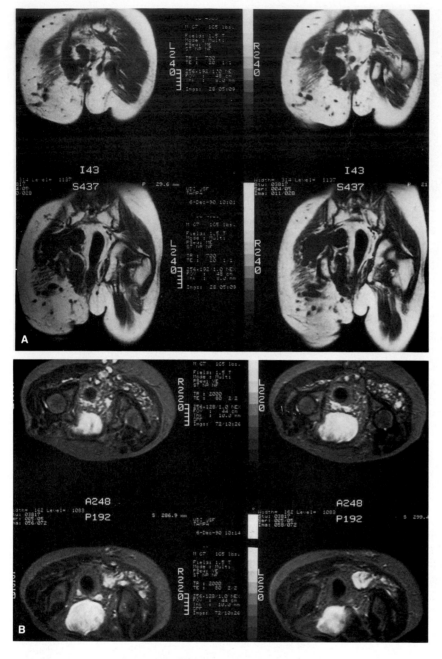

FIGURE 4-54. A 7-year-old boy with neurofibromatosis. (**A**) MR images (SE 700/20) reveal multiple, irregularly marginated, lobulated masses with many subcutaneous neurofibromas. (**B**) MR images (SE 2000/80). The neurofibromas increase in signal intensity in an irregular pattern. (From Greenfield GB, Arrington JA, Kudryk BT: MRI of soft tissue tumors. Skeletal Radiol 22:77–84, 1993)

normal. The usual age at diagnosis is from 6 to 25 years. People of African descent are most often affected. One or more joints may be involved, with a predilection for the paraarticular regions of the hips, elbows, and shoulders. Tumors along the linea aspera of the femur have been reported. Pain, swelling, ulceration, and disability often occur, although some lesions may be painless. Small, calcified nodules in the periarticular tissues of the large joints progress to form large, solid, lobulated tumors with a linear, lacy calcific distribution (Fig. 4-56). The joint itself is not involved. Fluid levels

may be detected. Solid and cystic calcific masses of various sizes are seen on CT scans. The regional bone marrow may be involved, demonstrating increased attenuation and spotty calcification. High signal intensity is seen on T2-weighted MR images for paraarticular masses and involved marrow despite the large amount of calcification.[154] This pattern is caused by the large, granulomatous, foreign-body response. In the elbow, the lower dorsal humerus is characteristically flattened. Similar calcific tumors can be seen in hyperparathyroidism and other causes of metastatic calcification.[159]

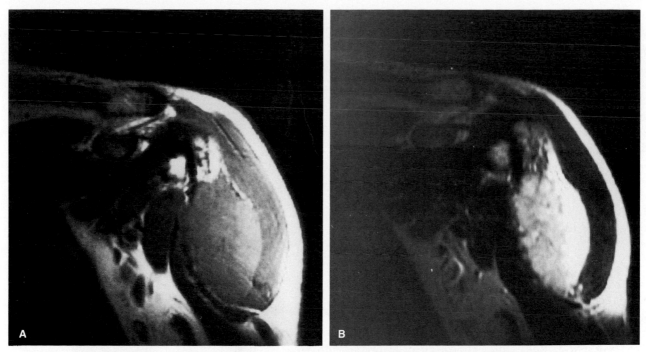

FIGURE 4-55. A 20-year-old man with a mass in his shoulder. (**A**) MR image (SE 600/20). A well-circumscribed mass is seen within the deltoid muscle. It is of intermediate signal intensity with several low-density streaks within it. (**B**) MR image (SE 2000/80). There is an increase in signal intensity of the mass. The outer margin remains smooth, but the inner margin is irregular. Biopsy revealed a soft-tissue Ewing sarcoma. (From Greenfield GB, Arrington JA, Kudryk BT: MRI of soft tissue tumors. Skeletal Radiol 22:77–84, 1993)

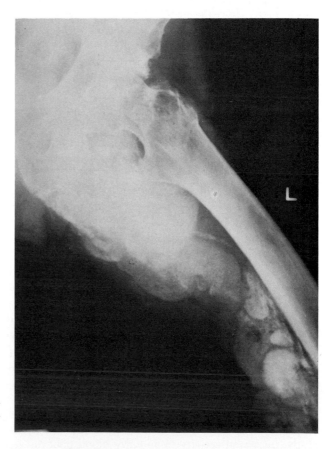

FIGURE 4-56. Tumoral calcinosis of the left thigh. Very extensive soft-tissue calcification has occurred. (Courtesy of Dr. Dharmashi V. Bhate, Veterans Administration Hospital, Hines, IL.)

Myositis Ossificans

Myositis ossificans is a benign, heterotopic, soft-tissue ossification that may result from several different causes.[160] The pathogenesis is unknown, and there is no primary inflammation of skeletal muscle, despite the name. The condition is a metaplasia of intramuscular connective tissue. Young adults are usually affected, and it is rare in children. It is not premalignant. The ectopic bone may lie longitudinally along the axis of muscle and may also be attached to the bone. The adjacent periosteum may react. In the early stages, a radiolucent zone of soft tissue separates the lesion from the underlying periosteal reaction and cortex. Bone erosion and blending of the new bone with the cortex may occur.

MYOSITIS OSSIFICANS CIRCUMSCRIPTA. Myositis ossificans circumscripta is localized ossification after direct acute or chronic trauma.[161–163] The symptoms are a persistent soft-tissue mass, pain, and tenderness after an injury. It begins as an ill-defined cloud of calcification 2 to 6 weeks after the onset of symptoms. Flocculent densities within the mass and local periosteal reaction are seen after about 1 month. After 6 to 8 weeks, a lacy pattern of bony trabeculation appears that is circumscribed by a cortex (Fig. 4-57). At about 6 months, it matures to a bony appearance, and the mass reduces in size. The ectopic bone may lie parallel to the bone shaft (Fig. 4-58). Localized myositis ossificans must be differentiated from parosteal sarcoma, which also has a thin, radiolucent line separating tumor from cortex, except at its origin from bone. In myositis ossificans, the hallmark is that more mature bone is seen peripherally.

Myositis ossificans about the elbow joint is common. An example caused by chronic trauma is rider's bone, or ossification of the adductor longus muscle. Drug-induced myositis ossificans circumscripta due to injections into the antecubital vein has been reported.[164] Hemophiliacs may develop myositis ossificans resulting from intramuscular hematomas.[165]

Arteriography during the active stage shows a diffuse blush of fine vessels. In the mature stage, the lesions are avascular.[166]

CT shows the progress of ossification from an early attenuation value lower than muscle to a calcific density. The zone phenomenon is demonstrated, with ossification about the periphery of the mass and central decreased attenuation, usually seen after 4 to 6 weeks. Later, complete ossification may be seen.[167] Ultrasound can demonstrate calcification within a soft-tissue mass.[168]

Radionuclide scanning with technetium diphosphonate, using the three-phase bone scan technique, may show regional soft-tissue hyperemia in the flow study, increased activity in an early blood pool image,

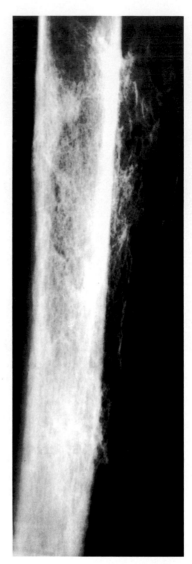

FIGURE 4-57. Myositis ossificans. A veil-like envelope of fine new bone surrounds a portion of the femoral shaft. The new bone is organized into cortex and trabeculae and lies along the muscle axis.

and generalized increase in soft-tissue activity in the involved region on static images.[169]

The MRI appearance depends on the age and maturation of the lesion.[170,171] Acute and subacute lesions may display a mass effect or no changes on T1-weighted images, or they may produce a pattern of edema and hemorrhage with high signal intensity on T2-weighted images. Fluid levels secondary to hemorrhage may sometimes be seen. Adjacent bone marrow edema may also be revealed. Mature lesions show low-signal-intensity margins corresponding to the calcific zone seen on plain films. The calcifications are of low signal intensity on T1-weighted and T2-weighted images. The central pattern varies, sometimes showing the signal characteristics of fat and sometime producing intermediate signal intensity (Fig. 4-59). Mature lesions may be seen

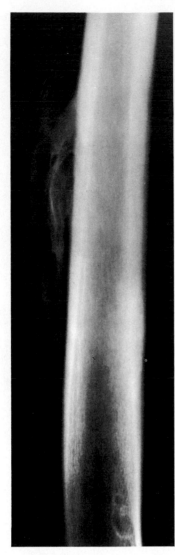

FIGURE 4-58. Posttraumatic myositis ossificans. An area of ectopic bone at the anterior aspect is visible; the superior portion is beginning to blend with the cortex. The long axis of the ectopic bone lies parallel to the muscle plane. A hole from a traction device can be seen in the distal femoral shaft.

as an irregular signal void on all sequences (Fig. 4-60), sometimes with areas containing fat. Active lesions enhance with gadolinium infusion.

Myositis ossificans may also result from neurologic disease and may be caused by a variety of conditions, including diseases of the brain, spinal cord including trauma, compression of the cauda equina, peripheral neuropathy, and tetanus.[172] Extensive soft-tissue ossification, particularly in the paraarticular regions, leads to joint ankylosis. Disuse osteoporosis and bone erosions are seen. The ossification may blend with the cortex. Ossification may form rapidly. Myositis ossificans develops below the level of the neurologic lesion. Pressure erosions develop at bony prominences, such as the trochanters and ischia in paraplegics, and should not be confused with a trochanterectomy, which is some-

times done to alleviate decubitus ulcers. Increased radionuclide uptake occurs in the heterotopic osseous tissue.

FIBRODYSPLASIA OSSIFICANS PROGRESSIVA. Fibrodysplasia ossificans progressiva (i.e., myositis ossificans progressiva) is a mesodermal disorder in which congenital anomalies, such as hypoplasia of the thumbs, and inflammatory foci in the fascia and ligaments occur. These foci progress to fibrosis and ossification (Fig. 4-61), which may be extensive (Fig. 4-62).

Pseudomalignant Osseous Soft-Tissue Tumor

Pseudomalignant osseous soft-tissue tumor is a rare bone-forming, soft-tissue mass that occurs in young adults and adolescents.[173–177] Some consider this entity to be localized myositis ossificans. Females are affected more often than males. There is a predilection for the hands and feet, with tumors arising from the periosteum or fibrous septa. The tumor grows slowly, usually attaining a maximum size of up to 3 cm. The lesion exhibits a zone phenomenon with a periphery of mature bone, which can be detected on CT or, under favorable circumstances, on conventional x-ray films. This differentiates the tumor from an osteosarcoma. There may be periosteal reaction of adjacent bone. MR images may show low signal intensity on T1-weighted images and inhomogeneous signal intensity on T2-weighted images of the tumor. There is no antecedent trauma, as is usually present with localized myositis ossificans. The lesion is benign and self-limiting.

Soft Tissue Osteosarcoma

Soft tissue osteosarcoma is a malignant mesenchymal tumor producing osteoid matrix and is not attached to bone.[160,178–180] It is rare, occurs in the adult age group, and may develop de novo or may occur as a late complication of radiation therapy. Some of these tumors arising in organs may represent malignant growth of a single component of a teratoma. It is most common in the thigh, but it has been reported in the rest of the extremities, neck, trunk, heart, lungs, pulmonary artery, pleura, kidney,[181] breast,[182] uterus,[183,184] and retroperitoneum. The extremities, most commonly the lower extremities, are the site of involvement in 90% of cases. The tumor commonly recurs and metastasizes.

Patients with soft tissue osteosarcoma are usually older than those with osteosarcoma of bone. Although the range is 8 to 70 years of age, the disease is rare in the first two decades of life.

A soft-tissue mass as large as 10 cm in diameter may have various degrees of streaky or amorphous calcification, but a large percentage of these tumors show no calcification. There may be spiculation at its periph-

(text continues on page 317)

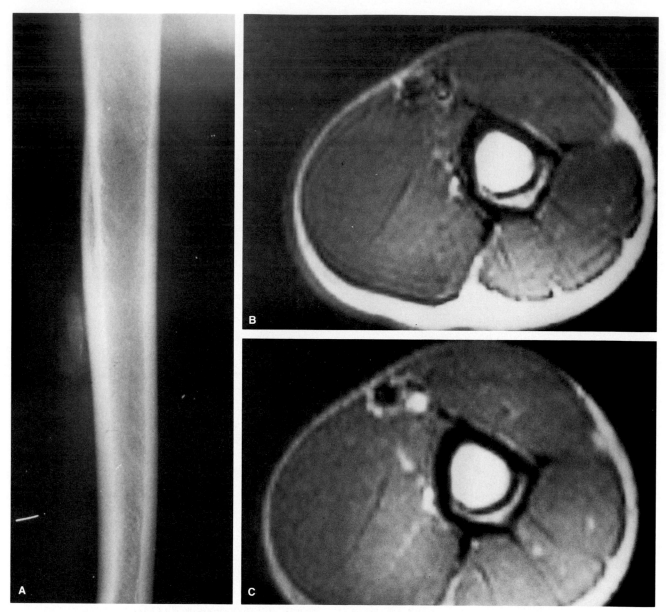

FIGURE 4-59. Myositis ossificans in a 20-year-old man. (**A**) A lateral view of the humerus shows a focus of ossification in the soft tissues adjacent to the cortex. (**B**) The axial MR (SE 660/15) section of the humerus shows an ossific rim around the posterior cortex of the humerus with a strand of ossification extending into the intermuscular septum. The central portion has lower signal intensity than the medullary fat. (**C**) MR image (SE 1700/20). The calcific rim is separate from the cortex, with several extensions into the intermuscular septa. (**D**) MR image (SE 1700/80). The central portion is increased somewhat in signal intensity. (**E**) MR image (SE 1700/80). There is an area of high signal intensity outside of the calcific rim of the soft tissues.

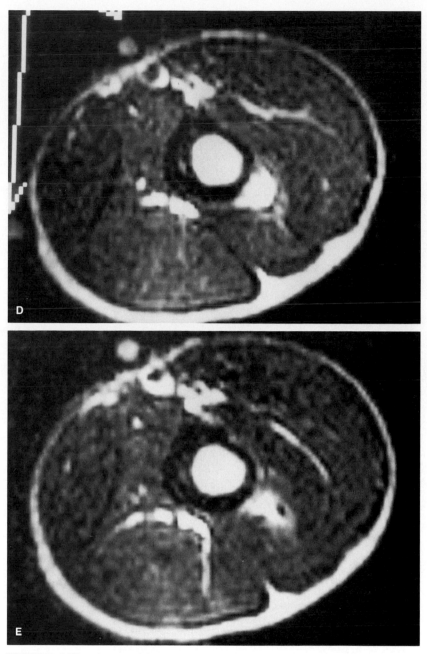

FIGURE 4-59. *(Continued)*

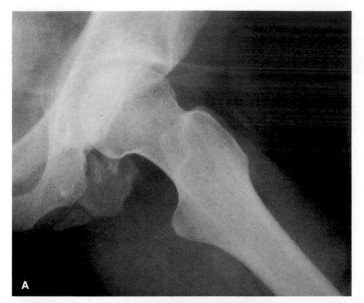

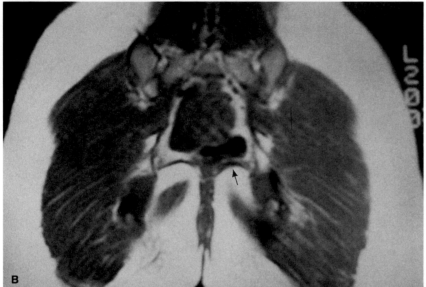

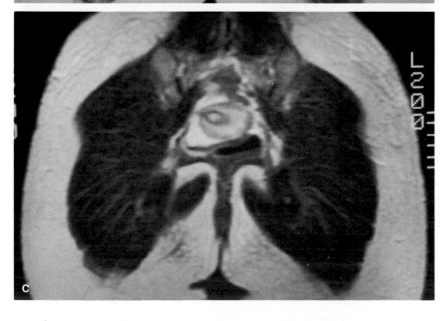

FIGURE 4-60. Myositis ossificans in a 16-year-old girl. (**A**) A lateral view of her left hip shows mature myositis ossificans in the region of the ischiac bone. (**B**) MR image (SE 650/16). The ossification is seen as a signal void. (**C**) MR image (FSE 4000/102 Ef). The ossification remains as a signal void.

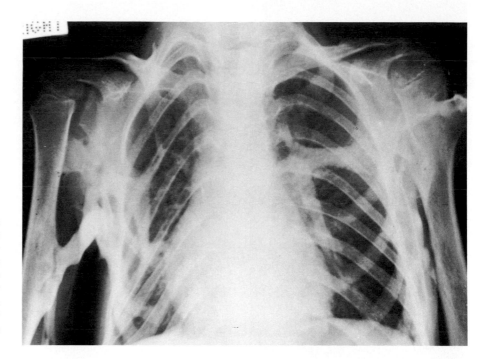

FIGURE 4-61. Myositis ossificans progressiva of the chest. Extensive new bone formation in the soft tissues has caused severe limitation of arm motion. The exostosis at the left proximal humerus is caused by blending of the ossific foci with the cortex of the bone. (Courtesy of Dr. Harvey White, Children's Memorial Hospital, Chicago, IL.)

ery (Fig. 4-63). The adjacent bone may be secondarily invaded. Radionuclide bone scans show increased isotope uptake, and angiography shows increased vascularity.

Bone-Forming Metastases

Bone-forming metastases have been reported for carcinoma of the colon, breast, and urinary tract.[185] These lesions are associated with bone destruction and adjacent soft-tissue ossification. Radionuclide bone scanning may show increased isotope uptake in calci-

fied and noncalcified soft-tissue metastases from osteosarcoma.[21] Uncalcified soft-tissue metastases have imaging characteristics similar to a primary soft tissue sarcoma (Fig. 4-64).[186]

Soft-Tissue Infections

Soft-tissue infections, particularly in HIV (human immunodeficiency virus)-positive and AIDS patients,[187] can take the form of cellulitis, myonecrosis, or pyo-

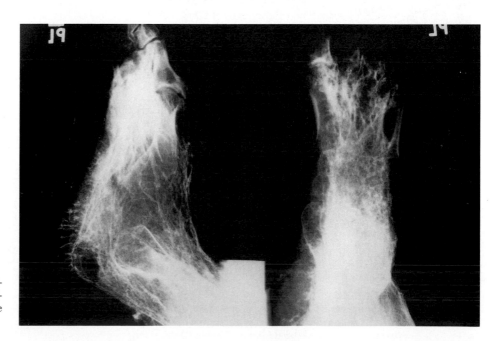

FIGURE 4-62. Myositis ossificans progressiva. Extensive ossification of the soft tissues of the foot has occurred.

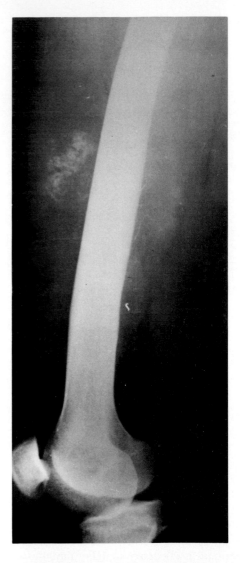

FIGURE 4-63. Soft tissue osteosarcoma. A soft-tissue mass in the midanterior thigh contains amorphous calcification with peripheral streaking. A thin calcific rim is at its inferior margin. (Courtesy of Drs. A. Pizarro and T. F. Kurtz, Veterans Administration Hospital, Hines, IL.)

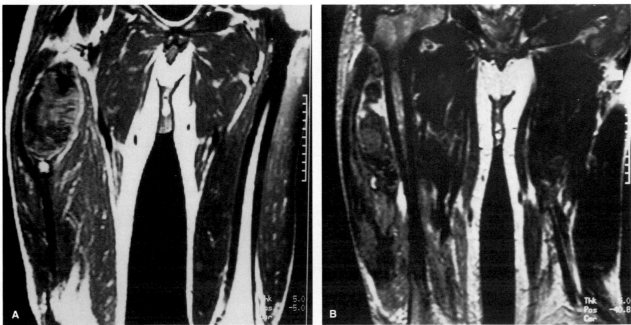

FIGURE 4-64. Soft-tissue metastasis. (**A**) MR image (SE 600/20). A well-circumscribed, inhomogeneous mass is detected in the thigh. (**B**) MRI (SE 2500/80). A mixed-signal-intensity tumor mass is delineated in the thigh. (From Greenfield GB, Arrington JA, Kudryk BT: MRI of soft tissue tumors. Skeletal Radiol 22:77–84, 1993)

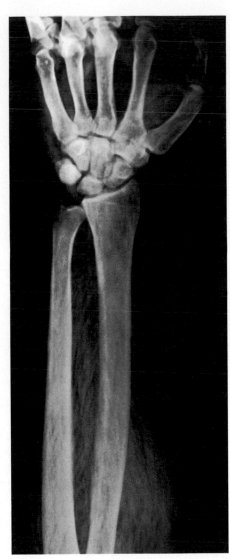

FIGURE 4-65. Advanced gas gangrene of the hand and forearm. There is extensive dissection of gas along the muscle fibers of the forearm.

myositis. CT is valuable for the diagnosis of cellulitis by showing tissue-density changes. The attenuation of subcutaneous fat approaches that of muscle with skin thickening and septal prominence and without a mass effect. Lymphedema may be concomitant, seen as a curvilinear and reticular pattern in the subcutaneous fat.

Myonecrosis may be nonclostridial or clostridial (Figs. 4-65 and 4-66), with gas dissecting along muscle fibers. Calcific myonecrosis has been reported in the calf as a late posttraumatic condition in which the muscle has been replaced by an enlarging fusiform mass with central liquefaction and peripheral calcification.[188] Pyomyositis is usually caused by *Staphylococcus aureus* (Fig. 4-67) but may also be opportunistic or tuberculous. It is rare outside of the tropics, except in immunocompromised patients. The muscle is enlarged and shows the low attenuation of edema on CT. A hematoma may mimic an abscess on CT scans, but MR images may help in differentiation. Abscesses may be seen as enlarged areas of low attenuation on CT and as well-circumscribed masses of high signal intensity on T2-weighted MR images (Fig. 4-68). Some muscle abscesses show a thin ring of high signal intensity on T1-weighted images, closely associated with a hypointense ring on T2-weighted images and encompassing a very-high-signal-intensity center (Fig. 4-69). The hypointense ring may represent the abscess pseudocapsule or the presence of hemosiderin. A central low-signal-intensity area may be caused by necrotic debris. The abscess is surrounded by a large high-signal-intensity region. Another appearance of an abscess is a focus of signal intensity isointense or of higher intensity than muscle, but without a rim, on T1-weighted images, which increases in intensity on T2-weighted images.[63] The abscess margin and surrounding tissue enhance after infusion of gadolinium (Fig. 4-70). Particularly in myositis, the entire muscle compartment may show as

(text continues on page 326)

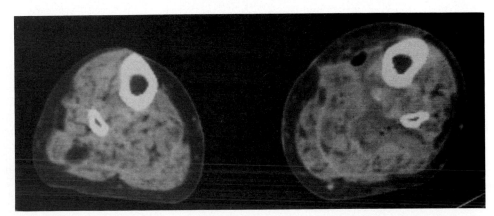

FIGURE 4-66. Gas within the deep musculature of the left leg and a larger gas collection at the margin of the subcutaneous tissue are seen on this CT scan. This patient is diabetic.

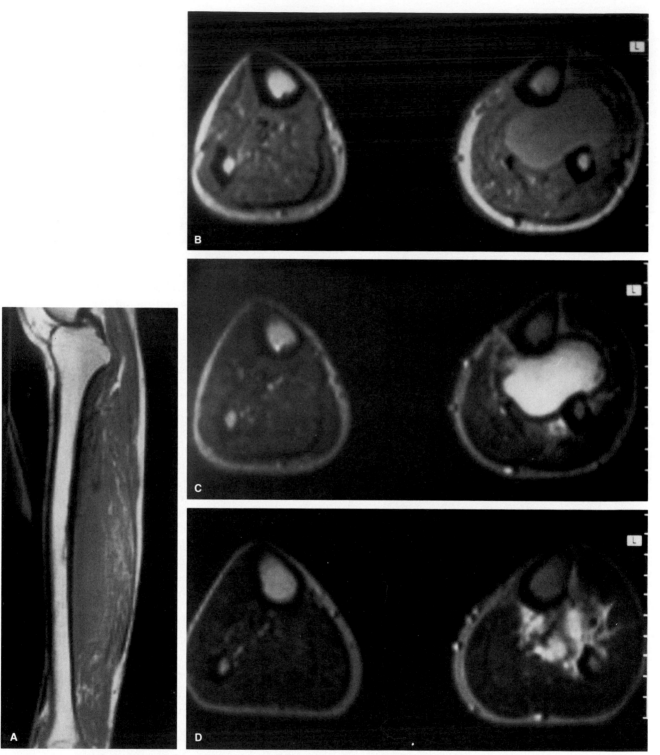

FIGURE 4-67. Pyomyositis in a patient with AIDS. **(A)** The T1-weighted sagittal MR scan shows a smooth soft-tissue mass posterior to the major portion of the tibia, displacing the musculature. The abscess is isodense with muscle. **(B)** The proton density axial image shows a well-circumscribed mass that has destroyed the interosseous membrane. This finding indicates an inflammatory lesion rather than a neoplasm. The signal intensity is slightly increased. **(C)** The T2-weighted MR image shows a marked increase in the signal intensity of the abscess. A low-signal-intensity margin is seen. **(D)** A T2-weighted MR image at a different level shows heterogeneous signal intensity and the invasive appearance of the margin. The lesion contains several low-density streaks. (Courtesy Dr. Mike Vermess, Tampa, FL.)

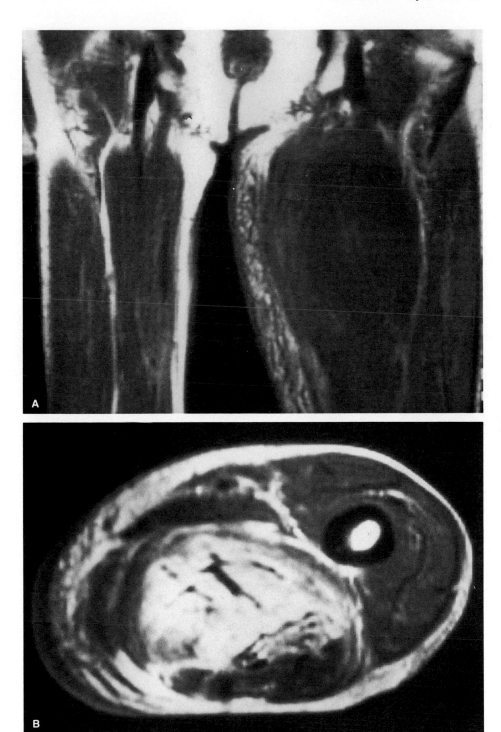

FIGURE 4-68. Abscess of the thigh in a 73-year-old man. (**A**) The T1-weighted MR image shows a large soft-tissue mass in the left thigh with a heterogeneous signal intensity. Lymphedema of the subcutaneous tissues is also seen. (**B**) A proton density axial image shows a large, heterogeneous mass in the medial musculature. Low-signal-intensity streaks are seen within the mass. The mass has increased in signal intensity, and inflammatory changes in the subcutaneous tissues are again seen. (**C**) The T2-weighted image shows an additional increase in signal intensity. Dilated, high-signal-intensity lymphatics are seen in the subcutaneous tissues. (**D**) Digital subtraction angiography shows displacement of the vessels but no tumor stain. This large abscess resolved completely after 6 weeks of antibiotic therapy. *continued*

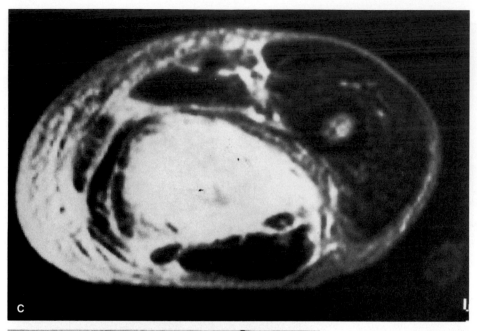

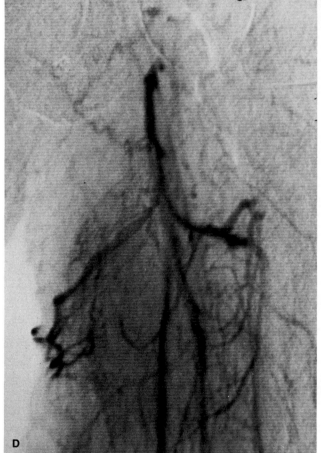

FIGURE 4-68. *(Continued)*

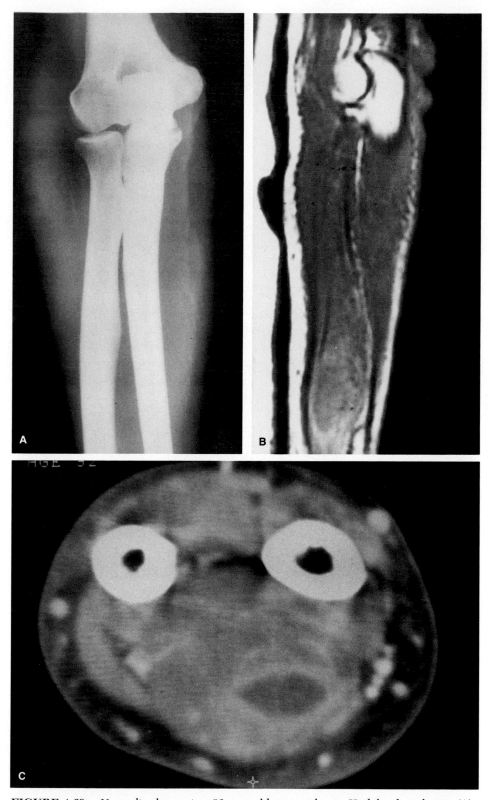

FIGURE 4-69.   *Nocardia* abscess in a 92-year-old man with non-Hodgkin lymphoma. (**A**) The anteroposterior view demonstrates soft-tissue irregularities around the elbow and forearm. (**B**) MR image (SE 600/14). The abscess of the forearm is basically isointense with muscle and shows some signal heterogeneity. (**C**) Enhanced CT. The abscess has a central necrotic area with an enhancing margin. (**D**) MR image (SE 850/16). The abscess is isointense with muscle and heterogeneous. (**E**) MR image (FSE 7000/102 Ef). The abscess is increased in signal intensity and shows a low-signal-intensity margin and a slightly lower-intensity central area.   *(continued)*

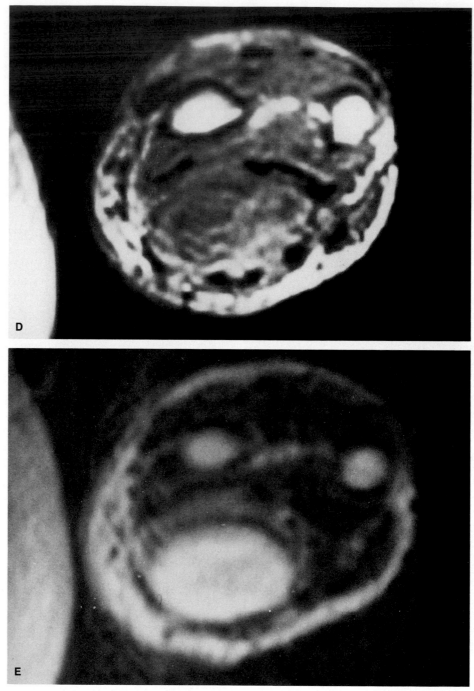

FIGURE 4-69. *(Continued)*

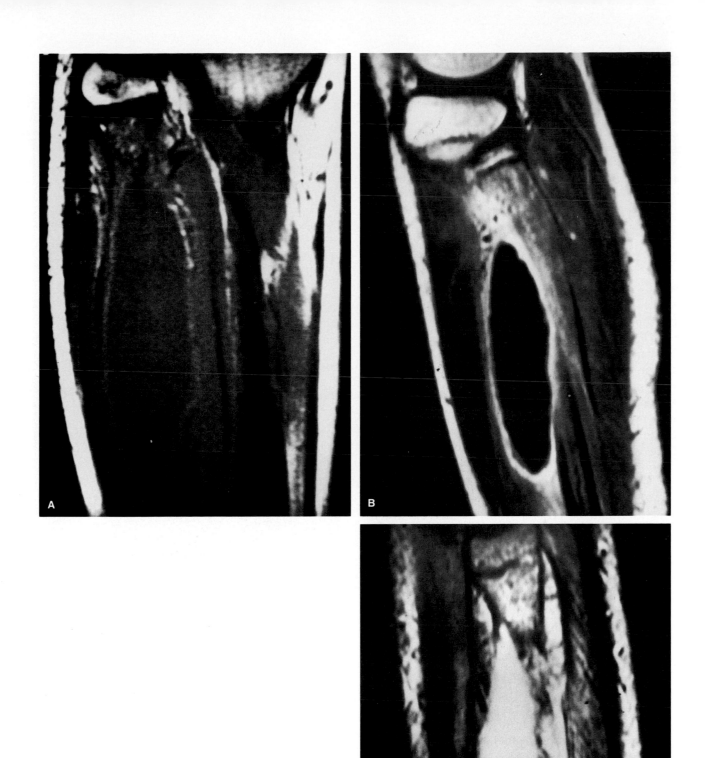

FIGURE 4-70. Abscess of the calf in a 12-year-old girl. (**A**) MR image (SE 400/17). An ovoid mass displaces the musculature. The lesion is isointense with muscle. (**B**) MR image (SE 400/11). After injection of 8 mL of Magnevist, enhancement occurs around the rim of the abscess and in the surrounding soft tissues. A reticular pattern is seen in the subcutaneous tissues. (**C**) MR image (SE 2000/70). Homogeneous high signal intensity is seen on this T2-weighted image.

high signal intensity without defined end margins on T2-weighted images.

Arteriography is helpful in differentiating tumor from abscess because of the lack of tumor stain and vessel encasement in the latter (see Fig. 4-67). Radionuclide scanning with ^{99m}Tc pyrophosphate demonstrates necrotic muscle. Ultrasound is useful in the detection and follow-up of pyomyositis.[189]

Soft-Tissue Edema

Muscle edema may be associated with malignant or benign musculoskeletal tumors. The distribution may be peritumoral or involve the entire extent of one or more muscles.[190] High signal intensity and a mass effect may be seen on T2-weighted images. Benign bone tumors, such as osteoid osteoma and chondroblastoma, and eosinophilic granuloma, myositis ossificans, hematoma, and infection may produce this feature. Massive involvement of a muscle with edema secondary to a malignant bone tumor indicates a poorer prognosis, and this condition is seen in patients with tumors that have penetrated the bony cortex and invaded the muscle.

Edema of a limb can have an obstructive or inflammatory basis. Obstructive edema may be caused by venous or lymphatic occlusion.[191] In venous occlusion, there is edema of the musculature and of the subcutaneous fat with prominence of the fibrous septa, causing a coarsened reticular pattern on plain films, CT scans, and MR images. Venous occlusion can be demonstrated by phlebography or cavography.

Lymphedema may be primary or secondary. Lymphangiography is most helpful for differentiation. *Primary lymphedema* (Fig. 4-71) is caused by a congenital lymphatic abnormality without central obstruction. This condition can be divided into four components: aplasia of lymphatics (rare), dermal backflow, hypoplasia of lymphatic channels, and varicose channels (frequently associated with dermal backflow). Lymphangiography shows sparse, dilated lymphatics with filled dermal and accessory lymphatic channels and extravasation of contrast material into interstitial tissues, perineural spaces, and veins. CT shows dilated lymphatic channels (Fig. 4-72), a coarse reticular pattern in an enlarged subcutaneous compartment, or both patterns. Absence of an obstructing mass proximally or in the retroperitoneum or pelvis excludes secondary lymphedema.

Secondary lymphedema results from lymphatic obstruction, which may be caused by filariasis, inflammation, lymphadenopathy, surgery (particularly postmastectomy; see previous discussion of the Stewart-Treves syndrome), radiation therapy, trauma, or tumor.

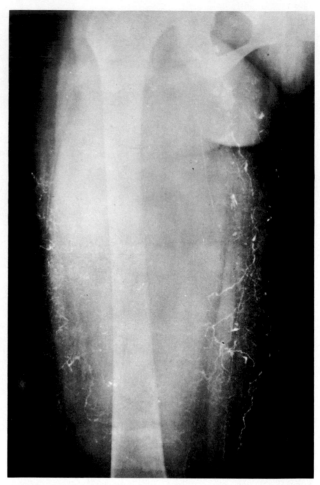

FIGURE 4-71. Primary lymphedema as seen on a lymphangiogram. There is filling of dermal lymphatic channels without evidence of central lymphatic obstruction. Lymphatic varicosities may be seen. (From Love L, Kim SE: Clinical aspects of lymphangiography. Med Clin North Am 51:227–248, 1967)

The lymphangiogram shows numerous filled lymphatic channels to the point of obstruction (Fig. 4-73). Collateral lymphatics are also visualized.

MR images can demonstrate dermal and subcutaneous lymphangiectasis as subcutaneous channels or lakes, subcutaneous edema, and increased fat.[192] It can visualize lymph nodes and trunks and soft-tissue masses at the site of obstruction. A honeycomb pattern is seen with a marked increase in signal intensity on T2-weighted images, where the dilated lymphatic channels can be seen in the subcutis against the low signal intensity of the subcutaneous fat. On T1-weighted images, the dilated lymphatic channels are seen as low-signal-intensity areas against a high-signal-intensity subcutis background, and on T2-weighted images, they increase in signal intensity (Fig. 4-74). Dilated veins are seen distal to the lesion.

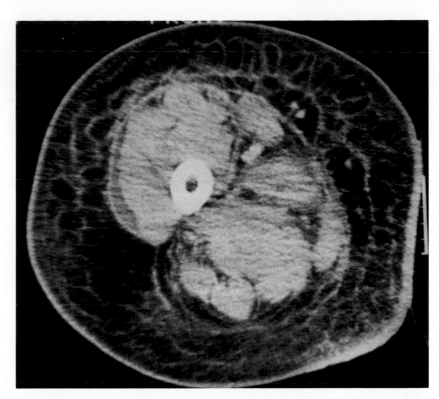

FIGURE 4-72. Lymphedema. The CT scan shows dilated lymphatic channels and prominent subcutaneous septa. A fluid collection is present around the muscles.

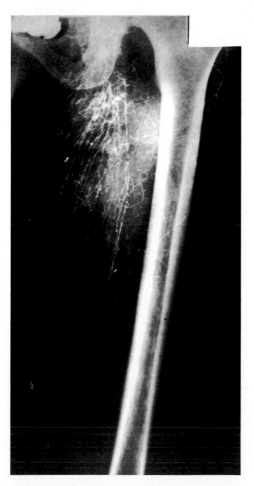

FIGURE 4-73. Secondary lymphedema. There is a central obstruction at the inguinal chain, with numerous filled lymphatics and collateral lymphatics. (From Love L, Kim SE: Clinical aspects of lymphangiography. Med Clin North Am 51:227–249, 1967)

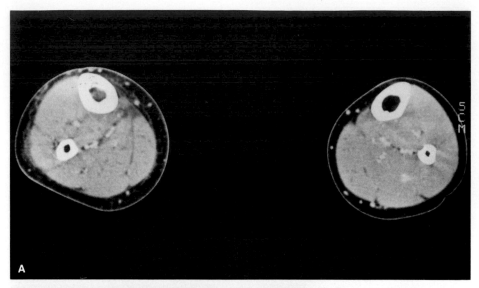

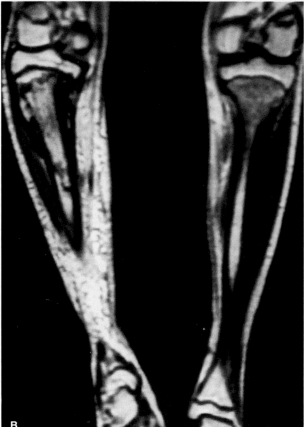

FIGURE 4-74. A 14-year-old boy with treated osteosarcoma of the right proximal tibia and lymphedema. (**A**) Enhanced CT shows dilated lymphatic channels in the subcutaneous tissues. The subcutaneous veins are enhanced. (**B**) MR image (FSE 4200/16 Ef). Low-signal-intensity, dilated lymphatic channels are seen in the subcutaneous tissue. A proximal metaphyseal osteosarcoma is depicted with a pathologic fracture. (**C**) MR image (FSE 4200/95 Ef). The dilated lymphatic channels in the subcutaneous tissue are high signal intensity against a lower-signal-intensity fatty background.

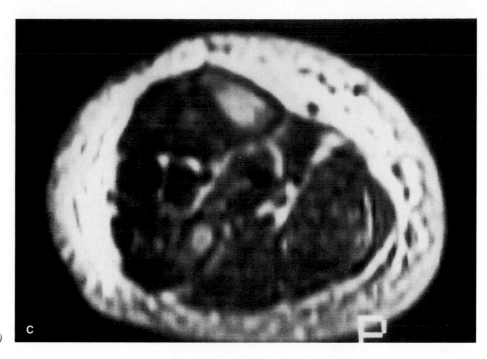

FIGURE 4-74. *(Continued)*

References

1. Martin RG et al: MD Anderson Hospital and Tumor Institute: Tumors of Bone and Soft Tissue. Chicago, Year Book Medical Publishers, 1965
2. Goodman AH, Briggs RC: Deep leiomyoma of an extremity. J Bone Joint Surg [Am] 47:529–532, 1965
3. Lange TA, Austin CW et al: Ultrasound imaging as a screening study for malignant soft-tissue tumors. J Bone Joint Surg 69:100–105, 1987
4. Choi H, Varma DGK, Fornage BD et al: Soft-tissue sarcoma: MR imaging vs sonography for detection of local recurrence after surgery. AJR Am J Roentgenol 157:353–358, 1991
5. Egund N, Ekelund L, Sako M et al: CT of soft-tissue tumors. AJR Am J Roentgenol 137:725–729a, 1981
6. Haaga JR, Alfidi RJ: Computed Tomography of the Whole Body, vol II. St. Louis, CV Mosby, 1983
7. Schultz SR, Bree RL et al: CT detection of skeletal muscle metastases. J Comput Assist Tomogr 10:8–83, 1986
8. Kirchner PT, Simon MA: The clinical value of bone and gallium scintigraphy for soft-tissue sarcomas of the extremities. J Bone Joint Surg [Am] 66:319, 1984
9. Binkovitz LA, Berquist TH, McLeon RA: Masses of the hand and wrist. AJR Am J Roentgenol 154:323–326, 1990
10. Wetzel LH, Levine E: Soft-tissue tumors of the foot: Value of MR imaging for specific diagnosis. AJR Am J Roentgenol 155:1025–1030, 1990
11. Aisen AM, Martel W et al: MRI and CT evaluation of primary bone and soft-tissue tumors. AJR Am J Roentgenol 146:749–756, 1986
12. Bohndorf VK, Reiser M et al: Wert der Kernspintomographie vor Chirurgischer Therapie und Radiatio Peripherer Weichteiltumoren. Fortschr Geb Rontgenstr 146:130–135, 1987
13. Demas BE, Heelan RT et al: Soft-tissue sarcomas of the extremities: Comparison of MRI and CT in determining the extent of disease. AJR Am J Roentgenol 150:615–620, 1988
14. Petasnick JP, Turner DA et al: Soft-tissue masses of the locomotor system: Comparison of MR imaging with CT. Radiology 160:125–133, 1986
15. Greenfield GB, Warren DL, Clark RA: MR imaging of periosteal and cortical changes of bone. RadioGraphics 11:611–623, 1991
16. Kransdorf MJ, Jelinek JS, Moser RP et al: Soft-tissue masses: Diagnosis using MR imaging. AJR Am J Roentgenol 153:541–547, 1989
17. Greenfield GB, Arrington JA, Kudryk BT: MRI of soft tissue tumors. Skeletal Radiol 22:77–84, 1993
18. Totty WG, Murphy WA et al: Soft-tissue tumors: MR imaging. Radiology 160:135–141, 1986
19. Sundaram M, McGuire MH et al: High signal intensity soft tissue masses on T1 weighted pulsing sequences. Skeletal Radiol 16:3–36, 1987
20. Berquist TH, Ehman RL, King BF et al: Value of MR imaging in differentiating benign from malignant soft-tissue masses: Study of 95 lesions. AJR Am J Roentgenol 155:1251–1255, 1990
21. Crim JR, Seeger LL, Yao L et al: Diagnosis of soft-tissue masses with MR imaging: Can benign masses be differentiated from malignant ones? Radiology 185:581–586, 1992
22. Sundaram M, McLeod RA: MR imaging of tumor and tumorlike lesions of bone and soft tissue. AJR Am J Roentgenol 155:817–824, 1990
23. Petterson H, Eliasson J, Egund B et al: Gadolinium-DTPA enhancement of soft tissue tumors in magnetic resonance imaging: Preliminary clinical experience in five patients. Skeletal Radiol 17:319–323, 1988
24. Arlen M, Marcove RC: Surgical Management of Soft Tissue Sarcomas. Philadelphia, WB Saunders, 1987
25. Enzinger FM, Weiss SW: Soft Tissue Tumors. 2nd ed. St Louis, CV Mosby, 1988
26. De Schepper AM, Ramon F: Medical imaging of soft-tissue tumors. University Hospital, Antwerp, Belgium, Monograph, 1993
27. Mahajan H, Kim EE, Wallace S et al: Magnetic resonance imaging of malignant fibrous histiocytoma. Magn Reson Imaging 7:283–288, 1989
28. Ros PR, Viamonte M, Rywlin AM: Malignant fibrous histiocytoma: Mesenchymal tumor of ubiquitous origin. AJR Am J Roentgenol 142:753–759, 1984
29. Spector DB, Miller J, Viloria J: Malignant fibrous histiocytoma. J Bone Joint Surg [Am] 61:190–193, 1979
30. Turculet V: Aspects radiologiques des tumeurs histiocytaires malignes des parties molles et osseuses. J Radiol 62:429–436, 1981
31. Fischer HJ, Lois JF et al: Radiology and pathology of malignant fibrous histiocytomas of the soft tissues: A report of ten cases. Skeletal Radiol 13:202–206, 1985

32. Panicek DM, Casper ES, Brennan MF et al: Hemorrhage simulating tumor growth in malignant fibrous histiocytoma at MR imaging. Radiology 181:398–400, 1991

33. Dorfman HD, Bhagavan BS: Malignant fibrous histiocytoma of soft tissue with metaplastic bone and cartilage formation: A new radiologic sign. Skeletal Radiol 8:145–150, 1982

34. Martell JR, Busnardo MS et al: Congenital fibrosarcoma of the forearm. J Bone Joint Surg 68:620–623, 1986

35. Quinn SF, Erickson SJ, Dee PM et al: MR imaging in fibromatosis: Results in 26 patients with pathologic correlation. AJR Am J Roentgenol 156: 539–542, 1991

36. Kransdorf MJ, Jelinek JS, Moser RP et al: Magnetic resonance appearance of fibromatosis. Skeletal Radiol 19:495–499, 1990

37. Hawnaur JM, Jenkins JPR, Isherwood I: Magnetic resonance imaging of musculoaponeurotic fibromatosis. Skeletal Radiol 19:509–514, 1990

38. Greenfield GB, Rubenstone AL, Lo M: Aggressive fibromatosis. Skeletal Radiol 2:4–46, 1977

39. Griffiths HJ, Robinson K, Bonfiglio TA: Aggressive fibromatosis. Skeletal Radiol 9:179–184, 1983

40. Ashby MA, Harmer CL et al: Case report. Infiltrative fibromatosis: A rare cause of fatal haemorrhage. Clin Radiol 37:193–194, 1986

41. Rhomberg VW, Taxer F: Hemihyperplasie von brustwirbelsegmenten und aggressive fibromatose. Fortschr Geb Rontgenstr 144:737–738, 1986

42. Francis IR, Dorovini-Zis K et al: The fibromatoses: CT-pathologic correlation. AJR Am J Roentgenol 147:1063–1066, 1986

43. Rubenstein WA, Gray G et al: CT of fibrous tissues and tumors with sonographic correlation. AJR Am J Roentgenol 147:1067–1074, 1986

44. Hudson TM, Vandergriend RA, Springfield DS et al: Aggressive fibromatosis: Evaluation by computed tomography and angiography. Radiology 150:495–501, 1984

45. Hudson TM, Bertoni F et al: Scintigraphy of aggressive fibromatosis. Skeletal Radiol 13:2–32, 1985

46. Sundaram M, Duffrin H et al: Synchronous multicentric desmoid tumors (aggressive fibromatosis) of the extremities. Skeletal Radiol 17:1–19, 1988

47. Abramowitz D, Zornoza J, Ayala AG et al: Soft-tissue desmoid tumors: Radiographic bone changes. Radiology 146:1–13, 1983

48. Broder MS, Leonidas JC, Mittay HA: Pseudosarcomatous fasciitis: An unusual cause of soft-tissue calcification. Radiology 107:173–174, 1973

49. Enzinger FM, Shiraki M: Musculoaponeurotic fibromatosis of the shoulder girdle (extraabdominal desmoid): Analysis of 30 cases followed up for 10 or more years. Cancer 20:1131–1140a, 1967

50. Kransdorf MJ et al: Fat-containing soft-tissue masses of the extremities. RadioGraphics 11:81–106, 1991

51. Milgram JW: Malignant transformation in bone lipomas. Skeletal Radiol 19:347–352, 1990

52. Jelinek JS, Kransdorf MJ, Shmookler BM et al: Liposarcoma of the extremities: MR and CT findings in the histologic subtypes. Radiology 186:455–459, 1993

53. Sundaram M, Baran G, Merenda G et al: Myxoid liposarcoma: magnetic resonance imaging appearances with clinical and histological correlation. Skeletal Radiol 19:359–362, 1990

54. Murphy WD, Hurst GC, Duerk JL et al: Atypical appearance of lipomatous tumors on MR images: High signal intensity with fat-suppression STIR sequences. JMRI 1:477–480, 1991

55. Kransdort MJ, Meis JM, Jelinek JS: Dedifferentiated liposarcoma of the extremities: Imaging findings in four patients. AJR Am J Roentgenol 161: 127–130, 1993

56. Bush CH, Spanier SS, Gillespy T: Imaging of atypical lipomas of the extremities. Skeletal Radiol 17:472–474, 1988

57. Orchis DD, Ozonoff MB: Infiltrating angiolipoma with phlebolith formation. Skeletal Radiol 15:464–467, 1986

58. Lachman RS, Finklestein J, Mehringer CM et al: Congenital aggressive lipomatosis. Skeletal Radiol 9:248–254, 1983

59. Lanploh JT et al: Lipoblastomatosis: A case report. J Bone Joint Surg [Am] 60:130–132, 1978

60. Kazerooni E, Hessler C: CT appearance of angiosarcoma associated with chronic lymphedema. AJR Am J Roentgenol 156:543–544, 1991

61. Gorham LW: Kaposi's sarcoma involving bone: With particular attention to angiomatous components of the tumor in relation to osteolysis. Arch Pathol 76:456, 1963

62. Steinbach LS, Tehranzadeh J, Fleckenstein JL et al: Human immunodeficiency virus infection: Musculoskeletal manifestations. Radiology 186:833–838, 1993

63. Fleckenstein JL, Burns DK, Murphy EK et al: Differential diagnosis of bacterial myositis in AIDS: Evaluation with MR imaging. Radiology 179:653–658, 1991

64. Hawnaur JM, Whitehouse RW, Jenkins JPR et al: Musculoskeletal haemangiomas: Comparisons of MRI with CT. Skeletal Radiol 19:251–258, 1990

65. Liu P, Daneman A et al: Computed tomography of hemangiomas and related soft-tissue lesions in children. J Can Assoc Radiol 37:248–255, 1986

66. Nelson MC, Stull MA, Teitelbaum GP et al: Magnetic resonance imaging of peripheral soft tissue hemangiomas. Skeletal Radiol 19:477–482, 1990

66a. Ehara S, Sone M, Tamakawa Y, et al: Fluid-fluid levels in hemangioma of soft tissue. Skeletal Radiol 23:107–109, 1994

67. Greenspan A, McGahan JP, Vogelsang P et al: Imaging strategies in the evaluation of soft-tissue hemangiomas of the extremities: Correlation of the findings of plain radiography, angiography, CT, MRI, and ultrasonography in 12 histologically proven cases. Skeletal Radiol 21:11–18, 1992

68. Cohen EK, Kressel HY et al: MR imaging of soft-tissue hemangiomas: Correlation with pathologic findings. AJR Am J Roentgenol 150:1079–1081, 1988

69. Kaplan PA, Williams SM: Mucocutaneous and peripheral soft-tissue hemangiomas: MR imaging. Radiology 163:163–166, 1987

70. Yuh WTC, Kathol MH et al: Hemangiomas of skeletal muscle: MR findings in five patients. AJR Am J Roentgenol 149:765–768, 1986

71. Buetow PC, Kransdorf MJ, Moser RP et al: Radiologic appearance of intramuscular hemangioma with emphasis on MR imaging. AJR Am J Roentgenol 154:563–567, 1990

72. Meyer JS, Hoffer FA, Barnes PD et al: Biological classification of soft-tissue vascular anomalies: MR correlation. AJR Am J Roentgenol 157:559–564, 1991

73. Engelstad BL, Gilula LA, Kyriakos M: Ossified skeletal muscle hemangioma: Radiologic and pathologic features. Skeletal Radiol 5:3–40a, 1980

74. De Smet, AA, Fisher DR, Heiner JP et al: Magnetic resonance imaging of muscle tears. Skeletal Radiol 19:283–286, 1990

75. Ekelund L, Rydholm A: The value of angiography in soft tissue leiomyosarcomas of the extremities. Skeletal Radiol 9:201–204, 1983

76. Herrlin K, Willen H, Rydholm A: Deep-seated soft tissue leiomyomas. Skeletal Radiol 19:363–365, 1990

77. Peterson KK, Renfrew DL, Feddersen RM et al: Magnetic resonance imaging of myxoid containing tumors. Skeletal Radiol 20:245–250, 1991

78. Genest P, Kim TH, Katsarkas A et al: Calcified synovial sarcoma of the oropharynx. Br J Radiol 56:580–582, 1983

79. Wright PH, Sim FH, Soule EH et al: Synovial sarcoma. J Bone Joint Surg [Am] 64:112–122, 1982

80. Azouz EM, Vicker DB, Brown KLB: Computed tomography of synovial sarcoma of the foot. J Can Assoc Radiol 35:85–87, 1984

81. Morton MJ, Berquist TH, McLeon RA et al: MR imaging of synovial sarcoma. AJR Am J Roentgenol 156:337–340, 1991

82. Dunn EJ, McGuaran MH, Nelson P, Greer RB: Synovial

chondrosarcoma: Report of a case. J Bone Joint Surg [Am] 56:811–813, 1974

83. Kaiser TE, Ivins JC, Unni KK: Malignant transformation of extra-articular synovial chondromatosis. Skeletal Radiol 5: 223–226, 1980

84. Milgram JW, Addison RG: Synovial osteochondromatosis of the knee: Chrondromatous recurrence with possible chondrosarcomatous degeneration. J Bone Joint Surg [Br] 58: 264–266, 1976

85. Hamilton A, Davis RI et al: Chondrosarcoma developing in synovial chondromatosis. J Bone Joint Surg 69:137–140, 1987

86. Hamilton A, Davis RI et al: Synovial chondrosarcoma complicating synovial chondromatosis. J Bone Joint Surg 69: 1084–1088, 1987

87. Davis S, Lawton G, Lowy M: Pigmented villonodular synovitis: Bone involvement of the fingers. Clin Radiol 26:357–361, 1975

88. Flandry F, Hughston JC et al: Current concepts review: Pigmented villonodular synovitis. J Bone Joint Surg 69:942–949, 1987

89. Jergesen HE, Mankin JH, Schiller AL: Diffuse pigmented villonodular synovitis of the knee mimicking primary bone neoplasm: A report of 2 cases. J Bone Joint Surg [Am] 60:825–829, 1978

90. Kindblom LG, Gunterberg G: Pigmented villonodular synovitis involving bone: A case report. J Bone Joint Surg [Am] 60:830–832, 1978

91. Goldman AB, DiCarlo EF: Pigmented villonodular synovitis diagnosis and differential diagnosis. Radiol Clin North Am 26:1327–1347, 1988

92. Crosby EB, Inglis A, Bullough PG: Multiple joint involvement with pigmented villonodular synovitis. Radiology 122:671–672, 1977

93. Eisenberg RL, Hedgecock MU: Bilateral pigmented villonodular synovitis of the hip. Br J Radiol 51:916, 1978

94. Gehweiler JA, Wilson JW: Diffuse biarticular pigmented villonodular synovitis. Radiology 93:845–852, 1969

95. Lapayouker MS, Miller WT, Levy WM, Harwick RD: Pigmented villonodular synovitis of the temporomandibular joint. Radiology 108:313–316, 1973

96. Wagner ML, Spjut HJ, Dutton RV et al: Polyarticular pigmented villonodular synovitis. AJR Am J Roentgenol 136: 821–823, 1981

97. Gagneri F, Taillan B et al: Three cases of pigmented villonodular synovitis of the knee. Fortschr Geb Rontgenstr 145:227–228, 1986

98. Butt WP, Hardy G, Chir B et al: Pigmented villonodular synovitis of the knee: Computed tomographic appearances. Skeletal Radiol 19:191–196, 1990

99. Kottal RA, Vogler JB et al: Pigmented villonodular synovitis: A report of MR imaging in two cases. Radiology 163:551–553, 1987

100. Spritzer CE, Dalinka MK et al: Magnetic resonance imaging of pigmented villonodular synovitis: A report of two cases. Skeletal Radiol 16:316–319, 1987

101. Campbell AJ, Wells IP: Pigmented villonodular synovitis of a lumbar vertebral facet joint. J Bone Joint Surg [Am] 64:145–146, 1982

102. Lowenstein MB, Smith JRV, Cole S: Infrapatellar pigmented villonodular synovitis: Arthrographic detection. AJR Am J Roentgenol 135:279–282, 1980

103. Spanier S: Case 46, presented at the meeting of the International Skeletal Society, Stockholm, 1992

104. Milgram JW: Synovial osteochondromatosis: A histopathological study of 30 cases. J Bone Joint Surg [Am] 59:792–801, 1977

105. Prager RJ, Mall JC: Arthrographic diagnosis of synovial chondromatosis. AJR Am J Roentgenol 127:344–346, 1976

106. Jaffe HL: Tumors and Tumorous Conditions of the Bones and Joints. Philadelphia, Lea & Febiger, 1958

107. Carey RPL: Synovial chondromatosis of the knee in childhood. J Bone Joint Surg [Br] 65:444–447, 1983

108. Pelker RR, Drennan JC, Ozonoff MB: Juvenile synovial

chondromatosis of the hip. J Bone Joint Surg [Am] 65:552–554, 1983

109. Dunn WA, Whisler JH: Synovial chondromatosis of the knee with associated extracapsular chondromas. J Bone Joint Surg [Am] 55:1747–1748, 1973

110. Lynn MD, Lee J: Periarticular tenosynovial chondrometaplasia: Report of a case at the wrist. J Bone Joint Surg [Am] 54:650–652, 1972

111. Bauer M, Johsson K: Synovial chondromatosis of the ankle. Fortschr a/d Gebeit Röntgenstrahlen 146:548–550, 1987

112. Holm CL: Primary synovial chondromatosis of the ankle. J Bone Joint Surg [Am] 58:878–880, 1970

113. Akhtar M et al: Synovial chondromatosis of the temporomandibular joint: Report of a case. J Bone Joint Surg [Am] 59:266–267, 1977

114. Silver CM, Simon SD, Litchman HM, Dychman J: Synovial chondromatosis of the temporomandibular joint: A case report. J Bone Joint Surg [Am] 53:777–780, 1971

115. Nokes ST, King PS et al: Temporomandibular joint chondromatosis with intracranial extension: MR and CT contributions. AJR Am J Roentgenol 148:1173–1174, 1987

116. Eisenberg KS, Johnston JO: Synovial chondromatosis of the hip joint presenting as an intrapelvic mass: A case report. J Bone Joint Surg [Am] 54:176–178, 1972

117. Pope TL Jr, Keats TE et al: Idiopathic synovial chondromatosis in two unusual sites: Inferior radioulnar joint and ischial bursa. Skeletal Radiol 16:205–208, 1987

118. Norman A, Steiner GC: Bone erosion in synovial chondromatosis. Radiology 161:749–752, 1986

119. Szypryt P, Twining P et al: Synovial chondromatosis of the hip joint presenting as a pathological fracture. Br J Radiol 59:399–401, 1986

120. Forrest J, Staple TW: Synovial hemangioma of the knee: Demonstration by arthrography and arteriography. AJR Am J Roentgenol 112:512–516, 1971

121. Larsen IJ, Landry RM: Hemangioma of the synovial membrane. J Bone Joint Surg [Am] 51:1210–1212, 1969

122. Burgan DW: Lipoma aborescens of the knee: Another cause of filling defects on a knee arthrogram. Radiology 101:583–584, 1971

123. Lee KR, Tines SC, Price HI et al: The computed tomographic findings of popliteal cysts. Skeletal Radiol 10:2–29, 1983

124. Krag DN, Stansel HC: Popliteal cyst producing complete arterial occlusion. J Bone Joint Surg [Am] 64:1369–1370, 1982

125. Bogumill GP, Bruno PD, Barrick EF et al: Malignant lesions masquerading as popliteal cysts. J Bone Joint Surg [Am] 63:474–477, 1981

126. Dungan DH, Seeger LL, Grand EG: Case report 707. Skeletal Radiol 21:52–55, 1992

127. Coleman BG, Arger PH, Dalinka MK et al: CT of sarcomatous degeneration in neurofibromatosis. AJR Am J Roentgenol 140:383–387, 1983

128. Patel YD, Morehouse HT: Neurofibrosarcomas in neurofibromatosis: Role in CT scanning and angiography. Clin Radiol 33:555–560, 1982

129. Curtis BH, Fisher RL, Butterfield WL, Saunders FP: Neurofibromatosis with paraplegia: Report of 8 cases. J Bone Joint Surg [Am] 51:843–861, 1969

130. Holt JF, Wright SM: Radiologic features of neurofibromatosis. Radiology 51:647–664, 1948

131. Holt JF: Neurofibromatosis in children. AJR Am J Roentgenol 130:615–639, 1978

132. Holt JF, Kuhns LR: Macrocranium and macrencephaly in neurofibromatosis. Skeletal Radiol 1:25–28, 1976

133. Hunt JC, Pugh DG: Skeletal lesions in neurofibromatosis. Radiology 76:1–20, 1961

134. Pitt MJ, Mosher JF, Edeiken J: Abnormal periosteum and bone in neurofibromatosis. Radiology 103:143–146, 1972

135. Allgayer VB, Reiser M, Kramann B: Typiche computertomographische befunde bei der neurofibromatose. Fortschr Geb Rontgenstr 140:669–672, 1984

136. Daneman A, Mancer K, Sonley M: CT appearance of thick-

ened nerves in neurofibromatosis. AJR Am J Roentgenol 141:899–900, 1983

137. Rockower S, McKay D, Nason S: Dislocation of the spine in neurofibromatosis. J Bone Joint Surg [Am] 64:1240–1242, 1982

138. Salerno NR, Edeiken J: Vertebral scalloping in neurofibromatosis. Radiology 97:509–510, 1970

139. Gupta SK, Tuli SM et al: Skeletal overgrowth with modelling error in neurofibromatosis. Clinical Radiol 36:643–646, 1985

140. Floyd A, Percy-Lancaster R: The elephant woman: Neurofibromatosis associated with pseudarthrosis of the humerus. J Bone Joint Surg 69:121–123, 1987

141. Beggs I, Shawa DG, Brenton DP et al: Case reports: An unusual case of neurofibromatosis: Cystic bone lesions and coarctation of the aortic arch. Br J Radiol 54:416–418, 1981

142. Mandell GA, Herrick WC et al: Neurofibromas: Location by scanning with Tc-99m DTPA. Radiology 157:803–806, 1985

143. Mandell GA, Harcke HT et al: SPECT imaging of para-axial neurofibromatosis with technetium-99m DTPA. J Nucl Med 28:1688–1694, 1987

144. Stull MA, Moser RP, Kransdorf MJ et al: Magnetic resonance appearance of peripheral nerve sheath tumors. Skeletal Radiol 20:9–14, 1991

145. Redd RA, Peters VJ, Emery SF et al: Morton Neuroma: Sonographic evaluation. Radiology 171:415–417, 1989

146. Rose JS, Hermann G, Mendelson DS et al: Extraskeletal Ewing sarcoma with computed tomography correlation. Skeletal Radiol 9:234–237, 1983

147. O'Keeffe F, Lorigan JG, Wallace S: Radiological features of extraskeletal Ewing sarcoma. Br J Radiol 63:456–460, 1990

148. Baldursson H, Evans EB, Dodge WF, Jackson WT: Tumoral calcinosis with hyperphosphatemia: A report of a family with incidence in 4 siblings. J Bone Joint Surg [Am] 51:913–925, 1969

149. Bishop AF, Destouet JM, Murphy WA et al: Tumoral calcinosis: Case report and review. Skeletal Radiol 8:269–274, 1982

150. D'Aboville M, Gaussin G, Regouby Y et al: Calcinose tumorale chez une femme blanche. J Radiol 64:429–432, 1983

151. Hug I, Guncaga J: Tumoral calcinosis with sedimentation sign. Br J Radiol 47:734–736, 1974

152. Palmer PES: Tumoural calcinosis. Br J Radiol 39:518–525, 1966

153. Yaghmai I, Mirbod P: Tumoral calcinosis. AJR Am J Roentgenol 111:573–578, 1971

154. Martinez S, Vogler JB, Harrelson JM et al: Imaging of tumoral calcinosis: New observations. Radiology 174:215–522, 1990

155. Seeger LL, Butler DL, Eckardt JJ et al: Tumoral calcinosis-like lesion of the proximal linea aspera. Skeletal Radiol 19:579–583, 1990

156. Sissons HA, Steiner GC, Bonar F et al: Tumoral calcium pyrophosphate deposition disease. Skeletal Radiol 18:79–87, 1989

157. Chew FS, Crenshaw WB: Radiologic-pathologic conferences of the Massachusetts General Hospital. Idiopathic tumoral calcinosis. AJR Am J Roentgenol 158:330, 1992

158. Kirk TS, Simon MA: Tumoral calcinosis. J Bone Joint Surg [Am] 63:1167–1169, 1981

159. Clarke E, Swischuk LE, Hayden CK: Tumoral calcinosis, diaphysitis, and hyperphosphatemia. Radiology 151:643–646, 1984

160. Kransdorf MJ, Meis JM: From the archives of the AFIP. Extraskeletal osseous and cartilaginous tumors of the extremeties. RadioGraphics 13:853–884, 1993

161. Kegal VW: Kausistischer beitrag zum krankheitsbild der myositis ossificans localisata. Fortschr Geb Rontgenstr 135:613–614, 1981

162. Norman A, Dorfman HD: Juxtacortical circumscribed myositis ossificans: Evolution and radiographic features. Radiology 96:301–306, 1970

163. Paterson DC: Myositis ossificans circumscripta. J Bone Joint Surg [Br] 52:296–301, 1970

164. Chung BS: Drug-induced myositis ossificans circumscripta. JAMA 226:469, 1973

165. Vas W, Cockshott WP, Martin RF et al: Myositis ossificans in hemophilia. Skeletal Radiol 7:2–31, 1981

166. Yaghmai I: Myositis ossificans: Diagnostic value of arteriography. AJR Am J Roentgenol 128:811–816, 1977

167. Amendola MA, Glazer GM, Agha FP et al: Myositis ossificans circumscripta: Computed tomographic diagnosis. Radiology 149:775–779, 1983

168. Kramer KL, Kurtz AB, Rubin C et al: Ultrasound appearance of myositis ossificans. Skeletal Radiol 4:1–20, 1979

169. Drane WE: Myositis ossificans and the three phase bone scan. AJR Am J Roentgenol 142:179–180a, 1984

170. Kransdorf MJ, Meis JM, Jelinek JS: Myositis ossificans: MR appearance with radiologic-pathologic correlation. AJR Am J Roentgenol 157:1243–1248, 1991

171. De Smet AA, Norris MA, Fisher DR: Magnetic resonance imaging of myositis ossificans: Analysis of seven cases. Skeletal Radiol 21:503–507, 1992

172. Voss H: Uber die parostalen und para-artikulären knochenneubildungen bie organischen nervenkrankheiten. Fortschr Geb Rontgenstr 55:423–441, 1937

173. Chaplin DM, Harrison MHM: Pseudomalignant osseous tumour of soft tissue. J Bone Joint Surg [Br] 54:334–340, 1972

174. Goldman AB: Myositis ossificans circumscripta: A benign lesion with a malignant differential diagnosis. AJR Am J Roentgenol 126:3–40, 1976

175. Jeffreys TE, Stiles PJ: Pseudomalignant osseous tumor of soft tissue. J Bone Joint Surg [Br] 48:488–492, 1966

176. Schutte HE, van der Heul RO: Pseudomalignant, nonneoplastic osseous soft-tissue tumors of the hand and foot. Radiology 176: 149–153, 1990

177. Nash S, Rubenstein J, Morava-Protzner I: Case report 766. Skeletal Radiol 22:55–57, 1993

178. Fine G, Stout AP: Osteogenic sarcoma of the extraskeletal soft tissues. Cancer 9:1027–1043, 1956

179. Kauffman SL, Stout AP: Extraskeletal osteogenic sarcomas and chondrosarcomas in children. Cancer 16:432–439, 1963

180. Lorentzon R, Larsson SE, Boquist L: Extraosseous osteosarcoma. J Bone Joint Surg [Br] 61:205–208, 1979

181. Chaulieu C, Delgoffe C, Adolphe J et al: Sarcome osteogenique primitif du rein. J Radiol 61:623–625, 1980

182. Aubrey DA, Andrews GS: Mammary osteogenic sarcoma. Br J Radiol 58:472–474, 1971

183. Karpas CM, Merendino VS: Uterine osteogenic sarcoma: Histochemical studies and report of a case. Obstet Gynecol 24:629–633, 1964

184. Caputo MG, Reuter KL, Reale F: Primary osteosarcoma of the uterus. Br J Radiol 63:578–580, 1990

185. Chinn D et al: Heterotopic bone formation in metastatic tumor from transitional-cell carcinoma of the urinary bladder. J Bone Joint Surg [Am] 58:881–883, 1976

186. Munk PL, Gock S, Gee R et al: Case report 708. Skeletal Radiol 21:56–59, 1992

187. Magid D, Fishman EK: Musculoskeletal infections in patients with AIDS: CT findings. AJR Am J Roentgenol 158:603–607, 1992

188. Janzen DL, Connell DG, Vaisler BJ: Calcific myonecrosis of the calf manifesting as an enlarging soft-tissue mass: imaging features. AJR Am J Roentgenol 160:1072–1074, 1993

189. Belli L, Reggiori A, Cocozza E et al: Ultrasound in tropical pyomyositis. Skeletal Radiol 21:107–109, 1992

190. Hanna SL, Fletcher BD, Parham DM et al: Muscle edema in musculoskeletal tumors: MR imaging characteristics and clinical significance. J Magn Reson Imaging 1444–1449, 1991

191. Duewell S, Hagspiel KD, Zuber J et al: Swollen lower extremity: Role of MR imaging. Radiology 184:227–231, 1992

192. Case TC, Witte CL, Witte MH et al: Magnetic resonance imaging in human lymphedema: Comparison with lymphangioscintigraphy. Magn Reson Imaging 10:549–558, 1992

Imaging of Bone Tumors: A Multimodality Approach,
edited by George B. Greenfield and John A. Arrington,
J. B. Lippincott Company, Philadelphia © 1995.

c h a p t e r

FIVE

Metastatic Tumors, Differential Diagnosis, and Bone Marrow

IMAGING STRATEGIES FOR METASTASES TO BONE

The methods available for detecting bone metastases are radionuclide scan,[1] bone survey and directed conventional radiologic examination, computed tomography (CT), magnetic resonance imaging (MRI), angiography, and needle biopsy.

The radionuclide bone scan is the simplest and most cost-effective modality for detection of skeletal metastatic disease. Early detection with conventional radiography is not possible.

A bone scan is positive because it reflects osteogenic or repair activity in the lesion. Highly anaplastic tumors and multiple myeloma may not stimulate sufficient osteoblastic response to be imaged on the scan. For approximately 5% of metastases, the bone scan is negative despite a radiographically evident destructive lesion, indicating that osteogenesis within the lesion is not greater than that in the normal surrounding bone. Multiple myeloma may even show photopenic lesions.

The bone scan may be used to monitor the response of metastases to therapy. Occasionally, a lesion may show an additional increase in uptake after completion of chemotherapy. In some cases, this response has been identified as a transient process that represents repair and healing of the bone rather than progression of disease.

A pattern that may be seen with far-advanced, widespread metastatic bone disease is the superscan.[1a,1b] The kidneys are not visualized, and the blood background is free of radioactivity. The generalized bone-to-background ratio of counts is very high (Fig. 5-1). This pattern may also be seen in hyperparathyroidism. Another pattern that may be seen with extensive metastases from prostate carcinoma is the headless scan, due to the lack of involvement of the calvarium by osteoblastic metastases.

The radionuclide angiogram is another technique. The scintillation camera is centered over the radiographically identified abnormality at the time of intravenous injection of the radiopharmaceutical, and the degree of vascularity of the lesion can be ascertained. These methods have been combined in the three-phase scan. The perfusion, blood pool, and uptake are determined by timing.

Conventional radiographic examination for *detection* of bony metastases is indicated only for specific circumstances. If the patient has a primary tumor, such as a highly anaplastic carcinoma or myeloma, and the radionuclide bone scan is negative, a bone survey may be carried out. If a patient is symptomatic, a directed radiographic examination of that part should be performed regardless of the outcome of the bone scan. If there is any question about the pattern or cause of increased uptake of isotope, a directed examination should be performed. It is not possible to demonstrate early bony metastases on conventional radiographs.

CT is most valuable in the detection of metastatic bone disease, particularly in the central skeleton.[2–4] It is superior to conventional radiography because marrow attenuation changes can be seen, and it should be used when the bone scan is positive and conventional radiographs are normal (Fig. 5-2). Bone marrow tumor infiltration can also be demonstrated using quantitative CT. A positive CT number greater than 15 Hounsfield units indicates an abnormal marrow,[3] which is not specific for metastatic disease.

CT is also useful for determining the extent of a lesion and for evaluating involvement of major structures, but MRI is superior in these respects. CT is superior in showing bony detail.

MRI has the unique ability to show focal or diffuse bone marrow changes. Care must be taken in the interpretation of the marrow signal in children. In the infant, all marrow cavities contain red marrow, which begins to convert to yellow marrow soon after birth. This progresses from the periphery centrally. The epiphyses convert to yellow marrow very early in life. At maturity, the entire appendicular skeleton is composed of yellow marrow, which exhibits a homogeneous high signal intensity on T1-weighted spin echo images. The physeal scar is seen as a dark line. The central skeleton contains red marrow admixed with yellow marrow.

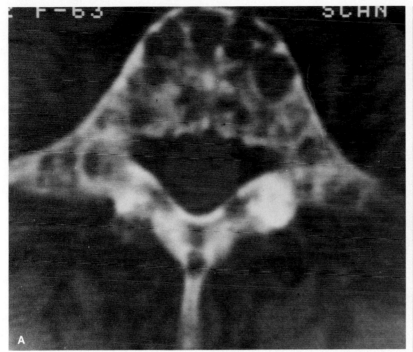

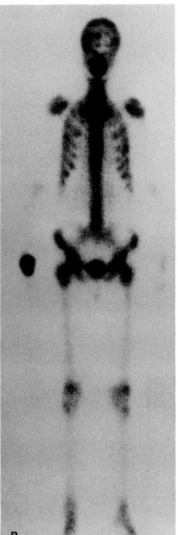

FIGURE 5-1. A 63-year-old woman with extensive metastases from an unknown primary tumor. (**A**) The CT scan shows extensive metastatic disease in the lumbar vertebrae. (**B**) The radionuclide bone scan shows the superscan phenomenon. There is increased isotope uptake in the skeleton without activity in the kidneys.

This yields a T1-weighted signal intensity lower than pure fat but higher than cellular tissue. T2-weighted images show lowering of the signal intensity, and fat-suppression images show a yet lower intensity. MRI age-related changes do not correlate with macrospecimens, because they are seen earlier. The adult pattern is seen after 24 years of age.[5] Marrow replacement alters the MR pattern. Conditions that can alter the MR pattern include histiocytosis X, leukemia, lymphoma, metastases, myelofibrosis, myeloma, osteomyelitis, primary bone tumors, and storage diseases. STIR imaging is particularly useful in cases of diffuse marrow infiltration, which are commonly seen with lymphoma, leukemia, and metastatic prostatic carcinoma. Because of the diffuse nature of the marrow infiltration, the signal appears homogeneous on standard T1-weighted and T2-weighted SE sequences. STIR imaging makes this pattern of pathologic marrow more obvious by suppressing the signal from yellow marrow and adding the

signal from the elongation of both T1 and T2 relaxation times of pathologic marrow.

On T1-weighted images, a pattern of lower signal intensity relative to marrow is usually seen. On T2-weighted images, the signal intensity of osteolytic or cellular metastases is increased, but osteoblastic lesions do not show an increase. All metastatic lesions appear as focal or diffuse low-signal-intensity areas contrasted against marrow fat on T1-weighted images (see Fig. 5-2),[6] except for hemorrhagic lesions. Nonneoplastic lesions also have this appearance. The extent of involvement of adjacent structures is much better shown by MRI than CT because of better soft-tissue contrast and multiplanar viewing.[7] CT is, however, superior to MRI in demonstrating cortical bone destruction and the pattern and extent of calcification.[8]

Bone marrow edema, with increased water content of the marrow, results in focal, patchy, or homogeneous

(text continues on page 338)

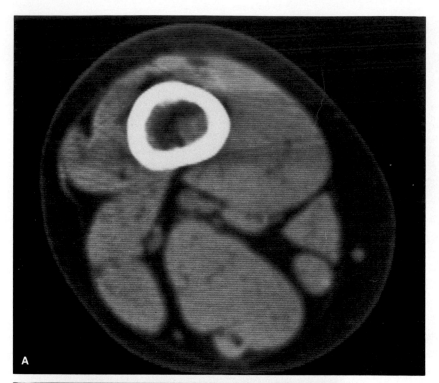

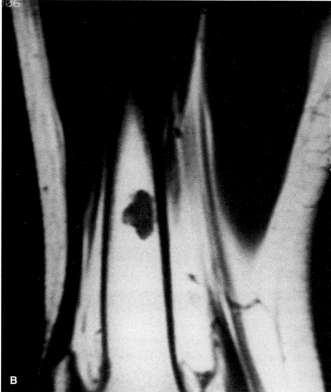

FIGURE 5-2. Metastasis from carcinoma of the breast to the femoral marrow cavity. The conventional radiographs showed no abnormalities. (**A**) The CT scan shows the high-attentuation tumor displacing the fatty marrow. The cortex is not destroyed. (**B**) The T1-weighted MR image shows focal replacement of high-signal-intensity fatty marrow by tumor. (**C**) The proton density image shows a low-signal-intensity tumor replacing higher-signal-intensity fat. (**D**) The T2-weighted MR image shows the tumor is increased in signal intensity while the fat is decreased. The tumor does not involve the cortex of the bone.

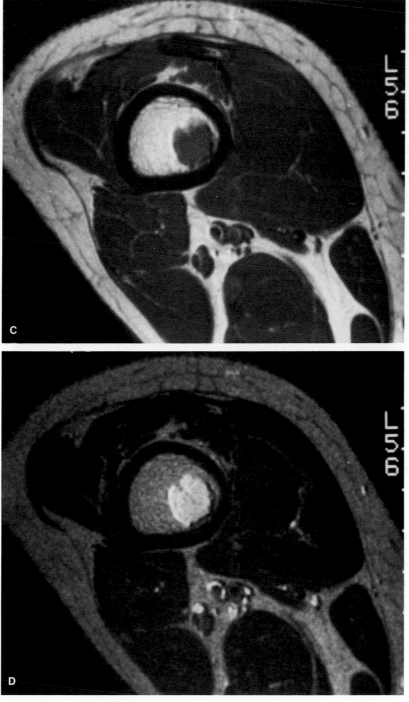

FIGURE 5-2.   *(Continued)*

low signal intensity on T1-weighted images and high signal intensity with T2 weighting. The cause may be trauma or reflex sympathetic dystrophy. Bone marrow infarction produces a variable picture, with some areas of low signal intensity with T1 weighting. Bone marrow ischemia results in conversion of red marrow to yellow marrow. MRI is the most sensitive means of detecting a bony lesion.

The angiographic features of hypervascular metastases reveal no characteristic findings. There is no way to differentiate a primary hypervascular bone tumor from a metastatic tumor by means of arteriography.[9] The vascularity of tumors metastatic to bone varies. The most vascular bone metastases are from carcinoma of the thyroid, gastrointestinal adenocarcinomas, hypernephroma, and melanoma. Bronchogenic carcinoma is moderately vascular, and osteoblastic prostatic carcinoma has normal or very low vascularity.

CT-directed needle biopsy has become an integral component in the diagnosis and treatment of musculoskeletal lesions. CT localization adds significantly to the safety of the procedure and greatly enhances the biopsy success rate. Percutaneous needle biopsies are most commonly performed on patients suspected of having systemic disease such as metastases, myeloma, or lymphoma. A successful percutaneous biopsy in this group of patients can save unnecessary surgery, because surgical resection usually is not possible, but treatment requires a definitive diagnosis.

A variety of needles are used and can be divided into small aspiration, small cutting, large cutting, and trephine needles. Complications correlate most closely with the experience of the radiologist, anatomic site, and needle size. Needle biopsies should not be done on suspected malignant cartilage tumors, because not enough tissue can be gotten to the pathologist and because of the danger of seeding.

METASTASES TO BONE AND DIFFERENTIAL DIAGNOSIS

Sclerosis of Bone

Osteoblastic Metastases

All carcinomas can yield osteoblastic metastases.[10-14] Lymphomas and leukemias may cause osteosclerotic reactions,[15-18] and mucinous carcinomas tend to do so. Cerebellar medulloblastoma also is known to cause osteosclerotic metastases.

The most frequently seen osteoblastic metastases in older men are from carcinoma of the prostate. Serum acid phosphatase and serum alkaline phosphatase levels are usually elevated, as is the prostate-specific antigen (PSA). Early metastases from carcinoma of the prostate are difficult to detect. The ^{99m}Tc diphosphonate bone scan is claimed to be the most sensitive means of detecting early prostatic carcinoma metastases,[19] although MRI is more sensitive in general. In the differential diagnosis, the serum acid phosphatase level is also elevated in Gaucher disease, and osteosclerotic lesions in adult Gaucher disease are common. Osteosclerotic lesions are commonly secondary to carcinoma of the lung,[20] particularly small cell carcinoma and

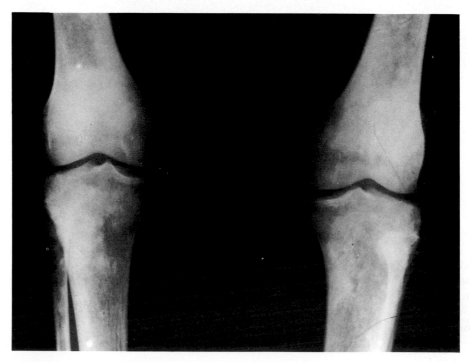

FIGURE 5-3. Osteoblastic metastases to the knees from carcinoma of the prostate. Ill-defined, patchy, sclerotic areas are present.

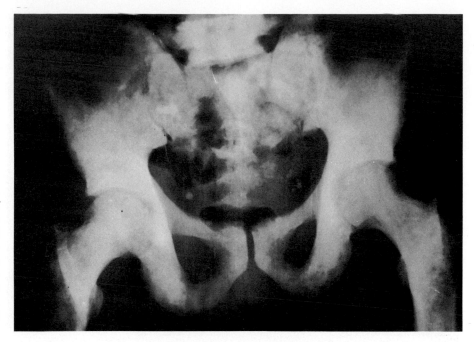

FIGURE 5-4. Osteoblastic metastases in the pelvis from carcinoma of the prostate. There is diffuse sclerosis of the pelvis, vertebrae, and upper femora, with loss of distinction between cortex and medulla in some areas. The fifth lumbar vertebral body is densely sclerotic. The caliber of the bone is not enlarged, in contrast to what is likely in Paget disease.

adenocarcinoma; breast, particularly after treatment; pancreas; malignant carcinoid; colon; and urinary bladder.[21]

In children, osteoblastic metastases secondary to cerebellar medulloblastoma, particularly after surgery, have been reported,[22,23] with a leukoerythroblastic anemia and diffuse osteosclerosis due to metastatic invasion of the bone marrow.[24]

Osteoblastic response to treatment of metastatic prostate carcinoma may occur.[25] Osteolysis in previously stable sclerotic areas indicate recurrence of malignancy.[26]

On plain films or CT, patchy or ill-defined areas of increased density are seen initially (Fig. 5-3). The lesions occur as discrete foci of various sizes with ill-defined margins. Less commonly, all of the bones are involved with a dense, uniform sclerosis (Fig. 5-4). Simple periosteal reaction or, more rarely, a spiculated pattern of periosteal new bone formation may occur (Fig. 5-5). These may fill in with new bone and increase the bone size (Figs. 5-6 and 5-7). The vertebrae may show sclerosis of a pedicle (Fig. 5-8). Sclerosis or enlargement of a pedicle may also result from stress due to a neural arch defect on either side, a variety of congenital, inflammatory, or neoplastic conditions, or after laminectomy, or sclerosis may be idiopathic.[27–30]

A dense vertebral body, or ivory vertebra, is usually caused by osteoblastic metastases, Hodgkin disease (Fig. 5-9), or the sclerotic stage of Paget disease. Lymphoma may show scalloping of the anterior margin of the vertebral body secondary to erosion from the lymphadenopathy that frequently occurs (Fig. 5-10), a feature not found in osteoblastic metastases. Reduction in density and restoration of the trabecular pattern

have been reported after radiation therapy.[31] NHL may also cause sclerotic vertebrae.

Calvarial osteoblastic metastases are extremely rare, even with widespread sclerotic lesions from car-

(text continues on page 342)

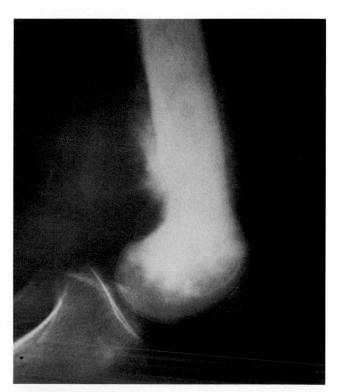

FIGURE 5-5. Lateral view of the knee of a patient with carcinoma of the prostate with osteoblastic metastases. The distal femur shows a sunburst pattern of spiculated periosteal new bone formation.

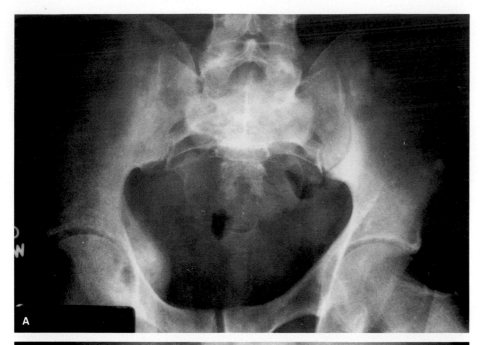

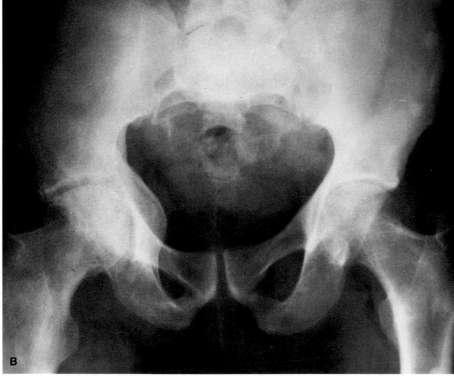

FIGURE 5-6. A 60-year-old man with osteoblastic metastases from carcinoma of the prostate. (A) An anteroposterior view of the pelvis shows osteosclerosis, spiculation, and a bony mass at the right ischiac bone. Patchy osteosclerosis is also seen throughout the pelvis. (B) One year after A. The bony mass has organized with a sharp margin and is seen as enlargement. The osteosclerotic densities are better formed.

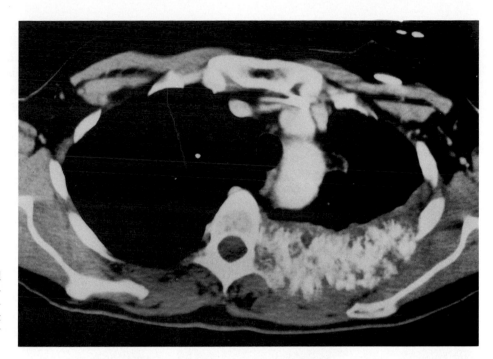

FIGURE 5-7. A 55-year-old woman with carcinoma of the colon. The CT scan shows an irregular, sclerotic metastasis to a left upper thoracic rib. The bony mass is markedly irregular.

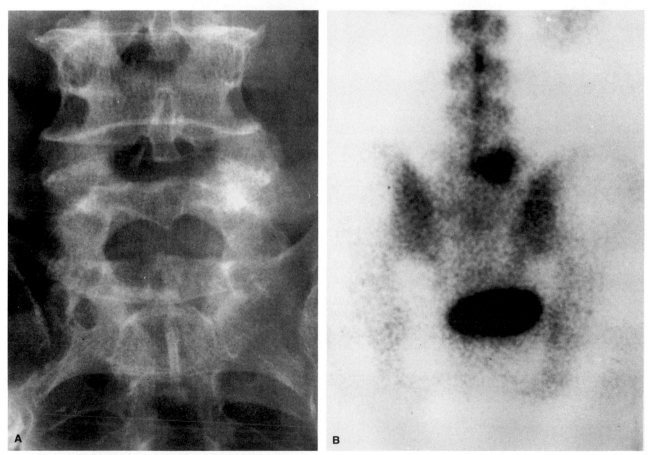

FIGURE 5-8. A 56-year-old man with carcinoma of the lung and osteoblastic metastasis to the left pedicle of the fifth lumbar vertebra. (**A**) The anteroposterior view of the lower lumbar spine shows osteosclerosis of the left pedicle of L5. The sclerosis extends to the superior articular process. (**B**) Radionuclide bone scan shows increased activity at the left side of L5.

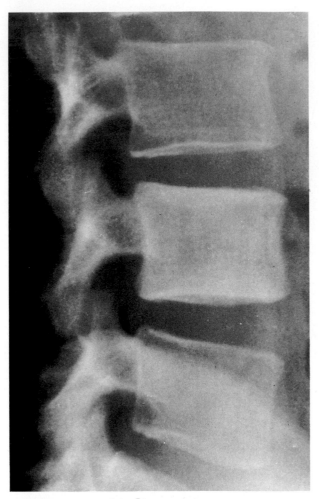

FIGURE 5-9. Hodgkin disease. Sclerosis of the body of the fourth lumbar vertebra occurred without changes in contour. This was the only bony lesion.

cinoma of the prostate. Prostatic carcinoma metastases to the sphenoid and zygomatic bones, simulating meningioma en plaque, have been reported.[32] Osteoblastic metastases from carcinoid tumors may produce bone expansion and periosteal spiculation.[33] Soft-tissue invasion is rare but may occur. Osteoblastic metastases distal to the knees are rare but occur more often with prostatic carcinoma than with other primary tumors (Fig. 5-11).

The radionuclide bone scan may range from minimal or no activity to a uniform symmetric increased bone uptake of isotope (i.e., superscan; see Fig. 5-1), with faint or absent renal activity. This finding may also occur in hyperparathyroidism. Carcinoma of the prostate has only a 7% incidence of cranial vault metastases, even though diffuse skeletal involvement may exist. The resulting radionuclide uptake distribution has been called the "headless bone scan."[34] After the start of treatment for advanced cancer of the prostate, the radionuclide bone scan occasionally shows apparent

progression of individual lesions despite clinical improvement. This is called the "flare phenomenon."[35] Bone scans are useful for monitoring tumor status in systemically treated patients with prostate cancer. However, because of the lack of sensitivity for response and paradoxically apparent worsening of the scan despite tumor regression in some patients, scans are not accurate enough to be used as the sole test in following these patients.[36] Osteoblastic metastases from prostate carcinoma often undergo healing reactions after successful endocrine treatment. This is characterized by intensification of osteosclerosis. In remission, the sclerosis usually remains unchanged but rarely may regress.[37]

CT findings consist of localized or generalized high-density regions, which are sometimes difficult to differentiate from reactive sclerosis in the spine.

Angiographically, osteoblastic metastases from carcinoma of the prostate have normal or very low vascularity.[9] MRI is more sensitive than radioscintigraphy for early detection. Focal or diffuse low signal intensity on T1-weighted images, which improve with chemotherapy, may be seen.[38]

MR images exhibit various appearances of metastases, depending on their histology.[39] They all show decreased signal intensity on T1-weighted images, reflecting replacement of marrow fat. Increased signal intensity of an osteolytic tumor on T2-weighted images may be seen, but an osteosclerotic bone metastasis is seen as low signal intensity (Fig. 5-12). The central skeleton, where red and mixed marrows occur in the adult, can present difficulties in evaluating metastases with MRI. Two signs that are helpful are bull's eyes and halos.[40] The bull's-eye sign refers to a focus of high signal intensity seen centrally within a bony lesion on T1-weighted images. This indicates that the area is not metastatic, but rather an island of hematopoietic marrow with a central fatty marrow focus. The halo sign, seen as a rim of high signal intensity around a lower-signal-intensity focus on T2-weighted images is an indicator of an osteoblastic metastasis.

Osteopoikilosis

Osteopoikilosis is a rare hereditary disorder of bone remodeling characterized by multiple, small, circumscribed, round or ovoid areas of increased bone density.[44] It is thought to be transmitted in an autosomal dominant manner. Laboratory studies show no abnormalities. It is asymptomatic, incidentally discovered on radiographs. It occurs in patients between 15 and 60 years of age, although prenatal and elderly cases have been reported. There are small foci of bone sclerosis that may be a few millimeters to several centi-

(text continues on page 346)

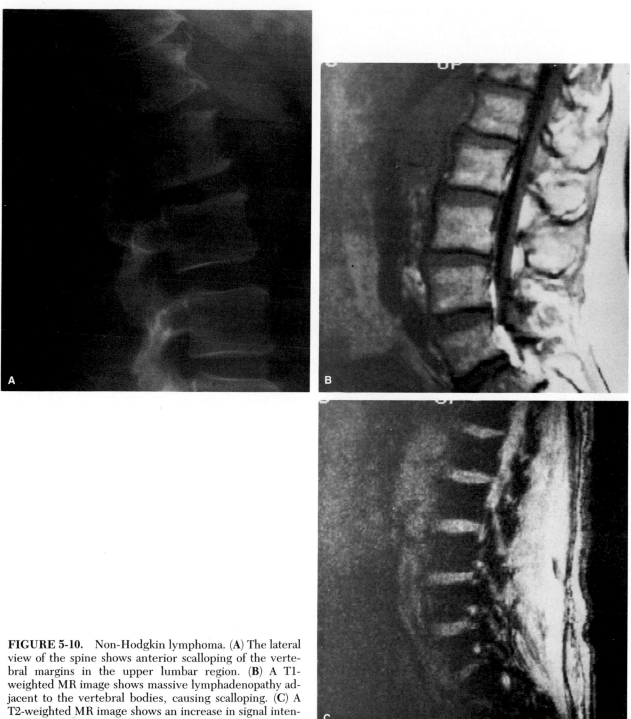

FIGURE 5-10.   Non-Hodgkin lymphoma. (**A**) The lateral view of the spine shows anterior scalloping of the vertebral margins in the upper lumbar region. (**B**) A T1-weighted MR image shows massive lymphadenopathy adjacent to the vertebral bodies, causing scalloping. (**C**) A T2-weighted MR image shows an increase in signal intensity of the lymphomatous mass.

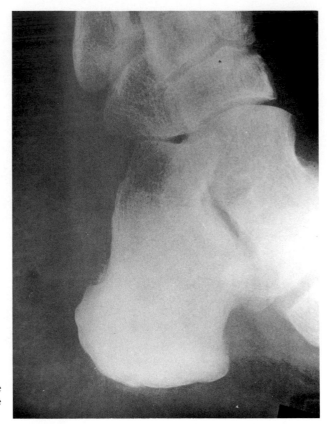

FIGURE 5-11. Osteoblastic metastases from carcinoma of the prostate cause diffuse sclerosis of the calcaneus without change in contour. This is an unusual site for metastasis.

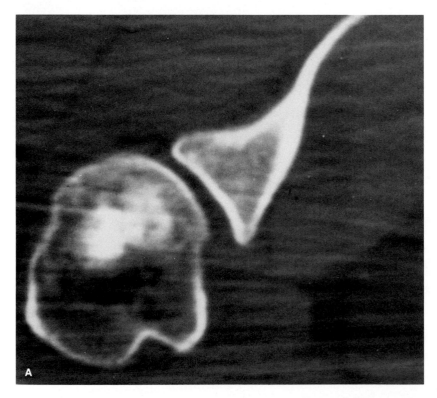

FIGURE 5-12. Osteoblastic metastases to the left humeral head from carcinoma of the prostate in a 60-year-old man. (**A**) The CT scan shows a dense osteosclerotic focus in the humeral head. (**B**) MR image (SE 3000/25). The metastatic focus is of low signal intensity replacing high-signal-intensity marrow fat. (**C**) MRI (SE 3000/80). The metastatic focus remains of low signal intensity, and the marrow fat is decreased in signal intensity.

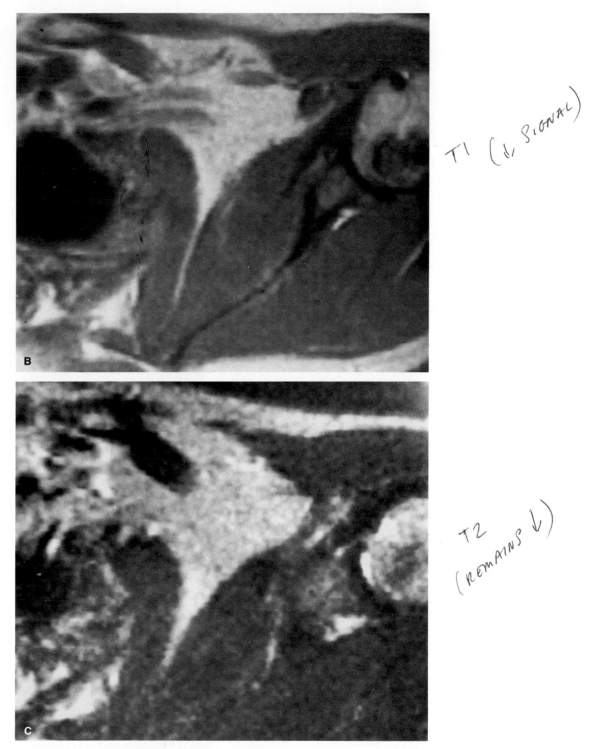

FIGURE 5-12.   *(Continued)*

meters in diameter. These are round or ovoid, and some contain radiolucent centers. They are thought not to progress, but disappearance and reappearance have been reported.

In the long bones, the lesions are seen at the ends but not on the shaft. The small bones and cuboid bones can be involved (Fig. 5-13). The pelvis is often involved, with the chief distribution about the acetabula (Fig. 5-14). The scapula may show involvement around the glenoid fossa. The skull, mandible, ribs, sternum, and vertebrae are rarely involved.

Bone Islands *No Skull*

Bone islands are solitary, small foci of dense bone within the spongiosa, which are asymptomatic and should be considered as normal variants.[42] Although usually stable, they can increase slowly in size until they are considerably larger than when originally discovered.

Bone islands are seen as well-circumscribed areas of increased density in tubular or flat bones (Fig. 5-15) and occur most commonly in the pelvis and upper femora. They may also be present in the spine.[43] The skull is not involved. The lesions are small, rarely exceeding 1 cm in size. The margins are characterized by spiculated radiations, or a brush border, but they may be smooth and sharp. Giant bone islands, up to 4 cm in diameter, have been reported.[44]

Differentiation from an osteoblastic metastasis can be helped by a normal radionuclide bone scan.[45] However, some bone islands show increased isotope uptake on a bone scan.[46]

Myelofibrosis *Get 2° Gout*

Myelofibrosis (i.e., myelosclerosis, agnogenic myeloid metaplasia, osteosclerotic anemia) is a hematologic disorder of unknown cause that is characterized by anemia, a leukemoid blood picture, progressive fibrosis of the bone marrow, marked splenomegaly, and bone involvement, which is usually osteosclerotic.[47,48]

Most patients are older than 50 years of age, although the range of patients' ages is between 34 and 85 years. The gender distribution is equal. The symptoms are related to anemia, a bleeding tendency, bone pain, and secondary gout. Splenomegaly, which may be massive, is consistently present. There is often elevation of the basal metabolic rate. A large percentage of patients have antecedent polycythemia vera.

Radiologically, the basic types of lesions are destructive bony lesions, extramedullary hematopoiesis, osteosclerosis, secondary gout, and splenomegaly. About half of patients develop osteosclerosis, which varies from mild to severe. There may be a coarsened trabecular or a ground glass appearance.

The sclerosis may be uniform or patchy (Figs. 5-16

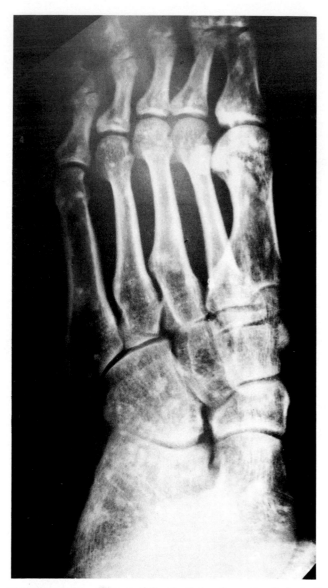

FIGURE 5-13. Osteopoikilosis of the foot. Small foci of bone sclerosis are evident in the tarsal bones and at the metaphyseal aspects of the metatarsals and the phalanges.

and 5-17), with the uniform appearance occurring most frequently. Irregular and thick periosteal new bone formation can be seen most often at the medial margins of the distal femora, the lateral margins of the proximal tibias, and the ankles. The changes at the knees and ankles are characteristic. Endosteal thickening of long bones also occurs. The ribs, spine, pelvis, humeri, and femora are the bones most frequently involved with osteosclerosis. Skull changes may be osteosclerotic, radiolucent, or mixed. The hands and feet are rarely involved.

Bony destructive changes are also sometimes seen. There may be discrete ovoid radiolucencies with the long axis of the lesion parallel to the long axis of the shaft, or a moth-eaten, ill-defined appearance.

Massive splenomegaly affects many of these pa-

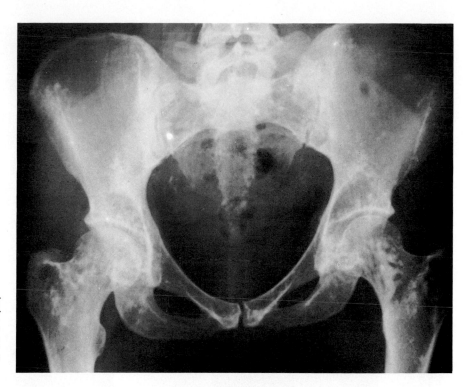

FIGURE 5-14. Osteopoikilosis of the pelvis. Multiple small areas of bone sclerosis are oriented bilaterally in the pelvis, femoral heads, femoral necks, and metaphyseal regions. The shafts are not involved.

tients. Extramedullary hematopoiesis may be seen in the liver, spleen, skin, paraspinal region, adrenals, lungs, choroid plexus, lymph nodes, and as an extrapleural mass adjacent to an area of rib destruction. Hyperuricemia may result in secondary gout with destructive bony lesions indistinguishable from those of primary gout.

An aggressive, rapidly progressive form called malignant myelosclerosis has been described. These lesions resemble bone metastases. Myelofibrosis has been associated with multiple myeloma,[49] and it has developed in cases of treated histiocytosis X. One case was associated with malignant lymphoma.[50]

Mastocytosis

Mastocytosis (i.e., urticaria pigmentosa) is a condition in which generalized visceral mast cell proliferation occurs, involving skin, bone marrow, liver, spleen, lungs, and lymph nodes.[51–54] Bone marrow involvement results in osteosclerosis.[55] Anemia, leukocytosis or leukopenia, and thrombocytopenia may occur, and symptoms due to the release of vasoactive substances include headache, flushing, bronchospasm, and diarrhea.[56]

Generalized or focal bone changes, with a mixture of osteosclerosis and osteoporosis, may be seen. There may be trabecular thickening or diffuse sclerosis alternating with areas of cystic rarefaction. The lesions are confined almost entirely to cancellous bone, with sclerosis obliterating the trabeculae. There may also be scattered, well-defined sclerotic foci (Fig. 5-18). The

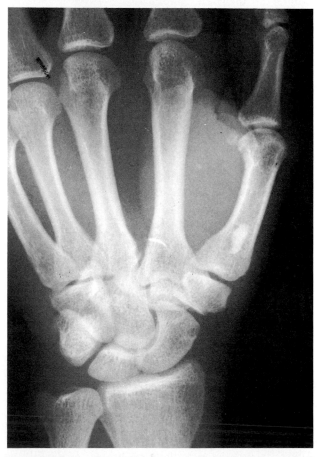

FIGURE 5-15. Bone island. A small, well-circumscribed area of increased density is present in the first metacarpal. Bone islands are similar to lesions seen in osteopoikilosis, but they are solitary.

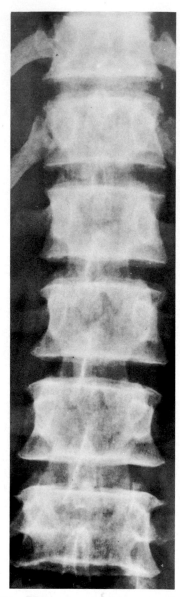

FIGURE 5-16. Myelosclerosis of the spine. Increased density of vertebral bodies is seen.

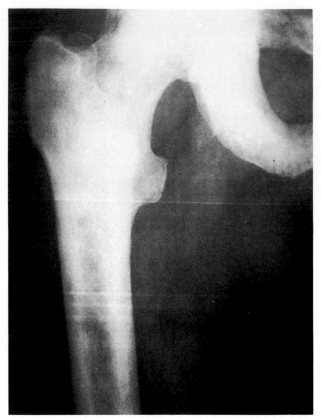

FIGURE 5-17. Myelosclerosis. Increased density is seen in the ischium and upper femur.

Tuberous Sclerosis HAMARTOMAS

Tuberous sclerosis is a rare disease caused by a defect of ectodermal development.[58] It is transmitted in an autosomal dominant manner and characterized by a clinical triad of adenoma sebaceum of the face, epilepsy, and mental deficiency. Multiple organs, particularly the central nervous system, are involved. Hamartomas are common, particularly in the kidney, and malignant change may occur. There is an increased incidence of congenital skeletal anomalies and congenital heart disease. Small nodules of gliosis are scattered throughout the cerebral cortex. Congenital tumors of the retina, called phakomas, also are present. The skin shows thickened plaques, café au lait spots, and subungual fibromas. The lungs may show an interstitial and honeycomb pattern.

The characteristic change in bone is patchy osteosclerosis. These may be round, ovoid, flame-shaped, or irregularly outlined foci. They vary in size from millimeters to several centimeters (Fig. 5-19). All bones may be involved with sclerotic lesions. There is frequent involvement of the pelvis, lumbar spine, and the cranial vault. The hands and feet may show cyst-like areas, particularly in the distal phalanges. Periosteal new bone formation may be seen. Widening of a rib

bones most often involved are the spine, ribs, pelvis, humeri, and femora. The skull may also be involved, showing stippling of the calvarium and thickening of the tables.

Mastocytosis with skeletal involvement has been reported in infancy. Most patients develop skin lesions during the first year of life. These appear as umbilicated papules, which may be discrete or coalescent. There may be hepatosplenomegaly and lymphadenopathy. The frequency of bone involvement in children is claimed to be 15%, with findings of osteosclerotic and osteolytic lesions, coarse trabeculation, undertubulation, and vertebral changes resembling Scheuermann disease.[57]

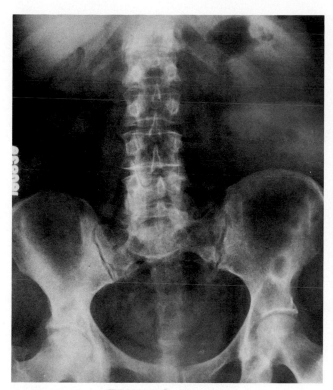

FIGURE 5-18. Mastocytosis. Osteosclerosis is scattered throughout the lumbar spine and pelvis with several radiolucent foci in the left side of the pelvis.

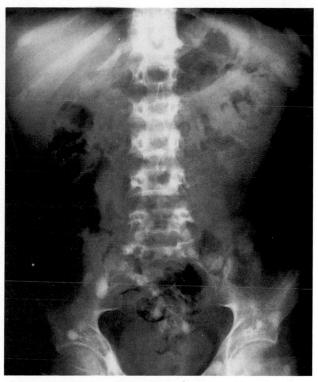

FIGURE 5-19. Tuberous sclerosis. Multiple, discrete, osteosclerotic foci of various sizes and shapes are scattered throughout the spine, ribs, and pelvis.

with osteosclerosis has been reported.[59] The spine may show sclerosis of the pedicles. Asymptomatic parents of patients may show signs of the disease.[60]

Paget Disease

Paget disease is seen as a spectrum of destruction and repair in which four stages may be discerned on imaging studies: stage 1, destructive or osteolytic; stage 2, combined destruction and repair; stage 3, osteosclerotic; and stage 4, malignant change. The combined stage is most commonly present, and the destructive and sclerotic stages are seen less frequently.

In the skull, the destructive stage is seen as a rarefied area called osteoporosis circumscripta. The area is well demarcated and can involve the major portion of the calvarium. The outer table is destroyed, but the inner table is spared (Fig. 5-20). Repair begins as sclerosis of the inner table. Thickening of the diploë and, later, of the outer table ensue. Irregular, patchy sclerosis in the thickened diploë, known as the cotton-wool appearance, follows (Fig. 5-21). MR images show thickening of the calvarium with high signal intensity on T1-weighted images (Fig. 5-22). Basilar invagination results from bone softening. In the sclerotic stage, diffuse sclerosis of the skull may be seen with loss of distinc-

tion between the tables and the diploë. Dental changes include loss of lamina dura, resorption of bone near the apices of the teeth, and hypercementosis. The paranasal sinuses and the petrous pyramids are frequently involved.

In the spine, the most common finding is a single vertebra involved in the combined stage. The vertebral body is enlarged with a rim of thickened cortex, giving a picture-frame appearance. The trabecular pattern is coarsened and may be vertically striated. The neural arch may be thickened. Rarely, the osteolytic stage of Paget disease in the spine may be seen, leading to compression fracture of a vertebral body.[61] Monostotic Paget disease of the vertebra may also be seen in the sclerotic stage.[62] Enlargement of the body and squaring of the anterior margin, when present, help to differentiate this condition from osteoblastic metastases. In Hodgkin disease, there may be erosion of the anterior margin of a sclerotic vertebral body due to pressure from contiguous enlarged lymph nodes, differentiating it from this condition.

The spine may be generally involved in polyostotic Paget disease. The destructive phase, pathologic fractures, and the combined stage may coexist (Figs. 5-23 and 5-24). The cervical spine is rarely involved. Serious

(text continues on page 352)

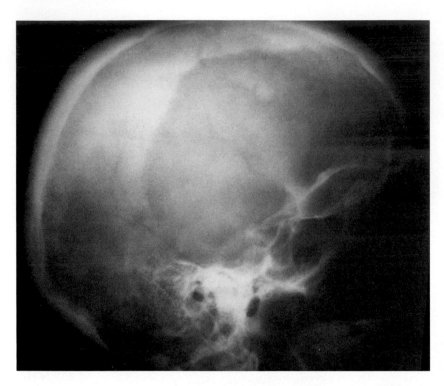

FIGURE 5-20. Paget disease, destructive stage. A lateral view of the skull shows osteoporosis circumscripta.

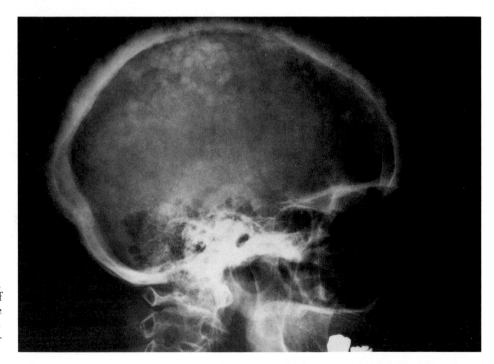

FIGURE 5-21. Paget disease, combined stage. A lateral view of the skull shows thickening of the calvarium and patchy sclerosis. This is the cotton-wool appearance.

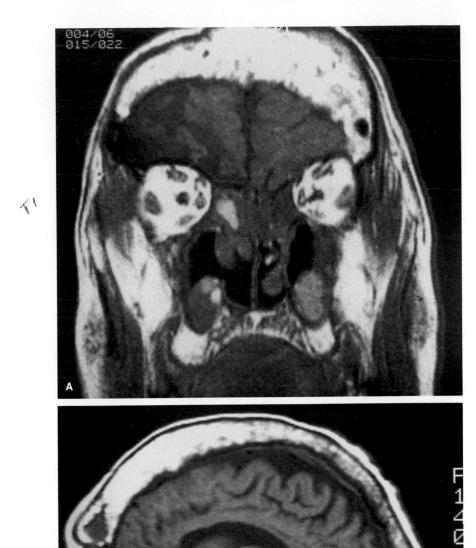

FIGURE 5-22.   Paget disease, combined stage. (**A**) The coronal MR (SE 600/20) section shows marked thickening of the calvarium with heterogeneous high signal intensity. (**B**) The sagittal MR (SE 600/20) image shows a thickening of the entire extent of the calvarium with a heterogenous high signal intensity. The inner and outer tables are intact and are seen as a low-signal-intensity margin.

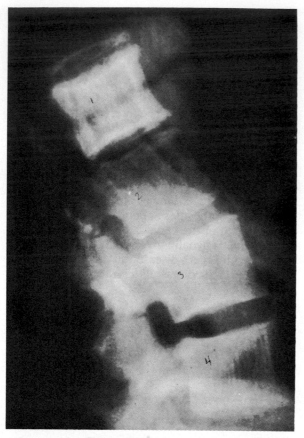

FIGURE 5-23. Paget disease. The lateral view of the spine shows the twelfth dorsal vertebral body and the upper four lumbar vertebral bodies. There is mixed involvement of the spine. The twelfth dorsal body is normal. The first lumbar vertebral body shows involvement in the combined phase of the disease, in which thickening of the anterior and posterior margins and of the vertebral end-plates gives it a picture-frame appearance. The second lumbar vertebral body is normal. The third lumbar vertebral body is involved in the sclerotic phase, characterized by a uniform increase in density of the body and squaring of the anterior margin, with a lack of normal convexity (compare with anterior margin of L1). The fourth lumbar vertebral body is involved in a transition between the combined phase and the sclerotic phase. It shows increased density of the vertebral body, with several prominent vertical trabeculae at the anterior aspect and squaring of its anterior margin.

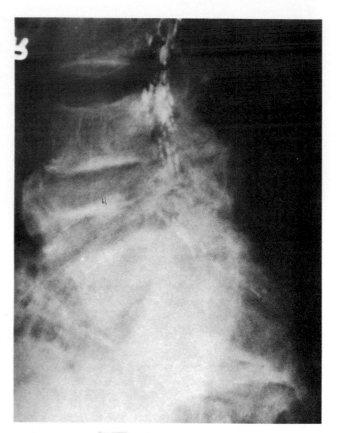

FIGURE 5-24. Paget disease, combined phase. The fourth lumbar vertebral body has collapsed. (Courtesy of Dr. Dharmashi V. Bhate, VA Hospital, Hines, IL.)

neurologic sequelae due to spinal stenosis may occur.[63] CT demonstrates spinal stenosis and severe facet joint arthropathy in a large percentage of patients.[64] The destructive stage may lead to vertebral body collapse with intact intervertebral spaces. The neural arches are also likely to be involved, differentiating this disease from metastases.

The pelvis is involved in two thirds of patients with Paget disease, and involvement is usually detected in the combined stage. It is rarely observed in the destructive stage. The involvement may be a small area, only one half of the pelvis, or general involvement. Cortical thickening, enlargement of bone, and coars-

ened trabecular pattern are present, as well as thickening of the pelvic rim. The latter is known as the rim sign (Fig. 5-25). There may be deformity and protrusion of the acetabulum. Uniform narrowing of the hip joint space with medial migration of the femoral head, known as Paget arthritis, is a common finding. When the pelvis is diffusely involved in the sclerotic stage, differentiation from osteoblastic metastases is difficult. Widening of the bone and thickening of the cortex help in differentiation.

Involvement of the long bones is commonly seen in the combined stage and rarely in the destructive stage. The destructive stage almost always begins at the end of a bone or at an apophysis, such as the greater trochanter or tibial tuberosity. The lesion extends along the shaft for some distance and ends in a sharply demarcated, angular configuration, producing the blade-of-grass appearance (Fig. 5-26). An ovoid, cyst-like, expansile radiolucency in the anterior tibial cortex may also be present.[65] The osteolytic stage has also been reported in the calcaneus, producing considerable expansion and deformity.[66]

In the combined stage, widening of the bone and thickening of the cortex occur with thickening of the trabeculae and disruption of the architectural pattern

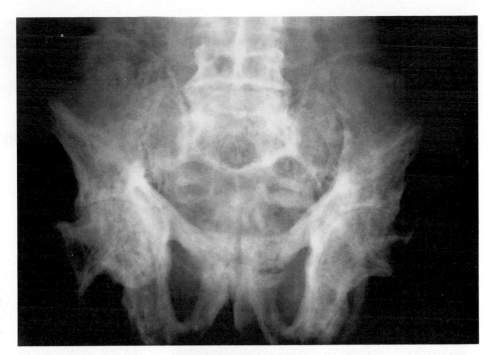

FIGURE 5-25. Paget disease, combined stage. The anteroposterior view of the pelvis shows thickening of the cortex, particularly of the pelvic rim. Coarsening of the trabecular pattern is evident. Narrowing of the joint space in both hips is seen, with medial migration of both femoral heads.

(Fig. 5-27). Contraction of the bone is a rare finding. Incomplete stress fractures resembling pseudofractures of osteomalacia (Figs. 5-28 and 5-29) and pathologic fractures of the transverse type occur in as many as 8% of cases. These most commonly involve the femur and tibia.[67] They tend to heal at the periosteal and endosteal surfaces, leaving only a midcortical residua. Softening of bone results in deformities, particularly the shepherd's-crook deformity of the upper femur and anterior bowing of the tibia. The fibula is least likely to be involved.

The ribs, singly or multiply, are uncommonly involved (Fig. 5-30). Widening and thickening of the bones occur. The clavicles and scapula may also be involved (Fig. 5-31). Rarely, the sternum, calcaneus, talus, patella (Fig. 5-32), and a metatarsal are involved. The hand may be affected, with the phalanges and metacarpals and even less frequently the carpals showing changes (Fig. 5-33).[68] Even the sesamoids may be involved (Fig. 5-34).

Malignant change, particularly in the form of osteosarcoma, occurs in widespread Paget disease with an incidence of 1% to 6% (Figs. 5-35 and 5-36).[69,70] Osteosarcoma accounts for half of all secondary neoplasms, and fibrosarcoma or malignant fibrous histiocytoma account for an additional quarter; the remainder are chondrosarcoma, reticulosarcoma, pleomorphic neoplasms, and unspecified types.[71] An osteosarcoma developing in Paget disease is most often osteolytic, but it can have a sclerotic appearance.

(text continues on page 358)

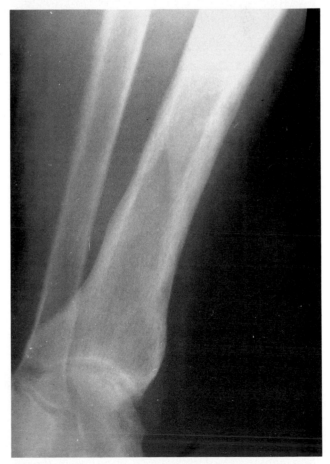

FIGURE 5-26. Paget disease, destructive stage. Radiolucency of the distal tibia with a sharply demarcated angular upper margin is seen extending to the end of the bone. This is the blade-of-grass appearance.

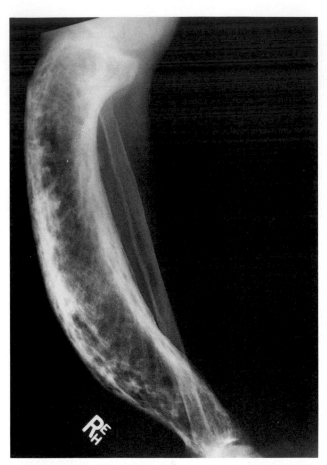

FIGURE 5-27. Paget disease. Marked widening and bowing of the tibia is noted with cortical thickening and accentuation of the trabecular pattern.

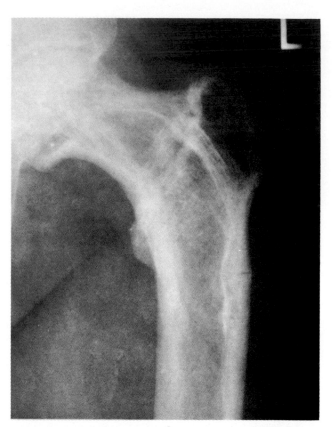

FIGURE 5-28. Paget disease of the femur. Pseudofractures are seen at the upper, outer cortex, as are cortical thickening and accentuation of the trabecular pattern.

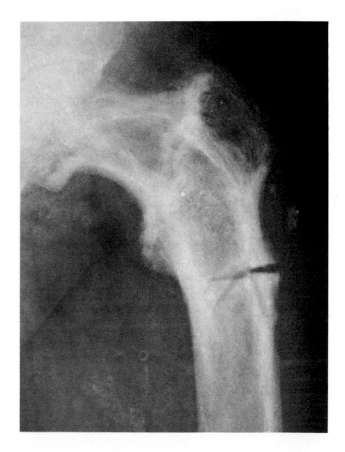

FIGURE 5-29. Paget disease of the femur in the same patient as in Figure 5-28. There is an incomplete fracture through the pseudofracture site. This progressed to a complete fracture with displacement of the fragments.

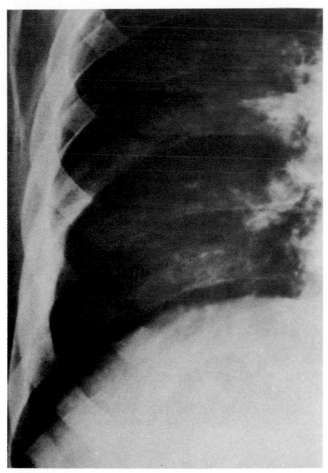

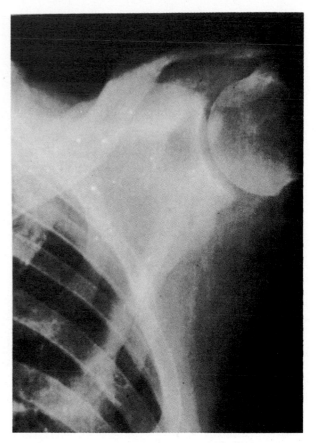

FIGURE 5-31. Paget disease of the left shoulder, sclerotic phase. Notice the uniform increase in density of the scapula and clavicle.

FIGURE 5-30. Paget disease with solitary rib involvement. The cortical thickening and widening of the bone is similar to changes seen in other bones in Paget disease. Increased density of the anterior aspect of the involved rib may also be seen.

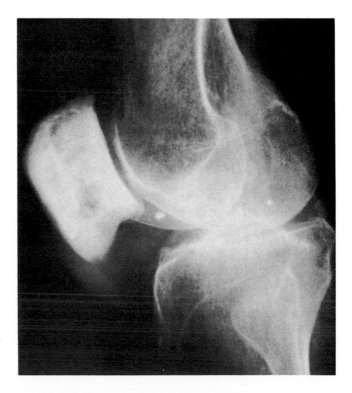

FIGURE 5-32. Paget disease of the patella. Marked sclerosis, cortical thickening, accentuation of the trabecular pattern, and enlargement of the patella are apparent.

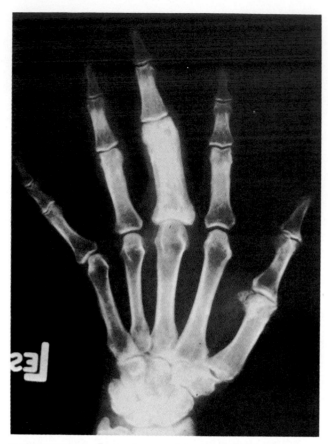

FIGURE 5-33. Paget disease of the hand. Sclerosis, accentuation of the trabecular pattern, and enlargement of the caliber of the proximal phalanx of the middle finger are seen on the radiograph.

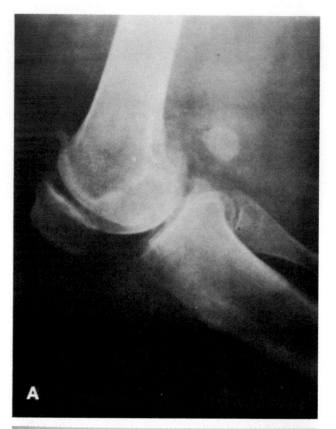

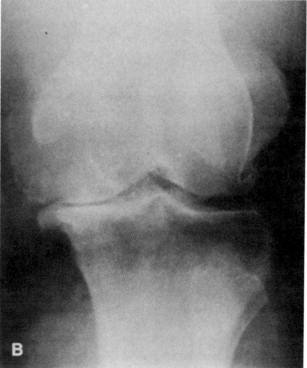

FIGURE 5-34. Paget disease of the knee. (**A**) Lateral and (**B**) anteroposterior views show thickening and enlargement of the cyamella, with a sclerotic cortex indicating involvement by Paget disease.

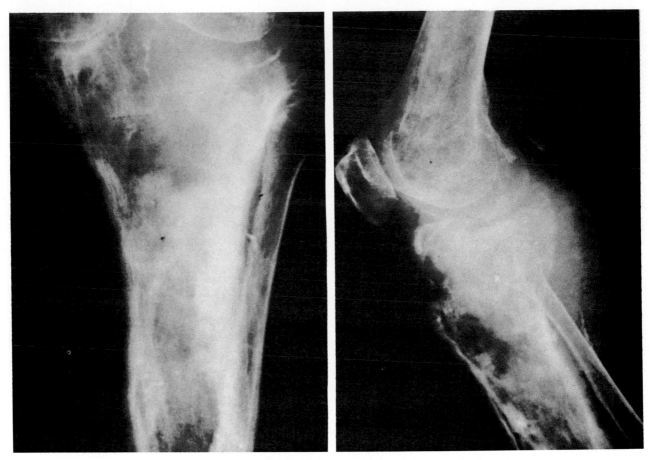

FIGURE 5-35.   Paget disease of the tibia. Malignant degeneration to osteosarcoma is shown on anteroposterior and lateral views. Cortical thickening and trabecular accentuation are characteristics of the combined phase. There is also a destructive process involving the proximal tibia, and the midlateral and lateral aspects of the articular surface have been destroyed. The ill-defined margin at the distal aspect is osteosarcoma. The destructive tumor is situated anteriorly at the proximal tibia. The margins of the tumor are poorly defined.

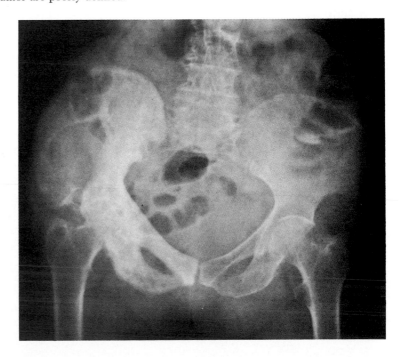

FIGURE 5-36.   Paget disease with malignant degeneration to osteosarcoma on the right side of the pelvis. Cortical thickening and trabecular accentuation are typical changes of the combined phase. A large destructive area in the right iliac bone is an osteosarcoma.

Giant cell tumors complicating Paget disease have a predilection for the skull and facial bones.[72,73] Benign giant cell tumors have shown extreme bone resorption at their periphery. Malignant giant cell tumors often follow a rapidly fatal course. Osteomyelitis superimposed on Paget disease may present a bizarre picture. Osteoblastic and osteolytic metastases may be superimposed on Paget disease.

Extramedullary hematopoiesis in Paget disease has been reported in the dorsal paraspinal region and in the pelvis.[74] It is thought that pathologic fractures lead to extrusion of marrow and resultant tumorous extramedullary hematopoiesis. Dysfunction of the spinal cord or cauda equina is a rare complication.[75]

The radionuclide bone scan is more sensitive in detecting early Paget disease than plain films. On the bone scan, a typical pattern consists of increased activity beginning at one end of a long bone and continuing a long distance or extending all the way to the opposite end.[76,77] Abnormal isotope uptake may be seen in any part of the skeleton with active disease (Fig. 5-37). Quiescent Paget disease may not show increased uptake.

CT shows cortical thickening, enlargement of bone, and increased trabecular pattern (Fig. 5-38). MR images show mixed signal intensity on spin echo pulse sequences with signal void in dense osteosclerotic regions and foci of high signal intensity on T2-weighted images (Fig. 5-39).

Destruction of Bone

Loss of bone substance may occur by resorption through the action of osteoclasts or by direct destruction of trabeculae by metastatic tumor cells.[53] Tissue culture studies with time-lapse motion pictures have shown dissolution of bone before an advancing osteoclastic front. Osteoclasts lyse mineral and organic matrix of bone.

Early bone destruction cannot be seen on conventional films. Later, it may be evident radiologically as a subtle alteration of bone texture or a barely perceptible decrease in bone density. A radionuclide bone scan is much more sensitive than conventional radiographs, except for myeloma and some anaplastic tumors. MRI is the most sensitive modality for detecting early bone lesions.

Bone destruction has several patterns of appearance, depending on the aggressiveness of the process. The simplest and the most benign are cyst-like dissolutions. These are small, well-marginated areas of radiolucency most commonly seen in the arthritides. They may contain synovial fluid, fibrous, or granulation tissue. In the next pattern, a larger focus can be seen, representing a lesion that grows slowly enough to destroy all of the bone in the involved area while progressing. This circumscribed osteolysis was called "geographic" by Lodwick.[78] Endosteal scalloping, with a large or multiple smaller endosteal excavations, also occurs. A more aggressive pattern appears as many moderate-sized radiolucencies that tend to become confluent, which has been called a moth-eaten pattern. In the most aggressive type of bone destruction, tiny infiltrative lesions tunnel through the cortex by means of the haversian system and cause myriad minute radiolucencies with no definite border between the involved regions and normal bone. This diffuse invasive pattern is called "permeative" and allows a large surrounding soft-tissue invasion without segmental destruction of bone. It is best seen on T2-weighted axial MR images.

Margination is an indication of aggressiveness. The margins may be ill defined or sharply defined, with irregular or smooth edges. A destructive area with a sharp, nonsclerotic margin is called a punched-out lesion. There may be a fine, thin wall or a thick, sclerotic wall surrounding the lesion. A sharp margin or abrupt transition indicates a more slowly growing lesion, and a wide zone of transition indicates an aggressive lesion.

If the growth rate of the lesion does not outpace the reparative ability of the bone, expansion results. Expansion indicates the rate of growth of a lesion and cannot differentiate malignant from benign tumors.

Loss of bone substance can also be caused by erosion from a malignant or benign process extrinsic to bone.

Several diseases are characterized by bone destruction: congenital scattered fibromatosis, cystic lymphangiomatosis of bone, gout, intraosseous hemangiomatosis, leukemia, lymphomas, massive osteolysis, multiple myeloma, osteolytic metastases, osteomyelitis, primary systemic amyloidosis, and reticuloses.

Osteolytic Metastases

All malignant extracranial tumors may yield osteolytic metastases to bone, which is a common site for metastases.[79] The usual route to the osseous system is hematogenous. Metastases to the spine may bypass the lungs by way of the Batson vertebral vein system. The spine is the most frequent site of skeletal metastases. Most patients who die of cancer have vertebral metastases. The neural arch is less often involved than the vertebral body. Lymphatic spread to bone is rare.

Most vertebral metastases are from carcinoma of the breast, carcinoma of the kidney, carcinoma of the

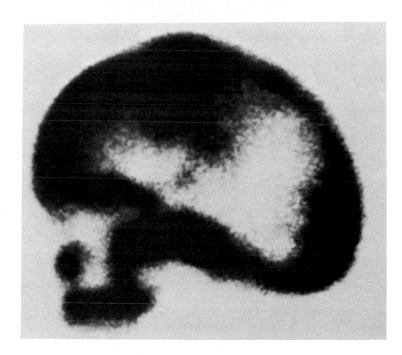

FIGURE 5-37. Technetium diphosphonate scan of the lateral view of the skull in a patient who has Paget disease. There is increased uptake in the entire calvarium.

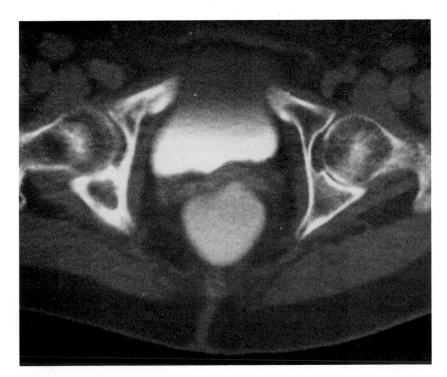

FIGURE 5-38. Paget disease. CT scan shows thickening of the cortex of the right ischium.

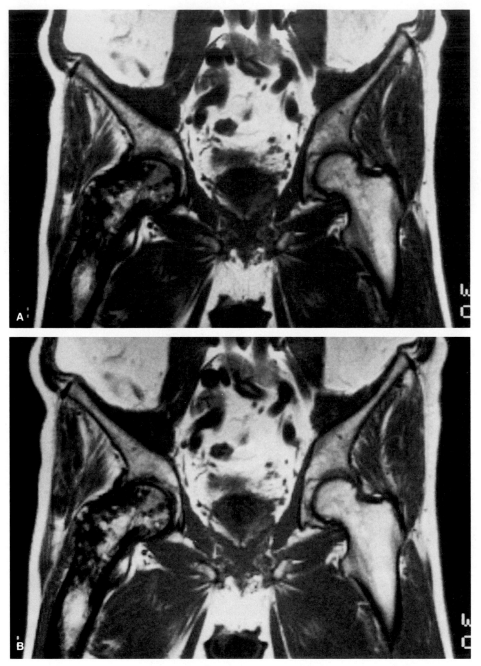

FIGURE 5-39. Paget disease in a 78-year-old man. (**A**) MR image (SE 550/10). Paget disease of the right proximal femur is seen as a deformity of the contour and multiple areas of signal void corresponding to osteosclerotic regions. (**B**) MR image (SE 2500/22). Areas of signal void, cortical thickening, and expansion of the proximal femoral metaphysis are seen. The fatty marrow signal is retained in the proximal shaft. (**C**) MR image (SE 2500/80). The areas of signal void remain. The fatty marrow signal in the diaphysis is suppressed, and there is heterogeneous high signal intensity at this site as well.

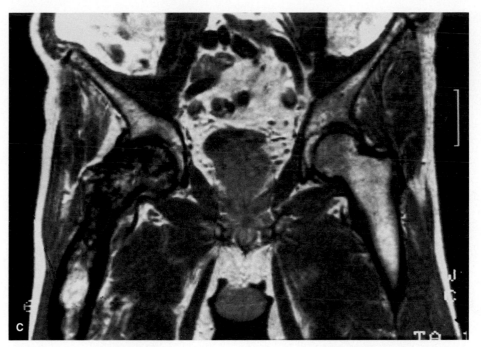

FIGURE 5-39.   *(Continued)*

lung, carcinoma of the prostate, carcinoma of the thyroid, and lymphoma. Autopsy material shows the following rates for all types of bone metastases.

Breast: 75%
Prostate: 70%
Lung: 40%
Kidney: 25%
Rectum: 13%
Pancreas: 13%
Thyroid: 12%
Stomach: 11%
Colon: 10%
Ovary: 10%

MRI allows more precise detection of osteolytic metastases, because it can image the bone marrow.

The level of spinal involvement varies with the primary tumor. Carcinoma of the breast and lung commonly metastasize to the thoracic spine, and prostatitic carcinoma usually involves the lumbosacral spine and pelvis. The breast drains chiefly by means of the azygous veins communicating with the Batson plexus in the thorax. The prostate drains by the pelvic veins, communicating with the paravertebral plexus at the lower spine. The lung primarily drains by the pulmonary veins to the left heart, and lung carcinomas metastasize throughout the skeleton. Colorectal tumors drain by means of the portal system, tending to involve the lung and liver earlier than bone.[80,81]

Most metastatic lesions are found in the red marrow of the spine (70%), pelvis (40%), femur and hip (25%), skull (15%), and the proximal humeri and ribs. Metastases distal to the knees and elbows rarely occur. Direct extension and invasion of bone also can occur. This is most commonly seen in carcinoma of the cervix extending to the pelvic rim or sacrum (Figs. 5-40 and 5-41).

The most probable cause of osteolytic metastases in a child is neuroblastoma; in an adult man, carcinoma of the lung; and in an adult woman, carcinoma of the breast. Carcinoma of the kidney, carcinoma of the thyroid, and melanoma also commonly cause osteolytic lesions that may have an expansile appearance. A small percentage of melanoma patients may present with metastases without the primary site being evident. Pain, edema, inflammatory signs, and pathologic fracture are common complaints. Paraplegia may result from spinal cord involvement.

A purely osteolytic metastasis does not cause reactive bone sclerosis. If this also occurs, the process is called mixed metastases. The lesions, single or multiple, develop from tumor embolic deposits in the spongiosa. They are seen less often in the cortex (Fig. 5-42). The latter occur secondary to a wide variety of tumors and may be more common than generally suspected.[82] These usually result from carcinoma of the lung or kidney but have also been reported in cases of melanoma, esophageal carcinoma,[83] and other primary tumors.[84] Patterns of cortical metastases range from small or large intracortical lesions to segmental destruction. The soft tissues or medullary cavity may be invaded.[85]

Metastatic tumors of bone are initially ill defined

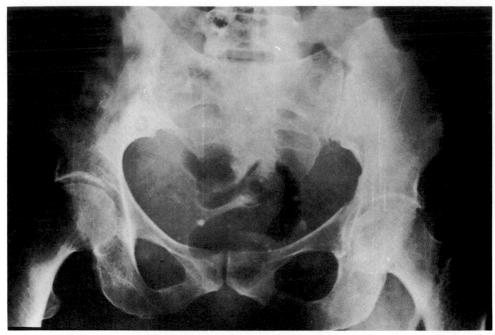

FIGURE 5-40. Destruction of the pelvis by direct extension from carcinoma of the cervix. The pelvic rim shows a destructive area.

and poorly marginated. They progress to destroy the compacta and may result in pathologic fractures. They can present as sharply circumscribed, geographic, destructive lesions (Fig. 5-43). A permeative pattern is also possible (Fig. 5-44). The soft tissues are rarely invaded. Button sequestra, or round central areas of residual bone within osteolytic lesions, are a rare finding (Fig. 5-45). The intervertebral disks and the joints are usually spared, because cartilage is resistant to tumor due to a vascular inhibiting factor. Periosteal reaction is uncommon.

The skull may show solitary or scattered foci in the calvarium or mottled destruction (Fig. 5-46). Metas-

tases to the nasal bones from breast carcinoma have been reported at a site of previous fractures.[86] The spine shows involvement of the bodies or pedicles and neural arch (Fig. 5-47), progressing to wedge or wafer-like compression of the bodies. Involvement of the pedicles helps to differentiate this process from multiple myeloma, in which the pedicles are not as often involved. This feature was described by Jacobson and is called the pedicle sign. Pathologic fractures of the odontoid process resulting from metastases from breast carcinoma have been described.[87] In the hip, nontraumatic avulsion of the lesser trochanter suggests metas-

(text continues on page 366)

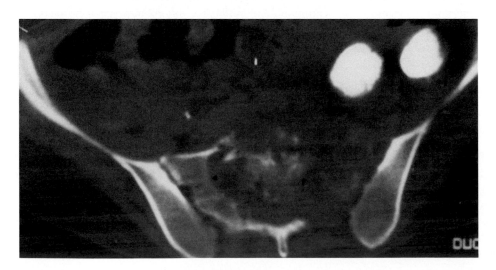

FIGURE 5-41. A 47-year-old woman with carcinoma of the cervix. The CT scan shows destruction of the sacrum, particularly at the sacral body and left sacral wing, secondary to direct invasion.

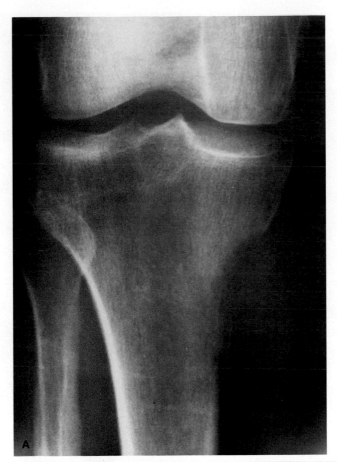

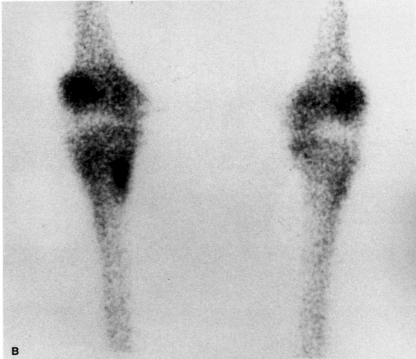

FIGURE 5-42.   A 38-year-old woman with carcinoma of the breast. (**A**) The anteroposterior view of the right knee shows a cortical or subperiosteal metastasis destroying the medial tibial metaphyseal cortex. (**B**) Radionuclide bone scan shows increased activity at the site of destruction.

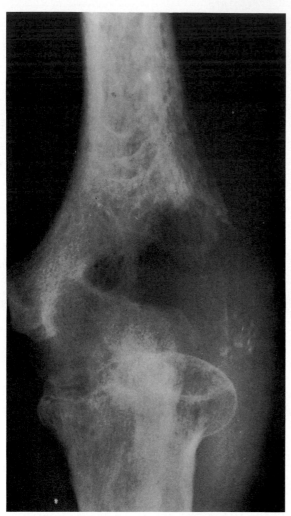

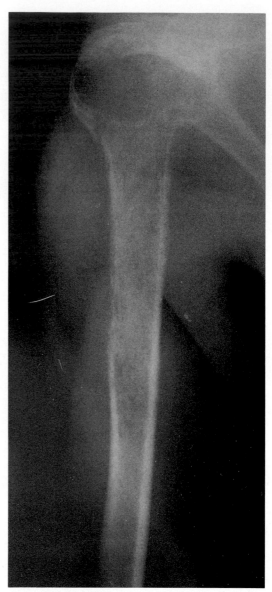

FIGURE 5-43. Metastases to the distal humerus from carcinoma of the lung. There is a geographic area of destruction of the lateral condyle of the distal humerus. Minimal or no periosteal new bone formation occurs. There is osteoporosis of the radial head, with a thin but intact cortical margin. The elbow joint cartilage serves as an effective barrier against the spread of the tumor, which does not involve the radius or ulna.

FIGURE 5-44. A 41-year-old woman with carcinoma of the breast. The anteroposterior view of the humerus shows permeative destruction of the proximal humerus extending down the shaft with a pathologic fracture at the humeral neck.

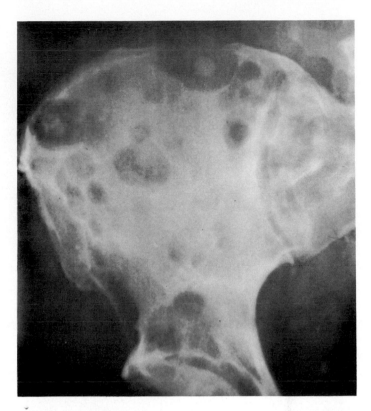

FIGURE 5-45. Osteolytic metastases to the pelvis from carcinoma of the breast. Well-circumscribed, punched-out, destructive lesions can be seen, several of which contain central round areas of residual bone called button sequestra.

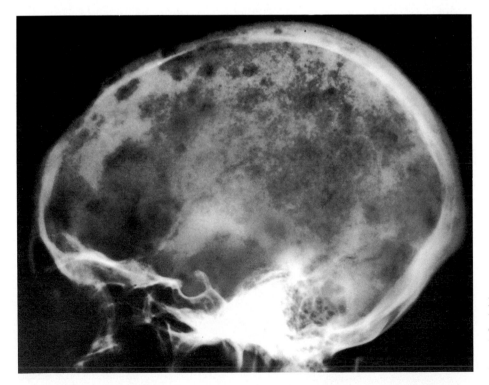

FIGURE 5-46. Osteolytic metastases to the skull from carcinoma of the breast. There has been extensive mottled destruction of the skull. Only several islands of bone density remain.

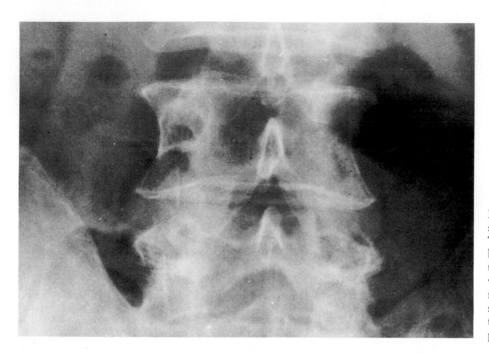

FIGURE 5-47. Metastases to the spine from carcinoma of the breast. The left pedicle of the fourth lumbar vertebra is destroyed, whereas the right pedicle is intact. The vertebral body is also intact. This is known as the one-eyed vertebra sign, with the pedicles of the vertebrae as the eyes and the spinous process as the nose.

tases.[88] In the sacrum, careful observation of sacral lines for destruction may be the only way to detect an occult lesion.[89]

In the peripheral skeleton, the feet (Fig. 5-48) are more often involved than the hands, and there may be multiple lesions. The incidence of metastases to the periphery is estimated at 2% to 4%.[90] Metastases are usually seen in the terminal phalanges (Fig. 5-49) and have been reported in tarsal bones and carpal bones (Fig. 5-50).[91] The source is usually carcinoma of the lung. The lesions are symptomatic and destructive, with no periosteal reaction. There may be destruction of the terminal phalanx with a thin layer of intact bone adjacent

to the articular surface.[92] The clinical presentation may simulate gout.[93]

Many different primary tumors from many sites have metastasized to the hand: breast, colon, kidney, lung, lymphosarcoma, oral cavity, parotid gland, prostate, and rectum.[94–97] Carcinomas of the gastrointestinal and genitourinary tracts may metastasize to the foot. This is retrograde spread of tumor emboli from the vertebral venous plexus down incompetent leg veins.[98]

Metastases from carcinomas of the kidney and thyroid may present as expansile, marginated, trabeculated lesions called blow-out metastases (Fig. 5-51).

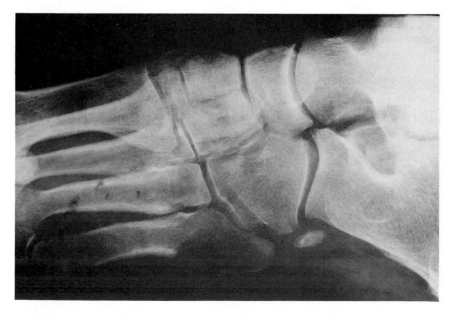

FIGURE 5-48. Metastases to the base of the fifth metatarsal from a melanoma. A destructive lesion is seen with neither new bone formation nor reactive sclerosis.

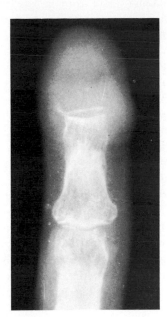

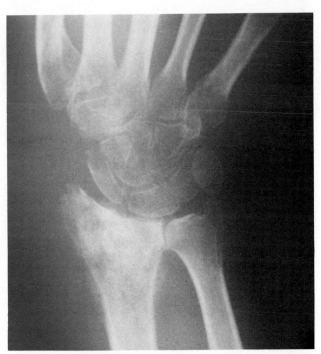

FIGURE 5-49. Metastases to the terminal phalanx from carcinoma of the lung. A soft-tissue mass and destruction of the major portion of the terminal phalanx can be seen, with a small, thin, intact sliver of bone at the base that is adjacent to the articular cartilage. (From Greenfield GB, Escamilla CH, Schorsch HA: The hand as an indicator of generalized disease. AJR Am J Roentgenol 99:736–745, 1967)

FIGURE 5-50. Metastasis to the wrist from carcinoma of the lung. Mixed sclerotic and destructive changes, and periosteal new bone formation are present in the distal radius. Destructive changes in the distal navicular bone and involvement of the lunate are seen on the radiograph. Regional osteoporosis of the carpal bones is associated with a large soft-tissue mass.

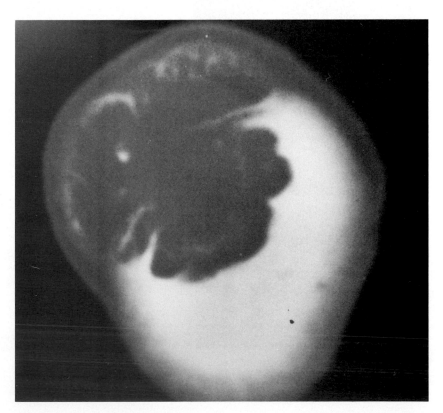

FIGURE 5-51. A 64-year-old man with carcinoma of the thyroid gland. CT scan shows a large, expansile, "blow-out" metastasis to the left parietal region.

Other tumors, including pheochromocytoma, melanoma, and carcinomas of the lung and breast[99] may rarely produce this finding. Hepatoma metastases have been reported as expansile, destructive lesions with associated soft-tissue masses, hypervascularity, and pathologic fractures.[100–102] Metastatic pheochromocytoma may show expansile or mixed sclerotic bony lesions.[103,104] Bronchogenic carcinoma has been reported to produce eccentric cortical metastases, with a focal cortical area of geographic bone destruction.[105]

The highest rate reported for bone metastases from carcinoma of the uterine cervix is 20%.[106] Bone metastases from squamous cell carcinoma of the larynx are rare. They are usually osteolytic but may be osteoblas-

tic.[107] Skeletal metastases from an intracranial angioblastic meningioma[108] and from an astrocytoma[109] have been reported. Metastases to bone from leiomyosarcoma rarely may occur with a lytic nonexpansile pattern.[110]

Metastatic neuroblastoma is similar to leukemia, producing extensive, permeative bony destruction (Fig. 5-52). A metaphyseal band of rarefaction, as in leukemia, also sometimes may be seen. The skull shows mottled destruction, splitting of the cranial sutures due to increased intracranial pressure, and perpendicular spicules of new bone formation. A vertebral body may be destroyed (Fig. 5-53).

Correlation of the radiographic appearance in breast cancer of metastatic bone lesions with the clinical course shows that an osteolytic bone pattern correlates clinically with progressive tumor growth, but a sclerotic bone pattern is associated with remission.[111]

CT shows bone destruction and an increase in marrow attenuation. MR images show marrow replace-

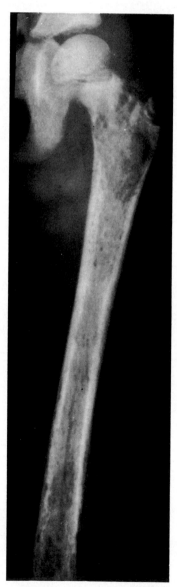

FIGURE 5-52. Metastatic neuroblastoma of the femoral shaft in a 5-year-old girl. Extensive mottled or permeative destruction of the shaft of the femur and periosteal new bone formation can be seen.

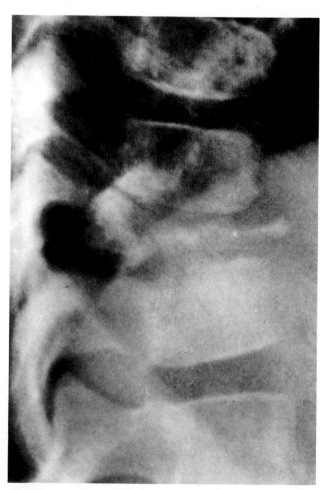

FIGURE 5-53. Metastatic neuroblastoma to the spine. There has been extensive destruction of the twelfth vertebral body, with wafer-like flattening. The intervertebral spaces are preserved, as in other metastatic processes.

ment and cortical destruction, with lower signal intensity of tumor on T1-weighted images, which increases with T2 weighting (Figs. 5-54 and 5-55).

A radionuclide bone scan usually shows increased isotope uptake in the involved areas, but a large, destructive lesion may show as a photopenic region surrounded by a margin of increased activity (Fig. 5-56). Certain anaplastic tumors, such as oat cell carcinoma metastases and myeloma, may not show increased activity.

A percutaneous bone biopsy of radionuclide scan-positive and radiographic-negative lesions is an accurate and safe procedure.[112]

Osteomyelitis

Osteomyelitis is most often caused by *Staphylococcus aureus.* Gram-negative, anaerobic,[113] and streptococcal osteomyelitis not infrequently occur. *Salmonella*

(text continues on page 372)

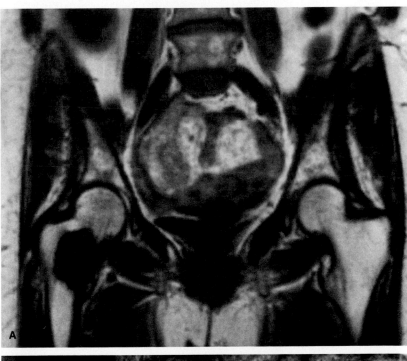

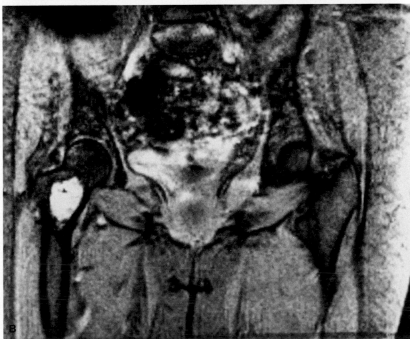

FIGURE 5-54. A 71-year-old woman with metastasis to the proximal femur from carcinoma of the breast. (**A**) The T1-weighted MR image shows a low-signal-intensity area in the intertrochanteric region of the right femur. (**B**) The T2-weighted MR image shows an increase in the signal intensity of the lesion.

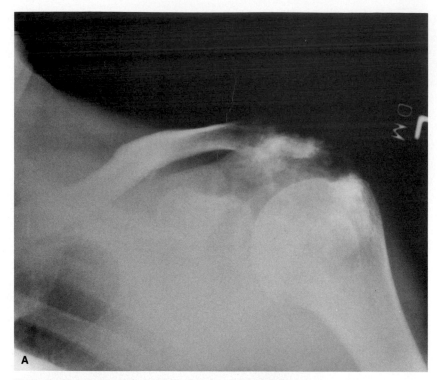

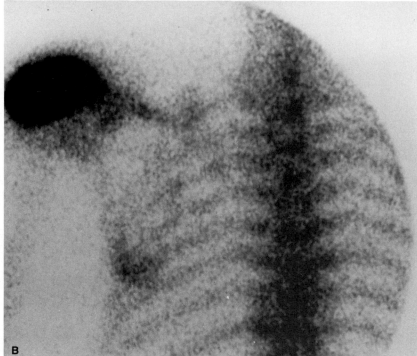

FIGURE 5-55. Metastasis from carcinoma of the prostate in a 72-year-old man. (**A**) The anteroposterior view of the shoulder shows expansion of the acromion process with a mixed sclerotic and destructive appearance. (**B**) The radionuclide bone scan shows increased activity in the left shoulder region. (**C**) The CT scan shows an expanded acromion process with a thin, permeated outer shell. (**D**) MR image (SE 600/20). The low signal intensity of the metastatic tumor at the acromion process is shown. (**E**) MR image (SE 2500/80). The tumor is heterogeneous in signal intensity, with increased signal intensity in its central portion.

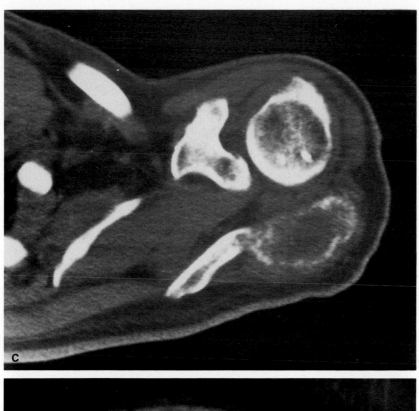

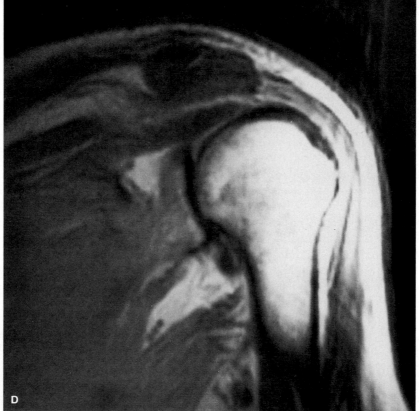

FIGURE 5-55.   *(Continued)*

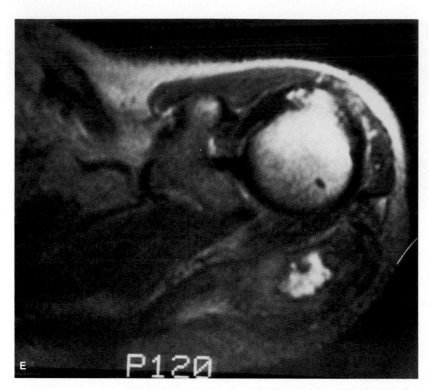

E   P120

FIGURE 5-55. *(Continued)*

osteomyelitis frequently occurs in sickle cell anemia. There is a high incidence of osteomyelitis as a complication of intravenous drug abuse,[114] and the most frequent causative organisms are *Pseudomonas aeruginosa* (Fig. 5-57),[115,116] *Klebsiella*, and *Aerobacter*. The common sites of involvement are the spine, the sacroiliac joints, symphysis pubis, bony protuberances, and sternoclavicular joints. Pneumococci, meningococci, *Brucella* organisms, fungi,[117] parasites, and viruses also occasionally invade bone. Tuberculosis and syphilis are reemerging as important diseases, and bone involvement in these conditions is well known. Tuberculosis is common in Asia and Africa. Osteomyelitis secondary to diabetes mellitus and diabetic gangrene are common. These must be differentiated from neurotrophic disease of the diabetic foot.[118] MRI can help in evaluating the diabetic foot, providing accurate information about the presence and extent of infection. Neurotrophic changes can be differentiated by low signal intensity on T1-weighted and T2-weighted images.[119] Compound fractures, penetrating wounds, and direct extension from soft-tissue infection are other mechanisms of bone involvement. Osteomyelitis of the iliac bone complicating Crohn disease has also been reported.[120]

ACUTE HEMATOGENOUS OSTEOMYELITIS. Acute hematogenous osteomyelitis usually affects infants and children, but it can affect adults, with a second age-related peak occurring in the sixth and seventh decades.[121–123] There is a period of about 10 days be-tween the onset of symptoms and bony changes becoming evident on conventional films, but deep soft-tissue swelling may be seen after about 3 days. Ultrasound has the potential to show fluid adjacent to bone.[124] MR and radionuclide bone scans show changes earlier, possibly after 24 hours. MRI is more specific and can differentiate osteomyelitis from soft-tissue infection.

The initial focus is most often found in the metaphysis (Fig. 5-58), and it may then extend to involve a portion or all of the medullary canal. In infants, persistent fetal vascular connections allow spread to the growth center, and the process may penetrate into an adjacent joint. Pus then spreads through the haversian system to the subperiosteal space. The periosteum is stripped from the cortex as the pressure from the pyogenic process increases. The cortex has two sources of blood supply: the nutrient artery and the periosteal plexus. The nutrient branches are occluded by bacterial emboli and by increased intramedullary pressure. The periosteal vessels are ruptured because of periosteal elevation. Deprived of both blood supplies, the bone dies. The periosteum forms new bone at its elevated site, enclosing the dead shaft. The dead bone is the sequestrum, and the shell of new bone is the involucrum. The latter is most pronounced in infancy. The uninvolved bone becomes osteoporotic. Defects in the involucrum, called cloaca, are sites of draining sinuses. The process may become chronic and continue indefinitely. The infection may localize to form an ab-

(text continues on page 376)

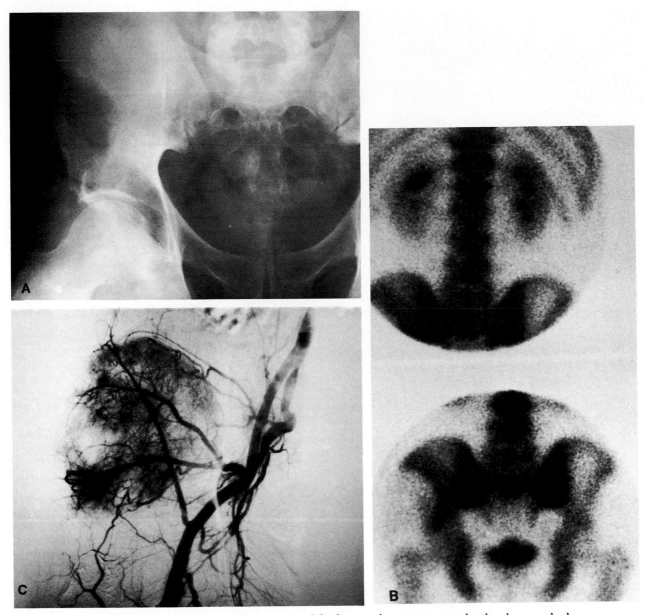

FIGURE 5-56. Squamous cell carcinoma of the lung with metastases to the iliac bone and adjacent soft tissues in a 46-year-old man. (**A**) Conventional radiograph of the pelvis shows a large destructive area at the outer aspect of the right iliac bone. (**B**) Technetium diphosphonate bone scan shows a defect in the outer aspect of the right iliac bone. (**C**) Arteriogram shows a large mass with displacement of vessels, tumor stain, and vascular irregularity and encasement.

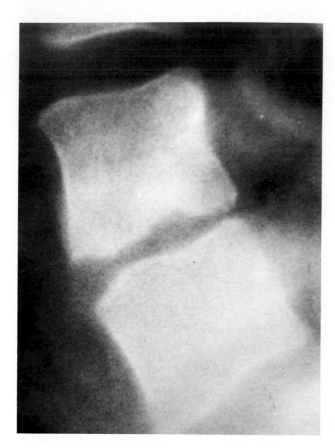

FIGURE 5-57. *Pseudomonas* osteomyelitis of the spine in a drug addict is shown on tomogram. There is narrowing of the intervertebral space with destructive changes at the contiguous vertebral margins.

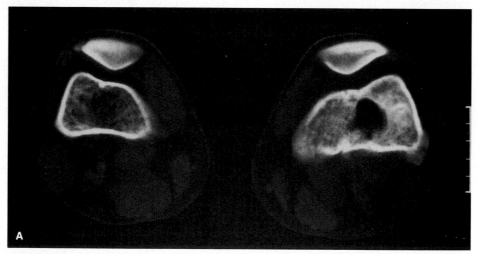

FIGURE 5-58. Osteomyelitis: Brodie abscess in the distal femoral metaphysis. (**A**) CT scan shows destruction with a sharp nonsclerotic margin. (**B**) MR image (SE 600/20). A large amount of marrow edema extends into the epiphysis and the diaphysis. The margin is outlined by relatively high signal intensity. (**C**) MR image (SE 2700/80). The abscess shows heterogeneous high signal intensity.

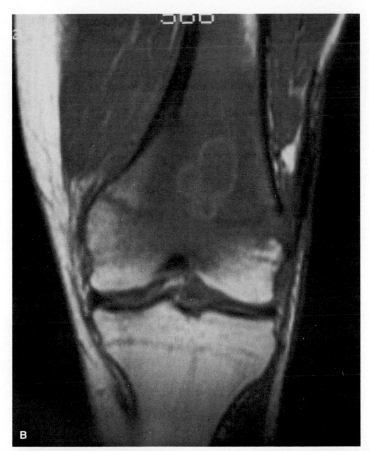

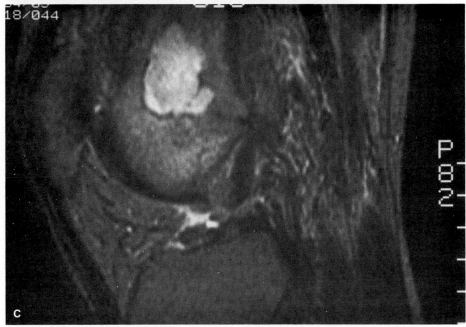

FIGURE 5-58.   *(Continued)*

scess, or a low-grade sclerosing osteitis may occur without suppuration.

In infants, osteomyelitis is usually caused by *Streptococcus*. The soft tissues and joints are involved more commonly than in older children. There is less tendency to form sequestra, and healing is more rapid.

There are no osseous changes seen on conventional films in the initial stages of the disease. The first sign is localized, deep soft-tissue swelling with displacement of the radiolucent plane away from the bone, followed by obliteration of intramuscular lucent planes. The shaft may be involved at an early stage with intracortical fissuring.[125] In infants or children, the earliest sign in bone is a metaphyseal area of destruction. Destructive changes may also be present in the epiphysis (Fig. 5-59) or shaft. Periosteal elevation with new bone formation follows. A subperiosteal abscess occasionally occurs. The periosteum usually shows a simple response, but rarely, it develops a laminated (Fig. 5-60) or spiculated appearance (Fig. 5-61). The cortex be-

comes sequestered, and multiple defects are seen. Local osteoporosis occurs, and as the sequestrum becomes separated by granulation tissue, it stands out as densely white. This relative radiodensity identifies a bone fragment as a sequestrum. Sequestra vary in size from the entire involucrum to small fragments extruded through a draining sinus (Fig. 5-62). Entities other than osteomyelitis may also be associated with sequestra (e.g., Gaucher disease, fibrosarcoma). Destruction of the epiphysis[126] and metaphysis leads to growth disturbances or bizarre residual deformities with malalignment.

Rarely, the initial focus of disease may be in the epiphysis. CT scans are valuable in these cases for differentiating an abscess from a chondroblastoma or osteoid osteoma. A sequestrum, a serpiginous tract, cor-

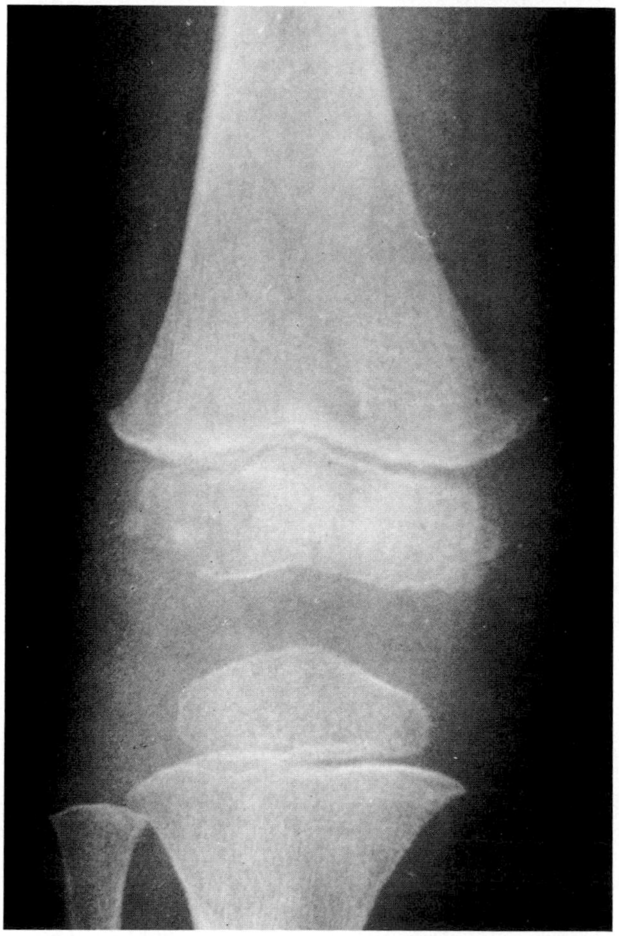

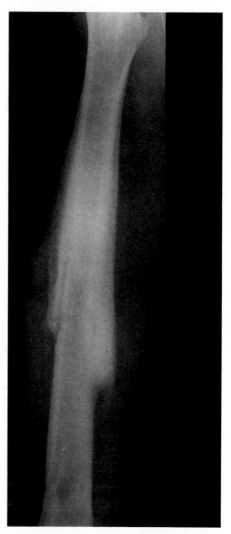

FIGURE 5-59. Pyogenic epiphysitis. A destructive area is seen at the lateral aspect of the distal femoral epiphysis. (Courtesy of Dr. Harvey White, Children's Memorial Hospital, Chicago, IL.)

FIGURE 5-60. Chronic osteomyelitis in a 13-year-old boy. A lateral view of the femur shows expansion of bone, reactive sclerosis, sequestration, and laminated periosteal new bone formation.

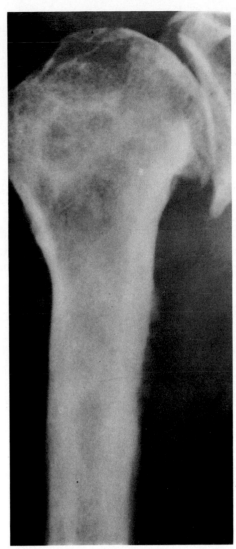

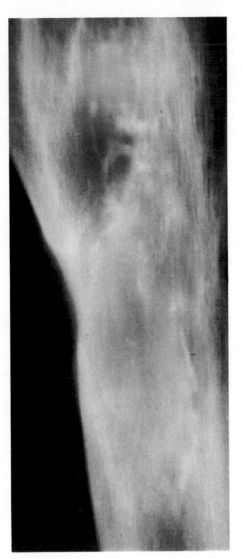

FIGURE 5-61. Osteomyelitis of the humerus. There is a spiculated type of periosteal elevation along the upper medial shaft. The spiculations are short and thick, unlike the fine, long spiculations commonly seen in osteosarcoma.

FIGURE 5-62. Tomogram showing osteomyelitis. Multiple, small, chalky white sequestra can be seen. There is a loss of cortex, indicating a cloaca through which pus and sequestra may extrude.

tical destruction, and adjacent soft-tissue swelling may be seen.[127]

In children, osteomyelitis is most common in the long bones femur, tibia, and humerus but has also been reported at unusual sites: in the bones of the thorax including the clavicle, in the spine, and in the foot. Nontubular bones may also be involved, particularly if multiple sites are affected. The most common flat bone to be involved is the pelvis, with a predilection for the sacroiliac area. This site of involvement is followed in frequency by the clavicle and the calcaneus.[128]

Osteomyelitis in adults has been reported at various sites, including the cranium. The infection may be localized to the metaphysis or diaphysis, and there is a greater tendency toward chronicity.

The flat bones have anatomic subdivisions analogous to long bones. Before skeletal maturation, areas adjacent to joints and apophyses have metaphyseal-type vascular anatomy.[129] These metaphyseal equivalents, such as the area adjacent to the sacroiliac joint or triradiate cartilage, account for a large percentage of hematogenous osteomyelitis in nontubular bones.

CT is particularly useful in assessing osteomyelitis of the spine.[130] The major findings are paravertebral soft-tissue swelling, abscess formation, bone erosions, disk involvement, and extension into the spinal canal. Needle biopsy may be done under CT control. The involved vertebral bodies and adjacent soft tissues may show lower Hounsfield units compared with normal cancellous bone and soft tissues.[131,132] Narrowing of the intervertebral disk with irregular destruction of the adjacent vertebral body end-plates develops.[133] Hypodensity of the intervertebral disk is a specific change in vertebral osteomyelitis.[134] CT can demonstrate gas in the medullary cavity of a bone involved with pyogenic osteomyelitis,[135] but an increase in marrow attenuation due to the inflammation is more typical. CT may also show fat-fluid levels in osteomyelitis. This indicates the presence of pus, particularly when associated with bone erosion.[136] CT is valuable in the detection of sequestra, and MRI helps in defining the extent of the process and in differentiating osteomyelitis from cellulitis.[137]

MRI is the best modality to demonstrate changes in bone marrow and soft tissue.[138,139] It may also show cortical destruction. Both T1-weighted and T2-weighted images are needed to evaluate osteomyelitis.

T2-weighted STIR images identify bright foci of active infection (Fig. 5-63).[140] A reduction in the normally bright signal of bone marrow on T1-weighted images and increased signal intensity on T2-weighted images indicate involvement (Fig. 5-64). A focal or a serpiginous area in the marrow cavity may be seen (Fig. 5-65). In sickle cell anemia, bone marrow ischemia may hasten conversion of red to yellow marrow. This can be seen as an irregular area of high signal intensity against a background of lower-signal-intensity red marrow on T1-weighted images. In the event of *Salmonella* osteomyelitis, high signal intensity on T2-weighted images in the medullary cavity and surrounding tissues identifies the inflammatory process (Fig. 5-66).

MRI has the ability to differentiate osteomyelitis from soft-tissue infection adjacent to bone and may be used to evaluate patients with positive bone scans and

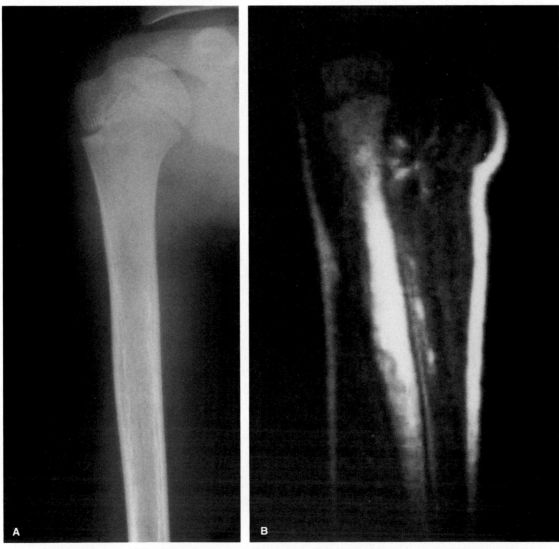

FIGURE 5-63. Sickle cell thalassemia with osteomyelitis of the humeral shaft. (**A**) The anteroposterior view of the humerus shows splitting of the cortex and minimal permeative changes. (**B**) The T2-weighted MR image shows high signal intensity in the medullary cavity and, to a lesser extent, in the surrounding soft tissue.

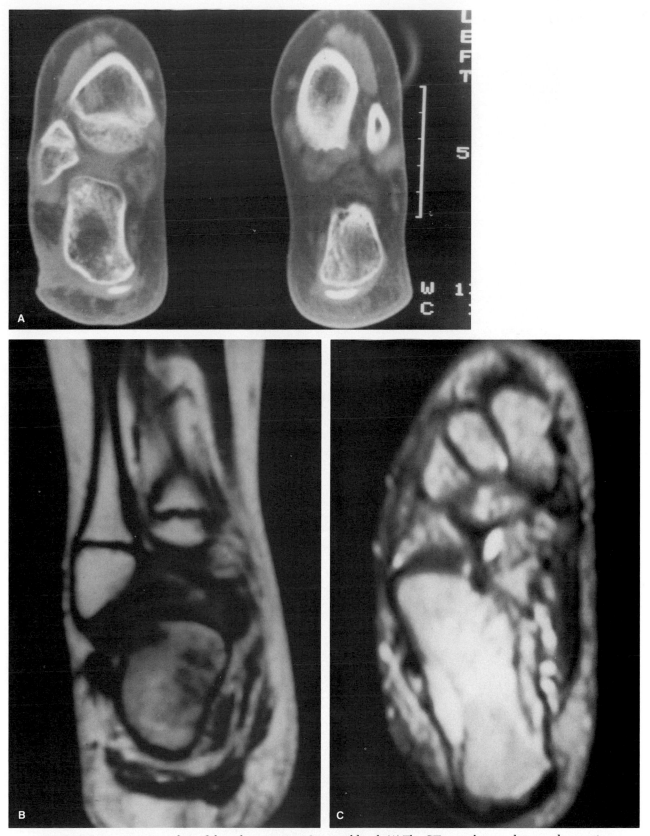

FIGURE 5-64. Osteomyelitis of the calcaneus in an 8-year-old girl. (**A**) The CT scan shows a discreet destructive area in the calcaneus with a surrounding soft-tissue reaction. The cortex is intact. Small sequestra are seen. (**B**) MR image (SE 810/15). Heterogeneous signal intensity depicts the calcaneus. (**C**) MR image (SE 2400/80). High signal intensity in the midcalcaneus corresponds to that seen on CT. The fatty marrow signal has been suppressed. High signal intensity is also seen in the surrounding soft tissues. (**D**) MR STIR image. The intense high signal intensity of the calcaneus is shown. (**E**) The lateral view of the calcaneus shows only minimal disruption of the trabecular pattern. *continued*

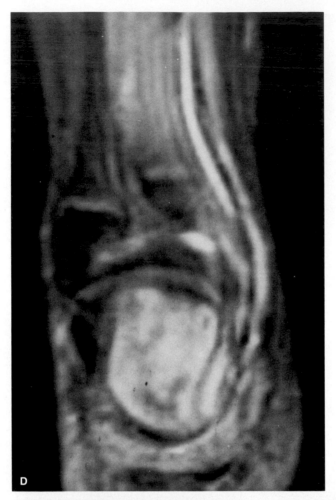

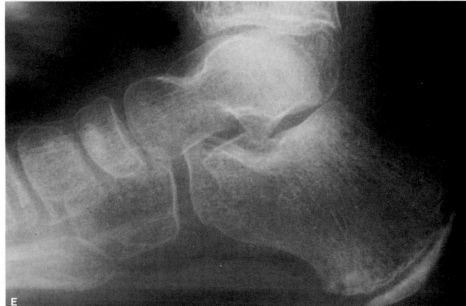

FIGURE 5-64. *(Continued)*

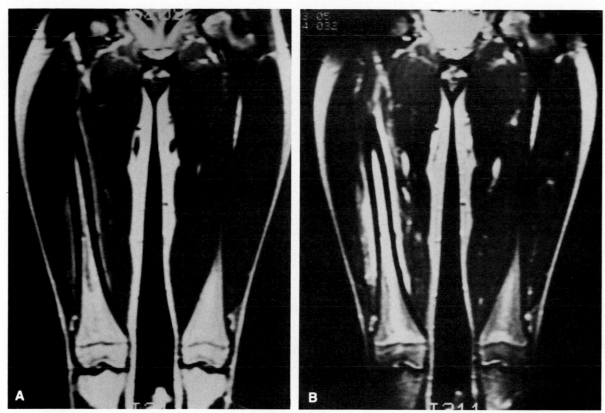

FIGURE 5-65. Osteomyelitis of the right femoral shaft. (**A**) T1-weighted MR image. A low-signal-intensity serpiginous area is seen in the femoral shaft, contrasted against high-signal-intensity marrow fat. (**B**) T2-weighted MR image. The low-signal-intensity area seen on the T1-weighted MR image shows high signal intensity. In addition, the high signal intensity of surrounding musculature indicates an inflammatory or edematous change. The distal metaphysis is involved. (Courtesy of Dr. Harold Posniak, Loyola University, Maywood, IL.)

improve the specificity of diagnosis.[141] Soft-tissue infection secondary to osteomyelitis can also be demonstrated. The MR appearance of vertebral osteomyelitis is characteristic,[142] with centering on the intervertebral space, showing bone destruction and involving the adjacent soft tissues. Abnormalities are seen on MR images earlier than on CT or radionuclide scans.[139–143]

Radioscintigraphy is an important modality,[144] because the bone scan may become positive 24 hours after the onset of osteomyelitis, but conventional x-ray film changes may not be apparent until 10 to 14 days later. The bone scan can help in early detection, differentiation of osteomyelitis from cellulitis, and identification of renewed activity in cases of chronic osteomyelitis.

The standard method employs ^{99m}Tc phosphate. Increased isotope uptake occurs in the involved area. It is reliable at all skeletal sites and in all age groups.[145]

The uptake of ^{99m}Tc depends on an intact blood supply. The isotope does not accumulate in foci of osteomyelitis around which thrombosis of arteries and capillaries has occurred. When this happens, the result

is a relatively normal or a cold, photon-deficient area on the radionuclide scan.[146] Eventually, an increased region of activity replaces the cold area as bone repair occurs and as the occlusion is replaced by a hyperemic response. The spectrum of the radionuclide uptake in osteomyelitis ranges from areas that are photon-deficient to those that have increased activity. Between these two extremes lies the normal amount of uptake. If the patient is imaged during the transient rise to the normal uptake range, a false-negative scan results. A subperiosteal abscess also shows a central, photopenic lesion. CT and radioscintigraphy are complementary in the surgical planning for this entity.[147]

If the results of the ^{99m}Tc bone scan are normal in patients with suspected osteomyelitis, a ^{67}Ga scan may be helpful. Gallium concentrates at a site of inflammation. Quantitative bone gallium scintigraphy has been reported as more specific for the diagnosis of osteomyelitis. Ratios of gallium and bone activity are used.[148] Another method uses leukocytes labeled with indium 111. This technique can detect acute osteomyelitis earlier than ^{99m}Tc bone scans,[149] and it has a high

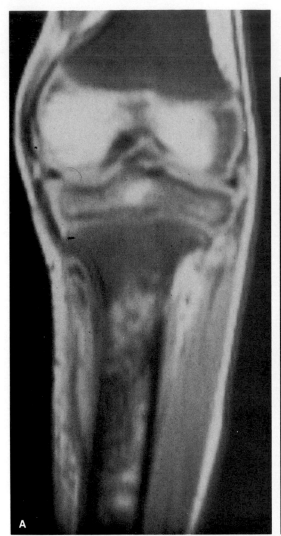

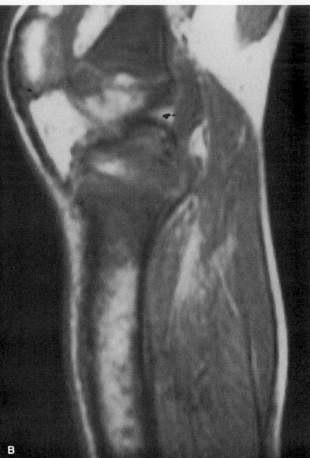

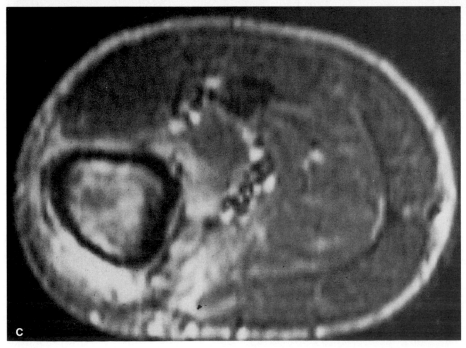

FIGURE 5-66. A 7-year-old boy with sickle cell anemia developed osteomyelitis in the proximal tibia. (**A,B**) The coronal and sagittal MR (SE 600/20) images show a normal fatty marrow signal in the distal femoral epiphysis and red marrow signal in the remainder of the bone. High signal intensity in the tibial shaft is caused by early conversion of red marrow to yellow marrow secondary to ischemia. The subperiosteal abscess and periosteal new bone formation are seen. (**C**) The axial MR (SE 2700/ 80) section shows a heterogeneous high signal intensity within the medullary cavity. The high signal intensity corresponds to the osteomyelitis, and the low signal intensity corresponds to the fatty marrow. The high signal intensity surrounding the bone reflects inflammatory changes.

degree of sensitivity.[150] In the presence of cellulitis, increased uptake of labeled leukocytes in adjacent bone strongly suggests osteomyelitis.[151]

The angiographic features of acute osteomyelitis are, in the early stages, hyperemia with a slight to moderate increase in blood flow. Hyperemia is seen only in the soft tissues in the absence of cortical destruction, but later, it is seen inside the bone. There is dilatation of arteries, veins, and capillaries, with early visualization of veins and uniform stain. With progression of the disease and development of necrosis, the angiographic appearance changes to areas of necrosis with interruption of smaller vessels. The peripheral portion of the lesion shows hyperemia.[9]

The spine may also be involved by tuberculosis, fungal infections, and brucellosis.[152,153] The midthoracic spine is more likely to be involved by tuberculosis, as is the lumbar spine by brucellosis. Brucellosis has also been reported to involve the distal femur.[154] Diabetes mellitus, rheumatoid arthritis, advanced age, and a cephalad level of involvement predispose patients to paralysis in cases of spinal infections.[155] Pyogenic osteomyelitis of the thoracic and lumbar spine is common, but only 12% of reported cases involve the cervical spine. It rarely affects the uppermost two cervical vertebrae, but when it does, it can progress to abscess formation, which may compress the spinal cord.[156] Spinal osteomyelitis may rarely be associated with intraosseous or intradiskal gas.[157]

Bacillary angiomatosis is an infectious disease occurring in patients who are positive for the human immunodeficiency virus (HIV). Cutaneous and multiple osteolytic lesions may be seen. CT, MR, and radionuclide bone scans help the diagnosis, because the skin lesions resemble Kaposi sarcoma. The lesions improve on antibiotic therapy.[158]

CHRONIC OSTEOMYELITIS. A bone involved with chronic osteomyelitis appears thickened, irregular, sclerotic, containing radiolucent areas, with periosteal new bone and a sequestered cortex (Fig. 5-67). Garré osteitis is a rare chronic sclerosing low-grade infection, resulting in sclerosis without destruction or sequestration (Fig. 5-68). In the spine, osteomyelitis causes vertebral destruction and collapse with an adjacent soft-tissue abscess. The intervertebral space is usually involved (Fig. 5-69), whereas it is usually spared in a neoplasm. Expansion of a vertebral body may occur (Fig. 5-70). In the atlantoaxial region, disappearance of the odontoid process has been reported.[158a]

The process may localize to form an abscess,[159] usually occurring at the end of a bone, but possibly in the shaft. This characteristically appears as a radiolucent area surrounded by a variable amount of sclerosis

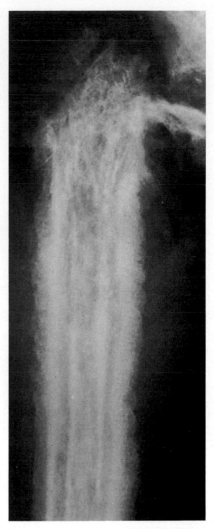

FIGURE 5-67. Chronic osteomyelitis of the femur. There is marked thickening of the femoral shaft with bone sclerosis and lace-like periosteal new bone formation. The sequestered cortex is central, giving a bone-within-a-bone appearance. Fracture of the femoral neck with destructive changes in the femoral head can also be seen.

and a central sequestrum (Fig. 5-71). Occasionally, an abscess that has never had an acute stage occurs. This is a subacute or Brodie abscess (Fig. 5-72).[160] It is characterized by the absence of pus and the presence of granulation tissue. It is surrounded by a thick, fibrous capsule and may have a sclerotic margin.

In 0.5% of patients with a history of long-standing chronic draining sinuses, a destructive area may rapidly appear at that site (Fig. 5-73), representing a squamous cell carcinoma.[161] This squamous cell carcinoma can metastasize.[162] Fibrosarcoma has also been reported.[163,164]

Chronic multifocal osteomyelitis, which occurs in children and young adults, must be differentiated from metastases and Ewing tumor.[165–168] Multiple scattered

(text continues on page 386)

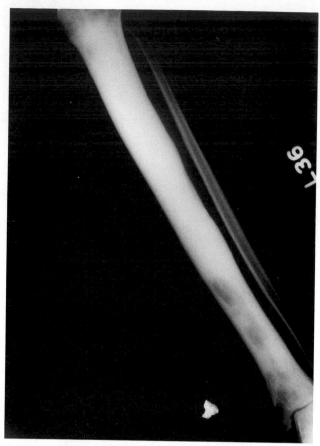

FIGURE 5-68. Garré osteomyelitis, showing a dense sclerosis of the tibia.

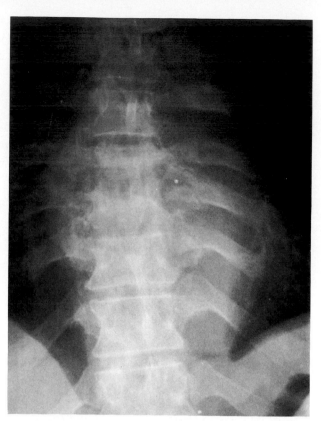

FIGURE 5-69. Osteomyelitis of the eighth and ninth thoracic vertebrae. The intervertebral space is destroyed, and the bodies are partially collapsed. A large, associated paraspinal mass is seen.

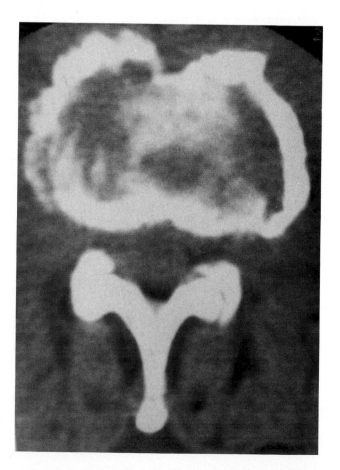

FIGURE 5-70. Chronic osteomyelitis of the spine. There is expansion of the vertebral body with a thickened, irregular margin of cortex. Destructive changes are seen centrally on CT scan.

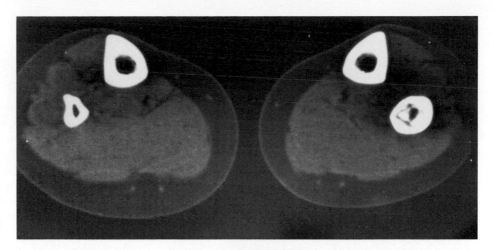

FIGURE 5-71. A 41-year-old woman with chronic osteomyelitis of the fibula. CT scan shows expansion and sequestration.

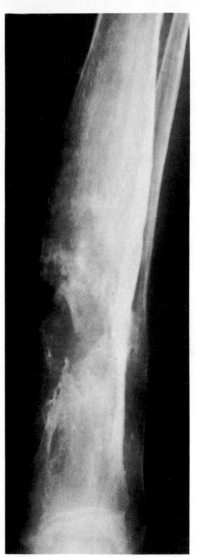

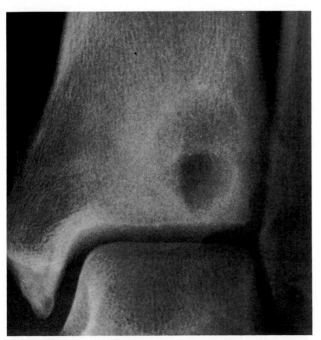

FIGURE 5-72. A Brodie abscess in the distal tibia is seen as a radiolucent lesion with slight surrounding reactive sclerosis.

FIGURE 5-73. Chronic osteomyelitis of the leg with the development of a large destructive area at the drainage site. There is marked widening of the shaft of the tibia and, to a lesser extent, of the fibula. An irregular area of bone destruction at the distal medial aspect of the tibia is associated with soft-tissue irregularity. There is localized cortical destruction. This appearance is due to the development of a squamous cell carcinoma at a chronic draining site.

permeative destructive areas associated with periosteal new bone formation are present in the skeleton (Fig. 5-74). Radionuclide bone scan shows multiple areas of increased activity, which may be symmetrically or asymmetrically distributed. Histology shows lymphocytes and plasma cells in otherwise normal tissue. The condition improves on antibiotic therapy.

CT can demonstrate more sequestra than conventional methods can.[169] An important advantage of CT is its ability to demonstrate involvement of the marrow cavity and abscesses in the soft tissues.[170]

Radionuclide scanning for determining activity and for monitoring response to treatment includes the use of ^{99m}Tc, ^{67}Ga, and ^{111}In techniques.[171–175]

MRI has advantages over other modalities in evaluating chronic, complicated osteomyelitis. Intraosseous and extraosseous sites display increased signal intensities on T2-weighted images. Sinus tracts and soft-tissue abscesses can be seen, allowing determination of disease activity.[176,177]

TUBERCULOUS OSTEOMYELITIS. Tuberculous (TB) osteomyelitis may occur with or without pulmonary tuberculosis. It is most common in patients younger than 30 years of age.[178]

The imaging findings resemble those of pyogenic osteomyelitis, except that osteoporosis is seen earlier and is more pronounced, sclerosis and periosteal reaction are less pronounced, and sequestration is less common. It has a predilection for the same sites that are involved by pyogenic infection.

The long bones may show a slowly enlarging, destructive lesion in any part of the bone (Figs. 5-75 and 5-76). TB granulomas of bone may mimic neoplasms. In the phalanges, an expansile lesion can occasionally be seen involving the entire bone, resulting in an ovoid configuration. This is called tuberculous spina ventosa (Fig. 5-77), which is similar to the dactylitis of syphilis. Spina ventosa most often occurs in children but has been reported in adults.[179] It can affect the metacarpals, metatarsals, ulnae, and humeri. Osteopenia, periosteal reaction, destruction, and pathologic fracture

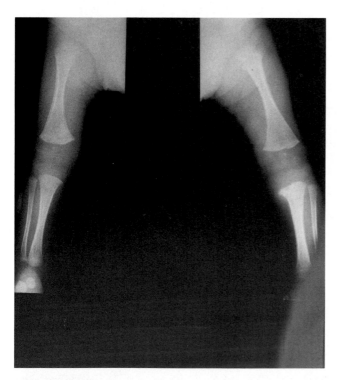

FIGURE 5-74. A 3-month-old infant with chronic multifocal osteomyelitis. The anteroposterior view of the lower extremities shows widespread periosteal new bone formation and destructive changes at the left proximal tibial metaphysis.

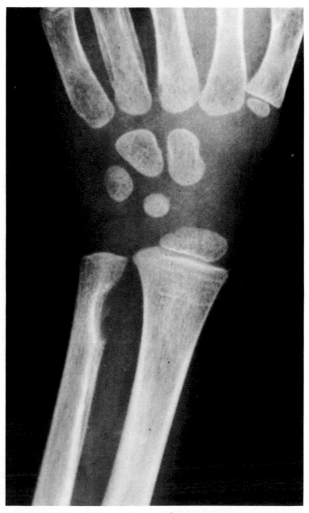

FIGURE 5-75. Tuberculosis. A destructive metaphyseal lesion is seen at the distal ulna. There is regional osteoporosis. Notice the slight degree of periosteal new bone formation proximal to the lesion and periosteal new bone formation in the fourth metacarpal.

can be seen in adults. Diffuse sclerosis with scattered areas of destruction and marked periostitis and honeycombing of bone with or without a pathologic fracture are other appearances. Chronic draining sinuses are common.

In the flat bones, punched-out cyst-like lesions with little or no reactive sclerosis are typical (Fig. 5-78). Disseminated bone TB with single or multiple cyst-like or aggressive osteolytic scattered lesions is a rare form that may be seen in children and adults. Hypercalcemia may be associated with the disease.[180] Cystic tuberculosis has been reported in the femur.[181] A medullary, ring-like calcification may be seen on CT scans.

There may be secondary infection of chronic draining sinuses, causing a mixed infection indistinguishable from pure pyogenic osteomyelitis.

One of the most common sites of involvement is the spine, leading to destruction of vertebral bodies and intervertebral spaces, and causing collapse, gibbus formation, atlantoaxial subluxation,[182] and reactive sclerosis. A paraspinal soft-tissue mass or psoas abscess, which may be densely calcified or noncalcified, is often

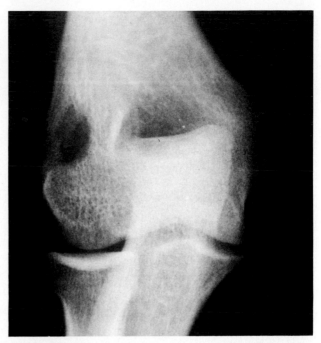

FIGURE 5-76. Tuberculosis. There is a destructive area with poorly defined margins in the lateral epicondyle of the distal humerus.

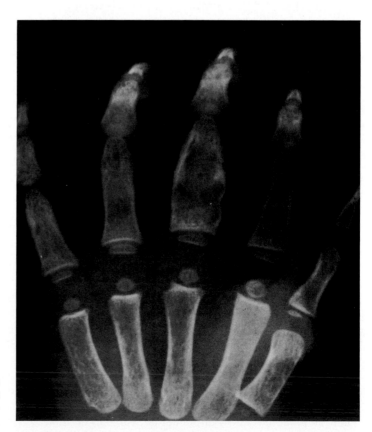

FIGURE 5-77. Tuberculosis of the fingers. Expansion of the third proximal phalanx with a thin cortex and lack of sclerotic reaction is called the spina ventosa tuberculosa.

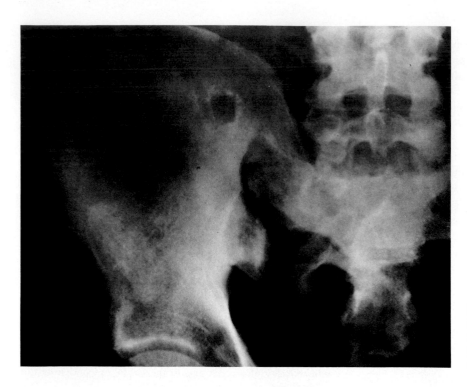

FIGURE 5-78. Tuberculosis of the flat bones. There is a destructive process of the right sacroiliac joint with no reactive sclerosis and a small, punched-out lesion in the ilium.

present. This is Pott disease (Fig. 5-79). Rarely, a TB psoas abscess can occur without vertebral lesions seen on plain films.[183] CT and MRI are useful in this case.[184] Less commonly, the anterior vertebral bodies may show destruction associated with an anterior cold abscess but without vertebral collapse (Fig. 5-80). This pattern may occur in the cervical region. Involvement of the pedicles occurs in about 2% of spinal cases.[185] The pedicles may be destroyed unilaterally or bilaterally, at one or multiple levels. On healing, the pedicles may be restored. TB of the ribs,[186] greater trochanter,[187] calcaneus,[188] patella,[189] and sphenoid bone[190] has also been reported. TB of the ribs usually presents with an extrapleural mass.[191]

Miliary TB may involve the skeleton. Multiple foci of increased activity on the ^{99m}Tc scan may mimic metastases. Some lesions may become photopenic after antituberculous therapy.[192]

Leukemia

Detectable skeletal involvement on plain films in leukemia occurs in 50% to 70% of cases of childhood leukemia and in as many as 10% of adult cases. MR images show earlier bone marrow leukemic changes and bone marrow infarction because of its unique ability to show marrow changes before bone destruction.[193,194] Primary infiltrating tumors of the marrow such as leukemia and lymphoma appear darker than normal marrow on T1-weighted images and show higher signal intensity on T2-weighted or T2-like images. The pattern, however, varies, and at times these changes may be difficult to demonstrate. CT has not proved to be useful in the early detection of diffuse and symmetric bone marrow disease.[195-197]

The age range of childhood leukemia includes congenital leukemia.[198-201] This may present with metaphyseal radiolucent bands, which are nonspecific findings in infancy and may also be seen with prematurity, malnutrition, and scurvy. Occasionally, sclerotic bands occur adjacent to the radiolucent bands. There may be widening of the medullary cavity with thinning of the cortex. Associated bilateral agenesis of the radii may rarely occur.

The peak age of incidence of childhood leukemia is between 2 and 5 years, with a smaller number of cases during the first year of life. Boys are affected more often than girls. The cell type is most commonly lymphocytic. There may be no circulating lymphocytes, a condition that is called aleukemic leukemia.

Bony changes include osteolysis, osteosclerosis, periosteal new bone formation, and transverse metaphyseal radiolucent bands. The bands usually constitute the earliest sign, and they may be deep and wide (Figs. 5-81 and 5-82). Horizontal radiolucent bands in the vertebral bodies adjacent to the end-plates may rarely be seen. A residual dense metaphysis has been reported in patients after chemotherapy.[202] Generalized osteopenia may also be present. The wide band may progress to an osteolytic lesion (Fig. 5-83). A moth-eaten, destructive pattern may develop at the metaphysis

(text continues on page 392)

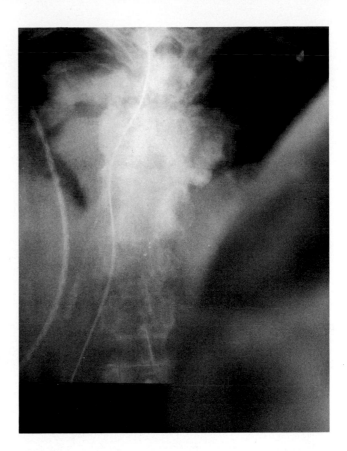

FIGURE 5-79. Pott disease. A calcified tuberculous abscess involves the major portion of the thoracic spine with marked kyphosis. Calcification tracks down the right psoas margin.

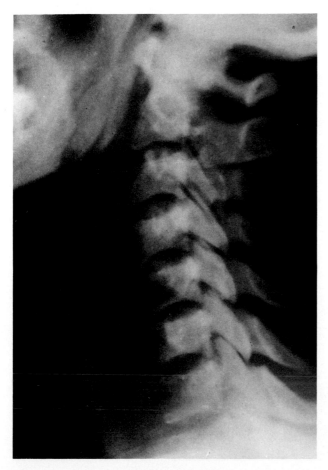

FIGURE 5-80. Tuberculosis of the cervical spine, with destruction of the anterior aspects of the vertebral bodies. There is no vertebral collapse, and the intervertebral spaces are preserved. A retrolaryngeal and retrotracheal abscess is seen on the radiograph. This represents the rare form of spinal tuberculosis with anterior involvement of the vertebral bodies.

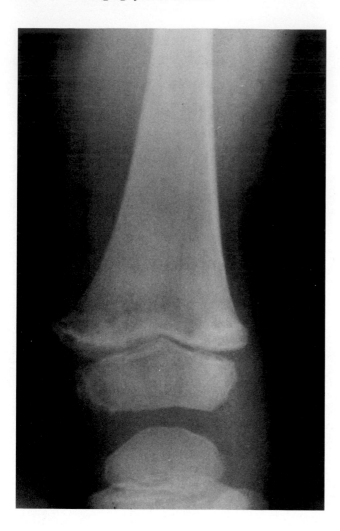

FIGURE 5-81. Leukemia. The anteroposterior view of the distal femur shows a submetaphyseal radiolucent band. The cortex is not destroyed.

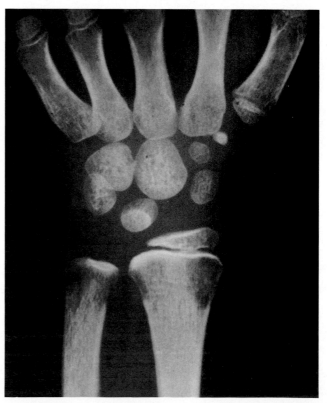

FIGURE 5-82. Leukemia of the wrist. A deep, wide metaphyseal band is seen. The cortex and the zone of provisional calcification remain intact.

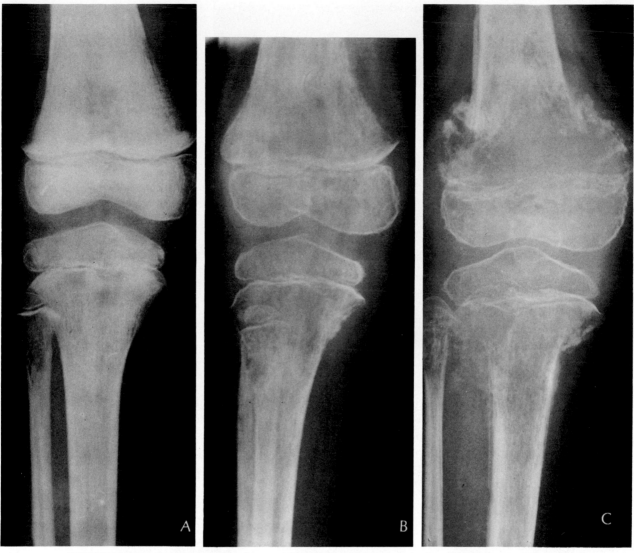

FIGURE 5-83.   Leukemia of the knees. (**A**) Wide bands of submetaphyseal radiolucency in the proximal tibial and fibular metaphyses. There is a rounded, ill-defined radiolucent lesion at the central metaphyseal aspect of the distal femur. Relative sclerosis at the distal femoral metaphyses can also be seen. (**B**) Three months after **A**, there is marked progression of destructive changes and loss of bone density. Soft-tissue atrophy can also be seen. The cortex is still intact in the major portion of the involved areas. (**C**) Six weeks after **B**, the lesions have progressed to severe destruction and periosteal new bone formation has taken place. Notice the moth-eaten appearance in the distal femur proximal to the major destructive lesion and the permeative destructive pattern in the proximal tibial shaft.

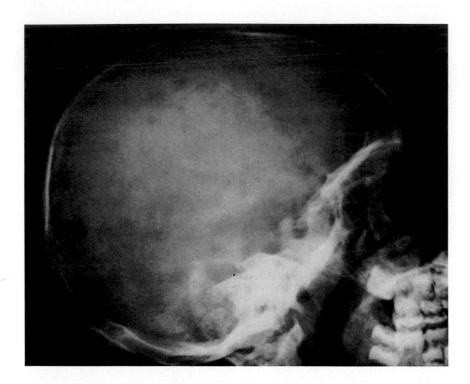

FIGURE 5-84. Leukemia of the skull. Multiple focal destructive lesions in the calvarium are seen; some are ill-defined and some appear as well-marginated or punched-out lesions.

and later extend along the diaphysis and to other bones. Ill-defined or sharp, punched-out radiolucencies may be seen in the skull and flat bones (Fig. 5-84). Osteosclerosis may be patchy or uniform (Fig. 5-85). Periosteal new bone formation commonly occurs in the long bones and ribs. This may be the presenting sign, without bony destruction or metaphyseal bands.

The meninges may be involved, resulting in increased intracranial pressure with splitting of the cranial sutures. Leukemia may be mimicked by neuroblastoma that has metastasized to bone. Differentiation is possible because of urinary vanillylmandelic acid (VMA) and vanilphenylethylamine, which are metabolic intermediary products in the case of neuroblastoma.

Adult leukemia produces fewer skeletal changes

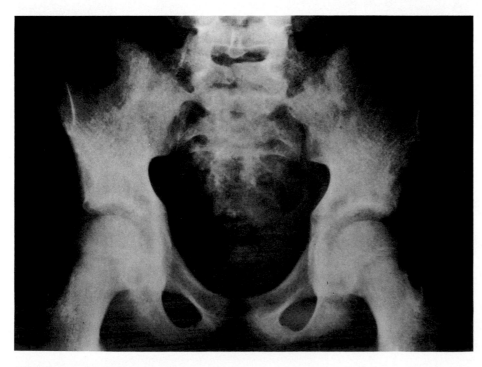

FIGURE 5-85. Leukemia of the pelvis. Osteosclerosis with coarsening of the trabecular pattern is seen on the radiograph.

than childhood leukemia. Osseous lesions occur rarely in acute leukemia. Most adults with bone lesions have chronic lymphatic leukemia. Bone lesions have been reported in 16% of patients with chronic myelogenous leukemia.[203]

Radiolucent bands are rare (Fig. 5-86). On plain films, generalized osteopenia is seen, most marked in the vertebrae, ribs, skull, and pelvis. Vertebral collapse sometimes follows. Cortical thinning and pathologic fractures, particularly of the ribs, may occur. Scattered osteolytic areas can occur in all bones, including the small bones of the hands and feet and the calvarium. The long axes of the lytic lesions are usually parallel to the axis of the shaft of a long bone. Periosteal new bone formation, cortical erosion, and joint effusions also may be seen. Osteosclerosis, patchy or generalized, is seen only rarely.

A radionuclide bone scan shows increased activity in the involved areas, but it may not convey the entire extent of the disease. MR images may show diffuse bone marrow changes. Low signal intensity is seen on T1-weighted images, with high signal intensity seen on

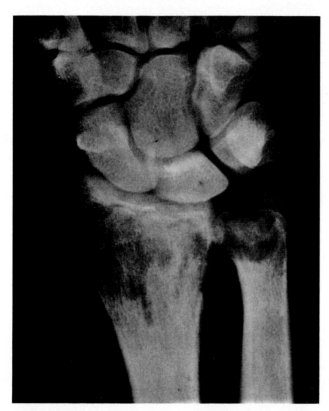

FIGURE 5-86. Adult leukemia of the wrist. Destructive changes in the metaphyses of the distal radius and ulna occurred after fusion of the epiphyseal growth center. This is an unusual finding. The bone density in adjacent areas is normal. The patient is a 50-year-old man with lymphocytic leukemia. (Courtesy of Dr. Miriam Liberson, West Side Veterans Administration Hospital, Chicago, IL.)

T2-weighted images. This may occur despite an entirely normal plain film examination (Fig. 5-87).

Several complications can occur. Secondary myeloid metaplasia may develop with bony sclerosis.[204] Leukemic acropachy, with clubbing of the fingers and bilateral symmetric destruction of the terminal phalanges is a rare manifestation.[205]

Chloroma

Chloroma (i.e., granulocytic sarcoma, myeloblastoma), a solid extramedullary tumor composed of early myeloid precursor cells, is an uncommon condition. It is most frequently seen in acute and chronic myelogenous leukemias, but it may also occur in polycythemia vera, hypereosinophilia, and myeloid metaplasia. The lesions are most commonly associated with bone and neural tissue, but they can occur almost anywhere. Femoral, sacral, rib, scapular, orbital, epidural, posterior mediastinal, and paravertebral locations have been described.[206,207] Bony destruction is usually seen (Fig. 5-88), but a sclerotic reaction may occur. They are named for their characteristic green color, which is caused by the enzyme myeloperoxidase. Not all chloromas have a green color. Although it rarely may be the initial manifestation of disease and precede the onset of leukemia by several months, it is usually found during the course of the disease.

Richter syndrome is a rare complication of chronic lymphocytic leukemia characterized by transformation into diffuse histiocytic lymphoma. The findings include hepatosplenomegaly, lymphadenopathy, and osteolytic lesions.[208]

Lymphoma

Lymphomas are divided into Hodgkin disease (HD) and non-Hodgkin lymphoma (NHL). HD involving bone is always secondary to generalized disease.[208a,209] NHL involving bone may be primary or secondary, according to defined criteria that include the initial involvement of only a single bone, only regional metastases, or the primary tumor preceding metastases by at least 6 months. Primary NHL of bone (i.e., reticulum cell sarcoma) is discussed in Chapter 2.

NHL is now usually classified by the Working Formulation (Table 5-1). This classification depicts the various types of lymphomatous cells as a malignant change during each stage of development of the normal lymphocyte. The histologic appearances are clinically classified as low grade, intermediate, and high grade. The three grades have different frequencies and patterns of bone involvement.

HD shows radiographic evidence of bone destruction in 20% of patients. In one series of patients with

(text continues on page 396)

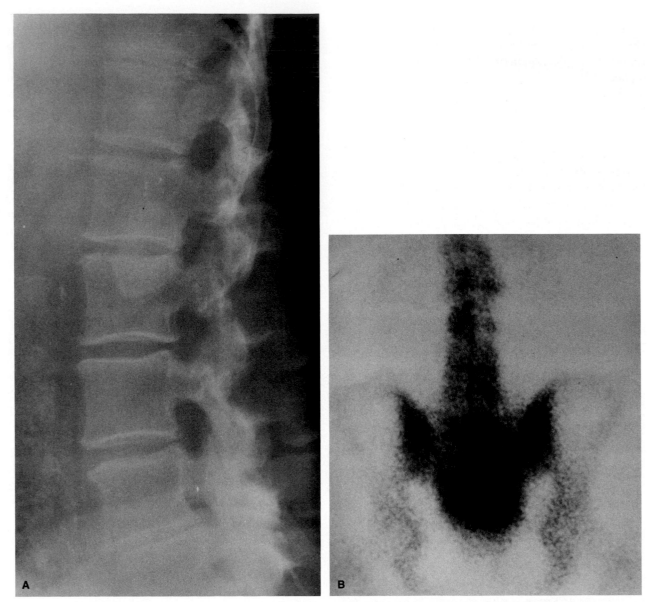

FIGURE 5-87. A 73-year-old woman with chronic lymphatic leukemia. (**A**) Lateral radiograph of the spine reveals the normal appearance of the vertebral bodies and paraspinal calcification. (**B**) Radionuclide bone scan shows several foci of increased activity in the lumbar spine. (**C**) A sagittal MR (SE 500/16) image of the lumbar spine shows diffuse replacement of bone marrow. (**D**) MR image (SE 2000/70). A heterogeneous high signal diffusely depicts all of the lumbar vertebral bodies.

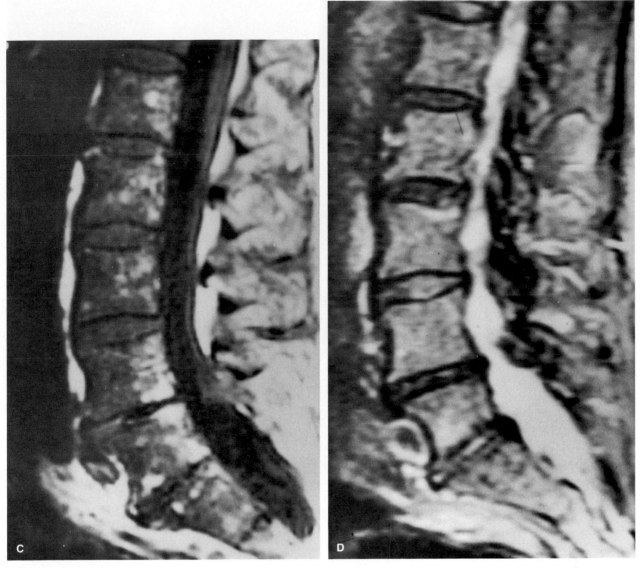

FIGURE 5-87. *(Continued)*

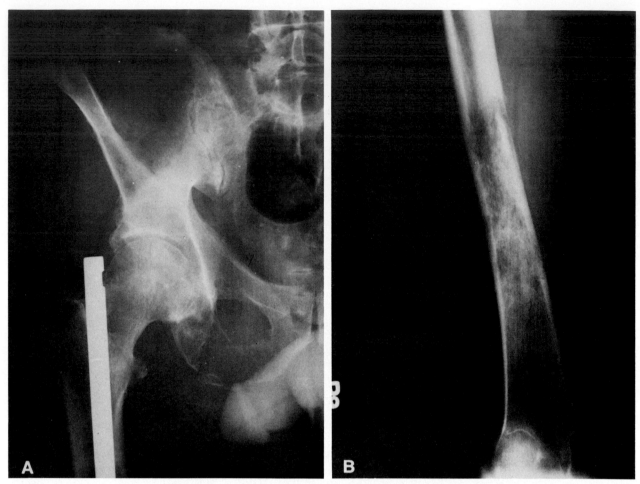

FIGURE 5-88. Granulocytic sarcoma. (**A**) A destructive lesion involves the right ischium. An intramedullary rod is in the right femur after a pathologic fracture. (**B**) The right femur before the fracture showed permeative destructive lesions in the midshaft, with cortical destruction and periosteal new bone formation. (Courtesy of Dr. Dharmashi V. Bhate, Veterans Administration Hospital, Hines, IL.)

mixed cellularity or lymphocytic depletion forms, 64% had bone destruction. In patients with lymphocytic predominance or nodular sclerosis, 11% had bone destruction.[210] The sites of involvement include the skull, face, extremities, spine, sacrum, ribs, and pelvis. The central skeleton is much more frequently involved than the extremities. The bony lesions usually are multiple. The patterns of bone destruction range from geographic to permeative in the more aggressive histologic types. The margins may be ill defined or sclerotic. Periosteal new bone formation of various patterns may be seen. Osteoblastic and mixed lesions are common (Figs. 5-89 and 5-90). The thoracolumbar spine is most often involved. The lesions are usually osteolytic or mixed sclerotic. Paravertebral masses and lymphadenopathy are common.

HD may also present as a solitary osteosclerotic or ivory vertebra (Fig. 5-91). Rarely, a soft-tissue mass may occur in the extremities (Fig. 5-92). Prevertebral lymph nodes may cause erosion to form a gouge defect, which results in a concave anterior margin of the body. This finding can help to differentiate HD from the third stage of Paget disease or an osteoblastic metastasis, both of which are densely osteosclerotic but without anterior erosion. This type of gouge defect may also be seen in NHL (see Fig. 5-10) and may also be caused by an aortic aneurysm (Fig. 5-93).

NHL shows bone or marrow involvement in 25% of cases during the course of the disease or treatment.[39] The findings include geographic (Fig. 5-94) and permeative (Fig. 5-95) destructive patterns; osteosclerosis (Fig. 5-96); soft-tissue invasion of bone (Fig. 5-97); and marrow changes. All bones may be involved, including the calvarium (Fig. 5-98). The three grades each have

TABLE 5-1.
National Cancer Institute Working Formulation
Classification of Non-Hodgkin Lymphoma

LOW GRADE

Diffuse
  Small lymphocytic cell type
Follicular
    Small cleaved cell type
    Mixed, small and large cell type

INTERMEDIATE GRADE

Follicular
  Large cell type
  Small cleaved cell type
Diffuse
  Mixed, small and large cell type
  Large cell type

HIGH GRADE

Diffuse
  Large immunoblastic cell type
  Lymphoblastic cell type
  Small non-cleaved cell type

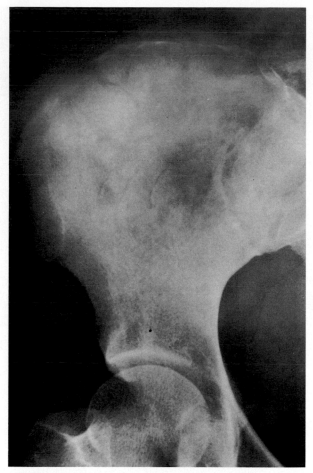

FIGURE 5-89. Hodgkin disease of the pelvis. Extensive destruction of the ilium has taken place. The destroyed area does not cross the sacroiliac joint or involve the sacral wing.

a different predominant type of osseous lesion. Low-grade NHL is sclerotic in most cases, with osteolytic and permeative destruction following. The intermediate grade is predominantly osteolytic with a permeative destructive pattern seen in only a small number of cases. Sclerotic lesions occur in a minority of cases, as do pathologic fractures. In high-grade NHL, osteolytic lesions are most frequent, with a minority showing permeative destruction. An ivory vertebra can also be seen in high-grade NHL (Fig. 5-99). Pathologic fractures and soft-tissue invasion of bone occur in a significant number of patients, but osteosclerotic reaction is uncommon. Any bone may be involved in any stage of the disease.

The spinal cord and nerve roots are involved in a small number of patients and may represent the initial manifestation of the disease. On myelography, an extradural mass or complete block may be found.[211]

Increased juxtaarticular activity may also be seen, associated with effusion, sclerosis, osteolysis, local osteoporosis, and epiphyseal involvement.[212,213] A radionuclide bone scan may reveal multiple asymptomatic lesions, frequently in the extremities. Increased uptake of isotope is often seen in the calvarium, and this picture may persist during remission.[214] Some lesions may be seen on MR images without increased uptake on the bone scan.

MRI can show a focal or diffuse marrow replacement pattern in the spine. Low signal intensity is seen on T1-weighted images, with variable signal intensity

on T2-weighted images of the lesions (Fig. 5-100). MRI contributes to a higher percentage of cases recognized with bone or marrow involvement. Soft-tissue tumors and lymphadenopathy, with or without invasion of bone, are best defined with MRI.

Burkitt tumor is a distinctive malignant lymphoma with rapid growth and large extranodal tumors.[215–218] It arises from B lymphocytes, with a peak incidence at about 6 to 7 years of age. Adults may also be involved. Association with the Epstein-Barr virus (EBV) has been established in the African form. The mechanism is postulated as chromosomal translocation. Burkitt lymphoma is endemic where malaria is endemic, and the association may be related to immunosuppression. EBV is also associated with B-cell lymphomas in HIV-positive patients.

Multifocal lesions with large extranodal tumors involve the skeleton and the gastrointestinal and genitourinary tracts. Two forms are described: the African or

(text continues on page 404)

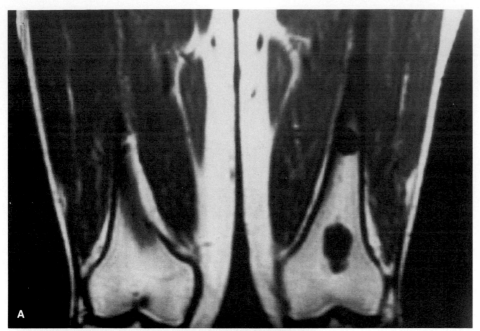

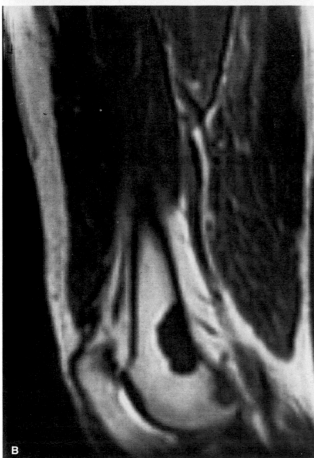

FIGURE 5-90. A 33-year-old man with Hodgkin disease and multiple skeletal lesions. (**A**) A coronal MR (SE 650/20) image shows two distinct low-signal-intensity foci in the distal left femur. (**B**) A sagittal MR (SE 600/20) image shows a well-defined, low-signal-intensity focus in the posterior femoral metaphysis. A small stripe of high signal intensity is seen adjacent to the lesion. (**C**) MR image (SE 2200/20). The lesion is of a low signal intensity in the posterior metaphysis. ,(**D**) MR image (SE 2200/80). The lesion remains low in signal intensity in this T2-weighted image, indicating that it is osteosclerotic.

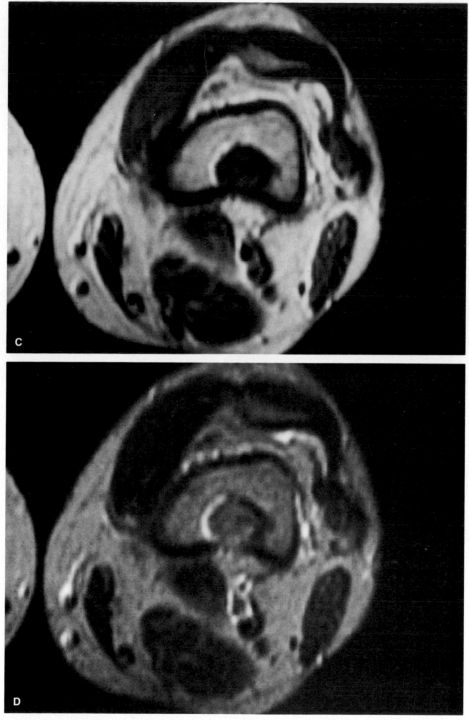

FIGURE 5-90.   *(Continued)*

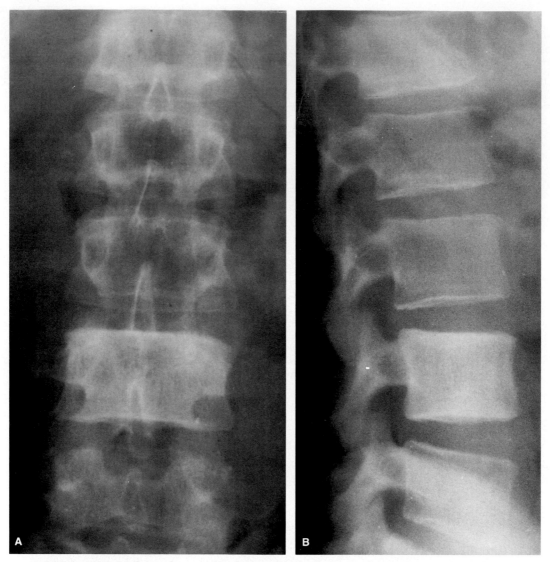

FIGURE 5-91. Hodgkin disease. (**A,B**) The anteroposterior and lateral views of the lumbar spine show a solitary ivory vertebra.

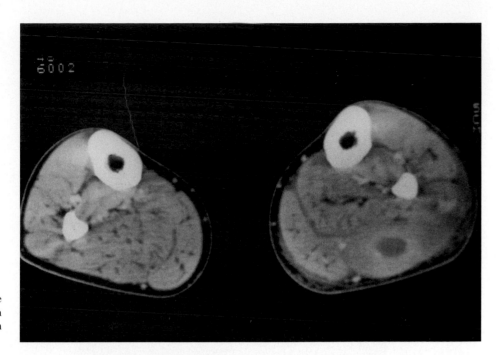

FIGURE 5-92. Hodgkin disease in a 55-year-old man. A CT scan shows a soft-tissue mass with central necrosis in the left calf.

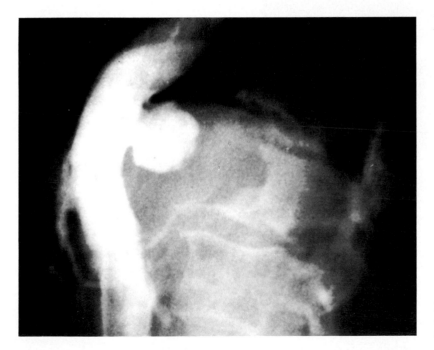

FIGURE 5-93. An aortogram shows erosion of the anterior aspect of a vertebral body by an abdominal aortic aneurysm.

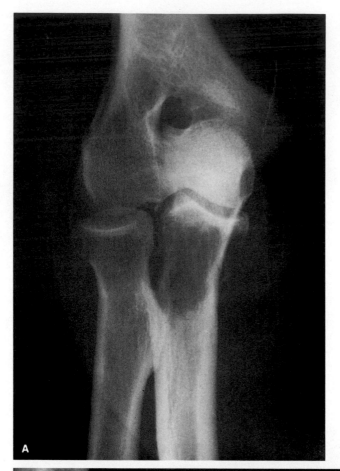

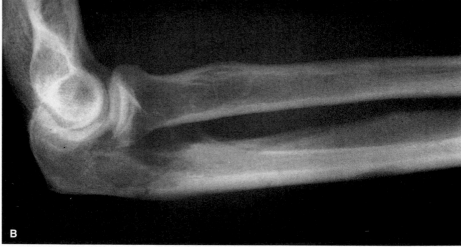

FIGURE 5-94. An 80-year-old man with intermediate-grade, diffuse, large cell non-Hodgkin lymphoma. (**A**) Anteroposterior and (**B**) lateral views of the right elbow show a poorly marginated expansile geographic area with a pathologic fracture. (**C**) Lateral view of the left ankle shows geographic destructive lesions in the distal tibia. (**D**) Radionuclide bone scan shows widespread foci of increased activity.

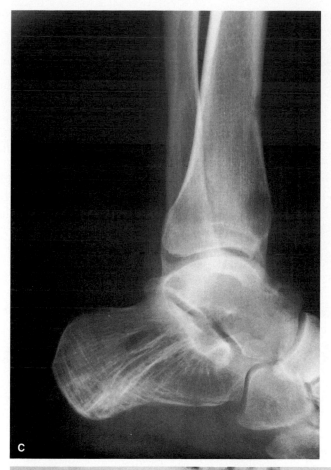

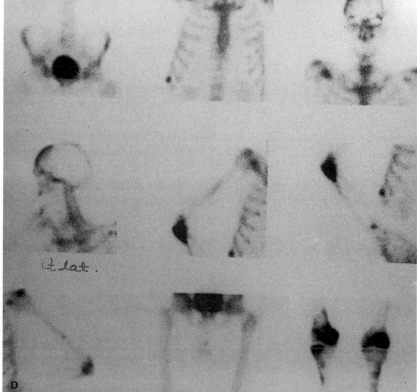

FIGURE 5-94.   *(Continued)*

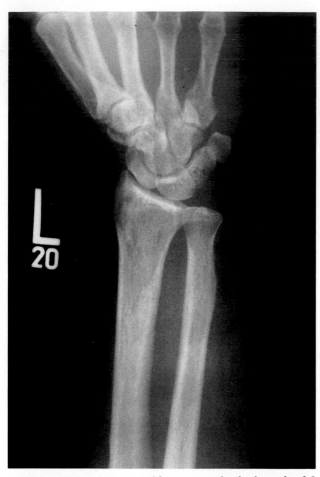

FIGURE 5-95. A 63-year-old woman with a high-grade, diffuse, small cell non-Hodgkin lymphoma. An anteroposterior view of the wrist and distal forearm shows permeative destructive changes in the distal radius and ulna. There is no periosteal new bone formation.

endemic and the American or nonendemic. The nonendemic form is rare. In the African form, jaw lesions are initially seen in about half of these patients. American Burkitt lymphoma has a 15% incidence of jaw tumors[38] but a higher incidence of abdominal tumors, pleural effusions, and peripheral lymph node involvement.[219]

Radiologically, the mandible or maxilla is frequently involved, with bony destruction, loss of the lamina dura, and displacement and loss of teeth (Fig. 5-101). Destructive lesions, ranging from small, multiple, osteolytic areas to large, destroyed areas are seen. A permeative pattern involving the metaphyses and diaphyses of the long bones and small bones occurs in a small percentage of patients. Usually the humerus, pelvis, femur, and tibia show lesions. It has been reported in the calvarium, ribs, spine, sternum, small bones, flat bones, and talus.[220] Pathologic fracture may

occur. Periosteal new bone formation, sometimes spiculated or laminated, may be seen. The bone lesions are relatively painless.

Histiocytosis X

Histiocytosis X (i.e., Langerhans cell histiocytosis) consists of three clinical syndromes with identical pathogenesis.[221,222] The syndromes, in decreasing order of severity, are acute or subacute disseminated histiocytosis X or Letterer-Siwe disease (LS), chronic disseminated histiocytosis X or Hand-Schüller-Christian disease (HSC), and eosinophilic granuloma (EG) of bone. The basis of this condition is the deposit of lipids, chiefly cholesterol and its esters, within histiocytes. The cause is unknown. The disease is generalized in LS. In HSC and EG, there are focal granulomas containing lipidized and nonlipidized histiocytes and eosinophils. An unidentified factor attracts the eosinophils. They may not be prominent, and rarely, they may be absent. Hyperlipidemia, hypercholesterolemia, and eosinophilia are rare.

There are four phases of histopathologic evolution[223]:

1. Proliferation of histiocytes, eosinophils, and inflammatory cells
2. Granulomatous phase, with intermingling of multinuclear giant cells
3. Xanthomatous phase, in which histiocytes are lipid-laden foam cells
4. Fibrous phase, with increased collagen and decreased cellularity.

Clinically, LS is usually seen in patients younger than 2 years of age, and it is characterized by a sudden onset and a rapidly progressive course that includes fever, hemorrhages, anemia, hepatosplenomegaly, and lymphadenopathy. Bone lesions may be absent, particularly if there is a rapid course.

HSC most commonly occurs in children younger than 5 years of age, but it may be seen up to adulthood. A triad of exophthalmos, diabetes insipidus, and skull lesions are the classical hallmark, but the concurrent presence of these three signs is found in fewer than 10% of cases. The mortality rate is 13%.

EG of bone usually occurs in patients younger than 10 years of age, but it may rarely affect patients of all ages.[224,225] It is most commonly monostotic, but disseminated bony lesions may also be seen. Bone pain, limitation of motion, local inflammatory signs, and fever may be present. The skull, ribs, mandible, spine, pelvis, sternum,[226] and extremities are most often involved. The epiphysis is not usually involved. The lesions may regress spontaneously over time, and they

(text continues on page 409)

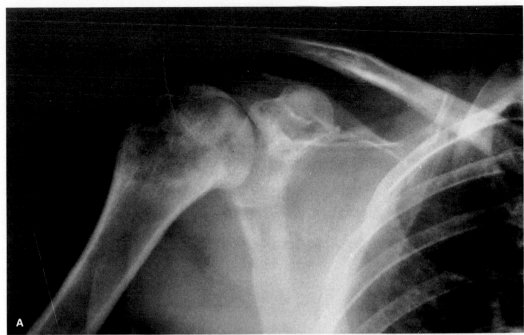

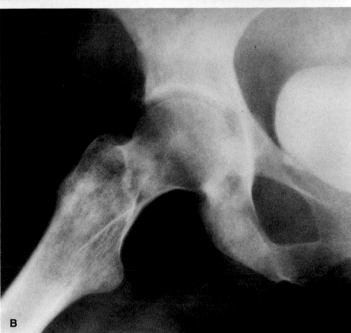

FIGURE 5-96. A 48-year-old woman with intermediate-grade, large cell non-Hodgkin lymphoma. (**A**) An anteroposterior view of the right shoulder shows patchy osteosclerosis of the proximal humerus and around the glenoid fossa. (**B**) A lateral view of the left hip shows patchy osteosclerosis around the proximal femur, the ischium, and the iliac bone.

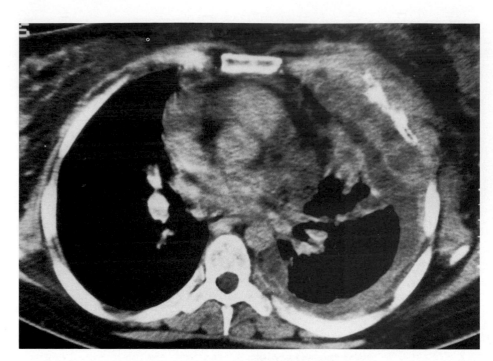

FIGURE 5-97. A 25-year-old woman with high-grade, immunoblastic non-Hodgkin lymphoma. A soft-tissue mass has surrounded and partially destroyed the rib. Pleural effusion is also seen.

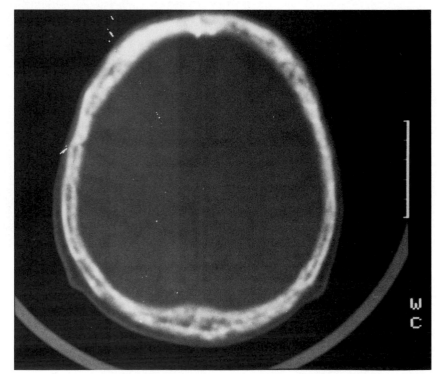

FIGURE 5-98. A 70-year-old man with intermediate-grade, diffuse, large cell non-Hodgkin lymphoma. CT scan of the head shows diffuse, mottled destruction of the calvarium.

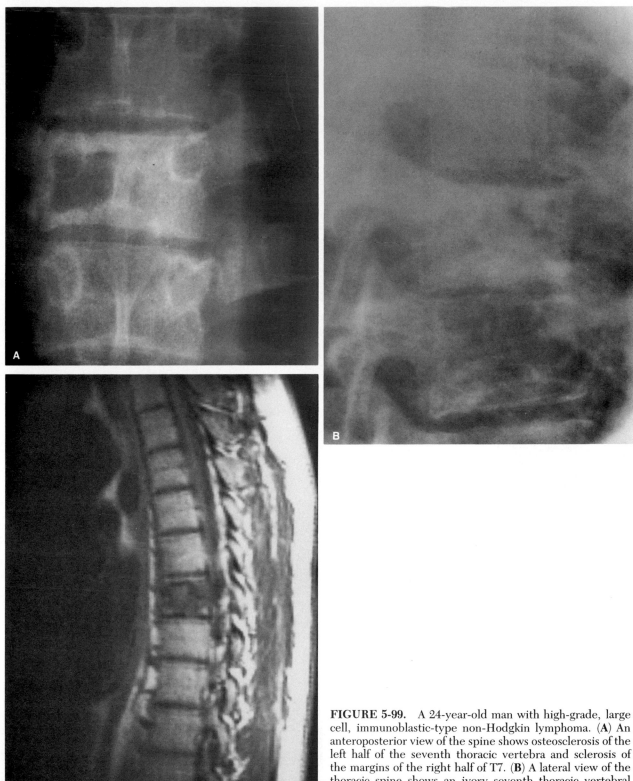

FIGURE 5-99. A 24-year-old man with high-grade, large cell, immunoblastic-type non-Hodgkin lymphoma. (**A**) An anteroposterior view of the spine shows osteosclerosis of the left half of the seventh thoracic vertebra and sclerosis of the margins of the right half of T7. (**B**) A lateral view of the thoracic spine shows an ivory seventh thoracic vertebral body. (**C**) MR image (SE 550/15) shows low signal intensity with linear areas of signal void in the seventh thoracic vertebral body.

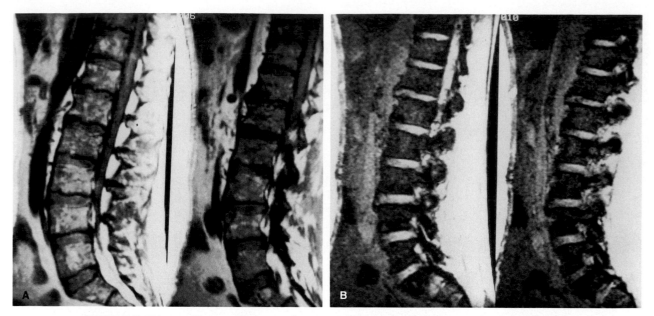

FIGURE 5-100. A 45-year-old man with intermediate-grade, diffuse, mixed cell non-Hodgkin lymphoma. (**A**) The T1-weighted MR image shows diffuse, mottled involvement of the lumbar spine and involvement of the meninges of the spinal cord. (**B**) The T2-weighted MR image shows a mottled pattern of the vertebral marrow without markedly high signal intensity. Spinal meningeal involvement is also seen.

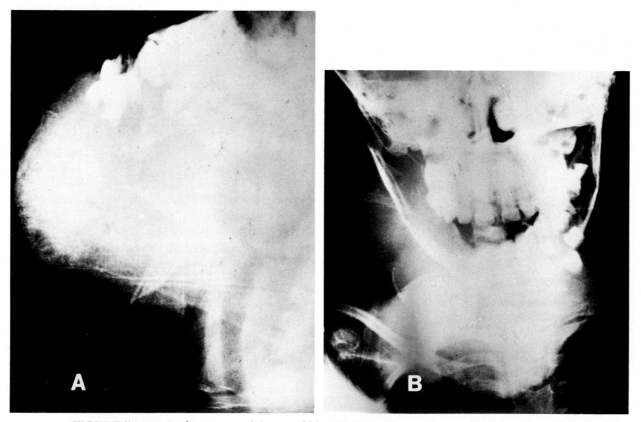

FIGURE 5-101. Burkitt tumor of the mandible. (**A**) A lateral view shows extensive soft-tissue swelling, mandibular destruction, and the appearance of floating teeth. (**B**) An anteroposterior view shows similar findings.

have reportedly healed after steroid injection.[227,228] Bone lesions are due to destruction by granulation tissue and are similar in all three forms of histiocytosis X.

Imaging studies initially show one or more small radiolucencies, which range from ill-defined to sharply marginated areas (Fig. 5-102). As the lesions enlarge, endosteal scalloping may occur (Fig. 5-103), producing a multilocular appearance or bone expansion. Some lesions show a characteristic marginal bevelling with undulating contours: a bevelled-edge or a hole-within-a-hole appearance, giving a three-dimensional effect (Fig. 5-104). Other cases may show poorly defined, patchy, destructive areas or a coarsened trabecular pattern. The cortex may be destroyed. Some lesions may originate in the cortex (Fig. 5-105). Periosteal reaction, usually solid but possibly laminated, may be seen. All

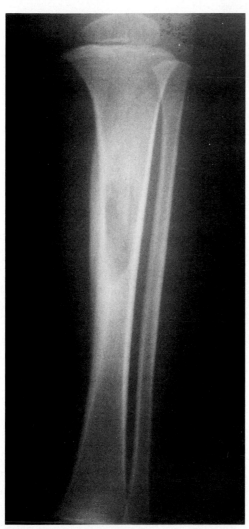

FIGURE 5-102. A 13-year-old girl with eosinophilic granuloma of the left tibial shaft. The anteroposterior view of the tibia shows a poorly marginated, radiolucent lesion with thick periosteal new bone formation medially.

portions of the long bones may be involved. Expansion of bone and pathologic fractures are rare. Reactive sclerosis, particularly after therapy, may also occur (Fig. 5-106). Sequestration within destructive areas may rarely be seen.

The skull is more commonly involved in disseminated disease. The lesions typically begin as small, intradiploic, punched-out areas and then unevenly expand and perforate the inner and outer tables. This creates the appearance of a double contour along the margin, called a bevelled edge (Fig. 5-107). More often, there is ill-defined or sharply defined margination. Extensive confluence later develops to produce the geographic skull (Fig. 5-108). A button sequestrum may rarely be seen. Destruction of the sella turcica, petrous bone, mastoids, base of the skull, paranasal sinuses, and orbits can occur. Orbital lesions are common, and they may involve the roof, lateral wall, and sphenoid wings. Healing results in a dense orbital sclerosis that should be differentiated from fibrous dysplasia.[229] Jaw lesions involving the teeth begin near the apices, destroying periodontal bone and giving the radiographic appearance of floating teeth (Fig. 5-109). The mandible may also be involved with a well-defined lesion with a bevelled edge (Fig. 5-110).

The pelvis is commonly involved, usually in the iliac bone. A bevelled edge or reactive sclerosis along the margin of a destructive lesion may be seen. The ribs may show expansile lesions, with or without pathologic fractures.

The spine may show involvement of the vertebral bodies or neural arches (Fig. 5-111). Multiple radiolucencies can be seen (Fig. 5-112), which proceed to vertebral body collapse and to a flat, thin, wafer shape. The regenerative phase follows with a residual vertebra plana. The intervertebral spaces are preserved. A wedge-like collapse may also occur. Calvé disease is due to eosinophilic granuloma rather than ischemic necrosis.

Radionuclide bone scans with ^{99m}Tc and with ^{67}Ga-citrate were compared with plain films of children with histiocytosis X. In 35% of patients, the bone scans were falsely negative with extensive radiographic evidence of skeletal disease. Only one case showed bone scan changes before radiographic abnormalities. None of the lesions was photopenic. The ^{99m}Tc-sulfur colloid bone marrow and ^{67}Ga-citrate whole-body scans were not useful.[230] A skeletal survey is superior to a bone scan for detecting bony lesions.[231]

MRI can best define the intraosseous and extraosseous extent of disease. Cortical destruction can be determined, and the extent of soft-tissue involvement can readily be seen. The lesions are seen as intermediate

(text continues on page 414)

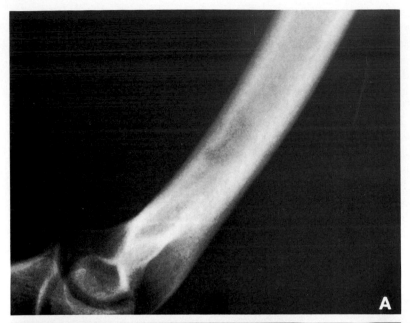

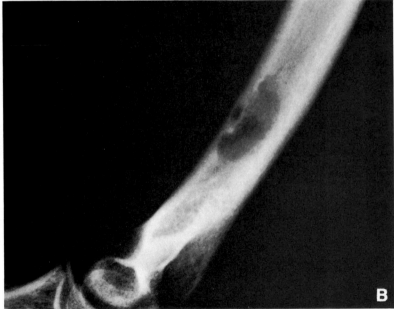

FIGURE 5-103. Eosinophilic granuloma of the distal humerus in a 15-year-old girl. **(A)** There is an ill-defined radiolucent lesion in the distal humeral shaft. **(B)** Seen 1 month later, the radiolucent area has become more defined and is larger. There is a scalloped margin without definitive sclerosis. No periosteal new bone formation has developed. (Courtesy of Dr. Chandra Modi, Walter Memorial Hospital, Chicago, IL.)

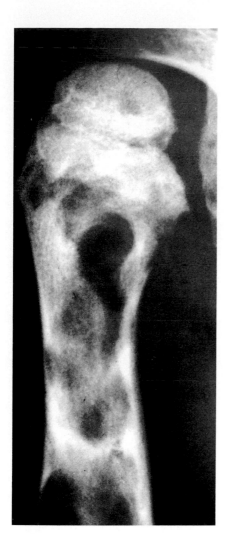

FIGURE 5-104. Hand-Schüller-Christian disease. There are multiple radiolucent lesions in the proximal humerus. The most proximal metaphyseal lesion has a double contour, giving a hole-within-a-hole or three-dimensional effect.

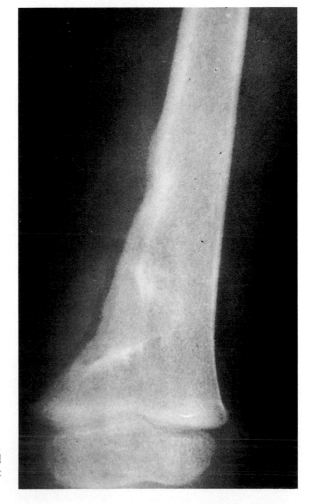

FIGURE 5-105. Eosinophilic granuloma originating in the cortex. There is extensive eccentric cortical destruction with a scalloped margin in the lower femoral shaft medially. A soft-tissue component is also shown.

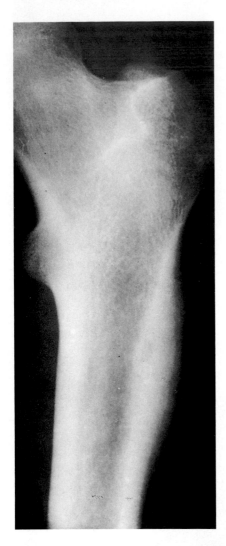

FIGURE 5-106. Eosinophilic granuloma of the proximal femur, simulating osteoid osteoma. Reactive bone sclerosis occurs at the outer aspect of the proximal femur, and the small radiolucent area represents the eosinophilic granuloma. (Courtesy of Dr. Marion Magalotti)

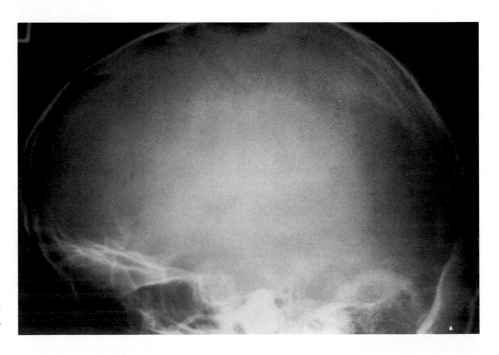

FIGURE 5-107. A 26-year-old man with eosinophilic granuloma. The lateral view of the skull shows a radiolucent defect with a "bevelled edge."

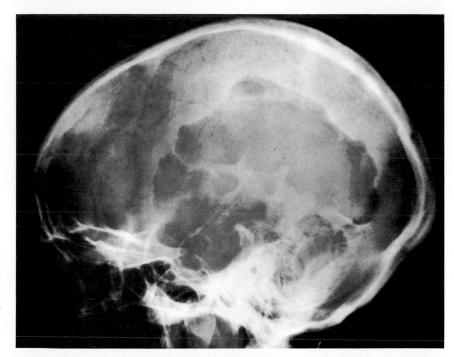

FIGURE 5-108. Hand-Schüller-Christian disease of the skull. The confluence of destructive lesions gives the geographic skull appearance. The major portion of the destroyed area has a beveled margin, indicating that the inner and outer tables are perforated unevenly.

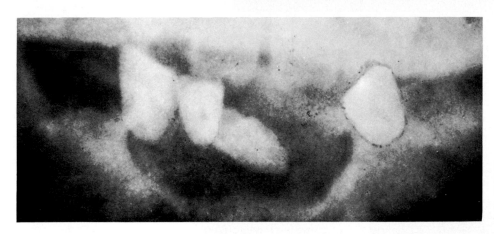

FIGURE 5-109. Hand-Schüller-Christian disease of the mandible. Periodontal destruction about the incisors gives the floating teeth appearance.

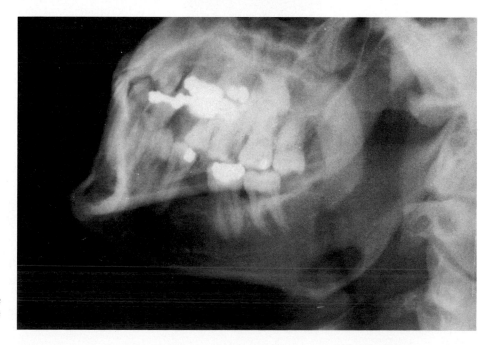

FIGURE 5-110. Eosinophilic granuloma of the angle of the mandible has a bevelled edge.

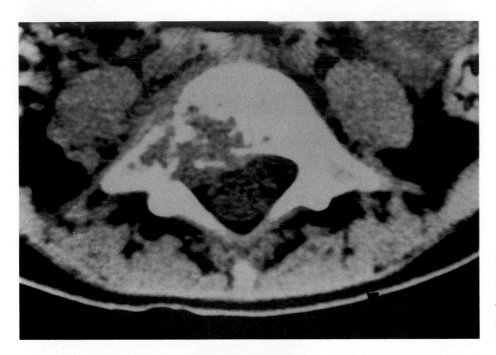

FIGURE 5-111. A 5-year-old boy with eosinophilic granuloma. CT scan shows destruction of the right half of the vertebral body. The lesion is irregularly marginated, and there is soft-tissue protrusion into the neural canal.

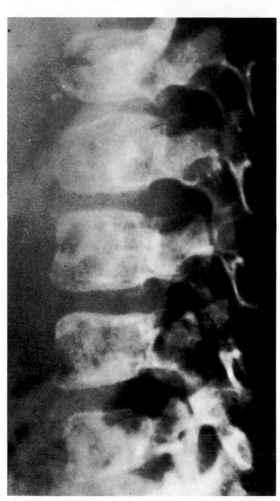

FIGURE 5-112. Hand-Schüller-Christian disease of the spine. There are multiple destructive lesions in the bodies of the lumbar vertebrae. Vertebral collapse has not yet occurred.

to high signal intensity on T1-weighted images and as high signal intensity on T2-weighted images. The higher signal intensity on T1-weighted images is seen in the xanthomatous phase, in which the histiocytes are lipid laden.[223] Enhancement occurs with gadolinium infusion (Fig. 5-113). Reactive changes in the adjacent soft tissues may be seen as high signal intensity on T2-weighted images (Figs. 5-114 and 5-115). This pattern may also be seen with osteoid osteoma and benign chondroblastoma.

Erdheim-Chester disease is a rare lipoid granulomatosis characterized by symmetric osteosclerotic or osteolytic lesions, principally in the diametaphyseal regions of the long bones.[232] An associated exophthalmos has been reported.[233] This entity may fall within the spectrum of histiocytosis X.[234] Expansile osteolytic lesions with cortical breakthrough have been reported in this condition that were histologically consistent with eosinophilic granuloma.[235]

Massive Osteolysis

Massive osteolysis (i.e., vanishing bone disease, Gorham disease) is a rare condition associated with hemangioma or lymphangioma, characterized by progressive resorption of large areas of bone.[236–242] The patients are usually younger than 30 years of age, although massive osteolysis has an age-related range of 14 months to 58 years. The onset is insidious, with pain and progressive weakness. Severe deformity may follow, and occasionally, pathologic fracture may occur. Progress may spontaneously be arrested[243] or may continue relentlessly to death, particularly in cases with

(text continues on page 420)

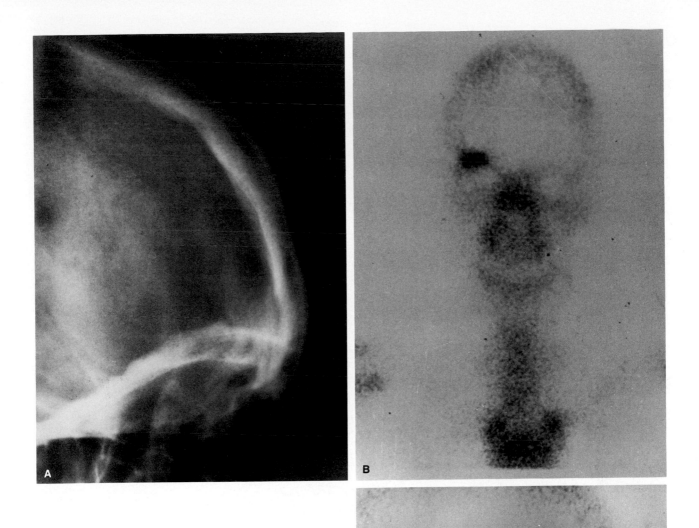

FIGURE 5-113. A 22-year-old woman with eosinophilic granuloma of the right orbital roof. (**A**) The lateral view of the skull shows a 1.5-cm ovoid radiolucent lesion with a bevelled edge. (**B,C**) Radionuclide bone scans show increased activity in the right supraorbital region. (**D**) A coronal CT scan shows bony destruction of a segment of the right orbital roof. (**E**) MR image (FSE 600/12 Ef) with infusion of Magnevist. A 1.0-cm, ring-like, enhancing lesion is seen in the right supraorbital region. (**F**) An axial MR (FSE 600/12 Ef) image after Magnevist infusion shows an ovoid, ring-like, enhancing lesion in the supraorbital plane. (**G**) An axial MR (FSE 4000/96 Ef) section in the supraorbital plane shows increased signal intensity of the lesion. At surgery, an eosinophilic granuloma approximately 1.0 cm in diameter was removed from between the orbital roof and the dura. *continued*

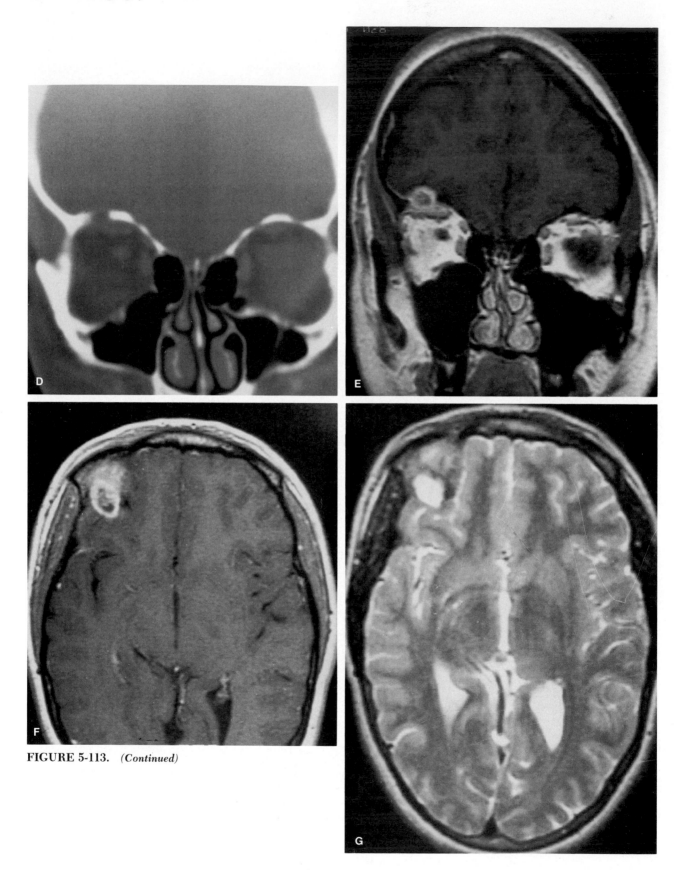

FIGURE 5-113. *(Continued)*

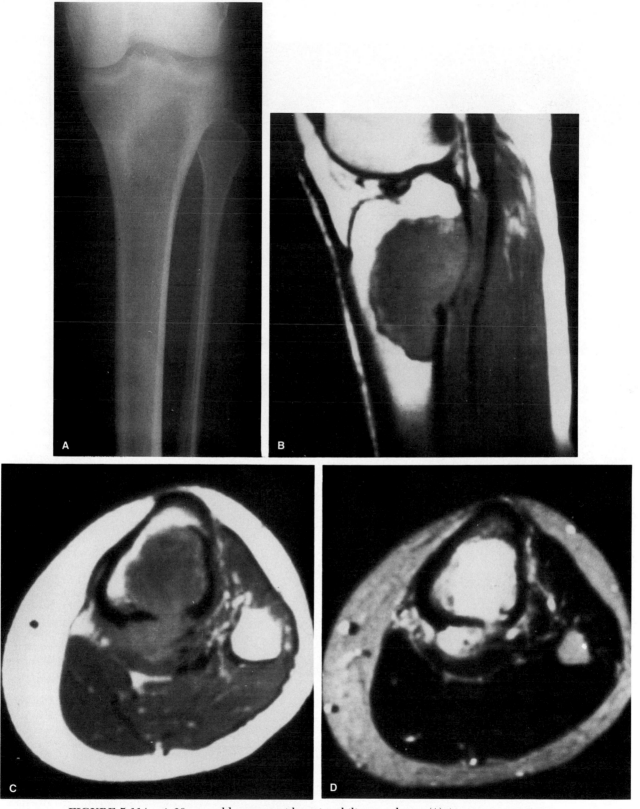

FIGURE 5-114. A 20-year-old woman with eosinophilic granuloma. (**A**) An anteroposterior radiograph of the tibia shows an ill-defined radiolucent lesion in the proximal tibial metaphysis. (**B**) A T1-weighted sagittal MR image shows a well-defined low-signal-intensity lesion replacing marrow fat. (**C**) A T1-weighted MR image shows the lesion has penetrated the cortex posteriorly and extended into the soft tissues. (**D**) A T2-weighted axial image shows high signal intensity of the lesion in and out of the bone. In addition, a high-signal-intensity soft-tissue reaction surrounds the bone.

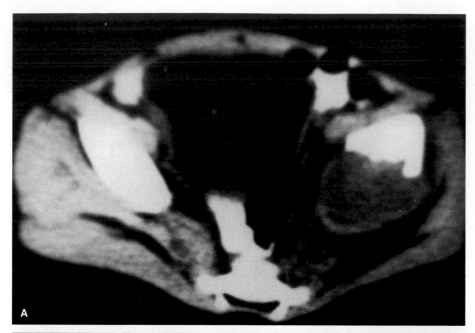

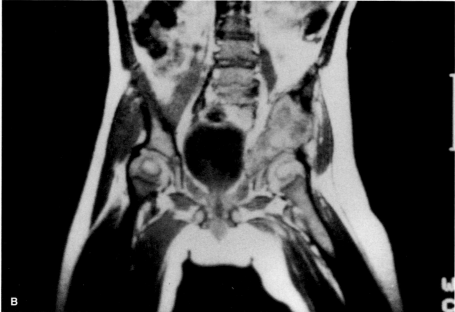

FIGURE 5-115. Eosinophilic granuloma of the iliac bone in an 18-month-old boy. (**A**) CT scan shows a mass destroying the major portion of the left iliac bone and irregular margination. (**B**) A coronal MR (SE 800/25) image shows irregular heterogeneous mass destroying the left iliac bone. (**C**) MR image (SE 3000/ 70). The mass has increased in signal intensity. A high-signal-intensity reaction is revealed in the soft tissues at the lateral aspect of the mass. (**D**) An anteroposterior view of the pelvis shows geographic destruction of the left iliac bone. The superior margin shows a bevelled edge.

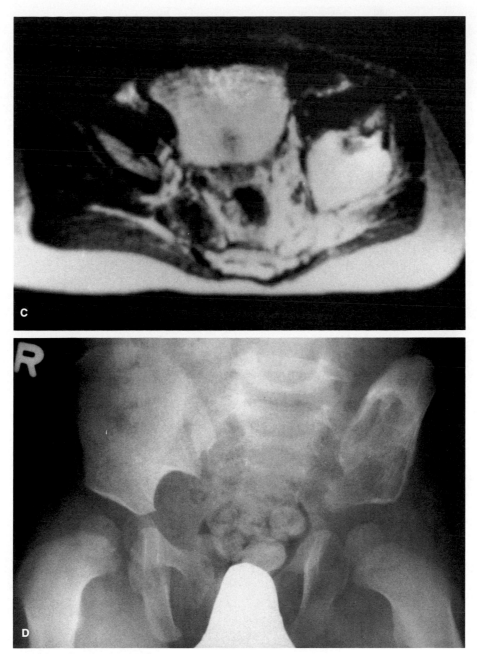

FIGURE 5-115.   *(Continued)*

rib cage involvement. Laboratory studies show nothing characteristic. At surgery, the bone is found to have vanished at the involved sites. Bone grafts are also resorbed. Cases have been reported of spontaneous reossification.[244]

Radiologically, extensive bone loss is seen. All bones may be affected, but most frequently, the shoulders, hips, pelvis, ribs, spine, and long bones are involved (Fig. 5-116). The process spreads across joints and intervertebral spaces to involve adjacent bones, resulting in massive areas of vanished bone. In a tubular bone, tapering of the margin of the lesion to a cone-like contour occurs. No osteosclerotic reaction nor periosteal reaction is seen. Neither soft-tissue debris nor phleboliths are present. Occasionally, cutaneous hemangiomas are associated with the condition. Skip areas do not usually occur.

Osteofibrous Dysplasia of the Tibia and Fibula

Osteofibrous dysplasia of the tibia and fibula has the histologic characteristics of fibrous tissue surrounding bone trabeculae bordered by active osteoblasts and a zonal architecture.[245,245a,245b] There are histologic similarities to adamantinoma of the tibia. The peak age of onset is from 1 to 3 years. It may be congenital or affect patients as old as 15 years of age.

Radiologically, bone enlargement, intracortical osteolytic lesions, thinning or disappearance of the external cortex, sclerosis, and narrowing of the medullary canal may be seen. There may be bowing of bone, pathologic fracture, or pseudoarthrosis (see Fig. 2-105). The lesions develop in childhood and are most often located in the diaphysis of the tibia, which is bowed anteriorly.

Medullary Bone Infarcts

Medullary infarction of bone may be associated with barotrauma, collagen diseases, idiopathic causes, infection, intraarterial chemotherapy,[246] leukemia, lymphoma, occlusive vascular disease, pancreatitis (Fig. 5-117),[247] posttransplantation states, sickle cell anemia, and storage diseases.

The sites most commonly involved are the distal femur and the proximal tibia. In infants with sickle cell anemia, dactylitis is common. Infarct-associated bone

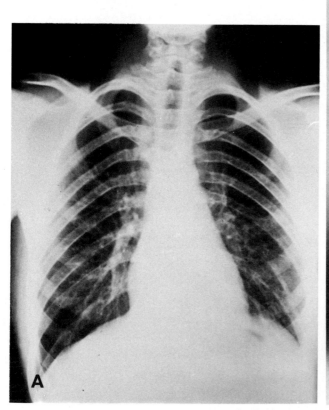

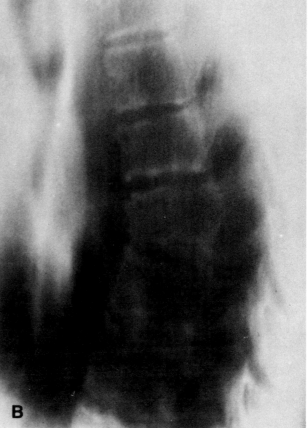

FIGURE 5-116. Massive osteolysis or vanishing bone disease. (**A**) Posteroanterior chest radiograph shows destruction of the left eighth and ninth ribs. (**B**) Tomogram of dorsal spine reveals partial collapse of the middorsal vertebrae and sharp gibbus formation. (Courtesy of Dr. Tom Hinckle, Beaumont, TX.)

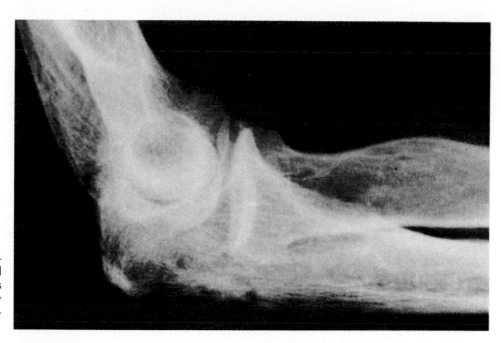

FIGURE 5-117. Acute pancreatitis of the left proximal ulna. The small patchy areas of radiolucency are caused by acute bone infarction secondary to fat necrosis.

sarcoma is rare, with only 37 fully documented cases in the literature. The type of tumor is osteosarcoma in 18% and malignant fibrous histiocytoma in 72% of patients. The long bones are principally involved.[248,249]

Radiologically, the immature infarcts show ill-defined bone rarefaction followed by mottled sclerosis.[246,250] MR images show foci of abnormal mixed signal centrally with a thin, serpiginous, low-signal-intensity margin.

A mature infarct appears as a densely calcified area in the medullary cavity, with serpiginous radiopaque streaks extending from the central region or sharply limited by a dense sclerotic zone (Fig. 5-118). CT shows calcification at the margin of the infarct. An infarct should be differentiated from an enchondroma, which shows amorphous punctate calcifications, is not surrounded by a sclerotic rim, and may cause endosteal scalloping or expand the bone. MR images of mature infarcts show low signal intensity on T1-weighted and T2-weighted images.

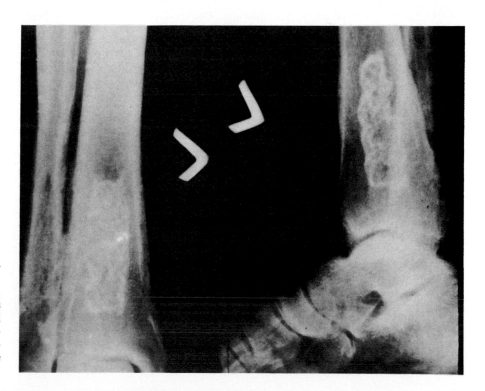

FIGURE 5-118. Mature metaphyseal infarct of the distal tibia. There is a well-circumscribed, dense area of calcification that is sharply delimited from normal bone. Notice the serpiginous anterior contour of the infarct. The periosteal reaction is caused by chronic stasis.

Cyst formation in a bone infarct is a rare occurrence (Fig. 5-119).[251] It is seen as an expansile, radiolucent, sharply demarcated lesion in an infarcted segment of bone. The cortex is thinned but intact.

A significant percentage of professional deep sea divers develop ischemic necrosis of bone (i.e., dysbaric osteonecrosis).[252] Medullary bone infarcts and ischemic necrosis of the femoral and humeral heads may be seen. This does not occur in recreational scuba divers who pay heed to diving tables.

Radionuclide bone scans may show increased uptake in the absence of radiographic findings or may show activity in long-standing bone infarcts.[253,254] Some lesions may not become visible on a radiograph. In the femoral or humeral heads, structural failure and collapse may subsequently occur.

Avascular necrosis of a vertebral body is seen as compression containing a horizontal intervertebral vacuum cleft. MR images show low signal intensity on T1-weighted images and high signal intensity on T2-weighted images at the cleft site.[255]

Brown Tumor of Hyperparathyroidism

As hyperparathyroidism progresses, one or rarely more expansile bone lesions may appear. They are located chiefly in the mandible, pelvis, ribs, and femora and rarely the orbit,[256] but any bone may be involved (Fig. 5-120). These lesions are osteoclastomas, also called brown tumors. Cysts result from hemorrhage and necrosis within the tumor. A radionuclide bone scan shows increased activity at the site of a brown tumor. A brown tumor may rarely be the initial manifestation of primary hyperthyroidism (Figs. 5-121 and 5-122). Periosteal reaction is sparse, and trabeculation is light. The tumors can be destructive, and pathologic fractures may occur. After removal of the causal parathyroid adenoma, a brown tumor often heals with the formation of dense bone. It is important to differentiate a cellular brown tumor from a cyst in a weight-bearing bone. A cyst will not heal after parathyroidectomy, and the patient will be at risk for a pathologic fracture. The two may be differentiated by arteriography or by dem-

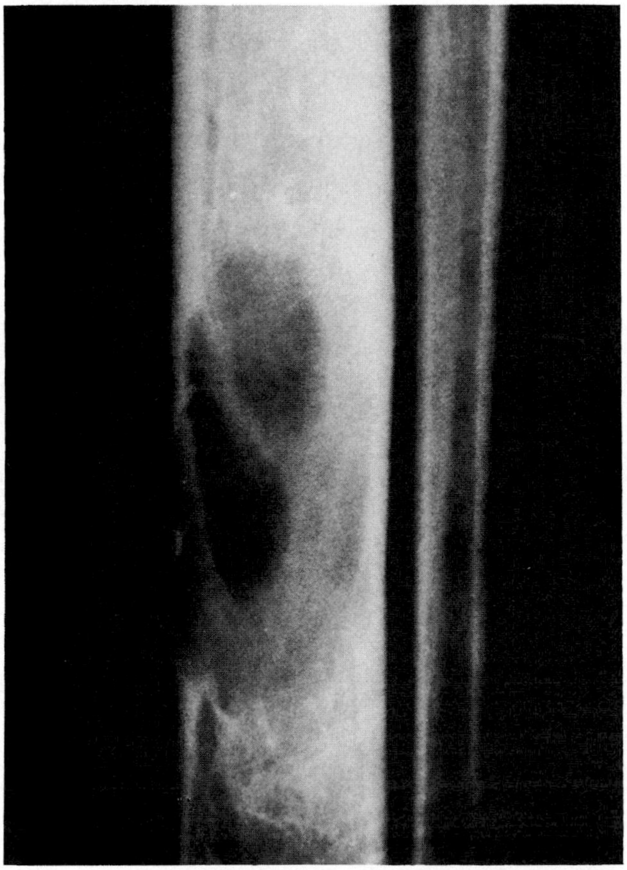

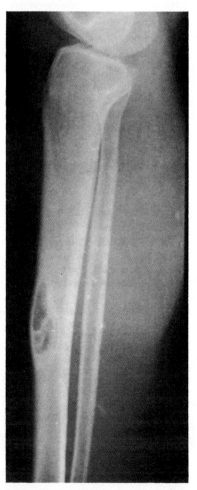

FIGURE 5-119. A radiograph of the tibial shaft shows a bone infarct with a 6-cm cyst, which has eroded the medial cortex. (Courtesy of Dr. Alex Norman, Hospital for Joint Diseases, Orthopedic Institute, New York, NY.)

FIGURE 5-120. Primary hyperparathyroidism. There is a slightly expansile, loculated, brown tumor in the midtibial shaft.

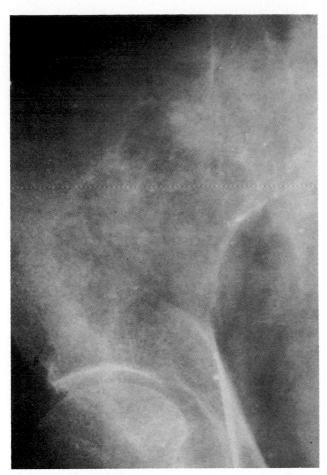

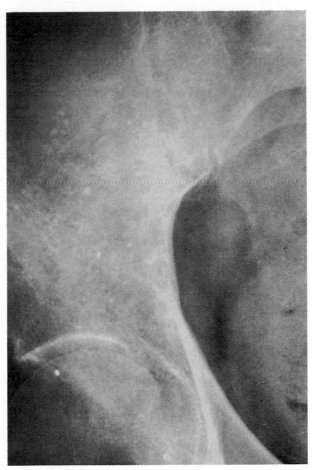

FIGURE 5-121. Primary hyperparathyroidism in a 60-year-old man who presented with right hip pain. There is a large, radiolucent, sharply demarcated, scalloped, lightly trabeculated lesion in the right pelvis. A small amount of cortical destruction of the pelvic rim is also seen. On biopsy, this lesion proved to be a brown tumor secondary to a parathyroid adenoma. There were no other skeletal signs of hyperparathyroidism; particularly, no subperiosteal bone resorption had occurred.

FIGURE 5-122. Same patient as in Figure 5-121, 1 year after removal of a large parathyroid adenoma. The previously seen radiolucent brown tumor has partially filled in with sclerotic bone. A residual coarsened trabecular pattern is present. The pelvic rim is now thickened in that region.

onstrating enhancement in the tumor on postinfusion CT.[257]

Multiple subchondral periarticular cysts may be associated with swollen joints in patients on long-term hemodialysis. These cysts can grow to large size, and some contain amyloid.[61] Skeletal metastases may occur, sometimes alongside a brown tumor, in the event of a parathyroid carcinoma.

Miscellaneous Rare Benign Syndromes Causing Widespread Lytic Lesions of Bone

INTRAOSSEOUS HEMANGIOMATOSIS. Intraosseous hemangiomatosis may cause multiple, widespread bone defects.[258] Diffuse skeletal hemangiomatosis showing osteosclerosis and osteolysis may also be seen.[259] Several skeletal abnormalities may be associated with hemangiomas, lymphangiomas, varicosities, and arteriovenous fistulae. These include enchondromas, bony hypertrophy, and osteolytic and sclerotic lesions. Associated syndromes include Maffucci syndrome, mixed sclerosing bone dystrophy with angiodysplasia, congenital angiectatic hypertrophy (i.e., Klippel-Trenaunay-Weber syndrome), and massive osteolysis (i.e., Gorham syndrome).

CYSTIC LYMPHANGIOMATOSIS. Cystic lymphangiomatosis in bone may show expansile lesions and multiple radiolucencies.[260–262] Children are usually affected. There is a relentless progression of osteolysis, and pathologic fractures may follow. Intraosseous lymphangiomatosis of the mandible has also been reported.[263] Mixed lymphangiomas and hemangiomas, called cystic angiomatosis, may also occur.

CONGENITAL SCATTERED FIBROMATOSIS. Congenital scattered fibromatosis is characterized by the presence of multiple fibromas in the subcutaneous tissues and viscera.[264,265] All bones show widespread osteolytic or expansile lesions, which at times may be calcified. The disease is usually fatal with visceral involvement. Association with extraskeletal congenital anomalies has been described.[266]

WEBER-CHRISTIAN DISEASE. Weber-Christian disease is a rare diffuse condition characterized by panniculitis and painful subcutaneous nodules.[267] Resulting from a disturbance in fat metabolism, multiple osteolytic lesions involve the calvarium, pelvis, and medullary bone. The appearance is similar to that of multiple myeloma. The spine is not involved.

SYSTEMIC LIPOMATOSIS OF BONE. Systemic lipomatosis of bone is a rare condition in which multiple osteolytic lesions with a predilection for the hands and feet may occur.[268]

MEMBRANOUS LIPODYSTROPHY. Membranous lipodystrophy is a rare condition in which multiple radiolucencies are found symmetrically distributed in the peripheral skeleton. The lesions contain a yellow lipid-like substance with a membranocystic structure. The hands, feet, and the long bones in the vicinity of the joints are chiefly involved. On plain films, cystic and expansile radiolucencies with irregular margins and light trabeculation are seen. Pathologic fractures may occur.

PRIMARY SYSTEMIC AMYLOIDOSIS. Primary systemic amyloidosis may rarely involve bone.[269–271] Multiple osteolytic areas are seen because of replacement of bone by amyloid. There is a predilection for the proximal humeral and femoral heads, simulating an appearance of ischemic necrosis. Soft-tissue swelling around the joints due to synovial amyloidosis may be seen. Amyloid arthropathy may also be seen in amyloidosis secondary to myeloma.[272] Infiltration of the bone marrow causes osteopenia and may lead to vertebral collapse (Fig. 5-123).

ELECTRICAL INJURY. Electrical injury may result in discrete areas of rarefaction in bones, as well as

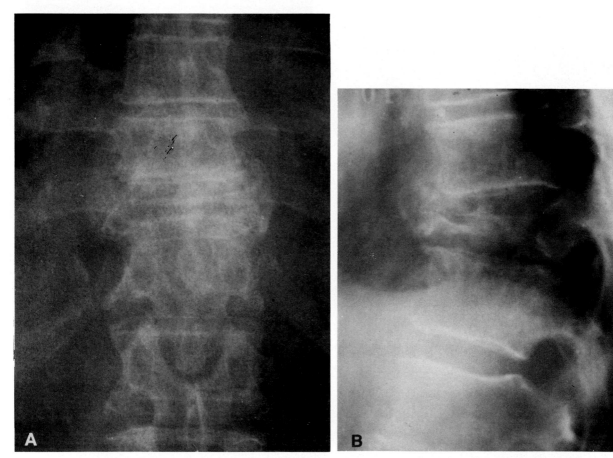

FIGURE 5-123. Primary amyloidosis. **(A)** Anteroposterior and **(B)** lateral radiographs of the lower dorsal spine reveal a wafer-like collapse of the eleventh dorsal vertebra with preservation of the intervertebral spaces. (Courtesy of Dr. Dharmashi V. Bhate, Veterans Administration Hospital, Hines, IL.)

periostitis, resorption of the phalangeal tufts, and fractures.[273] Small rounded densities or bone pearls result from the melting of bone by intense heat. Delayed effects may be manifested as extensive ischemic necrosis.[274] Growth and development are impaired if electrical injury involves the immature skeleton.[275]

KÜMMELL-VERNEUIL DISEASE. Kümmell-Verneuil disease produces the collapse of one or more vertebral bodies following a latent period after trauma, which may have been minor. The lower dorsal or lumbar spine is most often involved. Osteoporosis is followed by osteosclerosis.

SINUS HISTIOCYTOSIS. Sinus histiocytosis (i.e., Rosai-Dorfman disease) is a disease of unknown cause characterized by massive lymph node enlargement, particularly in the neck. The lymph nodes show sinusoidal dilatation with foamy histiocytes and lymphocytes. Clinically, the patients have adenopathy, fever, leukocytosis, and an elevated erythrocyte sedimentation rate. Orbital enlargement and multiple osteolytic bony destructive changes may be seen (Fig. 5-124).[66]

CONDENSING OSTEITIS OF THE CLAVICLE. Condensing osteitis of the clavicle is a rare, benign, painful condition for which the cause is unknown.[276–278] It occurs in young women and may be produced by chronic stress or inflammation at the sternoclavicular joint. Radiologically, unilateral osteosclerosis and enlargement of the sternal end of the clavicle are seen. The joint is usually not involved, but osteophytes may be present. This should not be mistaken for an osteoblastic metastasis.

DIFFERENTIAL DIAGNOSIS OF NONMALIGNANT MULTIPLE SKELETAL RADIONUCENCIES. The differential diagnosis of nonmalignant multiple skeletal radiolucencies includes aggressive fibromatosis, congenital scattered fibromatosis, cystic angiomatosis, cystic lymphangiomatosis, familial hypercholesterolemia, familial multiple nonosteogenic fibromas, fibrous dysplasia, histiocytosis X, hydatidosis, intraosseous hemangiomatosis, membranous lipodystrophy, primary systemic amyloidosis, sinus histiocytosis, and Weber-Christian disease.

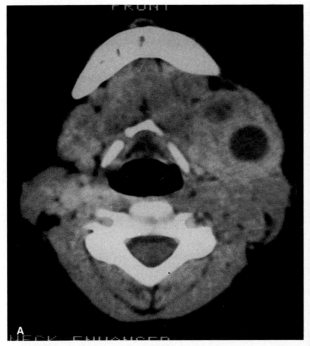

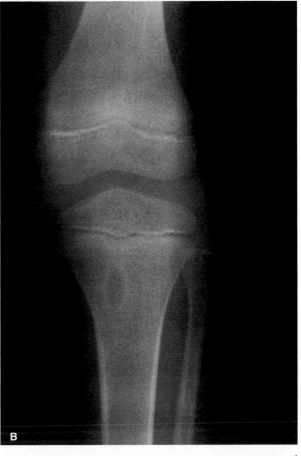

FIGURE 5-124. Sinus histiocytosis. (**A**) CT scan of the neck shows massive lymph node enlargement with central necrotic areas on the patient's left side. (**B**) An anteroposterior view shows an ovoid destructive lesion at the proximal tibial metaphysis and medially involving the epiphyseal ossification center. (**C**) A lateral view of the ankle shows well-marginated osteolytic lesions involving the talus, calcaneus, and cuboid bones.

continued

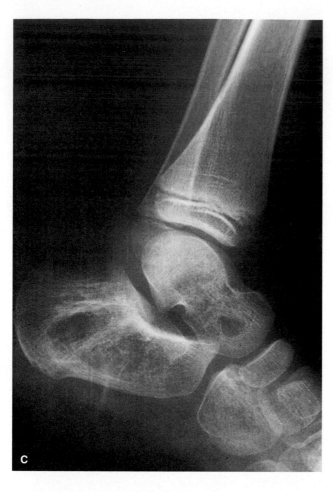

C

FIGURE 5-124. *(Continued)*

References

1. Kagan AR, Stecket RJ, Bassett LW et al: Radiologic contributions to cancer management. AJR Am J Roentgenol 147:305–312, 1986

1a. Fordham EW, Ali A, Turner DA, Charters JR: Atlas of Total Body Radionuclide Imaging. Vol. 1. Philadelphia, Harper & Row, 1982

1b. Licata AA, Farnand B, Gangemi R et al: Symmetrical bone scan in a patient with acute hypercalcemia. Arch Intern Med 143:1779–1781, 1983

2. Helms CA, Cann CE, Brunelle FO et al: Detection of bone marrow metastases using quantitative computed tomography. Radiology 140:745–750, 1981

3. Hermann G, Rose JS, Strauss L: Tumor infiltration of the bone marrow: Comparative study using computed tomography. Skeletal Radiol 11:17–21, 1984

4. Muindi J, Coombes RC, Golding S et al: The role of computed tomography in the detection of bone metastases in breast cancer patients. Br J Radiol 56:233–236, 1983

5. Moore SG, Dawson KL: Red and yellow marrow in the femur: Age-related changes in appearance at MR imaging. Radiology 175:219–223, 1990

6. Sugimura K, Yamasaki K et al: Bone marrow diseases of the spine: Differentiation with T1 and T2 relaxation times in MR imaging. Radiology 165:541–544, 1987

7. Weigert VF, Reiser M et al: Die darstellung neoplastisher wirbelveraenderungen durch die MR-tomographie. Fortschr Geb Rontgenstr 146:123–130, 1987

8. Beltran J, Noto AM et al: Tumors of the osseous spine: Staging with MR imaging versus CT. Radiology 162:565–569, 1987

9. Yaghmai I: Angiography of Bone and Soft Tissue Lesions. New York, Springer-Verlag, 1979

10. Kabela VM, Florianova M, Feit J et al: Nephroblastom bei einem erwachsenen mann mit multiplen osteoplastischen "knochenmetastasen." Fortschr Geb Rontgenstr 135:744–746, 1981

11. Neugut AI, Casper ES, Godwin RA et al: Osteoblastic metastases in renal cell carcinoma. Br J Radiol 54:1002–1004, 1981

12. Reidy JF: Osteoblastic metastases from a hypernephroma. Br J Radiol 48:225–227, 1975

13. Reyes J, Shimaoka K, Ghoorah J et al: Osteoblastic metastases from medullary carcinoma of the thyroid. Br J Radiol 53:1003–1006, 1980

14. Saha MM: Case of the spring season. Semin Roentgenol 18:69, 1983

15. Joffe N, Antonioli DA: Osteoblastic bone metastases secondary to adenocarcinoma of the pancreas. Clin Radiol 29:41–46, 1978

16. Peterson RT, Haidak DJ, Ferris RA et al: Osteoblastic bone metastases in Zollinger-Ellison syndrome. Radiology 118:63–64, 1976

17. Schatzki SC, McIlmoyle S, Lowis S: Diffuse osteoblastic metastases from an intracranial glioma. AJR Am J Roentgenol 128:321–323, 1977

18. Tsai FY, Lisella RS, Lee KF, Roach JF: Osteosclerosis of base of skull as a manifestation of tumor invasion. AJR Am J Roentgenol 124:256–264, 1975

19. Shaffer DL, Pendergrass HP: Comparison of enzyme, clin-

ical, radiographic, and radionuclide methods of detecting bone metastases from carcinoma of the prostate. Radiology 121:431–434, 1976

20. Napoli LD, Hansen HH, Muggia FM, Twigg HL: The incidence of osseous involvement in lung cancer, with special reference to the development of osteoblastic changes. Radiology 108:17–21, 1973
21. Evison G, Pizey N, Roylance J: Bone formation associated with osseous metastases from bladder carcinoma. Clin Radiol 32:303–309, 1981
22. Brutschin P, Culver GJ: Extracranial metastases from medulloblastomas. Radiology 107:359–362, 1973
23. Debnam JW, Staple TW: Osseous metastases from cerebellar medulloblastoma. Radiology 107:363–365, 1973
24. Bach M, Simpson WJ, Platts ME: Metastatic cerebellar sarcoma (desmoplastic medulloblastoma) with diffuse osteosclerosis and leukoerythroblastic anemia: A case report and review of the literature. AJR Am J Roentgenol 103:38–43, 1968
25. Pollen JJ, Schlaer WJ: Osteoblastic response to successful treatment of metastatic cancer of the prostate. AJR Am J Roentgenol 132:927–931, 1979
26. Pollen JJ, Reznek RH, Talner LB: Lysis of osteoblastic lesions in prostatic cancer: A sign of progression. AJR Am J Roentgenol 142:1175–1179, 1984
27. Hart KZ, Brower AC: Unilateral hypertrophy of multiple pedicles. AJR Am J Roentgenol 129:739–740, 1977
28. Maldague BE, Malghem JJ: Unilateral arch hypertrophy with spinous process tilt: A sign of arch deficiency. Radiology 121:567–574, 1976
29. Sherman FC, Wilkinson RH, Hall JE: Reactive sclerosis of a pedicle and spondylosis in the lumbar spine. J Bone Joint Surg [Am] 59:49–54, 1977
30. Yochum TR, Sellers LT, Oppenheimer DA et al: The sclerotic pedicle—how many causes are there? Skeletal Radiol 19:411–417, 1990
31. Hertz M, Solomon A, Aghai E: "Ivory vertebra" in Hodgkin's disease: Restoration of trabecular pattern after therapy. JAMA 238:2402, 1977
32. Kirkwood JR, Margolis T, Newton TH: Prostatic metastasis to the base of the skull simulating meningioma en plaque. AJR Am J Roentgenol 112:774–778, 1971
33. Peavy PW, Rogers JV, Clements JL, Burns JB: Unusual osteoblastic metastases from carcinoid tumors. Radiology 107:327–330, 1973
34. Massie JD, Sebes J: The headless bone scan: An uncommon manifestation of metastatic superscan in carcinoma of the prostate. Skeletal Radiol 17:111–113, 1988
35. Pollen JJ, Witztum KF, Ashburn WL: The flare phenomenon on radionuclide bone scan in metastatic prostate cancer. AJR Am J Roentgenol 142:773–776, 1984
36. Levenson RM, Sauer Brunn BJL, Bates MR et al: Comparative value of bone scintigraphy and radiography in monitoring tumor response in systemically treated prostatic carcinoma. Radiology 146:513–518, 1983
37. Amin R: Case reports: Regression of osteoblastic metastases from carcinoma of the prostate following therapy with tamoxifen. Br J Radiol 59:703–704, 1986
38. Algra PR, Postma T, Van Groeningen CJ, et al: MR imaging of skeletal metastases from neuroblastoma. Skeletal Radiol 21:425–480, 1992
39. Greenfield GB, Clark RA, Messina et al: Bone changes in non-Hodgkin lymphoma. Radiology 185(Suppl P):366, 1992
40. Schweitzer ME, Levine C. Mitchell DG et al: Bull's-eyes and halos: Useful MR discriminators of osseous metastases. Radiology 188:249–252, 1993
41. Green AE, Ellswood WH, Collins JR: Melorheostosis and osteopoikilosis. AJR Am J Roentgenol 87:1096–1111, 1962
42. Lagier R, Nussle D: Anatomy and radiology of a bone island. Fortschr Geb Rontgenstr 128:261–264, 1978
43. Resnick D, Nemcek AA Jr, Haghighi P: Spinal enostoses (bone islands). Radiology 147:373–376, 1983
44. Smith J: Giant bone islands. Radiology 107:35–36, 1973
45. Go RT, El-Khoury GY, Wehbe MA: Radionuclide bone image in growing and stable bone island. Skeletal Radiol 5:15–18, 1980
46. Greenspan A, Steiner G, Knutzon R: Bone island (enostosis): Clinical significance and radiologic and pathologic correlations. Skeletal Radiol 20:85–90, 1991
47. Jacobson HG et al: Agnogenic myeloid metaplasia. Radiology 72:716–725, 1959
48. Pettigrew JD, Ward HP: Correlation of radiologic, histologic, and clinical findings in agnogenic myeloid metaplasia. Radiology 93:541–548, 1969
49. Coughlin C, Greenwald ES, Schraft WC, Grossman S: Myelofibrosis associated with multiple myeloma. Arch Intern Med 138:590–592, 1978
50. Jennings WH, Yang-Chin L, Kiely JM: Concomitant myelofibrosis with agnogenic myeloid metaplasia and malignant lymphoma. Mayo Clin Proc 58:617–619, 1983
51. Barer M et al: Mastocytosis with osseous lesions resembling metastatic malignant lesions in bone. J Bone Joint Surg [Am] 50:142–152, 1968
52. Bendel WL, Race GJ: Urticaria pigmentosa with bone involvement. Case report and analysis of 21 cases from the literature. J Bone Joint Surg [Am] 45:1043–1056, 1963
53. Jaffe HL: Tumors and Tumorous Conditions of the Bones and Joints. Philadelphia, Lea & Febiger, 1958
54. Semerak VM: Urticaria pigmentosa mit skelettbeteiligung-mastozytosesyndrom. Fortschr Geb Rontgenstr 133:673–674, 1980
55. Huang TY, Yam LT et al: Radiological features of systemic mast-cell disease. Br J Radiol 60:765–770, 1987
56. Hills E, Dunstan CR, Evans RA: Bone metabolism in systemic mastocytosis. J Bone Joint Surg [Am] 63:665–669, 1981
57. Lucaya J et al: Mastocytosis with skeletal and gastrointestinal involvement in infancy. Radiology 131:363–366, 1979
58. Komar NN, Gabrielsen TO, Holt JF: Roentgenographic appearance of lumbosacral spine and pelvis in tuberous sclerosis. Radiology 89:701–705, 1967
59. Nathanson N, Anvet NL: An unusual x-ray finding in tuberous sclerosis. Br J Radiol 39:786–787, 1966
60. Cassidy SB, Pagon RA, Pepin M et al: Family studies in tuberous sclerosis. JAMA 249:1302–1304, 1983
61. Steinbach LS, Johnston JO: Case report 777. Skeletal Radiol 22:203–205, 1993
62. Durot JF, Gatfosse M et al: Diagnostic d'une vertebre d'ivoire. J Radiol 67:315–321, 1986
63. Feldman F, Seaman WB: The neurologic complications of Paget's disease in the cervical spine. AJR Am J Roentgenol 105:375–382, 1969
64. Zlatkin MB, Lander PH et al: Paget disease of the spine: CT with clinical correlation. Radiology 160:155–159, 1986
65. Seaman WB: The roentgen appearance of early Paget's disease. AJR Am J Roentgenol 66:587–594, 1951
66. Korber J, McCarthy S, Marsden W: Case report 782. Skeletal Radiol 22:222–225, 1993
67. Roy C, Bourjat P, Dirheimer Y, Wackenheim C: Fissures corticales de la maladie de Paget. J Radiol 64:525–527, 1983
68. Grundy M, Patton JT: Hand in Paget's disease. Br J Radiol 42:748–752, 1969
69. Ardran GM, Kemp FH: Radium poisoning: Two case reports. Br J Radiol 31:605–610, 1958
70. Hall FM: Incidence of bone sarcoma in Paget disease. Radiology 148:865, 1983
71. Price CHG, Goldie W: Paget's sarcoma of bone. J Bone Joint Surg [Br] 51:205–224, 1969
72. Hutter RVP, Foote FW, Frazell EL, Francis KC: Giant-cell tumors complicating Paget's disease of bone. Cancer 16:1044–1056, 1963
73. Schajowicz F, Slullite I: Giant-cell tumor associated with

Paget's disease of bone. J Bone Joint Surg [Am] 48:1340–1349, 1966

74. Kadir S, Kalisher L, Schiller AL: Extramedullary hematopoiesis in Paget's disease of bone. AJR Am J Roentgenol 129:493–495, 1977

75. Douglas DL, Duckworth T, Kanis JA et al: Spinal cord dysfunction in Paget's disease of bone. J Bone Joint Surg [Br] 63:495–503, 1981

76. Bassett LW, Gold RH, Webber MM: Radionuclide bone imaging. Radiol Clin North Am 19:675–702, 1981

77. Schlesinger A, Naimark A, Lee VW: Diaphyseal presentation of Paget disease in long bones. Radiology 147:83–84, 1983

78. Lodwick GS: Solitary malignant tumors of bone: The application of predictor variables in diagnosis. Semin Roentgenol 1:293–313, 1966

79. Forbes GS, McLeod RA, Hattery RR: Radiographic manifestations of bone metastases from renal carcinoma. AJR Am J Roentgenol 129:61–66, 1977

80. Erlemann VR, Roessner A et al: Tumoroese raumforderungen der wirbelsaeule. Fortschr Geb Rontgenstr 146:403–409, 1987

81. Harrington KD: Metastatic disease of the spine. J Bone Joint Surg 68:1110–1115, 1986

82. Hendriz RW, Rogers LF, Davis TM: Cortical bone metastases. Radiology 181:409–413, 1991

83. Frouge C, Metzger M et al: Metastase sous-periostee d'un adenocarcinome oesophagien. J Radiol 68:773–775, 1987

84. Coerkamp EG, Kroon HM: Cortical bone metastases. Radiology 169:525–528, 1988

85. Greenspan A, Norman A: Osteolytic cortical destruction: An unusual pattern of skeletal metastases. Skeletal Radiol 17:402–406, 1988

86. O'Connell D: Metastasis in the nasal bones. Clin Radiol 9:97–98, 1958

87. Lally JR, Cossrow JL, Dalinka MK: Odontoid fractures in metastatic breast carcinoma. AJR Am J Roentgenol 128:817–820, 1977

88. Phillips CD, Pope TL et al: Nontraumatic avulsion of the lesser trochanter: A pathognomonic sign of metastatic disease? Skeletal Radiol 17:106–110, 1988

89. Amorosa JK, Weintraub S et al: Sacral destruction: Foraminal lines revisited. AJR Am J Roentgenol 145:773–775, 1985

90. Pirschel J, Metzger HOFJ, Wismann C: Malignant metastases to the periphery of the skeleton. Fortschr Geb Rontgenstr 129:621–626, 1978

91. Cary PC, Helms CA, Genant HK: Metastatic disease to the carpus. Br J Radiol 54:992–994, 1981

92. Greenfield GB, Escamilla CH, Schorsch HA: The hand as an indicator of generalized disease. AJR Am J Roentgenol 99:736–745, 1967

93. Vaezy A, Budson DC: Phalangeal metastases from bronchogenic carcinoma. JAMA 239:226–227, 1978

94. Healey JH, Turnbull AD et al: Acrometastases. J Bone Joint Surg 68:743–746, 1986

95. Jarde O, Prigent F et al: Les metastases osseuses des doigts. J Radiol 67:621–624, 1986

96. Kerin R: Metastatic tumors of the hand. J Bone Joint Surg [Am] 65:1331–1335, 1983

97. Uriboro IMF, Morchio FJ, Marin JC: Metastases of carcinoma of the larynx and thyroid gland to the phalanges of the hand: Report of 2 cases. J Bone Joint Surg [Am] 58:134–135, 1976

98. Libson E, Bloom RA et al: Metastatic tumours of bones of the hand and foot. Skeletal Radiol 16:387–392, 1987

99. Mootoosamy IM, Anchor SC et al: Expanding osteolytic bone metastases from carcinoma of the breast: An unusual appearance. Skeletal Radiol 14:188–190, 1985

100. Golimbu C, Firooznia H et al: Hepatocellular carcinoma with skeletal metastasis. Radiology 154:617–618, 1985

101. Kuhlman JE, Fishman EK et al: Skeletal metastases from hepatoma: Frequency, distribution, and radiographic features. Radiology 160:175–178, 1986

102. Reed JD, Fishman EK, Kuhlman JE et al: Case report 535. Skeletal Radiol 18:161–163, 1989

103. Lynn MD, Braunstein EM et al: Bone metastases in pheochromocytoma: Comparative studies of efficacy of imaging. Radiology 160:701–706, 1986

104. Lynn MD, Braunstein EM et al: Pheochromocytoma presenting as musculoskeletal pain from bone metastases. Skeletal Radiol 16:552–555, 1987

105. Deutsch A, Resnick D: Eccentric cortical metastases to the skeleton from bronchogenic carcinoma. Radiology 137:49–52, 1980

106. Bassan JS, Glaser MG: Bony metastasis in carcinoma of the uterine cervix. Clin Radiol 33:623–625, 1982

107. Loughran CF: Bone metastases from squamous-cell carcinoma of the larynx. Clin Radiol 34:447–450, 1983

108. Jennings PG, Cook PL: Bony metastases from intracranial meningioma. Br J Radiol 56:421–422, 1983

109. Hornsby VPL: Bony metastases from malignant intra-cranial astrocytoma. Neuroradiology 27:426–429, 1985

110. Meltzer CC, Fishman EK, Scott WW: Computed tomography appearance of bone metastases of leiomyosarcoma. Skeletal Radiol 21:445–447, 1992

111. Barry WF Jr, Wells SA Jr, Cox CE et al: Clinical and radiographic correlations in breast cancer patients with osseous metastases. Skeletal Radiol 6:27–32, 1981

112. Mink J: Percutaneous bone biopsy in the patient with known or suspected osseous metastases. Radiology 161:191–194, 1986

113. Hall BB, Fitzgerald RH Jr, Rosenblatt JE: Anaerobic osteomyelitis. J Bone Joint Surg [Am] 65:30–35, 1983

114. Kido D, Bryan D, Halpern M: Hematogenous osteomyelitis in drug addicts. AJR Am J Roentgenol 118:356–363, 1973

115. Miskew DBW, Lorenz MA, Pearson RL et al: *Pseudomonas aeruginosa* bone and joint infection in drug abusers. J Bone Joint Surg [Am] 65:829–832, 1983

116. Salahuddin JI, Madhavan T, Fisher EJ et al: *Pseudomonas* osteomyelitis: Radiologic features. Radiology 109:41–47, 1973

117. Bryan CS: Vertebral osteomyelitis due to *Cryptococcus neoformans:* A case report. J Bone Joint Surg [Am] 59:275–276, 1977

118. Newman JH: Non-infective disease of the diabetic foot. J Bone Joint Surg [Br] 63:593–596, 1981

119. Beltran J, Campanini DS, Knight C et al: The diabetic foot: Magnetic resonance imaging evaluation. Skeletal Radiol 19:37–41, 1990

120. Ghahremani GG: Osteomyelitis of the ilium in patients with Crohn's disease. AJR Am J Roentgenol 118:364–370, 1973

121. Capitanio MA, Kirkpatrick JA: Early roentgen observations in acute osteomyelitis. AJR Am J Roentgenol 108:488–496, 1970

122. Nade S: Acute haematogenous osteomyelitis in infancy and childhood. J Bone Joint Surg [Br] 65:109–119, 1983

123. O'Brien T, McManus F, MacAuley PH et al: Acute haematogenous osteomyelitis. J Bone Joint Surg [Br] 64:450–453, 1982

124. Abiri MM, DeAngelis GA, Kirpekar M et al: Ultrasonic detection of osteomyelitis. Pathologic correlation in an animal model. Invest Radiol 27:111–113, 1992

125. Rosen RA, Morehouse HT, Karp HJ et al: Intracortical fissuring in osteomyelitis. Radiology 141:17–20, 1981

126. Roberts PH: Disturbed epiphyseal growth at the knee after osteomyelitis in infancy. J Bone Joint Surg [Br] 52:692–703, 1970

127. Azouz EM, Greenspan A, Marton D: CT evaluation of primary epiphyseal bone abscesses. Skeletal Radiol 22:17–23, 1993

128. Morrey BF, Bianco AJ, Rhodes KH: Hematogenous osteo-

myelitis at uncommon sites in children. Mayo Clin Proc 53:707–713, 1978

129. Nixon GW: Hematogenous osteomyelitis of metaphyseal-equivalent locations. AJR Am J Roentgenol 130:123–129, 1978

130. Whelan MA, Schonfeld S et al: Computed tomography of nontuberculous spinal infection. J Comput Assist Tomogr 9:280–287, 1985

131. Golimbu C, Firooznia H, Rafii M: CT of osteomyelitis of the spine. AJR Am J Roentgenol 142:159–163, 1984

132. Kattpuram SV, Phillips WC, Boyd R: CT in pyogenic osteomyelitis of the spine. AJR Am J Roentgenol 140:1199 1201, 1983

133. Price AC, Allen JH, Eggers FM et al: Intervertebral disk-space infection: CT changes. Radiology 149:725–729, 1983

134. Larde D, Mathieu T, Frija J et al: Vertebral osteomyelitis: Disk hypodensity on CT. AJR Am J Roentgenol 139:963–967. 1982

135. Ram PC, Martinez S, Korobkin M et al: CT detection of intraosseous gas: A new sign of osteomyelitis. AJR Am J Roentgenol 137:721–723, 1981

136. Rafii M, Firooznia H et al: Hematogenous osteomyelitis with fat-fluid level shown by CT. Radiology 153:493–494, 1984

137. Gold RH, Hawkins RA, Katz RD: Bacterial osteomyelitis: Findings on plain radiography, CT, MR, and scintigraphy. AJR Am J Roentgenol 157:365–370, 1991

138. Modic MT, Pflanze W et al: Magnetic resonance imaging of musculoskeletal infections. Radiol Clin North Am 24:247–258, 1986

139. Reiser VM, Kahn T et al: Ergebnisse der MR-tomographie in der diagnostik der osteomyelitis und arthritis. Fortschr Geb Rontgenstr 145:661–666, 1986

140. Tang JSH, Gold RH et al: Musculoskeletal infection of the extremities: Evaluation with MR imaging. Radiology 166:205–209, 1988

141. Unger E, Moldofsky P et al: Diagnosis of osteomyelitis by MR imaging. AJR Am J Roentgenol 150:605–610, 1988

142. Modic MT, Feiglin DH et al: Vertebral osteomyelitis: Assessment using MR. Radiology 157:157–166, 1985

143. Fletcher FD, Scoles PF, Nelson AD: Osteomyelitis in children: Detection by magnetic resonance. Radiology 150:57–60, 1984

144. Bassett LW, Gold RH, Webber MM: Radionuclide bone imaging. Radiol Clin North Am 19:675–702, 1981

145. Howie DW, Savage JP, Wilson TG et al: The technetium phosphate bone scan in the diagnosis of osteomyelitis in childhood. J Bone Joint Surg [Am] 65:431–437, 1983

146. Jones DC, Cady RB: "Cold" bone scans in adult osteomyelitis. J Bone Joint Surg [Br] 63:376–378, 1981

147. Allwright SJ, Miller JH, Gilsanz V: Subperiosteal abscess in children: Scintigraphic appearance. Radiology 179:725–729, 1991

148. Sorsdahl OA, Goodhart GL, Williams HT et al: Quantitative bone gallium scintigraphy in osteomyelitis. Skeletal Radiol 22:239–242, 1993

149. Raptopoulos V, Doherty PW, Goss TP et al: Acute osteomyelitis: Advantage of white cell scans in early detection. AJR Am J Roentgenol 129:1077–1082, 1982

150. Schauwecker DS: Osteomyelitis: Diagnosis with In-111-labeled leukocytes. Radiology 171:141–146, 1989

151. Jacobson AF, Harley JD, Lipskey BA: Diagnosis of osteomyelitis in the presence of soft-tissue infection and radiologic evidence of osseous abnormalities: Value of leukocyte scintigraphy. AJR Am J Roentgenol 157:807–812, 1991

152. Samra Y, Hertz M, Shaked Y et al: Brucellosis of the spine. J Bone Joint Surg [Br] 64:429–431, 1982

153. Sharif HS, Aideyan OA, Clark DC et al: Brucellar and tuberculous spondylitis: Comparative imaging features. Radiology 171:419–425, 1989

154. Keenan MA, Guttman GG: *Brucella* osteomyelitis of the

distal part of the femur. J Bone Joint Surg [Am] 64:142–144, 1982

155. Eismont FJ, Bohlman HH, Soni PL et al: Pyogenic and fungal vertebral osteomyelitis with paralysis. J Bone Joint Surg [Am] 65:19–29, 1983

156. Zigler JE, Bohlman HH et al: Pyogenic osteomyelitis of the occiput, the atlas, and the axis: A report of five cases. J Bone Joint Surg 69:1069–1073, 1987

157. Bielecki DK, Sartoris D et al: Intraosseous and intradiscal gas in association with spinal infection: Report of three cases. AJR Am J Roentgenol 147:83–86, 1986

158. Baron AL, Steinbach LS, LeBoit PE et al: Osteolytic lesions and bacillary angiomatosis in HIV infection: Radiologic differentiation from AIDS-related Kaposi sarcoma. Radiology 177:77–81, 1990

158a. Ahlback S, Collert S: Destruction of the odontoid process due to atlanto-axial pyogenic spondylitis. Acta Radiol [Diagn] 10:394–400, 1970

159. Laurent F, Diard F et al: Les osteomyelites circonscrites non tuberculeuses de l'enfant: A propos de 31 cases. J Radiol 65:545–553, 1984

160. Miller WB, Murphy WA, Gilula LA: Brodie abscess: Reappraisal. Radiology 132:15–23, 1979

161. Johnson LL, Kempson RL: Epidermoid carcinoma in chronic osteomyelitis: Diagnostic problems and management: Report of 10 cases. J Bone Joint Surg [Am] 47:133–145, 1965

162. Fitzgerald RH, Brewer NS, Dahlin DC: Squamous-cell carcinoma complicating chronic osteomyelitis. J Bone Joint Surg [Am] 58:1146–1148, 1976

163. Johnston RM, Miles JS: Sarcomas arising from chronic osteomyelitic sinuses. J Bone Joint Surg [Am] 55:162–168, 1973

164. Morris JM, Lucas DB: Fibrosarcoma within a sinus tract of chronic draining osteomyelitis: Case report and review of the literature. J Bone Joint Surg [Am] 46:853–857, 1964

165. Brown T, Wilkinson RH: Chronic recurrent multifocal osteomyelitis. Radiology 166:493–496, 1988

166. Cyrlak D, Pais MJ: Chronic recurrent multifocal osteomyelitis. Skeletal Radiol 15:32–39, 1986

167. Wiener MD, Newbold RG et al: Chronic recurrent multifocal osteomyelitis: Case report. AJR Am J Roentgenol 146:87–88, 1986

168. Reuland P, Feine U, Handgretinger R et al: Case report 756. Skeletal Radiol 21:478–481, 1992

169. Wing VW, Jeffrey RB Jr et al: Chronic osteomyelitis examined by CT. Radiology 154:171–174, 1985

170. Janson VR, Khr J, Lackner K et al: CT: Diagnostik der chronischen osteomyelitis. Fortschr Geb Rontgenstr 134:517–522, 1981

171. Alazraki N, Fierer J et al: Chronic osteomyelitis: Monitoring by ^{99m}Tc phosphate and ^{67}Ga citrate imaging. AJR Am J Roentgenol 145:767–771, 1985

172. Al-Sheikh W, Sfakianakis GN et al: Subacute and chronic bone infections: Diagnosis using In-111, Ga-67 and Tc-99m MDP bone scintigraphy, and radiography. Radiology 155:501–506, 1985

173. Kim EE, Pjura GA et al: Osteomyelitis complicating fracture: Pitfalls of 111In in leukocyte scintigraphy. AJR Am J Roentgenol 148:927–930, 1987

174. Maurer AH, Millmond SH et al: Infection in diabetic osteoarthropathy: Use of indium-labeled leukocytes for diagnosis. Radiology 161:221–225, 1986

175. Tumeh SS, Aliabadi P et al: Chronic osteomyelitis: Bone and gallium scan patterns associated with active disease. Radiology 158:685–688, 1986

176. Mason MD, Zlatkin MB, Esterhai JL et al: Chronic complicated osteomyelitis of the lower extremity: Evaluation with MR imaging. Radiology 173:355–359, 1989

177. Quinn SF, Murray W, Clark RA et al: MR imaging of chronic osteomyelitis. J Comp Assist Tomography 12:113–117, 1988

178. Poppel MH, Lawrence LR, Jacobson HG, Stein J: Skeletal

tuberculosis: A roentgenographic survey with reconsideration of diagnostic criteria. AJR Am J Roentgenol 70:936–963, 1953

179. Feldman F, Auerbach R, Johnston A: Tuberculous dactylitis in the adult. AJR Am J Roentgenol 112:460–479, 1971

180. O'Connor BT, Steel WM, Sanders R: Disseminated bone tuberculosis. J Bone Joint Surg [Am] 52:537–542, 1970

181. Mazas-Artasona L, Led A, Espinosa H et al: Case report 737. Skeletal Radiol 21:323–325, 1992

182. Fang D, Leong JCY, Fang HSY: Tuberculosis of the upper cervical spine. J Bone Joint Surg [Br] 65:47–50, 1983

183. Berges O, Sassoon C, Roche A et al: Abcès du psoas d'origine tuberculeuse sans spondylodiscite visible. J Radiol 62:467–470, 1981

184. Roos AD, Meerten ELVPV et al: MRI of tuberculous spondylitis. AJR Am J Roentgenol 146:79–82, 1986

185. Bell D, Cockshott WP: Tuberculosis of the vertebral pedicles. Radiology 99:43–48, 1971

186. Wolstein D, Rabinowitz JG, Twersky J: Tuberculosis of the rib. J Can Assoc Radiol 25:307–309, 1974

187. Lynch AF: Tuberculosis of the greater trochanter. J Bone Joint Surg [Br] 64:185–188, 1982

188. Richter VR, Köhler G, Michels P: Tuberkulöse kalkaneusherde, ihre behandlung und differential-diagnose. Fortschr Geb Rontgenstr 135:583–587, 1981

189. Shah P, Ramakantan R: Tuberculosis of the patella. Br J Radiol 63:363–364, 1990

190. Witcombe JB, Gremin BJ: Tuberculous erosion of the sphenoid bone. Br J Radiol 51:347–350, 1978

191. Brown TS: Tuberculosis of the ribs. Clin Radiol 31:681–684, 1980

192. Rust RJ, Park HM, Robb JA: Skeletal scintigraphy in miliary tuberculosis: Photopenia after treatment. AJR Am J Roentgenol 137:877–879, 1981

193. Reither VM, Kaiser W et al: Bedeutung der kernspintomographie fuer die diagnostik von knochenmarkserkrankungen im kindesalter. Fortschr Geb Rontgenstr 147:647–653, 1987

194. Van Zanten TEG, Golding RP et al: Nuclear magnetic resonance imaging of bone marrow in childhood leukaemia. Clin Radiol 39:77–81, 1988

195. Dewes VW, Ruhlmann J et al: MR Tomographie bei Lymphatischen und Leukemischen Knochenmarkinfiltrationen. Fortschr Geb Rontgenstr 147:654–661, 1987

196. McKinstry CS, Steiner RE et al: Bone marrow in leukemia and aplastic anemia: MR imaging before, during, and after treatment. Radiology 162:701–707, 1987

197. Porter BA, Shields A et al: Magnetic resonance imaging of bone marrow disorders. Radiol Clin North Am 24:269–290, 1986

198. Bernhard WG, Gore I, Kilby RA: Congenital leukemia. Blood 6:990–1001, 1951

199. Nixon GW, Gwinn JL: The roentgen manifestations of leukemia in infancy. Radiology 107:603–609, 1973

200. Silberstain MJ et al: Bone changes in a neonate with congenital leukemia. Radiology 131:370, 1979

201. Simmons CR, Harle TS, Singleton EB: The osseous manifestations of leukemia in children. Radiol Clin North Am 6:115–130, 1968

202. Rosenfeld NS, McIntosh S: Prospective analysis of bone changes in treated childhood leukemia. Radiology 123:413–415, 1977

203. Schabel SI, Tyminski L, Holland DR et al: The skeletal manifestations of chronic myelogenous leukemia. Skeletal Radiol 5:145–149, 1980

204. De Boeck M, Peeters O, Camp BV et al: Monocytic leukaemia associated with myeloid metaplasia, resembling metastatic bone disease. Skeletal Radiol 11:9–12, 1984

205. Glatt W, Weinstein A: Acropachy in lymphatic leukemia. Radiology 92:125–126, 1969

206. Stork JT, Cigtay OS, Schellinger D et al: Recurrent choloromas in acute myelogenous leukemia. AJR Am J Roentgenol 142:777–778, 1984

207. Hermann G, Feldman F, Abdelwahab IF et al: Skeletal manifestations of granulocytic sarcoma (chloroma). Skeletal Radiol 20:509–512, 1991

208. Cohen LM, Hill MC et al: CT manifestations of Richter syndrome. J Comput Assist Tomogr 11:1007–1008, 1987

208a. Edeiken-Monroe B, Edeiken J, Kim EE: Radiologic concepts of lymphoma of bone. Radiol Clin North Am 28:841–864, 1990

209. Malloy PC, Fishman EK, Magid D: Lymphoma of bone, muscle, and skin: CT findings. AJR Am J Roentgenol 159:805–809, 1992

210. Braunstein EM: Hodgkin disease of bone: Radiographic correlation with the histological classification. Radiology 137:643–646, 1980

211. Burgener FA, Hamlin DJ: Radiologic manifestation of histiocytic lymphoma in the skeletal and central nervous system. Fortschr Geb Rontgenstr 134:50–55, 1981

212. Nghiem HV, Ellis BI, Haggar AM et al: Juxta-articular large cell lymphoma. Skeletal Radiol 19:353–357, 1990

213. Giudici MAI, Eggli KD, Moser RP et al: Case report 730. Skeletal Radiol 21:260–265, 1992

214. Orzel JA, Sawaf NW et al: Lymphoma of the skeleton: Scintigraphic evaluation. AJR Am J Roentgenol 150:1095–1099

215. Alford BA, Coccia PF, c'Heureuz PR: Roentgenographic features of American Burkitt's lymphoma. Radiology 124:763–770, 1977

216. Beltran G, Baez A, Correa P: Burkitt's lymphoma in Colombia. Am J Med 40:211–216, 1966

217. Ferris RA, Hakkal HG, Cigtay OS: Radiologic manifestations of North American Burkitt's lymphoma. AJR Am J Roentgenol 123:614–620, 1975

218. Fowles JV, Olweny CLM, Katongole-Mbidde E et al: Burkitt's lymphoma in the appendicular skeleton. J Bone Joint Surg [Br] 65:464–471, 1983

219. Dunnick NR: Radiographic manifestations of Burkitt's lymphoma in American patients. AJR Am J Roentgenol 132:1–6, 1979

220. Bloom RA, Peylan-Ramu N, Okon E: Case report 755. Skeletal Radiol 21:474–477, 1992

221. Ennis JT, Whitehouse G, Ross FGM, Middlemiss JH: The radiology of bone changes in histiocytosis. Clin Radiol 24:212–220, 1973

222. Lichtenstein L: Histiocytosis X (eosinophilic granuloma of bone, Letterer-Siwe disease, and Schüller-Christian disease): Further observations of pathological and clinical importance. J Bone Joint Surg [Am] 46:76–90, 1964

223. DeSchepper AMA, Ramon F, Van Marck E: MR imaging of eosinophilic granuloma: Report of 11 cases. Skeletal Radiol 22:163–166, 1993

224. Fowles JV, Bobechko WP: Solitary eosinophilic granuloma in bone. J Bone Joint Surg [Br] 52:238–243, 1970

225. Ochsner SF: Eosinophilic granuloma of bone: Experience with 20 cases. AJR Am J Roentgenol 97:719–726, 1966

226. Peer A, Witz E et al: Solitary eosinophilic granuloma of sternum: Case report with review of the literature. Br J Radiol 58:1173–1176, 1985

227. Cohen M, Zornoza J, Cangir A et al: Direct injection of methylprednisolone sodium succinate in the treatment of solitary eosinophilic granuloma of bone. Radiology 136:289–293, 1980

228. Ruff S, Chapman GK, Taylor TKF et al: The evolution of eosinophilic granuloma of bone: A case report. Skeletal Radiol 10:37–39, 1983

229. Nesbit ME, Wolfson JJ, Kieffer SA, Peterson HO: Orbital sclerosis in histiocytosis X. AJR Am J Roentgenol 110:123–128, 1970

230. Siddiqui AR, Tashjian JH, Lazarus K et al: Nuclear medicine studies in evaluation of skeletal lesions in children with histiocytosis. Radiology 140:787–789, 1981

231. Crone-Munzebrock W, Brassow F: A comparison of radiographic and bone scan findings in histiocytosis X. Skeletal Radiol 9:170–173, 1983

232. Kolar J, Kucera V et al: Erdheim-Chester disease. Fortschr Geb Rontgenstr 141:698–701, 1984

233. Rozenberg I, Wechsler J et al: Erdheim-Chester disease presenting as malignant exophthalmos. Br J Radiol 59:173–177, 1986

234. Waite RJ, Doherty PW et al: Langerhans cell histiocytosis with the radiographic findings of Erdheim-Chester disease: Case Report. AJR Am J Roentgenol 150:869–871, 1988

235. Strouse PJ, Ellis BI, Shifrin LZ et al: Case report 710. Skeletal Radiol 21:64–67, 1992

236. Abrahams J, Ganick D, Gilbert E et al: Massive osteolysis in an infant. AJR Am J Roentgenol 135:1084–1086, 1980

237. Blundell G, Midgley RL, Smith GS: Massive osteolysis: Disappearing bones. J Bone Joint Surg [Br] 40:494–501, 1958

238. Cadenat H, Combelles R, Fabert G, Clovet M: Ostéolyse cryptogénétique de la mandibule. J Radiol 59:509–512, 1978

239. Kery L, Wouters HW: Massive osteolysis: A report of 2 cases. J Bone Joint Surg [Br] 52:452–459, 1970

240. Patrick JH: Massive osteolysis complicated by chylothorax successfully treated by pleurodesis. J Bone Joint Surg [Br] 58:347–349, 1976

241. Sacristan HD, Portal LF, Castresana FG, Pena DR: Massive osteolysis of the scapula and ribs: A case report. J Bone Joint Surg [Am] 59:405–406, 1977

242. Sage MR, Allen PW: Massive osteolysis. J Bone Joint Surg [Br] 56:130–135, 1974

243. Kolar J, Zidková H, Vohralik M et al: Langristige teilremission des gorhamschen syndroms. Fortschr Geb Rontgenstr 134:214–215, 1981

244. Campbell J, Almond HGA, Johnson R: Massive osteolysis of the humerus with spontaneous recovery. J Bone Joint Surg [Br] 57:238–240, 1975

245. Bloem JL, van der Heul RO, Schuttevaer HM: Fibrous dysplasia vs adamantinoma of the tibia: Differentiation based on discriminant analysis of clinical and plain film findings. AJR Am J Roentgenol 156:1017–1023, 1991

245a. Campanacci M: Osteofibrous dysplasia of long bones: A new clinical entity. Ital J Orthop Traumatol 2:221–237, 1976

245b. Campanacci M, Laus M: Osteofibrous dysplasia of the tibia and fibula. J Bone Joint Surg [Am] 63:367–375, 1981

246. Ollivier L, LeClere J, Vanel D et al: Femoral infarction following intraarterial chemotherapy for osteosarcoma of the leg: a possible pitfall in magnetic resonance imaging. Skeletal Radiol 20:329–332, 1991

247. Haller J, Greenway G, Resnick D et al: Intraosseous fat necrosis associated with acute pancreatitis: MR imaging. Radiology 173:193–195, 1989

248. Torres FX, Kyriakos M: Bone infarct-associated osteosarcoma. Cancer 70:2418–2430, 1992

249. Dorfman HD, Norman A, Wolff H: Fibrosarcoma complicating bone infarction in a caisson worker: A case report. J Bone Joint Surg [Am] 48:528–532, 1966

250. Munk PL, Helms CA, Holt RG: Immature bone infarcts: Findings on plain radiographs and MR scans. AJR Am J Roentgenol 152:547–549, 1989

251. Norman A, Steiner GC: Radiographic and morphological features of cyst formation in idiopathic bone infarction. Radiology 146:335–338, 1983

252. Ohta Y, Matsunaga H: Bone lesions in divers. J Bone Joint Surg [Br] 56:3–16, 1974

253. Gregg PJ, Walder DN: A study of old lesions of caisson disease of bone by radiography and bone scintigraphy. J Bone Joint Surg [Br] 62:214–221, 1980

254. MacLeod MA, McEwan AJB, Pearson RR, Houston AS: Functional imaging in the early diagnosis of dysbaric osteonecrosis. Br J Radiol 55:497–500, 1982

255. Naul LG, Peet GJ, Maupin WB: Avascular necrosis of the vertebral body: MR imaging. Radiology 172:219–222, 1989

256. Holzer NJf et al: Bone tumor of the orbit. J Am Med Assoc 238:1758–1759, 1977

257. Doppman JK et al: Differential diagnosis of brown tumor vs cystic osteitis by arteriography and computed tomography. Radiology 131:339–340, 1979

258. Christ VF, Siemes HD, Stiens R: Pelvine knochenangiome. Fortschr Geb Rontgenstr 140:79–83, 1984

259. Köster VR, Jansen H: Generalisierte hämangiomatose des skeletts mit organbefall. Fortschr Geb Rontgenstr 134:69–74, 1981

260. Brower AC, Culver JE, Keats TE: Diffuse cystic angiomatosis of bone: Report of 2 cases. AJR Am J Roentgenol 118:456–463, 1973

261. Hayes JT, Brody GL: Cystic lymphangiectasis of bone: A case report. J Bone Joint Surg [Am] 43:107–117, 1961

262. Schajowicz F et al: Cystic angiomatosis (hamartous haemolymphangiomatosis) of bone. J Bone Joint Surg [Br] 60:100–106, 1978

263. Ellis GL, Brannon RB: Intraosseous lymphangiomas of the mandible. Skeletal Radiol 5:253–256, 1980

264. Baer JW, Radkowski MA: Congenital multiple fibromatosis: A case report with a review of the world literature. AJR Am J Roentgenol 118:200–205, 1973

265. Heiple KG, Perrin E, Masamichi A: Congenital generalized fibromatosis: A case limited to osseous lesions. J Bone Joint Surg [Am] 54:663–669, 1972

266. Campanacci M, Laus M, Boriani S: Multiple nonossifying fibromata with extraskeletal anomalies: A new syndrome? J Bone Joint Surg [Br] 65:627–632, 1983

267. Doel G: Bone involvement in Weber-Christian disease. Br J Radiol 36:140–142, 1963

268. Döhler R, Poser HL, Harms D et al: Systemic lipomatosis of bone. J Bone Joint Surg [Br] 64:84–87, 1982

269. Gardner H: Bone lesions in primary systemic amyloidosis. Br J Radiol 34:778–783, 1961

270. Grossman RE, Hensley GT: Bone lesions in primary amyloidosis. AJR Am J Roentgenol 101:872–875, 1967

271. Weinfeld A, Stern MH, Marx LH: Amyloid lesions of bone. AJR Am J Roentgenol 108:799–805, 1970

272. Tagliabue JR, Stull MA, Lack EE et al: Case report 610. Skeletal Radiol 19:448–452, 1990

273. Brinn LB, Moseley JE: Bone changes following electrical injury. AJR Am J Roentgenol 97:682–686, 1966

274. Barber JW: Delayed bone and joint changes following electrical injury. Radiology 99:49–53, 1971

275. Ogden JA, Southwick WO: Electrical injury involving the immature skeleton. Skeletal Radiol 6:187–192, 1981

276. Greenspan A, Gerscovich E, Szabo RM et al: Condensing osteitis of the clavicle: A rare but frequently misdiagnosed condition. AJR Am J Roentgenol 156:1011–1015, 1991

277. Abdelwahab IF, Hermann G, Ramos R et al: Case report 623. Skeletal Radiol 19:387–389, 1990

278. Gerscovich EO, Greenspan A, Szabo RM: Benign clavicular lesions that may mimic malignancy. Skeletal Radiol 20:173–180, 1991

Bone Marrow Imaging

Stephanie D. Holman Ferris
Martin L. Silbiger

Analysis of the bone marrow is an integral part of the evaluation of musculoskeletal neoplasia. The marrow is a dynamic organ that has an orderly development and responds uniquely to various physiologic stresses. It is virtually always involved regionally in cases of bone neoplasia and systemically in primary marrow neoplasia. There also may be local involvement in cases of soft-tissue neoplasia. The degree of involvement is important in staging, planning treatment options, and prognosis.

Bone marrow imaging in assessing neoplastic disease requires a modality able to demonstrate the anatomy of the region studied and provide as much physiologic information as possible. Although plain radiography, CT, and scintigraphy play important roles in the imaging of skeletal neoplasia, MRI is the imaging modality of choice for evaluating bone marrow response states. MRI is extremely sensitive to changes in the marrow pattern and provides the most precise anatomic localization of histologic change available with current imaging techniques.[1]

There is considerable overlap in the appearance of normal marrow, primary hematologic abnormalities, and changes secondary to osseous diseases and external insult. Many pathologic states demonstrate characteristic disease patterns of distribution with respect to the bone marrow.[2] A basic working knowledge of the anatomy and physiology of bone marrow, its imaging characteristics secondary to normal aging, and patterns of response to various physiologic demands is crucial when evaluating the marrow for neoplastic involvement.

ANATOMY AND PHYSIOLOGY

The first detectable hematopoietic activity begins in the fetal yolk sac in the first weeks after conception and progresses to the liver and spleen early in fetal development. Bone marrow appears in the fourth fetal month, is the dominant hematopoietic organ at 6 months, and becomes the sole hematopoietic organ at birth.[3] All skeletal marrow is "red" or cellularly active at birth. The cellular elements—erythrocytes, leukocytes, and megakaryocytes—are supported by primary and bridging bony trabeculae combined with fat, reticulum cells, nerves, and vascular sinusoids. The trabeculae are constantly remodeled in response to growth and skeletal stress. Stem cells and blood cell lines at various stages of maturation coexist in the marrow, replenishing the peripheral blood as needed. Reticulum cells consist of macrophages and nondifferentiated cells of uncertain function. Lymph nodules without discrete lymph vessels are present. Marrow fat cells are smaller and have increased metabolic activity relative to body fat. Vascular sinusoids anastomose around them extensively. Marrow fat functions as more than filler material, providing nutritional and structural support. Fat cells shrink during periods of increased marrow activity, but in quiescent periods, the number and volume of fat cells increases.[1,4–6]

During growth and with aging, the red marrow converts to yellow or fatty marrow. Several mechanisms for initiation of this process have been described.[7–9] Physiologic factors, including intramedullary temperature, oxygen tension changes, and vascular changes, have been studied. The nutrient artery and its branches in a long bone containing red marrow are larger than in a bone that contains yellow marrow. With yellow marrow conversion, proliferated fat cells surround diminished-caliber capillaries, venules, and veins. These vessels become relatively sparsely distributed, decreasing the effective vascularity.

In general, marrow conversion occurs from the periphery of the skeleton centrally and from diaphysis to metaphysis in an individual long bone. Conversion occurs most rapidly in the periphery and progresses more slowly centrally. Marrow conversion is normally complete in the phalanges at 1 year of age. By 7 years of age, fat can be macroscopically detected in the distal epiphyses of all long bones except the femora and humeri.[3,8] Similar changes occur in the skull. The clivus and calvarium contain red marrow in virtually all newborns. This red marrow distribution converts to yellow marrow in 95% of persons studied by 25 years of age.[10] If red marrow persists in the adult skull, it is most likely seen in the parietal bone. The culmination of the conversion process into the adult marrow distribution usually occurs macroscopically by 25 years of age. Red marrow persists in vertebral bodies, sternum, ribs, pelvis, and the proximal femoral and humeral shafts. There is variable retention of red marrow in the skull, in the facial bones, and rarely, in the calcaneus. The extent of marrow in long bone shafts varies. Rests of red marrow are present microscopically even in the quite fatty yellow marrow of elderly persons.[3]

Cartilaginous epiphyses and apophyses lack marrow until ossification begins. In normal persons, if red marrow exists in these regions, it is so rapidly converted to yellow marrow that it is easier to think of these as containing only yellow marrow.[1,11] Microscopic changes in cellularity continue to occur throughout life. Red marrow cellularity in the axial skeleton may be greater than 75% at 25 years of age but may decline to 50% at 70 years of age.[3,5] Ultimately, a red-yellow marrow balance is achieved for each person. Variations exist from person to person and from bone to bone. However, marrow distribution in the extremities is grossly symmetric bilaterally,[3] and vertebral bodies appear similar to one another within the same person.[12] The changes within the regional marrow pattern for a person may provide important clues to marrow involvement by a neoplastic process or other pathology. An unusual but symmetric marrow pattern may also exclude a diagnosis of skeletal pathology in a person with a normal but unusual extent of persistent red marrow. A number of cases have been reported with normal variations that were mistaken for pathology.[13,14]

IMAGING METHODS

MRI is superior in bone marrow imaging because of its greater sensitivity, the ability to obtain multiplanar images, greater spatial resolution, and better contrast discrimination than other modalities. Plain films offer a good, inexpensive skeletal overview but 30% to 50% of bony trabeculae must be lost before abnormalities may be detected. Early histologic marrow changes remain undetected. This is unacceptable, because current therapeutic regimens for neoplastic disease require precision in defining the extent of the abnormality. MRI is a much more sensitive diagnostic tool and provides highly reproducible follow-up studies. Scintigraphy may provide physiologic information about the marrow or surrounding bone. Erythroid elements, reticuloendothelial elements, and bone remodeling can be independently assessed, but the extent of anatomic detail is low.[15] CT provides excellent anatomic detail of cortical and trabecular bone, with excellent in-plane spatial resolution.[16] Some information about the intramedullary space is also obtained. Plane selection for images is limited, and significant radiation exposure is possible if an extensive anatomic region is studied.

MAGNETIC RESONANCE CHARACTERISTICS

Marrow Characteristics

Red marrow contains approximately 40% water, 40% fat, and 20% protein, and yellow marrow contains approximately 15% water, 80% fat, and 5% protein.[2] These features plus the mineral matrix affect the signal characteristics of marrow on MR images. Fat is responsible for the greatest fraction of marrow signal on T1-weighted spin echo images. Predominantly hydrophobic methyl groups possess efficient spin-lattice relaxation, resulting in a short T1 relaxation time and high signal intensity.[17] Fat has a moderate signal intensity on T2-weighted images because of its less efficient spin echo relaxation.[18] In general, adult yellow marrow appears similar to extraosseous adipose tissue and shows the signal characteristics of fat on various MR pulse sequences.

Fat is also the major contributor to the signal characteristics of red marrow. However, protein and water content are increased in red marrow. This yields an overall signal intensity with longer T1 and T2 relaxation times than for yellow marrow.[18] Generally, red marrow is similar in intensity to skeletal muscle on T1-weighted sequences. Variable T2 relaxation times result in the red marrow signal in usually following water on T2-weighted spin echo images but becoming suppressed, as with fat on gradient echo images.

Mineral, with no mobile protons to produce signal, makes a slightly negative contribution to marrow signal. An age-related progressive decrease in T1 and T2 relaxation times occurs after the fourth decade, mainly attributed to increasing fatty component of marrow. With no appreciable histologic difference in cellularity, women tend to show this effect more than men. This is attributed to more rapid bone and mineral loss in older women.[12]

Age-Related Changes in Marrow Signals

It is important to realize that the interpreter may not infer a percentage of marrow cellularity by the signal intensity of MR images. Correlation with previous histologic studies indicates that, at 5 years of age, increasing signal intensity in the long bone diaphyses may reflect as little as 10% fatty conversion. At 10 years of age, 20% marrow fat gives the MR appearance of yellow marrow, and histologically, this marrow remains hematopoietically active.[11]

The pattern of marrow conversion with respect to age is also important when reviewing MR examinations. The earliest changes of marrow conversion during childhood are seen as a relative brightening of the epiphyses.[11,19] Inhomogeneous, sometimes geographic signal increases are seen in the diaphyses, proceeding to the metaphyses, with a gradual brightening of the marrow on T1-weighted sequences. This pattern persists throughout adolescence, with coalescence of increased signal regions until only islands of decreased signal are seen within a bright background, representing rests of red marrow in predominantly yellow marrow. A geographic pattern sometimes persists into adulthood. Recognition of this normal variation may prevent a diagnosis of pathology, and changes in the expected marrow pattern may alert the interpreter to the presence of an abnormal process. The recognition of solitary or multiple discrete lesions is much easier than recognition of a diffuse marrow process in which symmetry of the marrow pattern is preserved, particularly in the childhood and young adult years when the distribution of the red marrow is relatively expanded.

In the spine, red marrow normally persists in vertebral bodies throughout life. Focal areas of increased signal intensity on T1-weighted images are normal and commonly seen.[19] In young persons, this is seen as a band along the basivertebral vein. Bands of yellow marrow are commonly seen near the vertebral endplates in persons of increasing age, usually in the cervical and lumbar spine. These changes may represent mechanical stress and are associated with degenerated disks. Diffuse, spotty areas of increased signal intensity throughout the vertebral bodies is another common pattern seen, especially in older persons.[20] This pattern has also been described in younger persons with inflammatory disease of the spine, although it is nonspecific. Similar spotty changes have been seen in the pelvis, commonly in the acetabulum in older persons. Although the general pattern may vary from person to person, a characteristic regional marrow pattern emerges, lending itself to comparison with areas of interest.

Characteristics of Bone Pathology

Most active bone lesions contain increased amounts of cellular water. Lesions tend to appear dark on T1-weighted images against a background of relatively increased fat signal intensity and bright on T2-weighted images, in which fat signal intensity is suppressed. This is particularly apparent when the abnormality is situated in yellow marrow or the relatively less cellular red marrow of older persons. Unique MR pulse sequences may be used to improve lesion detection and red-yellow marrow differentiation in certain cases. Chemical shift imaging takes advantage of the different resonant frequencies of fat and water in biologic tissue.[21,22] A dark interface becomes apparent at the border of tissues with excess water. STIR imaging, a form of inversion recovery, acts to dampen the fat signal. Tissues differing in T1 and T2 relaxation times from fat have increased signal intensity relative to fat.[23] Although this sequence may provide the most contrast between a lesion and normal yellow marrow, anatomic detail may be limited in this sequence, because its signal-to-noise ratio is less than that observed in T1-weighted imaging.

Gradient echo imaging often provides an alternative to STIR and T2 imaging using much shorter scan times. Contrast between marrow and pathologic process is obtained, and there is greater anatomic detail than that seen with STIR images.[22,24] Cartilaginous changes are particularly well seen.

Fast spin echo imaging has allowed rapid image acquisition. It can be combined with fat suppression to afford excellent definition of bone marrow abnormalities and permit exquisite visualization of the surrounding soft tissues that may be involved in neoplasms and other diseases affecting the bone marrow.[25]

MR contrast is often not routinely administered during the imaging of skeletal neoplasm, but it may be helpful in certain clinical settings when neoplastic disease or postsurgical scar are suspected.[26–28] In spinal imaging, contrast enhancement has proven valuable in demonstrating the extradural and intradural spread of underlying malignant disease.

Marrow Reconversion

Reconversion of yellow to red marrow occurs on hematologic demand, following a reverse order of conversion.[3] The process is, like conversion, generally symmetric but not necessarily uniform within a given bone. Reconversion begins as heightened cellular activity within the appendicular skeleton and progresses to the axial skeleton, where areas of yellow marrow reconvert to red marrow microscopically and grossly with accompanying MR signal changes. The appearance may range from islands of decreased signal in a bright background to diffusely decreased signal throughout the skeleton on T1-weighted images, depending on the severity of the process.[29] When the marrow space is replaced with tumor, as in widespread skeletal metastatic disease or in primary hematologic malignancy, the red marrow must expand, sometimes greatly, into the axial skeleton to keep up with hematologic demand. This may make precise definition of tumor site difficult on T1-weighted images alone. Nonneoplastic conditions, such as chronic anemia, commonly accompany neoplastic conditions and may cause or exacerbate red marrow expansion.

Myeloid Depletion

Myeloid depletion is evidenced by signal changes of fatty marrow in areas expected to contain red marrow signal. The degree of signal change is influenced by the severity and duration of the inciting process.[30–35] Systemic changes in oncology patients may be seen with the administration of chemotherapy and with the development of aplastic anemia. Changes may be detectable only by obtaining serial quantitative signal measurements or may be grossly visualized on MR images. Local changes are commonly seen in patients who have undergone radiation therapy. Portions of the bone marrow included in the radiation field demonstrate myeloid depletion with a fatty signal change evident within weeks of treatment. Local changes may be also seen after intraarterial chemotherapy.

Marrow recovery from these processes, if it occurs, follows the same pattern as reconversion, beginning in the axial skeleton and spreading to the periphery.[3] Islands of decreased red marrow signal appear in a background of yellow marrow, enlarge and eventually coalesce. In the spine, the vertebral bodies may take on a mottled appearance. In younger patients, the periphery of the vertebral bodies may be spared, demonstrating evidence of rapid repair as red marrow regenerates around end-plate sinusoids.[36] If there is sufficient destruction of the marrow vascularity to preclude regeneration after radiation therapy, as is commonly the situation, the degree of contrast and sharpness of definition between the irradiated marrow and nonirradiated marrow is often quite striking.

Patterns of Neoplastic Involvement of Bone Marrow

Marrow infiltration or replacement represents the broadest category of bone marrow disorders, and neoplasia is the most commonly imaged marrow replacement process. There is some overlap in the MR appearance of marrow neoplasia and other infiltrative disorders, such as inflammation, edema, lipidoses, and histiocytoses.[29,37] The clinical setting is important in reaching the correct diagnosis.

Neoplastic processes involving the marrow usually exhibit long T1 values and variably increased signal intensity on T2-weighted images.[31,37–42] These lesions may be quite conspicuous in fatty marrow. Normal red or hyperplastic marrow may be more difficult to differentiate from pathology. In this situation, fat suppression techniques may be used to bring out subtle differences. If uncertainty persists, a biopsy can be performed using the images obtained to plan a high-yield site.

The skeletal distribution of neoplastic disorders follows red marrow distribution.[3] Hematogenous spread of metastatic disease would be favored in red marrow because of increased vascularity. Some primary malignancies are thought to originate in the red marrow. These include all forms of leukemia, myeloma, histiocytic lymphoma, and Ewing sarcoma. The distribution of disease provides prognostic clues; the more widely spread in the appendicular skeleton, the more the red marrow in the axial skeleton is involved, implying expansion of the marrow space.

Leukemic patients have been monitored throughout their disease course, and disease progress and response to therapy have been reported quantitatively.[43,44] MRI is the most sensitive examination for the detection of myelomatous involvement of the bone marrow, demonstrating disease despite normal plain films and radionuclide studies.[1,37,39]

The appearance of primary bone tumors varies with respect to type and location. The regional bone marrow is virtually always involved and often to a greater degree than is suggested by plain films, radionuclide studies, or CT scans. The specific appearance of primary bone tumors is described elsewhere in this book.

The appearance of metastases varies from solitary or multiple, discrete lesions in a background of normal red marrow to a diffuse, mottled pattern in disseminated disease, with possible expansion of the red marrow. The latter pattern can be reminiscent of primary hematologic malignancy.

In the spine, compression fractures secondary to metastasis are difficult to differentiate from osteoporotic compression fractures. More complete replacement of the vertebral fatty marrow signal in vertebrae involved with neoplasm may be seen than for benign compression fractures, but this is not foolproof. We have seen patients in which compression fractures in a cancer patient were proven to be benign only after months of healing occurred and the marrow signal reverted to a more normal pattern.

Normal regional marrow patterns may be helpful in providing a background for the visualization of neoplastic involvement of the bone marrow, particularly if attention is paid to the expected pattern with respect to age. Multiple examples of disease affecting the bone marrow are shown in Figures 5-125 through 5-132.

(text continues on page 444)

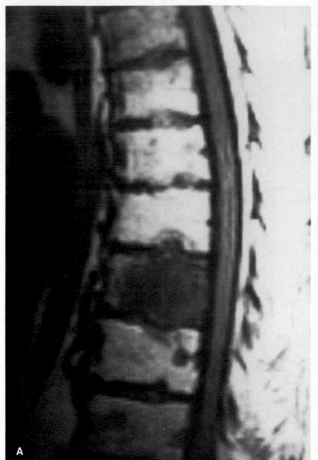

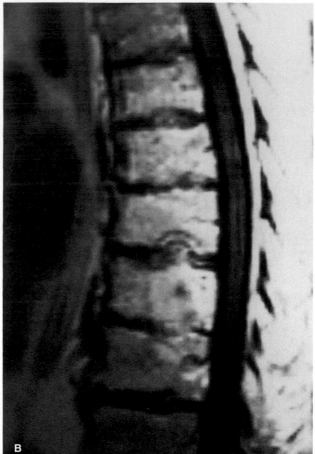

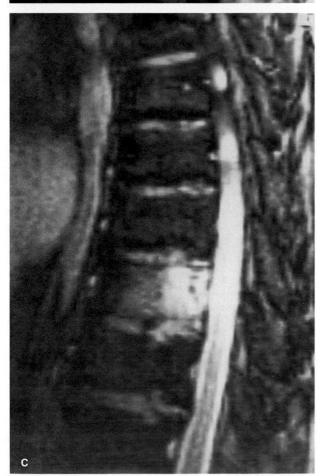

FIGURE 5-125. (**A**) T1-weighted sagittal MR image shows marrow permeation of the vertebral body T10 before cortical destruction. Decreased signal intensity without collapse is characteristic of malignant marrow involvement. (**B**) Contrast-enhanced views may mask the extent of involvement. (**C**) T2-weighted images often best show the extent of marrow involvement. The patient had carcinoma of the lung.

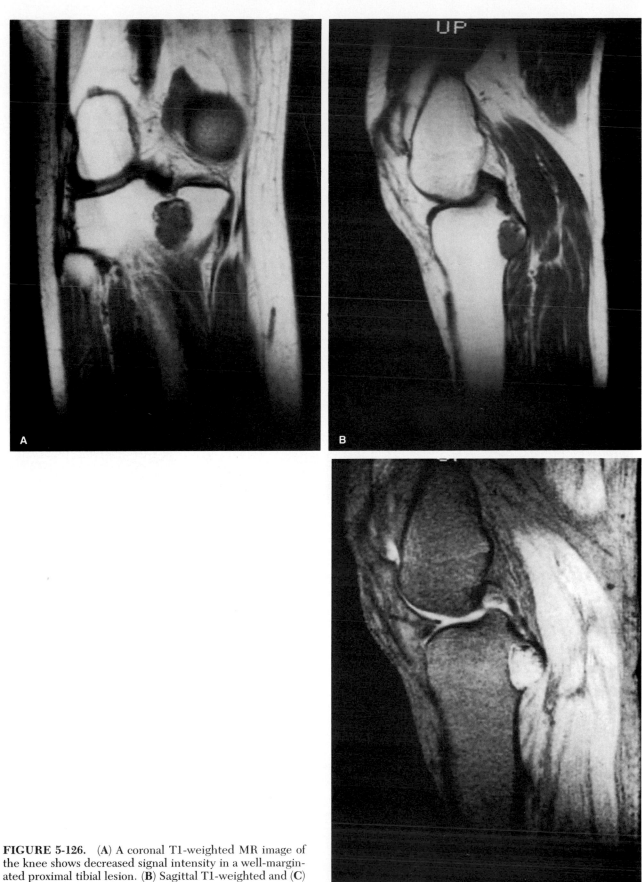

FIGURE 5-126. (**A**) A coronal T1-weighted MR image of the knee shows decreased signal intensity in a well-marginated proximal tibial lesion. (**B**) Sagittal T1-weighted and (**C**) T2-weighted images show the well-marginated edge of a benign, fluid-filled bone cyst.

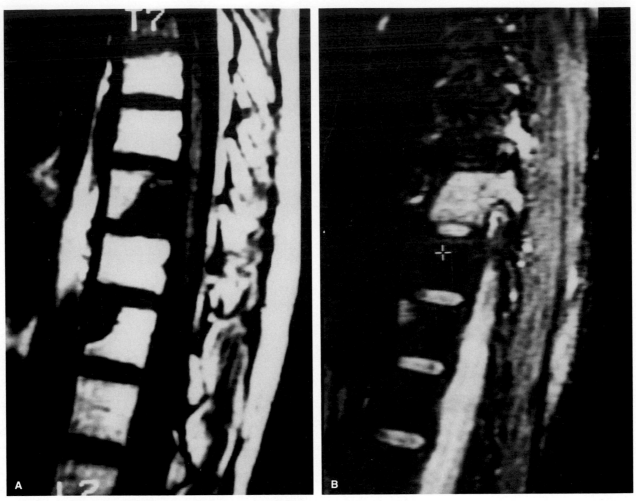

FIGURE 5-127. A midline sagittal T2-weighted MR image of a patient with metastatic carcinoma of the lung involving the vertebral bodies T10 and T12 with marrow permeation. (**B**) A parasagittal fat-suppressed image shows extension of the tumor into the pedicle and facets at T10. Unexpected involvement of the facet at T9 was demonstrated. Fat-suppressed images sensitively demonstrate tumor extension in the bone marrow.

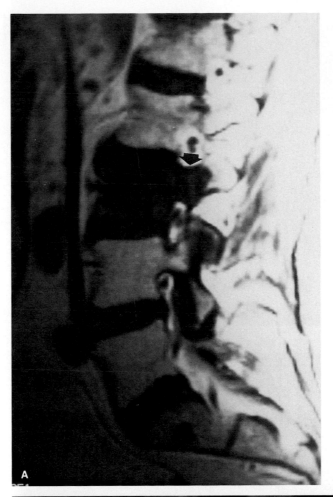

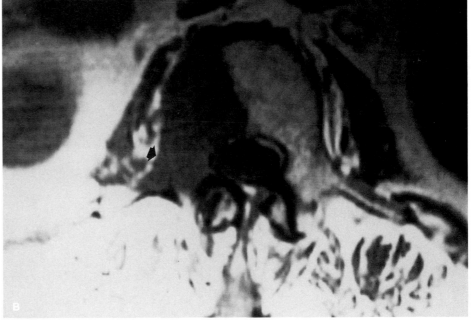

FIGURE 5-128. (**A**) Sagittal and (**B**) axial T1-weighted images of the lumbar spine show pedicle marrow permeation at L3 in a patient with metastatic renal cell carcinoma (*arrows*). Posterior element involvement is often critical in differentiating benign from malignant disease. MR is much more sensitive than standard radionuclide imaging in demonstrating pedicle involvement.

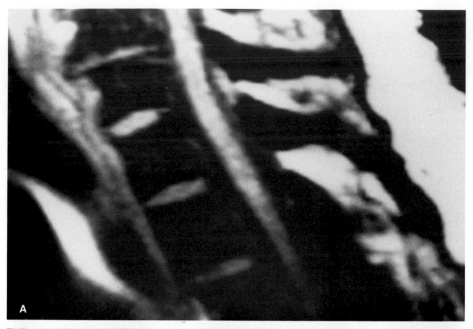

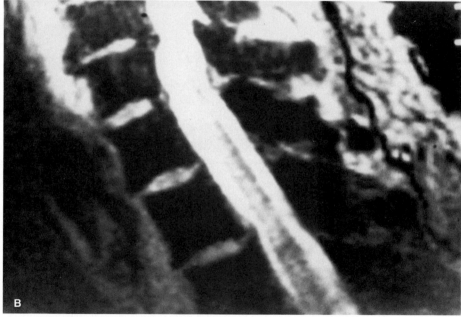

FIGURE 5-129. (**A**) Diffuse fibrotic replacement of normal bone marrow is seen as a signal decrease on T1-weighted and (**B**) T2-weighted images. Sagittal views of the cervical spine demonstrate diffuse fibrotic replacement in a patient with transfusion-dependent myelofibrosis.

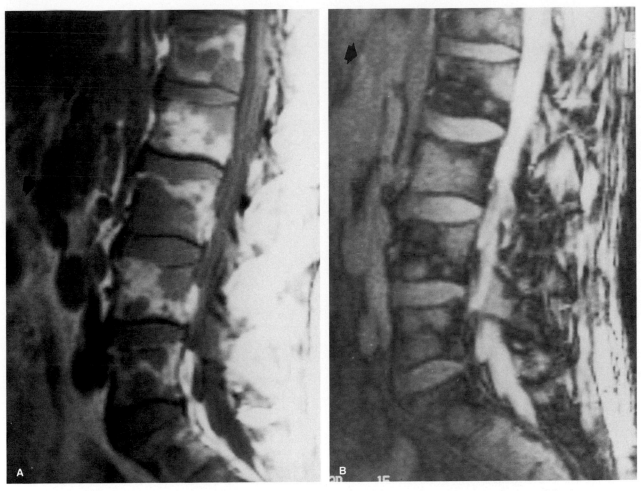

FIGURE 5-130.   Sagittal lumbar spine MR images show widespread metastatic carcinoma of the breast involving multiple vertebral bodies and paraaortic lymph nodes (*arrows*). (**A**) T1-weighted and (**B**) gradient echo MR images demonstrate the extensive spread of the disease. Gradient echo images are often more sensitive than standard T2-weighted studies in showing the soft-tissue component of malignant disease.

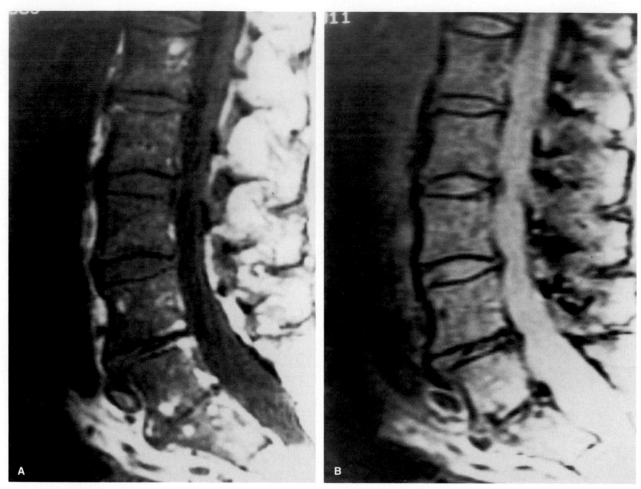

FIGURE 5-131. Widespread, diffuse, infiltrative marrow malignancy such as leukemia can be difficult to assess on T1-weighted images alone. (**A**) A sagittal MR image of the lumbar spine shows spotty, bright fatty depositions and a marrow pattern that is not unusual. This type of image is nondiagnostic. (**B**) A T2-weighted image shows a diffuse signal increase caused by proven leukemic infiltration.

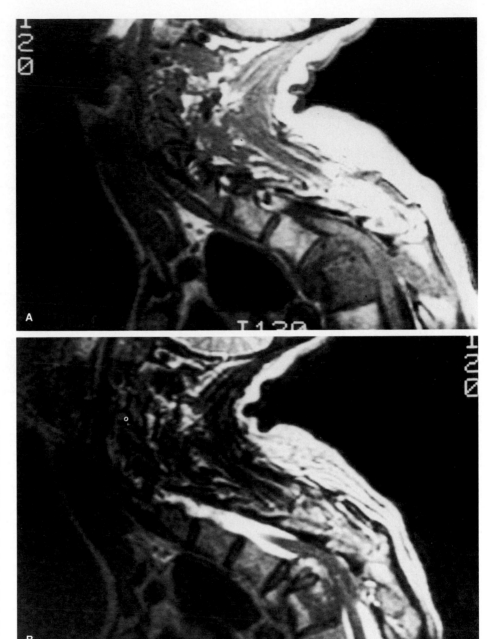

FIGURE 5-132. Although marrow involvement in malignant disease is important and often well shown on T1-weighted images, paravertebral extension is best shown with other imaging sequences. Lung carcinoma with direct extension into the spine and thecal sac and with paravertebral extension is seen in this sagittal study of the upper thoracic spine. (**A**) Although the T1-weighted image shows the disease well, (**B**) the T2-weighted study shows the soft-tissue extension and relations among the bone, spinal cord, and tumor much better.

References

1. Vogler JB III, Murphy WA: Bone marrow imaging. Radiology 168:679–693, 1988
2. Vogler JB III, Murphy WA: Diffuse marrow diseases. *In* Berquist TH, ed. MRI of the Musculoskeletal System. 2nd ed. New York, Raven, 1990:491–516
3. Kricun ME: Red-yellow marrow conversion. Its effect on the location of some solitary bone lesions. Skeletal Radiol 14:10–19, 1985
4. Trubowitz S, Davis S, eds: The bone marrow matrix. *In* The Human Bone Marrow: Anatomy, Physiology, and Pathophysiology. Boca Raton, FL, CRC Press, 1982:43–75
5. Custer RP, Ahlfeldt FE: Studies on the structure and function of bone marrow. II. Variations in cellularity in various bones with advancing years of life and their relative response to stimuli. J Lab Clin Med 17:960–962, 1932
6. Custer RP: Studies on the structure and function of bone marrow. I. Variability of the hemopoietic pattern and consideration of method for examination. J Lab Clin Med 17:951–959, 1932
7. Huggins C, Blocksom BH Jr: Changes in outlying bone marrow accompanying a local increase of temperature within physiological limits. J Exp Med 64:253–274, 1936
8. Piney A: The anatomy of the bone marrow. Br Med J 2:792–795, 1922
9. Tribukait B: Experimental studies on the regulation of erythropoiesis with special reference to the importance of oxygen. Acta Physiol Scand 58(Suppl 208):1–48, 1963
10. Okada Y, Aoki S, Barkovich AJ et al: Cranial bone marrow in children: Assessment of normal development with MR imaging. Radiology 171:161–164, 1989
11. Moore SG, Dawson KL: Red and yellow marrow in the femur: Age-related changes in appearance at MR imaging. Radiology 175:219–223, 1990
12. Dooms GC, Fisher MR, Hricak H et al: Bone marrow imaging: Magnetic resonance studies related to age and sex. Radiology 155:429–432, 1985
13. Deutsch AL, Mink JH, Rosenfelt FP, Waxman AD: Incidental detection of hematopoietic hyperplasia on routine knee MR imaging. AJR Am J Roentgenol 152:333–356, 1990
14. Schuck JE, Czarnecki DJ: MR detection of probable hematopoietic hyperplasia involving the knees, proximal femurs, and pelvis. AJR Am J Roentgenol 153:655–656, 1990
15. Datz FL, Taylor A Jr: The clinical use of radionuclide bone marrow imaging. Semin Nucl Med 15:239–259, 1985
16. Genant HK, Wilson JS, Bovill EG et al: Computed tomography of the musculoskeletal system. J Bone Joint Surg [Am] 62:1088–1101, 1980
17. Wehrli FW, MacFall JR, Shutts D et al: Mechanisms of contrast in NMR imaging. J Comput Assist Tomogr 8:369–380, 1984
18. Mitchell DG, Burk DL Jr, Vinitskis S, Rifkin MD: The biophysical basis of tissue contrast in extracranial MR imaging. AJR Am J Roentgenol 149:831–837, 1987
19. Ricci C, Cova M, Kang YS et al: Normal age-related patterns of cellular and fatty bone marrow distribution in the axial skeleton: MR imaging study. Radiology 177:83–88, 1990
20. Hajek PC, Baker LL, Goobar JE et al: Focal fat deposition in axial bone marrow: MR characteristics. Radiology 162:245–249, 1987
21. Wismer GL, Rosen BR, Buxton R et al: Chemical shift imaging of bone marrow: Preliminary experience. AJR Am J Roentgenol 145:1031–1037, 1985
22. Winkler ML, Ortendahl DA, Mille TC et al: Characteristics of partial flip angle and gradient reversal imaging. Radiology 166:17–26, 1988
23. Bydder GM, Young IR: MR imaging: Clinical use of the inversion recovery sequence. J Comput Assist Tomogr 9:659–675, 1985
24. Hendrick RE, Kneeland JB, Stark DD: Maximizing signal-to-noise and contrast-to-noise ratios with FLASH imaging. Magn Reson Imaging 5:117–127, 1987
25. Prorok RJ, Sawyer AM: Signa Advantage Applications Guide, vol IV. Milwaukee, General Electric, 1992
26. Sze G, Krol G, Zimmerman RD, Deck MDF: Malignant extradural spinal tumors: MR imaging with Gd-DTPA. Radiology 167:217–223, 1988
27. Hueftle MG, Modic MT, Ross JS et al. Lumbar spine: Postoperative MR imaging with Gd-DTPA. Radiology 167:817–824, 1988
28. Ross JS, Delamarter R, Hueffle MG et al. Gadolinium-DTPA-enhanced MR imaging of the postoperative lumbar spine: Time course and mechanism of enhancement. AJNR Am J Neuroradiol 10:37–46, 1969
29. Porter BA, Shields AF, Olson DO: Magnetic resonance imaging of bone marrow disorders. Radiol Clin North Am 1986;24:269–289
30. Kaplance PA, Asleson RJ, Klassen LW, Duggan MJ: Bone marrow patterns in aplastic anemia: Observations with 1.5 T MR imaging. Radiology 164:441–444, 1987
31. Cohen MD, Klatte EC, Baehner R et al: Magnetic resonance imaging of bone marrow disease in children. Radiology 151:715–718, 1984
32. Olson DO, Shields AF, Scheurich CJ et al. Magnetic resonance imaging of the bone marrow in patients with leukemia, aplastic anemia and lymphoma. Invest Radiol 21:540–546, 1968
33. Kangarloo H, Dietrich RB, Taira RT et al: MR imaging of bone marrow in children. J Comput Assist Tomogr 10:205–209, 1986
34. McKinstry CS, Steiner RE, Young AT et al: Bone marrow in leukemia and aplastic anemia: MRI imaging before, during and after treatment. Radiology 162:701–707, 1987
35. Casamassima F, Ruggerio C, Caramella D et al: Hematopoietic bone marrow recovery after radiation therapy: MRI evaluation. Blood 73:1677–1681, 1989
36. Stevens SK, Moore SG, Kaplan ID: Early and late bone marrow changes after irradiation: MR evaluation. AJR Am J Roentgenol 154:745–750, 1990
37. Nyman R, Rehn S, Glimelius B et al: Magnetic resonance imaging in diffuse malignant bone marrow diseases. Acta Radiol 28:199–205, 1987
38. Zimmer WD, Berquist TH, McLeod RA: Bone tumors: Magnetic resonance imaging versus computed tomography. Radiology 155:709–718, 1985
39. Daffner RH, Lupetin AR, Dash N et al: MRI in the detection of malignant infiltration of bone marrow. AJR Am J Roentgenol 146:353–358, 1986
40. Hanna SL, Fletcher BD, Fairclough DL et al: Magnetic resonance imaging of disseminated bone marrow disease in patients treated for malignancy. Skeletal Radiol 20:79–84, 1991
41. Boyko OB, Cory DA, Cohen MD et al: MR imaging of osteogenic and Ewing's sarcoma. AJR Am J Roentgenol 148:317–322, 1987
42. Bloem JL, Taminiau AHM, Eulderink F et al: Radiologic staging of primary bone sarcoma: MR imaging, scintigraphy, angiography, and CT correlated with pathologic examination. Radiology 169:805–810, 1988
43. Moore SG, Gooding CA, Brasch RC et al: Bone marrow in children with acute lymphocytic leukemia: MR relaxation times. Radiology 160:237–240, 1986
44. Rosen BR, Fleming DM, Kushner DC et al: Hematologic bone marrow disorders: Quantitative chemical shift MR imaging. Radiology 169:799–804, 1988

Imaging of Bone Tumors: A Multimodality Approach,
edited by George B. Greenfield and John A. Arrington,
J. B. Lippincott Company, Philadelphia © 1995.

chapter

SIX

SOME CLINICAL CONSIDERATIONS

Osteosarcoma

Jaime Estrada

Osteosarcomas originate from primitive, mesenchymal, bone-forming cells in the metaphysis of long bones in adolescents and young adults.[1,2] In young adults, osteosarcomas are the third most common malignancies, exceeded only by leukemias and lymphomas.[3] We measure success in the treatment of patients with osteosarcomas of the extremities in terms of disease-free survival, which has approached 70% past 3 years of follow-up in several patient series, and in terms of the number of limb-salvage procedures being performed on these patients. Through the use of preoperative chemotherapy, the surgical treatment of osteosarcomas of the extremities has evolved from amputations and disarticulations to sophisticated reconstructive surgical procedures with excellent functional results.[4]

CLINICAL PRESENTATION AND NATURAL HISTORY

Patients with osteosarcomas of the extremities usually present with a history of pain in the affected extremity that may vary from 3 to 6 months. Patients often refer the pain to the joint adjacent to the affected bone, such as the knee join in cases of distal femur or proximal tibial tumors. Initial physical examinations may be inconclusive, and plain radiographs often fail to reveal a bone lesion. Common findings in the history of patients with tumors close to the knee joint include negative results for arthroscopic examinations. Further tumor growth causes worsening of the pain, enlargement of the affected body part, and radiographic changes characteristic of an expansile, permeative bone lesion, often with invasion of soft tissues.

Between 10% and 20% of new patients have macroscopic, radiologically visible metastatic disease at presentation. Most metastatic lesions occur in the lungs, and a small fraction of the patients present with bone metastasis with or without coexistent lung lesions.[5]

DIAGNOSTIC STUDIES

Initial Evaluation

The initial clinical evaluation should include a careful review of malignancies in the family members, because deletions or abnormalities of the *P53* gene, first described in members of families with the Li-Fraumeni syndrome, predispose to bone and soft tissues sarcomas, breast cancer, leukemias, brain tumors, and other malignancies at an early age.[6] In addition, the loss of heterozygosity at the retinoblastoma gene loci (*RB1*) in chromosome 13 also occurs in osteosarcoma cells, implicating the loss of this gene in the generation of osteosarcomas in the same manner that homozygosity for the allele in a retinoblast cell leads to retinoblastoma.[7,8] These findings may explain the several observations suggesting a relation between osteosarcoma and hereditary retinoblastoma. For example, more than 98% of patients with retinoblastoma who develop second non ocular tumors have bilateral disease, although the bilateral form of retinoblastoma occurs in only 25% of cases.[9] In hereditary retinoblastoma patients, osteosarcomas occur 2000 times more frequently in the skull after radiotherapy and 500 times more frequently in the extremities than would be expected in the general population.[10] Patients with retinoblastoma have developed secondary osteosarcomas in the extremities at sites distant from orbital irradiation. Osteosarcomas have been seen in patients who did not receive radiation as treatment for their retinoblastomas. Remarkably, the actuarial risk for the development of second tumors among patients with bilateral retinoblastomas is 90% at 30 years.[11]

Radiologic Evaluation

Plain films of the involved bone are still the most useful study for evaluating a suspected malignant bone tumor. Permeative destruction of the trabecular bone pattern with ill-defined margins and a lack of endosteal reaction are characteristic findings. Periosteal new bone formation and lifting of the cortex with formation of a Codman triangle is commonly seen. A soft-tissue mass is frequently observed as the tumor erodes the cortex and invades the adjacent soft tissues. Osteosarcomas may appear osteosclerotic, lytic, or mixed sclerotic and lytic, reflecting the degree of ossification and mineralization of the osteoid produced by the tumor.[12,13]

The initial imaging evaluation to determine the extent of the primary tumor should also include computerized tomography (CT) and magnetic resonance imaging (MRI) of the tumor area, a CT examination of the chest, and a bone scan. CT is useful in evaluating the extent of soft-tissue infiltration and the destruction of the bone cortex. CT is particularly valuable for imaging centrally located lesions, such as those arising in or near the pelvis or trunk.[14] The value of CT imaging for extremity lesions is limited by the small size of the distal extremity structures, the paucity of fat, and bone-related artifacts. MRI is clearly superior for the imaging of distal lesions because of its better contrast resolution.[15]

MRI is more sensitive in detecting intramedullary tumor than CT because of the very high contrast discrimination between tumor and marrow fat. MRI has two additional advantages over CT in the evaluation of bone tumors: the absence of beam-hardening CT artifact and the ability to obtain coronal, sagittal, oblique, and off-axis images. For example, the entire medullary canal of the femur can be imaged by MR using several coronal cuts. CT of this area can be done only transaxially and would require more cuts.[16] Complete visualization of the intramedullary tumor extent is essential for the initial staging and for planning the definitive surgical procedure in patients with osteosarcomas of the extremities.

The presence of metastases at diagnosis is an extremely important prognostic feature with a major impact in the initial management of the patient. Routine posteroanterior and lateral chest radiographs can detect most of the lung metastases during the initial evaluation, but CT is the examination of choice to screen patients for lung lesions, particularly pleural-based nodules that can be missed in as many as 20% of the plain chest radiographs.[17]

Because bony metastases occur in as many as 10% of patients at presentation, scanning with methylene diphosphonate labeled with technetium 99m is also indicated in the initial screening. Radionuclide bone scanning is highly sensitive for detection of metastatic bone lesions and skip lesions in patients with osteosarcomas. The uptake of the radionuclide extends slightly beyond the limits of the tumor, which helps in defining a safe margin to use in planning surgery of the primary tumor.[18]

Two-plane (i.e., anteroposterior and lateral) arteriography is an extremely useful diagnostic tool, because it provides accurate pictures of the main tumor feeders, the degree of neovascularization, and capillary stain after the contrast injection. This information serves as a baseline for evaluating the response of the tumor to chemotherapy. In general, a decrease in the tumor neovascularity and stain after a chemotherapy treatment provides evidence of the chemosensitivity of the tumor.[19] After the arteriography, the major tumor artery is catheterized to deliver cisplatin intraarterially, a component of our treatment program, following published chemotherapy protocols.[20] The information gained from the arteriography is also useful to the surgeon in planning the limb-salvage procedure at the end of the chemotherapy program.

Follow-Up Studies

Patients with osteosarcomas should be followed with monthly chest radiographs for the first 2 years from diagnosis, because most of the recurrences occur during this time. CT scans of the lungs should be performed routinely every 3 to 4 months during this period as an adjunct to the plain chest radiographs and whenever a suspicious abnormality appears on plain films. After 2 years, plain radiographs and CT scans can be done with decreasing frequency for at least 5 years of follow-up. Radionuclide bone scans should also be obtained every 3 to 4 months during the first 2 years. Any abnormality in the bone scan should be followed with plain radiographs, even in an asymptomatic patient. Attention should be paid to the stump area for evidence of local recurrences, particularly in patients who have undergone limb-salvage procedures.

TREATMENT OF OSTEOSARCOMAS

Local control of osteosarcoma of the extremities was historically achieved by amputation. However, as many as 80% of the patients treated with surgery only succumbed to metastatic disease within 2 years of diagnosis.[21,22] The use of combination chemotherapy after the surgical resection of the tumor has been responsible for the increase in the 5-year disease-free survival from 20% to approximately 65% in several patient series.[23,24] The effectiveness of adjuvant chemotherapy after surgical ablation of the primary tumor in patients with osteosarcomas proved that micrometastatic disease was treatable with chemotherapy in most cases.[25]

The primary antitumor effect of induction or presurgical chemotherapy, also known as neoadjuvant therapy, is currently under investigation. Even short courses of chemotherapy given preoperatively produce tumor regressions that allow more limited resections. Limb-sparing procedures using autologous grafts, vascularized grafts, allografts, and custom metal prosthesis are routinely performed in these patients after induction chemotherapy.[26-28] Chemotherapy is continued adjuvantly after the surgery in most treatment programs. Induction chemotherapy may effectively eliminate micrometastatic disease present at the time of diagnosis and decrease the chances of the spread of viable tumor cells during the resection of the primary tumor.[22]

The main objective of our program for newly diagnosed osteosarcoma patients is to test the hypothesis that a relatively short, intensive course of induction chemotherapy using the six most active, non–cross-resistant agents can become the primary treatment modality for these patients. High-dose methotrexate-cisplatin-doxorubicin (Adriamycin) cycles alternate with ifosfamide-etoposide cycles to achieve maximum tumor cell kill and to minimize or prevent the development of multidrug resistance according to the Goldie and Coldman model.[29] The end point of the program is the surgical resection of the tumor, which permits evaluation of the efficacy of this approach by measuring the amount of tumor necrosis, residual tumor, and fibrosis by the pathologist in the surgical specimen. The response of the tumor to induction chemotherapy measured in terms of percent tumor necrosis after resection of the tumor appears to be the most significant prognostic parameter for patients with nonmetastatic osteosarcomas of the extremities. For the most part, patients with 90% or more tumor necrosis are the long-term survivors.[19] In the long term, the response is usually measured in terms of incidence of metastatic disease and relapse-free survival of the treated patients.

Chemotherapy

The five active agents used in our induction chemotherapy treatment program for newly diagnosed patients with osteosarcomas of the extremities are doxorubicin, cisplatin, high-dose methotrexate, etoposide, and ifosfamide. These agents, used singly and in various combinations, have consistently shown the highest response rates in patients with untreated osteosarcomas.[30-34] Although little information exists about the use of ifosfamide and etoposide in osteosarcoma pa-

tients, this combination is used because of the theoretical potentiation effect of etoposide on ifosfamide, based on its inhibition of the DNA topoisomerase II.[35] Evidence supporting this approach was recently provided by Miser and colleagues[36] in a phase II study in patients with Ewing and other sarcomas that showed a very high response rate with this combination.

A controversy exists about the effectiveness of intraarterial and that of intravenous cisplatin in the treatment of these patients. In the only prospective study published, Winkler and associates[37] found no difference in terms of percent of tumor necrosis between intraarterially and intravenously administered cisplatin in a group of 109 patients with high-risk osteosarcomas of the extremities. Although it involves greater technical requirements, we prefer to administer cisplatin intraarterially, because the information obtained from the arteriograms before each dose of cisplatin permits more accurate monitoring of the response to the treatment.

Evaluation of Tumor Response During Therapy

Conventional osteosarcomas have been classified as osteoblastic, chondroblastic, and fibroblastic, depending on the predominant matrix pattern of the tumor. This pattern is usually apparent on plain radiographs. An osteoblastic osteosarcoma may appear osteosclerotic or completely lytic, depending on the degree of calcification of the osteoid produced by the tumor. Serial radiographs of the affected bone are the most useful study to follow the response of the tumor to induction chemotherapy. The tumor changes with therapy may vary according with the type of osteosarcoma, but a good response is characterized by an increase in the calcification of the tumor matrix and osteoid.[19,38] This is usually associated with reduction in the tumor size and clear delineation of the tumor extent due to calcification of the tumor margins. Tumor response during treatment can also be evaluated with serial arteriograms that may show a decrease in the tumor neovascularity with pruning of the vessels and disappearance of the vascular lakes characteristic of the typical untreated osteosarcoma.[19,38] These radiologic changes are usually associated with improvement in the patient's pain, attitude, and function of the affected extremity.

Failure to show radiographic or clinical evidence of response after the first cycle of chemotherapy should alert the treating team to the development of drug resistance or the presence of an inherently drug-resistant tumor. Immediate surgical ablation of the primary tumor should be considered at that point. In our experience, a poor clinical and radiologic response to initial induction chemotherapy carry a grave prognosis for these patients.

Historically, osteosarcomas have been considered highly radioresistant tumors,[38] but preliminary evidence suggest that radiation therapy in combination with cytotoxic radiosensitizers, such as cisplatin, may have a role in the treatment of patients with tumors considered nonresectable because of the inherent surgical morbidity, such as pelvic osteosarcomas.[39]

Multidisciplinary Sarcoma Team

The current gains in the outcome of patients with bone malignancies have been possible only through the collaborations of the orthopedic surgeon, who usually sees the patient first, and the oncologist, radiologist, radiotherapist, and pathologist in a multidisciplinary team approach. The expertise of chemotherapy-certified nurses, physical therapists, social workers, and radiology technicians is also essential for the comprehensive care of patients with bone malignancies.

An important component of the treatment program is the multidisciplinary sarcoma conference, during which new patients are presented and the various clinical, radiologic, and pathologic evaluations of patients undergoing treatment are discussed. Decisions concerning the surgical options at the end of the treatment are reached, and the pathologic evaluation of the response after the surgery is reviewed. These conferences greatly contribute to the patient care and the teaching of students and residents.

The success in the treatment of patients with osteosarcomas of the extremities can be attributed for the most part to the development of effective combination-chemotherapy programs, initially used after surgical resection of the tumors and currently used in a presurgical or neoadjuvant setting. Sarcoma-treating teams have pioneered the approach of organ conservation or limb sparing in the treatment of patients with bone malignancies. This concept is being applied to the treatment of other types of solid tumors in children and adults. Presurgical chemotherapy and conservative surgical procedures have made limb preservation a realistic goal for most patients with osteosarcomas of the extremities.

References

1. Sissons H: The WHO classification of bone tumors. Recent Results Cancer Res 54:104–108, 1976
2. Dahlin DC, Unni KK: Osteosarcoma. *In* Dahlin DC, Unni KK, eds. Bone Tumors. General Aspects and Data on 8,542 Cases. Springfield, IL, Charles C. Thomas, 1986:269–307
3. Young JL, Ries LG, Silverberg E et al: Cancer incidence, survival, and mortality for children younger than 15 years. Cancer 58:598, 1986
4. Link MP, Eilber F: Osteosarcoma. *In* Pizzo PA, Poplack DG, eds. Principles and Practice of Pediatric Oncology. Philadelphia, JB Lippincott, 1989:689–711
5. Dahlin D, Unni K: Osteosarcoma of bone and its important recognizable varieties. Am J Surg Pathol 1:61–72, 1977
6. Hollstein M, Sidransky D, Vogelstein B, Harris CC: P53 mutations in human cancers. Science 253:49–53, 1991
7. Dryja T, Rapaport J, Epstein J et al: Chromosome 13 homozygosity in osteosarcoma without retinoblastoma. Am J Hum Genet 38:59–66, 1986
8. Friend S, Bernards R, Rogelj S et al: A human DNA segment with properties of the gene that predisposes to retinoblastoma and osteosarcoma. Nature 323:643–646, 1986
9. Abramson D, Ellsworth R, Kitchin F, Tung G: Second nonocular tumors in retinoblastoma survivors. Ophthalmology 91:1351–1355, 1984
10. Murphee A, Benedict W: Retinoblastoma: Clues to human oncogenesis. Science 223:1028–1033, 1984
11. Abramson D, Ellsworth R, Kitchin F, Tung G: Second nonocular tumors in retinoblastoma survivors. Ophthalmology 91:1351–1355, 1984
12. Unni KK: Osteosarcoma of bone. Contemp Issues Surg Pathol 11:107–133, 1988
13. Kesselring F, Penn W: Radiological aspects of "classic" primary osteosarcoma: Value of some radiologic investigations. Diagn Imaging 51:78–92, 1982
14. McLeod RA, Stephens DH, Beabout JW et al: Computed tomography of the skeletal system. Semin Roentgenol 13:235–247, 1978
15. Richardson ML, Kilcoyne RF, Gillespy T et al: Magnetic resonance imaging of musculoskeletal neoplasms. Radiol Clin North Am 24:259–267, 1986
16. McLeod RA, Berquist TH: Bone tumor imaging: Contribution of CT and MRI. Contemp Issues Surg Pathol 11:1–34, 1988
17. Neifeld J, Michaelis L, Doppman J: Suspected pulmonary metastases: Correlation of chest x-ray, whole lung tomograms and operative findings. Cancer 39:383–387, 1977
18. McKillop J, Etcubanas E, Goris M: The indications for and limitations of bone scintigraphy in osteogenic sarcoma. Cancer 48:1133–1138, 1981
19. Raymond AK, Chawla SP, Carrasco CH et al: Osteosarcoma chemotherapy effect: A prognostic factor. Semin Diagn Pathol 4:212–236, 1987
20. Jaffe N, Knapp J, Chuang VP et al: Osteosarcoma: Intraarterial treatment of the primary tumor with *cis*-diammine-dichloroplatinum II (CDP): Angiographic, pathologic and pharmacologic studies. Cancer 51:402–407, 1983
21. Dahlin DC, Coventry MB: Osteogenic sarcoma: a study of 600 cases. J Bone Join Surg [Am] 49:101–110, 1967
22. Goorin AM, Abelson HT, Frei E: Osteosarcoma: Fifteen years later. N Engl J Med 313:1637–1643, 1985
23. Rosen G, Marcove RC, Huvos AG et al: Primary osteogenic sarcoma: eight year experience with adjuvant chemotherapy. J Cancer Res Clin Oncol 106(Suppl):55–67, 1983
24. Link MA, Goorin AM, Miser AW et al: The effect of adjuvant chemotherapy on relapse-free survival in patients with osteosarcoma of the extremity. N Engl J Med 314:1600–1606, 1986
25. Schabel FM Jr: Concepts for systemic treatment of micrometastases. Cancer 35:15–24, 1975
26. Enneking WF, Shirley PD: Resection-arthrodesis for malignant and potentially malignant lesions about the knee using intramedullary rod and local bone grafts. J Bone Joint Surg [Am] 59:223–236, 1977
27. Mankin H, Doppelt S, Sullivan R, Tomford W: Osteoarticular and intercalary allograft transplantation in the manage-

ment of malignant tumors of bone. Cancer 50:613–630, 1982

28. Lewis MM: The use of an expandable and adjustable prosthesis in the treatment of childhood malignant bone tumors of the extremity. Cancer 57:499–502, 1986

29. Goldie JH, Coldman AJ: A mathematical model for relating the drug sensitivity of tumors to their spontaneous mutation rate. Cancer Treat Rep 63:1727–1733, 1979

30. Cortes EP, Holland JF, Wang JJ, Sinks LF: Doxorubicin in disseminated osteosarcoma. JAMA 221:1132–1138, 1972

31. Baum ES, Gaynon P, Greenberg L et al: Phase II study of *cis*-dichlorodiammineplatinum (II) in childhood osteosarcoma: Children's Cancer Study Group Report. Cancer Treat Rep 63:1621–1627, 1979

32. Jaffe N, Farber S, Traggis D et al: Favorable response of metastatic osteosarcoma to pulse high dose methotrexate with citrovorum factor rescue and radiation therapy. Cancer 31:1367–1373, 1973

33. Pratt C, Howarth C, Ransom J et al: High dose methotrexate used alone and in combination for measurable primary and metastatic osteosarcoma. Cancer Treat Rep 64:11–20, 1980

34. Marti C, Kroner T, Remagen W et al: High-dose ifosfamide in advanced osteosarcoma. Cancer Treat Rep 69:115–117, 1985

35. Miser JS, Kinsella TJ, Triche TJ et al. Ifosfamide with mesna uroprotection and etoposide: an effective regimen in the treatment of recurrent sarcomas and other tumors of children and young adults. J Clin Oncol 5:1191–1198, 1987

36. Clark PI, Slevin ML: The clinical pharmacology of etoposide and teniposide. Clin Pharmacokinet 12:223–252, 1987

37. Winkler K, Bielack S, Delling G et al: Effect of intraarterial versus intravenous cisplatin in addition to systemic doxorubicin, high dose methotrexate, and ifosfamide on histologic tumor response in osteosarcoma (Study COSS-86). Cancer 66:1703–1710, 1990

38. Jenkin R, Alt W, Fitzpatrick P: Osteosarcoma: An assessment of management with particular reference to primary irradiation and selective delayed amputation. Cancer 30:393–400, 1972

39. Estrada-Aguilar J, Greenberg H, Walling AK et al: Primary treatment of pelvic osteosarcoma. Report of five cases. Cancer 69:1137–1145, 1992

Surgical Treatment for Osteosarcoma

George Douglas Letson

Osteosarcoma is the most common primary malignant bone tumor in children and young adults. It accounts for approximately one third of all malignant bone neoplasms. The treatment of this disease has changed dramatically over the years, from amputative surgery alone to a combination of chemotherapy and limb-sparing surgery. The survivorship of patients with osteogenic sarcoma has increased from approximately 20% with surgery alone to 60% with chemotherapy and surgery.[1] With the addition of chemotherapy to surgery, survivorship has increased, and ablative surgery has changed to more functional and reconstructive surgery. Patients can now expect to live despite their disease, and they can expect to have their limb retained with a reasonably good functional and excellent cosmetic result.

The treatment of osteogenic sarcomas should be considered in two phases: surgical eradication of the primary tumor and chemotherapy.[2] Neoadjuvant chemotherapy may be performed before surgery, or chemotherapy may follow surgical eradication. There are different schools of thought about performing the surgery before chemotherapy or using neoadjuvant chemotherapy followed by surgical eradication of the tumor. The advantage of neoadjuvant chemotherapy is to change some tumors that were deemed nonresectable before chemotherapy into tumors that are resectable after the initiation of chemotherapy.

Preoperative chemotherapy gives time to make custom prostheses, which are needed in many patients for the reconstruction after a surgical resection. Other advantages are that the response of the tumor to the chemotherapy can be evaluated after surgical resection and the chemotherapeutic regimen could be altered if there is poor response. However, if there is a poor response to the chemotherapy, there could be an increased chance of metastatic spread. The advantage of immediate surgery is that early, complete resection of the tumor may decrease the chance of metastatic disease, although most patients probably have microscopic metastatic disease at presentation. After surgery, the patient can begin rehabilitation while starting chemotherapy. Emotionally, the patient does not have to wait several months in anticipation of extensive surgery.

SURGICAL APPROACHES

The surgical treatment options for osteogenic sarcomas are amputation, rotationplasty, and limb sparing, which may consist of resection, allograft arthrodesis, autograft bone reconstruction, or metallic reconstruction. The treatment of the primary osteogenic sarcoma is a surgical treatment, and this must be done by obtaining at least a wide or radical margin at the time of resection. Reconstruction is a secondary procedure that should be done when possible.

Amputation

The treatment of choice for primary osteogenic sarcoma in the past has been amputation. Originally, this was done by whole-bone amputations through the joint or bone above the tumor.[3,4] This was thought to be necessary because of the reported high incidence of intramedullary skip metastasis.[5] However, later studies reviewing the local recurrence rate for patients having transmedullary amputations for primary osteogenic sarcoma were approximately equal to that of patients having disarticulation or whole-bone amputations.[1,6,7] It is thought that the surgical amputation should be at least 5 to 10 cm proximal to the margin of the tumor, but there are no clinical studies that support how close surgery can be to the tumor and still provide a safe margin for amputation. With chemotherapy, the local recurrence rates for cross-bone amputation have been exceptionally low, approximately 5% to 10%.[1,6,7]

After amputation, the patient can be treated with an immediate-fit prosthesis that can be applied while the patient is still in the hospital. With advances in the the design in permanent prostheses, the functional status of these patients is very good, and the patients can actually participate in more athletic activities than is possible after limb-sparing procedures. The major disadvantage is the obvious cosmetic effect of having an amputation of an extremity.

Rotationplasty

Rotationplasty or turniplasty was initially described in 1930 for the treatment of nonneoplastic bone diseases by Borggrede.[8,9] It was popularized by van Ness in 1950. In 1982, Kotz and colleagues described the use of the rotationplasty for the treatment of osteogenic sarcoma in the lower extremities of children who were not suitable for the more conventional limb-sparing operation.[9] This technically difficult operation is designed for adolescents who, because of their continued growth, would not be candidates for a reconstruction that would not allow for this growth. This procedure is also suitable for patients who, because of the size and extent of the tumor, are not candidates for a limb-sparing procedure.

This procedure is a viable alternative as long as the sciatic nerve can be dissected free from the tumor. The procedure is designed for osteogenic sarcomas of the distal part of the femur and entails a double amputation (Figs. 6-1 through 6-3). The first amputation occurs through the proximal femur, and the second amputation occurs through the proximal tibia. The sciatic nerve is dissected free of the tumor, and the popliteal artery is dissected free or tied off.

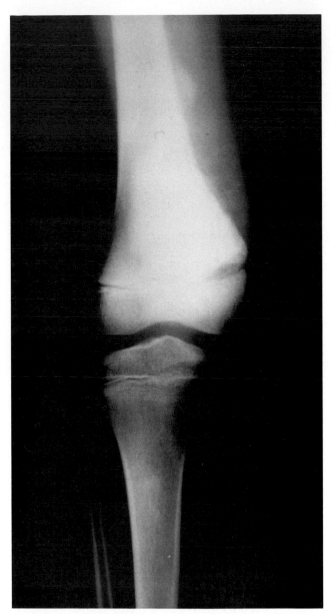

FIGURE 6-1. Osteosarcoma of the distal femur in an adolescent. (Courtesy of Mark Gebhardt, M.D., Boston, MA.)

After amputation of the distal femur, the entire leg is externally rotated 180 degrees, and the tibia is brought up to the proximal femur. This is usually fixed with plates and screws. The redundant vessel and nerve are then coiled up and buried into muscle, and the vessel is surgically reunited with the femoral artery in the proximal thigh. The ankle joint and heel then function as a knee joint. Cosmetically, this operation is not an attractive alternative, but functionally, the procedure offers some of the best results after resection from a malignant neoplasm, and patients may resume participation in many sports.

that has made limb sparing an option for the treatment of osteogenic sarcoma. However, there have been many other new developments, especially in the field of radiology, that have made this surgery possible. The sarcoma can be localized much better today than 20 years ago. Before surgery, a determination can be made of how much bone and soft tissue must be resected at the time of surgery. We can preoperatively determine to what extent the tumor is involved with the limb or if a neurovascular structure is fixed to the tumor, allowing a decision about whether limb sparing is possible to be made before surgery. After a determination is made that the patient is a candidate for a limb-sparing procedure, the physician must determine what the patient's cosmetic and functional expectations are. Although a patient meets all the criteria for a limb-sparing procedure, it may not be the procedure of choice for him or her. The cosmetic results may be far superior to any of the other surgical options, but the functional results may be far different from the expectations of the patient.

Many surgical options are possible for a patient who is a candidate for a limb-sparing procedure. The patient may elect to have an allograft arthrodesis for an osteogenic sarcoma of the distal femur or proximal tibia. This will gives far more stability to the reconstruction and lessens the chance for future complications. However, with the loss of motion within the knee, it makes some of the tasks of daily living much more difficult.

Autograft bone reconstructions offer many advantages over an allograft reconstruction. An autograft eliminates the possibility of transferring a viral or bacterial illness. The autograft also offers the advantage of much more rapid incorporation at the osteosynthesis site. The major disadvantage is the limited size of bone defect that an autograft can reconstruct. To use an autologous bone graft, there must be expendable bones, which are limited to the fibula, ribs, and the iliac crest. If the area to be reconstructed after a resection fulfills these limited requirements, this is an excellent option for reconstruction. However, this is rarely possible with osteogenic sarcomas.

Metallic replacements are an excellent choice for a limb-sparing procedure (Fig. 6-4). They have good functional results and have the advantage of offering immediate stability. The immediate stability of a metallic implant is a factor of the strength of the cement fixation of the prosthesis to the bone and the inherent strength of the metal. The stability of the reconstruction should be strong enough to support immediate weight bearing after surgery. There is no need to wait for healing or bone ingrowth to occur. The rehabilitation of these patients is very rapid. However, the du-

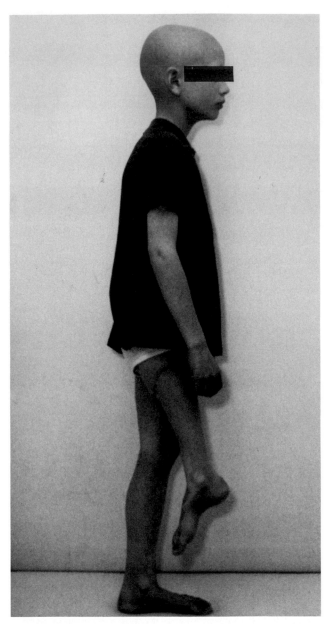

FIGURE 6-2. Rotationplasty was performed in an adolescent after osteosarcoma resection. The ankle functions as a knee. (Courtesy of Mark Gebhardt, M.D., Boston, MA.)

Limb Sparing

The limiting factor in a limb-sparing procedure is being able to obtain a wide surgical margin without compromising a major neurovascular bundle or sacrificing so much tissue that reconstruction is made impossible. The primary objective of the surgical procedure is for the patient to survive this disease, and by no means should any oncologic principles be compromised to establish better functional results.

It has been primarily the addition of chemotherapy

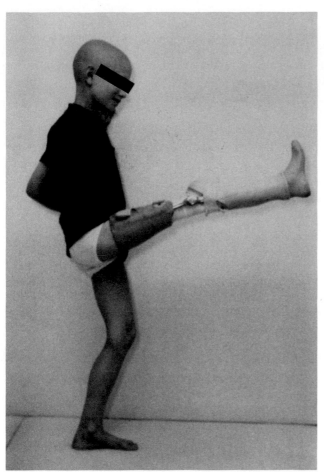

FIGURE 6-3. The patient shows how he can flex and extend his knee after rotationplasty. This would not be possible with a midthigh amputation. (Courtesy of Mark Gebhardt, M.D., Boston, MA.)

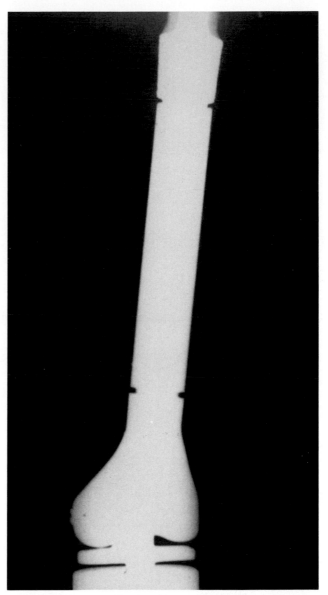

FIGURE 6-4. Metallic distal femoral replacement was performed after osteosarcoma resection and a limb-sparing procedure.

rability of these prosthesis may be only as long as 10 years, and once loosening or failure of the prosthesis occurs, the reconstruction options are poor and few due to the loss of additional bone.[10,11]

Osteoarticular allograft reconstruction is a valuable alternative that probably offers better long-term results but more early complications.[12,13] The osteoarticular joint reconstruction offers a more anatomic reconstitution of the joint (Figs. 6-5 through 6-7). However, the joint itself may need to have a surface replacement at a later date, and the patient's rehabilitation is much slower because he or she must wait for healing of the host allograft bone junction site. Healing at the osteosynthesis site may take 6 months to 1 year if the patient is undergoing chemotherapy. This may mean that the patient must be on crutches for this entire time. The benefit of this procedure is that, after bony union of the osteosynthesis site, the chance of late failure decreases. If the reconstruction fails, there is minimal loss of bone, and a secondary reconstruction is still possi-

ble. Another major advantage of the osteoarticular allograft is that the ligament and tendon origins and insertions remain on the graft, allowing reconstruction of the joint and muscles. This gives a much more functional reconstruction, and the patient is able to have better control of the limb.

Other alternatives include combinations of the previously described procedures. A metal joint replacement can be used with an allograft (Figs. 6-8 and 6-9). This can offer many of the advantages of both procedures. A patient can have a stable joint and also have the benefits of reconstruction of the muscles and tendons for better function. All of these procedures have

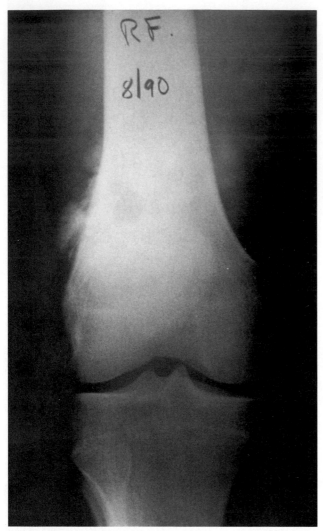

FIGURE 6-5. Distal femoral osteosarcoma in a young adult. (Courtesy of Dempsey Springfield, M.D., Boston, MA.)

benefits and pitfalls. The surgeon must weigh the risks and benefits of these procedures with the patient and select the procedure most beneficial for that patient.

ANATOMIC DETERMINANTS OF SURGICAL TREATMENT

Tibia

Osteosarcomas about the distal tibia should be treated by primary amputation. Although some patients may be considered for a limb-sparing procedure, it is not without added risk. In the distal tibia, much of the surface of the tibia is subcutaneous, and there is insufficient tissue to obtain a wide margin after resection. Because of the excellent functional results from a below-knee amputation, chances should not be taken

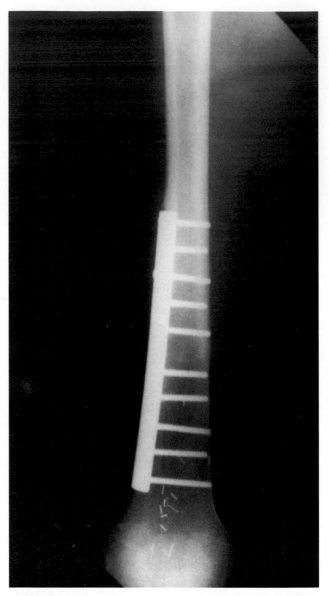

FIGURE 6-6. Osteoarticular allograft was performed after distal femoral resection with a limb-sparing procedure. (Courtesy of Dempsey Springfield, M.D., Boston, MA.)

with too narrow of a margin to allow a heroic reconstruction.

Proximal tibial osteosarcomas can be treated with a thigh-high amputation, knee disarticulation, or a proximal tibia resection with a limb-sparing procedure. There is more area for a soft-tissue coverage after a resection of the proximal tibia, and many patients with tumors may be candidates for a reconstruction of the leg. Another option for proximal tibial lesions that are in proximity to the joint is an arthrodesis. A distal femoral and proximal tibia resection can be performed, followed by a arthrodesis with an allograft or autogenous bone graft.

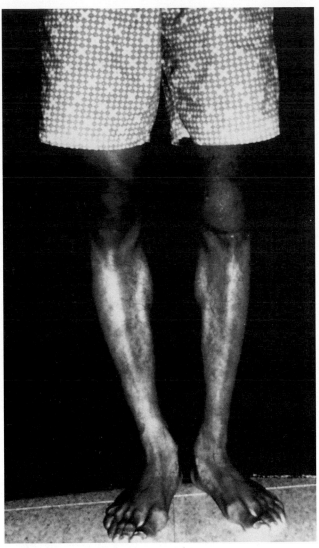

FIGURE 6-7. Postoperative photograph of patient after he underwent a limb-sparing distal femoral resection and osteoarticular allograft. (Courtesy of Dempsey Springfield, M.D., Boston, MA.)

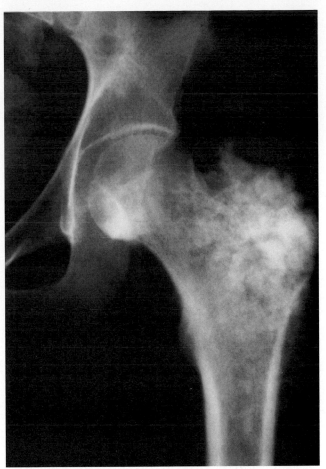

FIGURE 6-8. Proximal femoral osteosarcoma in a young adult. (Courtesy of Dempsey Springfield, M.D., Boston, MA.)

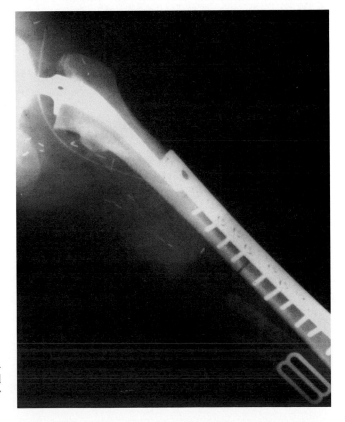

FIGURE 6-9. Combination allograft and prosthetic joint replacement were performed in a patient after a proximal femoral resection for osteosarcoma. (Courtesy of Dempsey Springfield, M.D., Boston, MA.)

Femur

The distal femur is the most common site for osteogenic sarcomas. Because the metaphyseal area of the distal femur is in close proximity to the joint, many of these sarcomas involve the knee joint itself, and extraarticular resections may be needed for a wide margin. If an extraarticular resection is performed, a reconstruction can be performed with an arthrodesis, a custom-made metallic implant, or a combination of allograft reconstruction with a total-knee replacement. In children younger than 10 years of age, a surgical option may be a rotationplasty, as was discussed earlier.

Lesions of the proximal femur usually necessitate an artificial hip replacement. Due to the many sizes and shapes of the hip joint and the possibility of instability due to incongruency, it is difficult to perform an osteoarticular allograft reconstruction of the proximal femur. There are advantages to using allograft for the proximal femur. A reconstruction of the abductor mechanism to the tendon on the allograft can be performed, and the capsule can be repaired to increase the joint stability. A good alternative is to use a combination of proximal femoral allograft and total hip replacement. The artificial hip replacement eliminates the difficulties in finding a exact femoral head size that will fit into the acetabulum, but there is still the advantage of having the tendons of the greater trochanter for reconstruction of the abductor mechanism. Allograft arthrodesis is another possibility, but hip arthrodeses in general are difficult to achieve, and the use of allograft increases the chance of nonunion.

Forearm

Osteosarcoma distal to the elbow is usually best treated by primary amputation, because there is a very limited margin of error for obtaining a wide margin in bones that are subcutaneous. There are also limited reconstructive capabilities distal to the elbow. There are few metallic implants made for the forearm that are functionally good. There are some reasonable results with allograft reconstructions of the radius and ulna, but these are also limited. The primary concern is to be able to perform a wide resection of this malignant neoplasm, and reconstruction may not be possible.

Humerus

Lesions of the distal humerus are probably best treated with an elbow arthrodesis with autogenous or allograft bone for the reconstruction. Artificial elbow joints have poor long-term functional results, and with a large amount of bone loss and muscle loss after a osteosarcoma resection, it is probably best to offer the patient stability to the elbow with an elbow fusion.

Lesions of the proximal humerus are best treated with an osteoarticular allograft reconstruction or a combination of metallic implant with a proximal humeral allograft. One of the main problems of reconstruction of the glenohumeral joint is the instability after resection and the pull of gravity that subluxates this joint after reconstruction. Metallic implants have no soft tissue for reconstructing the capsule nor for preventing subluxation of the glenohumeral joint. The advantage of using an allograft is that the surgeon has the allograft capsule to use for joint stability. The insertions of the rotator cuff muscles offer additional support and functional results after reconstruction.

Another option after resection of the proximal humerus is an arthrodesis of the glenohumeral joint. This can be performed with allograft or autogenous bone graft for the arthrodesis. These patients function fairly well with an arthrodesis, because some of the motion in the shoulder is translated through the scapula thoracic junction.

Scapula

The shoulder girdle is an unusual site for a primary osteogenic sarcoma. However, lesions that do arise within the scapula are probably best treated by a scapular resection and reconstruction of the proximal shoulder girdle to the thoracic wall. Other possibilities are for an allograft or metallic scapular replacement and reconstruction; however, the initial reports of these reconstruction attempts have been poor. The problem occurs because the scapula is not fixed to the axial skeleton and because the shoulder is the most mobile joint of the body.

Pelvis

Osteosarcomas about the pelvis are difficult areas to treat surgically. Lesions that are isolated within the ilium can be treated with a wide resection of the ilium with good functional results. However, lesions that are located within the acetabulum make treatment options difficult, and functional results poor. These lesions can be treated with a hemipelvectomy, but this offers the patient poor chances for adequate functional capabilities after the loss of a limb. Internal hemipelvectomies can be done in many cases. This involves removing part of the pelvis but retaining the limb. However, the difficulty lies within the reconstruction. Allograft hemipelvis reconstruction is fraught with many complications, such as neurovascular compromise, nonunion of the bone, and failure of the graft, and the functional results are fair. In addition to using an allograft pelvis, it is usually necessary to perform a hip replacement on the side of the reconstruction. It is possible to reconstruct the hemipelvis with a metallic implant, but these are fraught with many of the same complications and difficulties as using an allograft.

Spine

Primary osteosarcomas of the spine are the most difficult tumors to treat. It is almost impossible to obtain a wide resection of a vertebral body without compromising the spinal cord. Some of these tumors can be treated with an intralesional resection, followed by intraoperative radiation or brachytherapy. It may be possible to perform a complete vertebral body resection by using anterior and posterior approaches to the spine, but this is an extremely difficult procedure with potentially devastating complications.

Metastatic Disease

Patients who have metastatic osteogenic sarcoma should not be looked on as having end-stage disease. Patients may have continued long-term survival after chemotherapy and surgical removal of all metastatic lesions. The most common site for metastatic osteogenic sarcoma is the lung, and when these lesions occur, thoracotomy and removal of all gross tumor should be performed.[14] Any skip metastases should be considered as part of the primary tumor and should be resected en bloc with the involved sarcoma. Metastatic lesions that occur within the spine can be treated with an intralesional procedure to remove gross tumor, followed with intraoperative radiation or brachytherapy. For any patient with osteogenic sarcoma and metastatic disease, all gross tumor should be surgically removed whenever possible to have any chance of eradicating this tumor. Chemotherapy is effective in treating microscopic disease but has a poor chance of eliminating gross disease.

PROGNOSIS

The surgical treatment of osteogenic sarcoma has changed dramatically over the years, partly because of the advances of chemotherapy and radiology. In the past, isolated, surgical treatment of osteogenic sarcoma was thought to be fruitless because of the high rate of metastasis and eventual death. With the new chemotherapeutic regimens and new radiographic imaging studies, there can be an increase in the survival rates of these patients and in the rate of salvage of functional limbs with excellent cosmetic results. Between 60% and 70% of patients receiving the current mode of treatment can expect long-term survival and salvage of their affected limbs. However, it cannot be stressed enough that oncologic principles should never be sacrificed for improved functional results. The goal of the surgical oncologist is to preserve life.

References

1. Simon A: Current concepts review: Causes of increased survival of patients with osteosarcoma current controversies. J Bone Joint Surg [Am] 66:306–310, 1984
2. Gebhardt MC, Mankin MJ: Osteosarcomas: The treatment controversy, part II. Surg Rounds 2:25–42, 1988
3. Simon MA, Aschliman MA, Thomas N, Mankin HJ: Limb-salvage treatment versus amputation for osteosarcoma of the distal end of the femur. J Bone Joint Surg [Am] 68:1331–1337, 1986
4. Springfield DS, Schmidt R, Graham-Pole J et al: Surgical treatment for osteosarcoma. J Bone Joint Surg [Am] 70:1124–1130, 1988
5. Enneking WF, Kagan A: "Skip" metastases in osteosarcoma. Cancer 36:2192–2205, 1975
6. Wuisman P, Enneking WF: Prognosis for patients who have osteosarcoma with skip metastasis. J Bone Joint Surg [Am] 72:60–68, 1990
7. Campanacci M, Laus M: Local recurrence after amputation for osteosarcoma. J Bone and Joint Surg [Br] 62:201–207, 1980
8. Cammisa FP Jr, Glasser DB, Otis JC et al: The van Ness tibial rotationplasty: A functionally viable reconstructive procedure in children who have a tumor of the distal end of the femur. J Bone Joint Surg [Am] 72:1541–1547, 1990
9. Kotz R, Salzer M: Rotationplasty for childhood osteosarcoma of the distal part of the femur. J Bone Joint Surg [Am] 64:959, 1982
10. National Institutes of Health Consensus Conference: Limb-sparing treatment of adult soft-tissue sarcomas and osteosarcomas. JAMA 254:1791–1794, 1985
11. Horowitz SM, Lane JM, Otis JC et al: Prosthetic arthroplasty of the knee after resection of a sarcoma in the proximal end of the tibia: A report of sixteen cases. J Bone Joint Surg [Am] 73-A:286–293, 1991
12. Gebhardt MC, Roth YF, Mankin HJ: Osteoarticular allografts for reconstruction in the proximal part of the humerus after excision of a musculoskeletal tumor. J Bone Joint Surg [Am] 72:334–345, 1990
13. Tomford WW, Thongphasuk J, Mankin HJ et al: Frozen musculoskeletal allografts: A study of the clinical incidence and causes of infection associated with their use. J Bone Joint Surg [Am] 72:1137–1143, 1990
14. Schajowicz F: Tumors and Tumorlike Lesions of Bone and Joints. New York, Springer-Verlag, 1981

Orthopedic Perspective: What I Want From the Radiologist

Arthur K. Walling

The imaging of bone tumors requires a cooperative effort between the person ordering the tests and the radiologist performing the tests. The role that the radiologist plays depends to some degree on who orders the imaging tests. Often these tests are ordered by primary physicians, pediatricians, or general orthopedists, whose sophistication and knowledge of appropriate imaging is quite different from that of the musculoskeletal oncologist. *It is imperative that the radiologist have a clear understanding of what is desired from the imaging tests and has as much information about the patient as possible.* This allows him or her to suggest alternative or more appropriate imaging tests than may have been originally ordered.

CONVENTIONAL RADIOGRAPHY

Although the radiologic workup of a tumor or a tumor-like lesion may include the entire gamut of imaging modalities, the most important test for establishing the diagnosis is the plain radiograph. It is unfair to expect the radiologist to perform and evaluate more sophisticated imaging (e.g., bone scan, CT, MRI) without access to the plain films. If these are not provided, they should be repeated before additional studies so that they may guide the radiologist in the interpretation.

The plain x-ray interpretation should describe the site of the lesion (e.g., epiphysis, metaphysis, diaphysis), the effect of the lesion on the bone, the response of the bone to the lesion, and any distinguishing features of the matrix. These aspects should be included in the dictated report.

Site of the Lesion

Certain tumors have a predilection for specific bones and specific embryologic areas within the bone. These sites are often characteristic enough to suggest the diagnosis. A good example is the occurrence of chondroblastoma within the epiphysis with an open physeal plate. Other lesions can be virtually excluded from consideration based on location. A very small number of tumors are known to arise in a diaphyseal location.

Lesion Effect

Although not pathognomonic of any specific lesion, the type of destruction produced by the tumor provides information regarding the histology of the lesion. For instance, a permeative type of destruction is most characteristic of Ewing sarcoma and its round cell associates, but a geographic pattern suggests a giant cell tumor.

Bone Response

The margins of a lesion provide information about the rate of growth of the tumor. Slower growing (i.e., usually benign) lesions allow the bone to attempt containment and develop a reactive zone of new bone formation. More aggressive lesions have no reactive border. Periosteal reaction can be uninterrupted (i.e., solid layers of density indicating a long-standing and usually benign process) or interrupted (i.e., sunburst or onion skinning more commonly associated with aggressive growth). Soft-tissue extension beyond the cortex almost invariably indicates an aggressive lesion and most likely a malignant process.

Distinguishing Characteristics

The extracellular matrix produced by the lesion provides the information to categorize the lesion as bone forming or cartilage forming. For example, punctate or smoke-ring calcifications indicate a probable tumor of cartilage origin. Fibrous dysplasia has a fairly typical ground glass appearance.

Using these four features, the radiologist formulates and conveys his or her primary diagnosis and a differential diagnosis to be considered. This information dictates what, if any, additional staging studies are appropriate and which studies will help narrow the differential diagnosis.

RADIONUCLIDE IMAGING

Physicians often expect bone scans to provide a diagnosis, but they do not realize that bone scans, although sensitive, are quite nonspecific. The radiologist may need to explain that the appropriate use of a bone scan is to verify a lesion that may not readily be apparent on plain x-ray films, to rule out the presence of additional lesions, to determine the anatomic extent of a lesion, and to provide information about the intrinsic activity of a lesion.

I am often disappointed when a bone scan report states only that there is an area of uptake in the proximal femur. Useful information can be derived from the amount of activity (e.g., mild, moderate, marked) and whether or not the area of activity corresponds with the area seen on the plain x-ray film. The area of isotope uptake should be identified by whether it involves the periphery or the entire lesion and by areas of decreased density. If possible, the imaging should be performed in the anteroposterior and lateral planes.

Radionuclide imaging can also provide information about soft-tissue lesions. While at the University of Florida, Terry M. Hudson, my orthopedic radiologist, often made the point that uptake in a soft-tissue lesion did not differentiate benign from malignant disease, but soft-tissue lesions that showed no uptake during scanning were invariably benign.

COMPUTED TOMOGRAPHY AND MAGNETIC RESONANCE IMAGING

CT and MRI have very limited capabilities in diagnosis, and neither CT nor MRI is suitable for establishing the precise nature of a bone tumor. It is a common misconception among orthopedists that MRI can reliably differentiate benign from malignant lesions. The major indication for both tests remains anatomic detailing.

CT scanning provides information regarding the anatomic extent of lesions, the presence of soft-tissue extension, and the proximity of neurovascular structures. It has probably been underused with the advent of MRI. It remains superior to MRI in providing cortical detail and allowing characterization of tumor matrix, especially calcification and ossification. For soft-tissue lesions, CT can accurately depict lipomas (i.e., characteristic density of -90 to -100 HU), identify necrosis, and suggest inflammatory processes.

MRI also provides information regarding the extent and relations of important anatomic structures. Its primary advantage is its ability to provide axial information in addition to cross-sectional anatomy, and it is especially helpful in delineating the intramedullary extent of tumor in the coronal plane. Although T1-weighted and T2-weighted measurements are of limited value for histologic determination of musculoskeletal lesions, they are useful in determining areas of the lesion that may be best suited for biopsy, and this should be communicated in the written report.

With the increasing demand for fiscal accountability, the radiologist may need to remind the physician that a CT scan can provide the necessary information at a lower cost and that only if additional information is needed would he proceed to MRI.

ROLE OF THE RADIOLOGIST

The role of the radiologist is crucial to the proper diagnosis and eventual treatment of musculoskeletal tumors. This role is occasionally multifaceted and depends on who orders the tests. If the radiologist's expertise is called on by the primary practitioner, pediatrician, or general orthopedist, he or she may need to intervene and suggest better methods of evaluation than were originally ordered. It may require an adverse business decision—not every lesion deserves an MR scan. It may require the suggestion of a simple chest radiograph to rule out metastatic disease. If the imaging is ordered by an oncologist, decisions regarding which tests will provide the maximum information at the best economic value may need to be made. Both situations require communication.

In reporting the results of an imaging test, a thorough examination of all tests available should be done, and how these tests influence the results of the ordered examination should be communicated in the final report. The information should include all of the information that was previously discussed under the individual imaging sections and an appropriate differential diagnosis with supporting and refuting information from the imaging studies. If the radiologist's diagnosis differs from the surgeon's, it will lead to a reexamination of the surgical plan. The treatment of bone tumors is a combined effort, and the more information that can be derived from the imaging studies, the better the outcome is for all.

Radiotherapeutic Treatment of Soft Tissue Sarcoma

Harvey M. Greenberg

The goal of therapy in the treatment of soft tissue sarcoma is to control the local tumor and distant disease. Radiation therapy is frequently used as a major treatment modality in achieving local control. Before the 1960s, patients with sarcomas were often treated with simple excisions of tumors, with the likelihood of local failure. After the high local recurrence rate with the simple procedures was reported, there was a strong trend toward the use of other therapeutic approaches, including more aggressive surgery and often using amputation. This resulted in a marked improvement in local tumor control but at the expense of functional and cosmetic deficits, particularly in patients with extremity sarcomas.

For many years, radiation therapy was not thought to be an effective treatment modality for sarcomas. This was principally because radiation therapy is not uniformly effective in locally controlling large, unresected tumor masses. In the late 1960s, researchers at M. D. Anderson Cancer Center reported work indicating that a combination of local surgical excision followed by adequate radiation therapy treatment resulted in local control rates that were comparable to the most aggressive forms of surgical treatment. This combination is now generally agreed to be effective and can lead to highly successful functional and cosmetic results.

The idea of combining surgery and radiotherapy is now well accepted, although the precise techniques by which radiation therapy is administered for sarcomas are still evolving. Protocols using various combinations of surgery, external beam radiation therapy, intraoperative radiation therapy, or interstitial radiation therapy have been reported by single institutions or national collaborative groups.

Three-dimensional (3D) or conformal radiation therapy delivery promises further advances in more precisely treating the tumor and preserving normal tissues. Before the advances in diagnostic imaging techniques, the treatment of sarcomas with radiation therapy was associated with an unacceptably high likelihood of error in estimating accurate tumor volumes. Clinicians once used palpation and two-dimensional plain radiographs as their principal guides in defining radiation therapy portals. Advances in computerized tomography, nuclear medicine, and magnetic resonance imaging have made estimations of tumor volumes much more precise, allowing significant improvement in designing treatment portals.

Before discussing the newer imaging modalities in sarcoma treatment, the basic radiotherapeutic principles related to sarcoma treatment should be outlined. Many sarcomas, particularly those of the extremities, tend to grow in a longitudinal fashion, and wide surgical margins proximally and distally are usually advised. Sarcomas do not extend as much circumferentially. Radiation oncologists can generally avoid treating the entire cross section of an extremity and still achieve local control. The ability to spare soft tissues in this manner is especially important for weight-bearing extremities treated for soft tissue sarcoma.

Although compartmental resection was popularized as a surgical technique in the 1970s, the entire muscle compartment from origin to insertion usually is not at risk for tumor involvement. Modern radiotherapy techniques use treatment portals that encompass the palpable or radiographically evident disease plus a safety margin of at least 5 cm proximally and distally. For tumors that are exceptionally large or of high grade, clinicians may use safety margins as great as 10 cm. Because there is only a small likelihood of regional lymph node involvement by sarcomas, radiation therapy portals do not include draining lymph nodes. However, a biopsy should be performed on any palpable or clinically suspicious nodes to rule out involvement.

PRINCIPLES OF RADIATION TREATMENT

Although the exact details of radiotherapy treatment depend on individual factors such as site, grade, and the amount of tissue involved, there are basic principles that hold for any treatment site.

Patient Immobilization

To achieve local tumor control and a good functional result, the radiation treatment must be delivered in a precise manner. Patients must be strictly immobilized to prevent variation in the treatment setup on a day-to-day basis. A variety of devices allow daily treatments to be simple and reproducible to within a day-to-day variance of less than 5 mm. Such devices allow all normal tissues not at risk for tumor involvement to be effectively excluded in a reproducible way from the radiation therapy portal.

Shrinking Field Technique

A dose of 6500 to 7000 cGy commonly used in the treatment of soft tissue sarcomas produces substantial normal tissue morbidity if administered to a large radiation therapy portal. This morbidity can be minimized if the size of the portal is progressively reduced during the course of treatment. The initial portals should encompass all areas with a moderate probability of microscopic tumor involvement and should deliver between 4500 to 5000 cGy. After that dose is delivered, field portal reductions are designed to treat only those areas at highest risk for local recurrence; the high-risk areas should be treated to a total dose of 6500 to 7000 cGy.

Optimal Beam Shaping

Sarcomas can rarely be treated with simple fields in an optimal fashion. A combination of a customized blocking readily available in most radiation therapy centers and multiple field techniques lead to superior dose distributions and allow maximal shielding of normal tissues.

Site Individualization

The radiation therapy technique used to treat an individual patient is tailored according to the characteristics of the tumor and the anatomy of the site. Radiation oncologists must have a precise understanding of the patient's surgical anatomy, adequacy of the tumor excision, and adequacy of healing before initiation of radiation therapy treatment.

The radiation therapist must understand when preservation of function through the combination of radiation therapy and surgery is not appropriate. These situations include sarcomas that directly involve and cannot be resected from adjacent bone or the major neurovascular bundle. If resection after radiation therapy may lead to a cosmetically or functionally unsatisfactory result, amputation may prove to be a better choice.

IMAGING MODALITIES USED IN THE RADIOTHERAPEUTIC MANAGEMENT OF SARCOMAS

Plain Radiography

Plain radiographs of soft tissue sarcomas are of little value in diagnosis or treatment, except for tumors in the extremities. Extremity soft tissue masses may be seen on plain radiographs, as may bone permeation or erosion. These films are not often used for planning treatment. They may be useful in continuing follow-up, because they may show the response of tumor to treatment and may show improvement or deterioration in bone that has been irradiated.

Conventional Arteriography

Pretreatment arteriography may play a significant role in establishing the direct involvement of the neurovascular bundle by sarcoma. Although angiography can be useful in establishing tumor boundaries, its function has largely been supplanted by CT or MRI. Arteriography can play a significant role in therapy as a way of delivering chemotherapy or embolization techniques along with concurrent radiotherapy.

Nuclear Medicine

Traditional technetium-based bone scanning plays a significant role in the treatment of patients with sarcomas. A bone scan used as a survey technique can estab-lish the presence or absence of distant bony metastasis. Bone scanning may also help to establish whether extremity sarcomas are unifocal or multifocal within a bone. This distinction may be extremely important in establishing whether patients are candidates for limb preservation or should proceed to more aggressive techniques, such as amputation.

Bone scanning has value in the delivery of radiation therapy to patients with extremity sarcoma. If MRI is not available, bone scanning often represents the most sensitive technique for establishing the proximal and distal extent of tumor. Bone scanning, even with the most sophisticated 3D techniques, has not been proven to be of significant value in establishing treatment portals for conformal radiation therapy. In the posttreatment setting, serial bone scans are useful for establishing the emergence of metastatic disease in distant sites but are of equivocal value in establishing the recurrence of disease at the irradiated site. Irradiated bone often shows a mixture of increased photon and photon-deficient activity. Companion techniques, such as MRI, are often necessary to establish whether persistent disease remains in bone and adjacent soft tissue.

Computerized Tomography

In the diagnostic phase of patient evaluation, CT is valuable in establishing the presence of metastatic disease in soft tissues, particularly the lungs. At the primary site, CT is an effective modality for establishing the 3D parameters of the soft-tissue mass. Presurgical CT scans should uniformly be obtained as an adjunct to eventual radiation treatment planning.

CT scanning is the most commonly used form of 3D imaging for planning radiation therapy. A well-designed radiation oncology treatment unit has access to a CT scanner for the treatment planning process. For a typical sarcoma patient, the treatment planning process consists of defining the appropriate treatment position, fashioning of customized immobilization devices, and developing preliminary portals. The patient is then scanned at 5- to 10-mm intervals while in the treatment position using the customized immobilization device. This allows the radiation oncologist to obtain images that define the patient's 3D anatomy while in the appropriate treatment position. Information from the individual CT slices are fed into the treatment planning computer, and an optimal treatment plan is devised.

In the postoperative setting, CT scanning is the most commonly used modality for assessing recurrence and the effect of the various treatment modalities on affected soft tissues.

Magnetic Resonance Imaging

As MRI has become more widely available, it has become an important imaging technique in the treatment of sarcomas. Although MRI is not commonly used as a screening modality to evaluate distant bony or soft-tissue metastasis, it is effective at determining the extent of primary tumors and multifocality. MRI also appears to be the most accurate imaging technique for defining bone marrow involvement when obvious bony changes are not seen on plain films or on bone scans.

MRI has a limited role in radiation treatment planning. Anatomic distortions in the translation of MR data make anatomically based MR treatment planning less accurate than CT planning. After this problem is solved, clinicians will need to compare anatomic volumes delineated by MRI and CT to ascertain which is more accurate in determining tumor volumes.

In the posttreatment setting, MRI appears to be an extremely useful modality for delineating whether viable tumor is present in the treated site. Gadolinium contrast agents are particularly helpful in making this distinction.

Radiation oncologists rely heavily on diagnostic imaging techniques to delineate anatomic targets for the delivery of therapeutic radiation. The newer techniques, including CT and MRI, have been extremely helpful in accurately defining progressively limited tumor volumes. The coupling of more accurately defined tumor volumes with 3D treatment delivery techniques promises future therapy requiring that smaller amounts of normal tissue be exposed to therapeutic radiation. This should lead to an improved therapeutic ratio, with better local control of sarcomas and a reduced likelihood of treatment-related complications.

BIBLIOGRAPHY

IMAGING STUDIES

Radiology

Abdelwahab IF, Present DA et al: Tumorlike tuberculous granulomas of bone. AJR Am J Roentgenol 149:1207–1208, 1987

Abdelwhab IF, Norman A: Osteosclerotic sarcoidosis. AJR 150:161–162, 1988

Abel MS, Smith, GR: The case of the disappearing pelvis. Radiology 111:105–106, 1974

Abramson MN: Disseminated asymptomatic osteosclerosis with features resembling melorheosis, osteopoikilosis, and osteopathia striata: A case report. J Bone Joint Surg [Am] 50:991–996, 1968

Ahmed MJ, Omar YT et al: Soft tissue sarcoma in Kuwait: A review of 114 patients. Clin Radiol 38:2–29, 1987

Alho A, Connor JF, Mankin HJ et al: Assessment of malignancy of cartilage tumors using flow cytometry. J Bone Joint Surg [Am] 65:779–785, 1983

Allen BL, Jinkins WJ: Vertebral osteonecrosis associated with pancreatitis in a child: A case report. J Bone Joint Surg [Am] 60:985–987, 1978

Amin PH, Evans ANW: Essential osteolysis of carpal and tarsal bones. Br J Radiol 51:539–541, 1978

Anastasides KD, Otis JB et al: Vertebral malacoplakia: A case report. J Bone Joint Surg 69:458–462, 1987

Aoki J, Yamamoto I et al: Reactive endosteal bone formation. Skeletal Radiol 16:545–551, 1987

Aoki J, Yamamoto I et al: Sclerotic bone metastasis: Radiologic–pathologic correlation. Radiology 159:127–132, 1986

Arlart IP, Maier W, Leupold D et al: Massive periosteal new bone formation in ulcerative colitis. Radiology 144:507–508, 1982

Arlart VI, Gargon G: Periostale knochenneubildung bei colitis ulcerosa im jugendlichen alter. Fortschr Geb Rontgenstr 135:577–582, 1981

Ayala AG, Zornosa J: Primary bone tumors: Percutaneous needle biopsy. Radiology 149:675–679, 1983

Ayella RJ: Hemangiopericytoma. Radiology 97:611–612, 1970

Aymard A, Chevrot A et al: Fracture spontanee du sternum. J Radiol 68:593–595, 1987

Baudrillard JC, Lerair JM et al: Compression medullaire dorsale par chondrome sous-perioste vertebral. J Radiol 68:527–531, 1987

Beals RK, Bird CB: Carpal and tarsal osteolysis. J Bone Joint Surg [Am] 57:681–686, 1975

Bell RS, Goodman SB, Fornasier VL: Coccygeal glomus tumors:

A case of mistaken identity. J Bone Joint Surg [Am] 64:595–597, 1982

Berger PE, Heidelberger KP, Poznanski AK: Extravasation of calcium gluconate as a cause of soft-tissue calcification in infancy. AJR Am J Roentgenol 121:109–117, 1974

Bernardino ME, Jing BS, Thomas JL et al: The extremity soft-tissue lesion: A comparative study of ultrasound, computed tomography, and xeroradiography. Radiology 139:5–59, 1981

Bhate DV, Pizarro AJ, Greenfield GB: Idiopathic hypertrophic osteoarthropathy without pachyderma. Radiology 129:379–382, 1978

Blane CE, Perkash I: True heterotopic bone in the paralyzed patient. Skeletal Radiol 7:2–25, 1981

Blank N, Lieber A: The significance of growing bone islands. Radiology 85:508–511, 1965

Bléry M, Chagnon S, Picard A et al: Ostéites du crêne. J Radiol 61:677–781, 1980

Bliznak J, Staple TW: Radiology of angiodysplasias of the limb. Radiology 110:3–44, 1974

Bloon RA, Libson E et al: The periosteal sunburst reaction to bone metastases: A literature review and report of 20 additional cases. Skeletal Radiol 16:629–634, 1987

Boillat MA, Garcia J, Velebit L: Radiological criteria of industrial fluorosis. Skeletal Radiol 5:161–165, 1980

Bottomly JP, Bradley J, Whitehouse GH: Waldenstrom's macroglobulinemia and amyloidosis with subcutaneous calcification and lymphographic appearances. Br J Radiol 47:232–235, 1974

Braithwaite PA, Lees RF: Vertebral hydatid disease: Radiological assessment. Radiology 140:763–766, 1981

Brauner M, Hassan M et al: Nocardiose osseuse: A propos d'une observation chez un jeune enfant. J Radiol 66:699–701, 1985

Buirski G, Ratliff AHC et al: Cartilage cell containing tumours of the pelvis: A radiological review of 40 patients. Br J Radiol 59:197–204, 1986

Buirski G, Watt I: The radiological features of "solid" aneurysmal bone cysts. Br J Radiol 57:1057–1065, 1984

Buonocore E, Salomon A, Kerley HE: Pseudomyeloma. Radiology 95:41–46, 1970

Burgener FA, Landman S: The radiological manifestations of fibroxanthosarcomas. Fortschr Geb Roentgenstr 125:123–128, 1976

Burkhardt R, Frisch B, Schlag R et al: Carcinomatous osteodysplasia. Skeletal Radiol 8:169–178, 1982

Caffey J, Silverman FN: Pediatric X-ray Diagnosis, 5th ed. Chicago, Year Medical Book Publishers, 1967

Cahill BR: Osteolysis of the distal part of the clavicle in male athletes. J Bone Joint Surg [Am] 64:1053–1058, 1982

Campbell CJ, Papademetriou T, Bonfiglio M: Melorheostosis: A report of the clinical, roentgenographic, and pathological findings in 14 cases. J Bone Joint Surg [Am] 50:1281–1304, 1968

Capanna R, Springfield DS et al: Juxtaepiphyseal aneurysmal bone cyst. Skeletal Radiol 13:21–25, 1985

Capanna R, Van Horn J et al: Epiphyseal involvement in unicameral bone cysts. Skeletal Radiol 15:428–432, 1986

Cavanagh RC: Tumors of the soft tissues of the extremities. Semin Roentgenol 8:7–89, 1973

Chamberlain DS, Whitaker J, Silverman FN: Idiopathic osteoarthropathy and cranial defects in children. AJR Am J Roentgenol 93:408–415, 1965

Charneux F, Bretagne MC, Hoeffel JC et al: Tumeur rare du naso pharynx. J Radiol 62:335–337, 1981

Chevrot A, Pallardy G, Ledoux P, Lebard G: Skeletal manifestations of hyperthyroidism. J Radiol 59:167–173, 1978

Christie DP: The spectrum of radiographic bone changes in children with fluorosis. Radiology 136:85–90, 1980

Clarisse PDT, Staple TW: Diffuse bone sclerosis in multiple myeloma. Radiology 99:327–328, 1971

Claudon M, Bracard S et al: Spinal involvement in alveolar echinococcosis: Assessment of two cases. Radiology 162:571–572, 1987

Claudon M, Regent D et al: La trochanterite tuberculeuse: Interet de l'echographie et de la scanographie: A propos de trois observations. J Radiol 67:309–314, 1986

Comstock C, Wolson AH: Roentgenology of sporotrichosis. Am J Roentgenol 125:651–655, 1975

Condon RR, Allen RP: Congenital generalized fibromatosis. Radiology 76:444–448, 1961

Cone RO, Resnick D, Goergen TG et al: Condensing osteitis of the clavicle. AJR Am J Roentgenol 141:387–388, 1983

Crone M, Watt I: Case of the month: A lump on the thigh. Br J Radiol 60:1035–1036, 1987

Daffner RH, Martinez S, Gehweiler JA et al: Stress fractures of the proximal tibia in runners. Radiology 142:63–65, 1982

Daffner RH: Stress fractures: Current concepts. Skeletal Radiol 2:221–229, 1978

Dalinka MK, Chunn SP: Osteoblastoma—benign or malignant precursor? Report of a case. J Can Assoc Radiol 23:214–216, 1972

Dalinka MK, Dinnenberg S, Greendyke WH, Hopkins R: Roentgenographic features of osseous coccidioidomycosis and differential diagnosis. J Bone Joint Surg [Am] 53:1157–1164, 1971

Danigelis JA, Long RE: Anonymous mycobacterial osteomyelitis: A case report of a 6-year-old child. Radiology 93:353–354, 1969

DeSmet AA: Acro-osteolysis occurring in a patient with idiopathic multicentric osteolysis. Skeletal Radiol 5:29–34, 1980

Destouet JM, Kyriakos M, Gilula LA: Fibrous histiocytoma (fibroxanthoma) of a cervical vertebra. Skeletal Radiol 5:241–246, 1980

Dihlmann W: Hemispherical spondylosclerosis: A polyetiologic syndrome. Skeletal Radiol 7:99–106, 1981

Dillon E, Parkin GJS: The role of diagnostic radiology in the diagnosis and management of rhabdomyosarcoma in young persons. Clin Radiol 29:5–59, 1978

Dismukes WE et al: Destructive bone disease in early syphilis. JAMA 236:2646–2648, 1976

Dodds WJ, Steinbach HL: Gout associated with calcification of cartilage. N Engl J Med 275:745–749, 1966

Doe WF, Henry K, Doyle FH: Radiological and histological findings in 6 patients wiht alpha-chain disease. Br J Radiol 49:3–11, 1976

Donovan RM, Shah KJ: Unusual sites of acute osteomyelitis in childhood. Clin Radiol 33:222–230, 1982

Dorfman HD, Bhagavan BS: Malignant fibrous histiocytoma of soft tissue with metaplastic bone and cartilage formation: A new radiologic sign. Skeletal Radiol 8:145–150, 1982

Draper MW, Chafetz N, Weinberg GL et al: Distinct form of osteosclerosis in identical twins with mental retardation. AJR 1Am J Roentgenol 39:1205–1209, 1982

DuBois PJ, Orr DP, Meyersen EN, Barnes LE: Undifferentiated parotid carcinoma with osteoblastic metastases. AJR Am J Roentgenol 129:744–746, 1977

Edeiken B, de Santos LA: Percutaneous needle biopsy of the irradiated skeleton. Radiology 146:653–655, 1983

Edeiken-Monroe B, Edeiken J, Kim EE: Radiologic concepts of lymphoma of bone. Radiol Clin North Am 28:841–864, 1990

Ellis W: Multiple bone lesions caused by Avian–Battey mycobacteria. J Bone Joint Surg [Br] 56:323–326, 1974

Elson MW: The syndrome of exophthalmos, hypertrophic osteoarthropathy, and pretibial myxedema. AJR Am J Roentgenol 85:114–118, 1961

Engels EP, Smith RC, Krantz S: Bone sclerosis in multiple myeloma. Radiology 75:242–247, 1960

Erikson V, Hjelmstedt A: Roentgenologic aspects of BCG osteomyelitis. Radiology 101:575–578, 1971

Fink IJ, Lee MA et al: Case reports: Radiographic and CT appearance of intraosseous xanthoma mimicking a malignant lesion. Br J Radiol 58:262–264, 1985

Foley WD, Baum JK, Wheeler RH: Diffuse osteosclerosis with lymphocytic lymphoma: A case report. Radiology 117:553–554, 1975

Franck JL, Lhez JM, Arlet J: Une métastase osseuse exubérante d'origine prostatique. J Radiol 63:209–211, 1982

Frangione B, Franklin EC: Heavy chain diseases: Clinical features and molecular significance of the disordered immunoglobulin structure. Semin Hematol 10:53–64, 1973

Franquet T, Lecumberri F et al: Condensing osteitis of the clavicle. Skeletal Radiol 14:184–187, 1985

Freiberger R: Thoughts on the diagnosis of bone tumors. Radiology 150:276, 1984

Gehweiler JA, Capp MP, Chick EW: Observations on the roentgen patterns in blastomycosis of bone: A review of cases from the blastomycosis cooperative study of the Veterans Administration and Duke University Medical Center. Am J Roentgenol 108:497–510, 1970

Geoffroy J et al: Les lesions osteoarticulaires du pied chez le diabetique. J Radiol 59:557–562, 1978

Gilsantz V, Grunebaum M: Radiographic appearance of iliac marrow biopsy sites. AJR Am J Roentgenol 128:597–598, 1977

Gilula LA, Bliznak J, Staple TW: Idiopathic nonfamilial acrosteolysis with cortical defects and mandibular ramus osteolysis. Radiology 121:63–68, 1976

Glass TA, Mills SE et al: Giant cell reparative granuloma of the hands and feet. Radiology 149:65–68, 1983

Goergen TG, Resnick D, Riley RR: Posttraumatic abnormalities of the pubic bone simulating malignancy. Radiology 126:85–87, 1978

Goldman AB, Bullough P, Kammerman S, Ambos M: Osteitis deformans of the hip joint. AJR Am J Roentgenol 128:601–606, 1977

Gompels BM, Vataw ML, Martel W: Correlation of radiological manifestations of multiple myeloma with immunoglobulin abnormalities and prognosis. Radiology 104:509–514, 1972

Greaney RB, Gerber FH, Laughlin RL et al: Distribution and natural history of stress fractures in U.S. Marine recruits. Radiology 146:339–346, 1983

Greenfield GB, Escamilla CH, Schorsch HA: The hand as an indicator of generalized disease. AJR Am J Roentgenol 99:736–745, 1967

Greenfield GB: Radiology of Bone Diseases. 5th ed. Philadelphia, JB Lippincott, 1990

Greenspan A, Elguezbel A, Bryk D: Multifocal osteoid osteoma: A case report and review of the literature. AJR Am J Roentgenol 121:103–106, 1974

Greenspan A, Steiner G et al: Mixed sclerosing bone dysplasia coexisting with dysplasia epiphysealis hemimelica (Trevor-Fairbank disease). Skeletal Radiol 15:452–454, 1986

Greyson-Fleg RT, Reichmister JP et al: Post-traumatic osteochondroma. J Can Assoc Radiol 38:195–198, 1987

Grunow OH: Radiating spicules, a nonspecific sign of bone disease. Radiology 65:200–205, 1955

Guibert JL, Pastaud P, Bui BN et al: Aspects tomodensitometriques des sarcomes des parties molles des membres de l'adulte. J Radiol 64:489–494, 1983

Guilbeau JC, David M et al: Metastases osseuses des carcinomes bronchiques. J Radiol 67:79–82, 1986

Gyepes MT, D'Angio GJ: Extracranial metastases from CNS tumors in children and adolescents. Radiology 87:55–63, 1966

Hall FM, Gore SM: Osteosclerotic myeloma variants. Skeletal Radiol 17:101–105, 1988

Hardy R, Lehrer H: Desmoplastic fibroma vs desmoid tumor of bone. Radiology 88:899–901, 1967

Harris VJ, Ramilo J: Caffey's disease: A case originating in the 1st metatarsal and review of a 12-year experience. AJR Am J Roentgenol 130:335–337, 1978

Harverson G, Warren AG: Tarsal bone disintegration in leprosy. Clin Radiol 30:317–322, 1979

Haverbush TJ, Wilde AH, Hawk WA, Scherbel AL: Osteolysis of the ribs and cervical spine in progressive systemic sclerosis (scleroderma). J Bone Joint Surg [Am] 56:637–640, 1974

Heitzman ER, Bornhurst RA, Russell JP: Disease due to anonymous mycobacteria. AJR Am J Roentgenol 103:533–539, 1968

Hemingway SP, Leung A, Lavender JP: Familial vanishing limbs: Four generations of idiopathic multicentric osteolysis. Clin Radiol 34:585–588, 1983

Herold CJ, Wittich GR et al: Skeletal involvement in hairy cell leukemia. Skeletal Radiol 17:171–175, 1988

Himmelfarb E, Sebes J, Rainowitz J: Unusual roentgenographic presentations of multiple myeloma: Report of 3 cases. J Bone Joint Surg [Am] 56:1723–1728, 1974

Ho A, Williams DM et al: Unilateral hypertrophic osteoarthropathy in a patient with an infected axillary–axillary bypass graft. Radiology 162:573–574, 1987

Horner K, Forman GH et al: Atypical simple bone cysts of the jaws. I: Recurrent lesions. Clin Radiol 39:53–57, 1988

Horner K, Forman GH: Atypical simple bone cysts of the jaws. II: A possible association with benign fibro-osseous (cemental) lesions of the jaws. Clin Radiol 39:59–63, 1988

Howie JL: CT of osteoid osteoma of the femoral neck: The value of oblique reformatting. J Assoc Can Radiol 36:254–257, 1985

Hsieh CK: Echinococcus involvement of bone with x-ray examination. Radiology 14:562–575, 1930

Isley JK: Prognosis in osteitis condensans ilii. Radiology 72:234–237, 1959

Jacobson HG, Poppel MH, Shapiro JH, Grossberger S: The vertebral pedicle sign: A roentgen finding to differentiate metastatic carcinoma from multiple myeloma. AJR Am J Roentgenol 80:817–821, 1958

James AE et al: Roentgen findings in pseudoxanthoma elasticum (PXE). AJR Am J Roentgenol 106:642–647, 1969

Janecki CJ, Nelson CL, Dohn DF: Intrasacral cyst: Report of a case and review of the literature. J Bone Joint Surg [Am] 54:423–428, 1972

Jensen WN, Lasser EC: Urticaria pigmentosa associated with widespread sclerosis of the spongiosa of bone. Radiology 71:826–832, 1958

Johnson AC, James AE, Reddy ER, Johnson S: Relation of vascular and osseous changes in leprosy. Skeletal Radiol 3:36–41, 1978

Johnson GF: Osteoid osteoma of the femoral neck. AJR Am J Roentgenol 74:65–69, 1955 236. Johnson LC: A general theory of bone tumors. Bull NY Acad Med 29:164–171, 1953

Jurik AG, Graudal H et al: Sclerotic changes of the manubrium sterni. Skeletal Radiol 13:195–201, 1985

Jurik AG, Moller BN: Inflammatory hyperostosis and sclerosis of the clavicle. Skeletal Radiol 15:284–290, 1986

Jurik AG, Moller SH et al: Chronic sclerosing osteomyelitis of the iliac bone: Etiological possibilities. Skeletal Radiol 17:114–118, 1988

Kaibara N, Mitsuyasu M, Katsuki I et al: Generalized enchondromatosis with unusual complications of soft tissue calcifications and hemangiomas. Skeletal Radiol 8:43–46, 1982

Kanis JA, Thomson JG: Mixed sclerosing bone dystrophy with regression of melorheostosis. Br J Radiol 48:400–402, 1975

Karasick D, O'Hara EA: Juvenile aponeurotic fibroma. Radiology 123:725–726, 1977

Karlin CA, De Smet AA, Neff J et al: The variable manifestations of extraarticular synovial chondromatosis. AJR Am J Roentgenol 137:731–735, 1981

Karnel VF, Salomonowitz E et al: Digital subtraktionsangiographie: Eine wertvolle methode zum nachweis eines osteoidosteoms. Fortschritte a/d Gebiet Röntgenstrahlen 144:735–736, 1986

Kaufman RA et al: False negative bone scans in neuroblastoma metastatic to the ends of long bones. AJR Am J Roentgenol 130:131–135, 1978

Kenin A, Levine J, Spinner M: Parosteal lipoma: A report of 2 cases with associated bone changes. J Bone Joint Surg [Am] 41:1122–1126, 1959

Kenney PJ, Siegel MJ, McAlister WH: Congenital intraspinal neuroblastoma: A treatable simulant of myelodysplasia. Am J Roentgenol 138:166–167, 1982

Kim KS, Rogers LF, Lee C: The dural lucent line: Characteristic sign of hyperostosing meningioma en plaque. AJR Am J Roentgenol 141:1217–1221, 1983

Kirkpatrick DJ: Donovanosis (granuloma inguinale): A rare cause of osteolytic bone lesions. Clin Radiol 21:101–105, 1970

Kittredge RD, Finby N: The many facets of lymphangioma. AJR Am J Roentgenol 95:56–66, 1965

Klumper A: Congenital diaphyseal venous dysplasia. Fortschr Geb Rontgenstr 125:396–399, 1976

Kohler E, Babbitt D, Huizenga B, Good TA: Hereditary osteolysis: A clinical, radiological, and chemical study. Radiology 108:99–105, 1973

Koischwitz VD, Anders G: Die chondroplasia punctata. Fortschr Geb Rontgenstr 132:689–694, 1980

Konstantinov VD: Verlauf der purulenten sakroileitis im rontgenbild. Fortschr Geb Rontgenstr 140:195–199, 1984

Korber J, McCarthy S, Marsden W: Case report Skeletal Radiol 22:222–225, 1993

Krause VFJ: Hyperostosis sternocosto-clavicularis. Fortschr Geb Rontgenstr 147:350–352, 1987

Kricun ME: Red-yellow marrow conversion: Its effect on the location of some solitary bone lesions. Skeletal Radiol 14:10–19, 1985

Kumar R, Smissen EVD, Jorizzo N: Systemic sporotrichosis with osteomyelitis. J Can Assoc Radiol 35:83–84, 1984

Kumar R, Swischuk LE et al: Benign cortical defect: Site for an avulsion fracture. Skeletal Radiol 15:553–555, 1986

Kutzner J, Kohler H, Vehlinger E: Sternocostoclavicular hyperostosis. Fortschr Geb Rontgenstr 123:446–449, 1975

Lagier R, Mbakop A, Bigler A: Osteopoikilosis: A radiological and pathological study. Skeletal Radiol 11:161–168, 1984

Lamego CMB, Zerbini MCN: Bone-metastasizing primary renal tumors in children. Radiology 147:449–454, 1983

Lee SM, Lee RGL et al: Magnification radiograpy in osteomyelitis. Skeletal Radiol 15:625–627, 1986

Lehrer HZ, Maxfield WS, Nice CM: The periosteal "sunburst" pattern in metastatic bone tumors. AJR Am J Roentgenol 108:154–161, 1970

Leonard RCF, Owen JP, Proctor SJ et al: Multiple myeloma: Radiology or bone scanning? Clin Radiol 32:291–295, 1981

Lerner MR, Southwick WO: Keratin cysts in phalangeal bones:

Report of an unusual case. J Bone Joint Surg [Am] 50:365–372, 1968

Levin DC, Blazina ME, Levine E: Fatigue fractures of the shaft of the femur: Simulation of malignant tumor. Radiology 89:883–885, 1967

Lewall DB, Ofole S et al: Mycetoma. Skeletal Radiol 14:257–262, 1985

Lindell MM Jr, Shirkhoda A et al: Parosteal osteosarcoma: Radiologic–pathologic correlation with emphasis on CT. Am J Roentgenol 148:323–328, 1987

Linschied RL, Dahlin DC: Unusual lesions of the patella. J Bone Joint Surg [Am] 48:1359–1365, 1966

Lodwick GS: Solitary malignant tumors of bone: The application of predictor variables in diagnosis. Semin Roentgenol 1:293–313, 1966

Ludwig H, Kumpan W, Sinzinger H: Radiography and bone scintigraphy in multiple myeloma: A comparative analysis. Br J Radiol 55:173–181, 1982

Macpherson RI, Letts RM: Skeletal diseases associated with angiomatosis. J Can Assoc Radiol 29:90–100, 1978

Majid MA, Mathias PF, Seth HN, Thirumalachar MJ: Primary mycetoma of the patella. J Bone Joint Surg [Am] 46:1283–1286, 1964

Malghem J, Maldague B: Transient fatty cortical defects following fractures in children. Skeletal Radiol 15:368–371, 1986

Marchal AL, Bretagne MC, Fourchy E: Memoires originaux. J Radiol 64:675–679, 1983

Marsot-Dupuch K, Cauquil P, Muntlak H: Metastases osseuses d'un hemangiopericytome. J Radiol 65:41–45, 1984

Martel W, Abell MR, Duff IF: Cervical spine involvement in lipoid dermatoarthritis. Radiology 77:613–617, 1961

McCarthy J, Twersley J, Lion M: Thyroid acropachy. J Can Assoc Radiol 26:199–202, 1976

McNulty JG, Pim P: Hyperphosphatasia: A report of a case with a 30-year follow-up. AJR Am J Roentgenol 115:614–618, 1972

Melhem RE, Saber TJ: Erosion of the medial cortex of the proximal humerus. Radiology 137:77–79, 1980

Milgram JW: Intraosseous lipomas: Radiologic and pathologic manifestations. Radiology 167:155–160, 1988

Mok PM, Reilly BJ, Ash JM: Osteomyelitis in the neonate. Radiology 145:677–682, 1982

Mortensson W, Eklof O, Jorulf H: Radiologic aspects of BCG osteomyelitis in infants and children. Acta Radiol [Diagn] 17:845–855, 1976

Morton KS, Bartlett LH: Benign osteoblastic change resembling osteoid osteoma: A report of 3 cases with unusual radiologic features. J Bone Joint Surg [Br] 48:478–487, 1966

Moser RP Jr, Sweet DE et al: Multiple skeletal fibroxanthomas: Radiologic–pathologic correlation of 72 cases. Skeletal Radiol 16:353–359, 1987

Murphy FD, Blount WB: Cartilaginous exostosis following irradiation. J Bone Joint Surg [Am] 44:662–668, 1962

Murphy NB, Price CHG: The radiological aspects of chondromyxoid fibroma of bone. Clin Radiol 22:261–269, 1971

Murray RO, McCredie J: Melorheostosis and the sclerotomes: A radiological correlation. Skeletal Radiol 4:57–71, 1979

Murray RO: Iatrogenic lesions of the skeleton: Caldwell lecture, 1AJR Am J Roentgenol 126:5–22, 1976

Naji AF et al: So-called adamantinoma of long bones: Report of a case with massive pulmonary metastases. J Bone Joint Surg [Am] 46:151–158, 1964

Nakamura T, Yamada N et al: Autosomal dominant type of endosteal hyperostosis with unusual manifestations of sclerosis of the jaw bones. Skeletal Radiol 16:48–51, 1987

Nathanson I, Riddlesberger MM Jr: Pulmonary hypertrophic osteoarthropathy in cystic fibrosis. Radiology 135:649–651, 1980

Nessi R, Gattoni F, Mazzoni R et al: Lipoblastic tumours of somatic soft tissues: A xerographic evaluation of 67 cases. Skeletal Radiol 5:137–143, 1980

Ngan H, Preston BJ: Non-Hodgkin's lymphoma presenting with osseous lesions. Clin Radiol 26:351–356, 1975

Nguyen VD, London J et al: Ring sequestrum: Radiographic characteristics of skeletal fixation pin-tract osteomyelitis. Radiology 158:129–131, 1986

Nussbaum AR, Treves ST et al: Bone stress lesions in ballet dancers: Scintigraphic assessment. Am J Roentgenol 150:851–855, 1988

O'Connell DJ, Frank PH, Riddel RH: The metastases of meningioma: Radiologic and pathologic features. Skeletal Radiol 3:30–35, 1978

O'Reilly GV, Clark TM, Crum CP: Skeletal involvement in mycosis fungoides. AJR Am J Roentgenol 129:741–743, 1977

Ohuchida T, Nishitani H et al: "Adult T-cell leukemia/lymphoma" with bone demineralization. Skeletal Radiol 14:194–197, 1985

Omojola MF, Cockshott WP, Beatty EG: Osteoid osteoma: An evaluation of diagnostic modalities. Clin Radiol 32:199–204, 1981

Osborn AG et al: Case 3. RadioGraphics 11:139–140, 1991

Paling MR, Herdt JR: Radiation osteitis: A problem of recognition. Radiology 137:339–342, 1980

Paltiel HJ, Wilkinson RH, Kozakewich HPW: Case report 507. Skeletal Radiol 17:527–530, 1988

Pastakia B, Horvath K et al: Seventeen-year follow-up and autopsy findings in a case of massive osteolysis. Skeletal Radiol 16:291–297, 1987

Pastershank SP, Yip S, Sodhi HS: Cerebrotendinous xanthomatosis. J Can Assoc Radiol 25:282–286, 1974

Pear BL: The plasma cell in radiology. AJR Am J Roentgenol 102:908–915, 1968

Peison B, Benisch B: Malignant myelosclerosis simulating metastatic bone disease. Radiology 125:62, 1977

Pere P, Fagart JP et al: Les hyperostoses sterno-costo-claviculaires: Conceptions nosologiques. J Radiol 68:809–814, 1987

Peterson CC, Silbiger ML: Reiter's syndrome and psoriatic arthritis: Their roentgen spectra and some interesting similarities. AJR Am J Roentgenol 101:860–871, 1967

Pettersson H, Gillespy T III et al: Primary musculoskeletal tumors: Examination with MR imaging compared with conventional modalities. Radiology 164:237–241, 1987

Phillips WC, Kattapuram SV, Doseretz DE et al: Primary lymphoma of bone: Relationship of radiographic appearance and prognosis. Radiology 144:285–290, 1982

Picci P, Baldini N et al: Giant cell reparative granuloma and other giant cell lesions of the bones of the hands and feet. Skeletal Radiol 15:415–421, 1986

Pinckney L, Parker BR: Myelosclerosis and myelofibrosis in treated histiocytosis X. AJR Am J Roentgenol 129:521–523, 1977

Pirschel VJ: Zur differentialdiagnose primärer und sekundarer sternumtumoren. Fortschritte a/d Gebiet Röntgenstrahlen 135:197–203, 1981

Porter AR, Tristan TA et al: Florid reactive periostitis of the phalanges. AJR Am J Roentgenol 144:617–618, 1988

Poznanski AK, Fernbach S et al: Bone changes from prostaglandin therapy. Skeletal Radiol 14:20–25, 1985

Ramin D: Tertiary yaws: Skeletal changes in the spine and ribs. Fortschr Geb Rontgenstr 125:185–186, 1976

Reed MH, Shokeir MHK, Macpherson RI: Skeletal metastases from retinoblastoma. J Can Assoc Radiol 26:249–254, 1975

Reeder MM, Felson B with contributions by Theros EG, Parks HE, Greenfield GB: Gamuts in Radiology [Comprehensive lists of roentgen differential diagnosis]. Cincinnati, Audiovisual Radiology of Cincinnati, 1975

Reese EJ, Baker HL, Scanlon PW: The roentgenologic aspects of metastatic pheochromocytoma. AJR Am J Roentgenol 115:783–793, 1972

Resnick D, Conne RO: The nature of humeral pseudocysts. Radiology 150:27–28, 1984

Resnick D, Greenway GD, Bardwick PA et al: Plasma-cell dyscrasia with polyneuropathy, organomegaly, endocinopathy, M-protein, and skin changes: The POEMS syndrome. Radiology 140:17–22, 1981

Resnick D, Pineda CJ et al: Osteomyelitis and septic arthritis of the hand following human bites. Skeletal Radiol 14:263–266, 1985

Rhea JT, Weber AL: Giant-cell granuloma of the sinuses. Radiology 147:135–137, 1983

Rich PJ, King W III: Benign cortical hyperostosis underlying soft-tissue tumors of the thigh. AJR Am J Roentgenol 138:419–422, 1982

Robinson AE, Thomas RL, Monson DM: Aneurysmal bone cyst of the rib: A report of 2 unusual cases. AJR Am J Roentgenol 100:526–529, 1967

Rodde A, Becker S et al: Chordomes du rachis cervical: Aspects radiologiques caracteristiques: A propos de 2 observations. J Radiol 68:587–591, 1987

Rong SH, Nie ZQ: Hydatid disease of bone. Clin Radiol 36:301–305, 1985

Ros PR, Viamonte M, Rywlin AM: Malignant fibrous histiocytoma: Mesenchymal tumor of ubiquitous origin. Am J Roentgenol 142:753–759, 1984

Rosen RS, Jacobson G: Fungus disease of bone. Semin Roentgenol 1:370–391, 1966

Ross P: Gardner's syndrome. AJR Am J Roentgenol 96:298–301, 1966

Rossleigh MA, Smith J et al: Case reports: A photopenic lesion in osteosarcoma. Br J Radiol 60:497–499, 1987

Roth SI: Squamous cysts involving the skull and phalanges. J Bone Joint Surg [Am] 46:1442–1450, 1964

Rudwan MA, Sheikh NA: Aspergilloma of paranasal sinuses: A common cause of unilateral proptosis in Sudan. Clin Radiol 27:497–502, 1976

Russell WJ, Bizzozero OJ, Omori Y: Idiopathic osteosclerosis. Radiology 90:70–76, 1968

Sartoris DJ, Clopton P et al: Vertebral-body collapse in focal and diffuse disease: Patterns of pathologic processes. Radiology 160:479–483, 1986

Sartoris DJ, Pate D et al: Plasma cell sclerosis of bone: A spectrum of disease. J Can Assoc Radiol 37:25–34, 1986

Sartoris DJ, Schreiman JS et al: Sternocostoclavicular hyperostosis: A review and report of 11 cases. Radiology 158:125–128, 1986

Satin R, Usher MS, Goldenberg M: More causes of button sequestrum. J Can Assoc Radiol 27:288–289, 1976

Scalley JR, Collins J: Thymoma metastatic to bone: Report of a case diagnosed by percutaneous biopsy. Radiology 96:423–424, 1970

Scanlon GT, Clemett AR: Thyroid acropachy. Radiology 83:1039–1042, 1964

Schanche AF, Bierman SM, Sopher RL, O'Loughlin BJ: Disseminated lipogranulomatosis, early roentgen changes. Radiology 82:675–678, 1964

Schey WL, Shkolnik A, White H: Clinical and radiographic considerations of sacrococcygeal teratomas: An analysis of 26 new cases and review of the literature. Radiology 125:189–195, 1977

Schoener VE, Gutgesell H: Osteochondrosarkom der mamma. Fortschr Geb Roentgenstr 135:714–717, 1981

Schwaighofer VB, Pohl-Markl H et al: Der diagnostische stellenwert des ultraschalls beim malignen melanom. Fortschr Geb Roentgenstr 146:409–411, 1987

Schwarz E, Fish A: Reticulohistiocytoma: A rare dermatologic disease with roentgen manifestations. AJR Am J Roentgenol 83:692–697, 1960

Schwimer SR, Bassett LW, Mancuso AA et al: Giant cell tumor of the cervicothoracic spine. Am J Roentgenol 136:63–67, 1981

Scott I, Connell DG et al: Regression of aneurysmal bone cyst following open biopsy. J Can Assoc Radiol 37:198–200, 1986

Shogry MEC, Armstrong P: Case report 630. Skeletal Radiol 19:465–467, 1990

Singleton EB, Rosenberg HS, Dodd GD, Dolan PA: Sclerosing osteogenic sarcomatosis. Am J Roentgenol 88:483–490, 1962

Singson RD, Berdon WE et al: "Missing" femoral condyle: An unusual sequela to neonatal osteomyelitis and septic arthritis. Radiology 161:359–361, 1986

Smart MJ: Traumatic osteolysis of the distal ends of the clavicles. J Can Assoc Radiol 23:264–266, 1972

Smith J, Ahuja SC, Huvos AG, Bullough P: Parosteal (juxtacortical) osteogenic sarcoma: A roentgenological study of 30 patients. J Can Assoc Radiol 29:167–174, 1978

Smith J, McLachlan DL, Huvos AG, Higinbotham NL: Primary tumors of the clavicle and scapula. AJR Am J Roentgenol 124:113–123, 1975

Smith J: Radiation-induced sarcoma of bone: Clinical and radiographic findings in 43 patients irradiated for soft tissue neoplasms. Clin Radiol 33:205–221, 1982

Soffa DJ, Sire DJ, Dodson JR: Melorheostosis with linear sclerodermatous skin changes. Radiology 114:577–578, 1975

Som PM, Lawson W, Cohen BA: Giant-cell lesions of the facial bones. Radiology 147:129–134, 1983

Spagnoli I, Gattoni F, Viganotti G: Roentgenographic aspects of non-Hodgkin's lymphomas presenting with osseous lesions. Skeletal Radiol 8:39–41, 1982

Spiers FW, King SD, Beddoe AH: Measurements of endosteal surface area in human long bones: Relationship of sites of occurrence of osteosarcoma. Br J Radiol 50:769–776, 1977

Staple TW, Melson GL, Evens RG: Miscellaneous soft-tissue lesions of the extremities. Semin Roentgenol 8:117–127, 1973

Steinbach LS, Johnston JO: Case report Skeletal Radiol 22:203–205, 1993

Stevens J, Love S, Davis C et al: Capillary haemangioblastoma of bone resembling a vertebral haemangioma. Br J Radiol 56:571–575, 1983

Stewart JR, Dahlin DC, Pugh DG: Pathology and radiology of solitary bone tumors. Semin Roentgenol 1:268–292, 1966

Stringer DA, Hall CM: Juvenile hyaline fibromatosis. Br J Radiol 54:473–478, 1981

Swischuk LE, Jorgenson F, Caden D: Wooden splinter induced "pseudotumors" and "osteomyelitis-like" lesions of bone and soft tissue. Am J Roentgenol 122:176–179, 1974

Symeonides P: Bursal chondromatosis. J Bone Joint Surg [Br] 48:371–373, 1966

Taber DS, Libshitz HI, Cohen MA: Treated Ewing's sarcoma: Radiographic appearance in response, recurrence, and new primaries. Am J Roentgenol 140:753–758, 1983

Teplick JG et al: Ghost infantile vertebrae and hemipelves within adult skeleton from thorotrast administration in childhood. Radiology 129:657–660, 1978

Theros E: Plasma cell granuloma of pelvis and femora: RPC case of the month from AFIP. Radiology 95:679–686, 1970

Toland J, Phelps PDD: Plasmacytoma of the skull base. Clin Radiol 22:93–96, 1971

Torrance DJ: "Negative" bone density in a case of multiple myeloma. Radiology 70:864–865, 1958

Torrance DJ: "Negative" bone density in a case of multiple myeloma. Radiology 70:864–865, 1958

Torres-Reyes E, Staple TW: Roentgenographic appearance of thyroid acropachy. Clin Radiol 21:95–100, 1970

Tumeh SS, Aliabadi P et al: Disease activity in osteomyelitis: Role of radiography. Radiology 165:781–784, 1987

Tyler T, Rosenbaum HD: Idiopathic multicentric osteolysis. AJR Am J Roentgenol 126:23–31, 1976

Unni KK: Case report 457. Skeletal Radiol 17:129–132, 1988

Valderrama JAF, Matthews JM: The haemophilic pseudotumour or haemophilic subperiosteal haematoma. J Bone Joint Surg [Br] 47:256–265, 1965

Vallance R, Hamblen DL et al: Vascular complications of osteochondroma. Clin Radiol 36:639–642, 1985

Vandevoort PLM, Rosenbusch G: Ossifizierende lymph kontenmetastasen eines osteosarcoms. Fortschritte a/d Gebiet Röntgenstrahlen 126:492–494, 1977

Vanek J: Idiopathic osteolysis of Hadju–Cheney. Fortschr Geb Rontgenstr 128:75–79, 1978

Vanel D, Couanet D, Piekarski JD et al: Radiological findings in 23 pediatric cases of malignant histiocytosis. Eur J Radiol 3:60–62, 1983

Vermess M, Pearson KD, Einstein AB, Fahey JL: Osseous manifestations of Waldenstrom's macroglobulinemia. Radiology 102:497–504, 1972

Vilar J, Lezana AH, Pedrosa CS: Spiculated periosteal reaction in metastatic lesions of bone. Skeletal Radiol 3:230–233, 1979

Vinstein AL, Franken EA: Hereditary multiple exostoses: Report of a case with spinal cord compression. AJR Am J Roentgenol 112:405–407, 1971

Weigert VF, Pfaendner K et al: Rasch wachsende aneurysmatische knochenzyste in roentgenbild und MRT. Fortschritte a/d Gebiet Röntgenstrahlen 147:454–456, 1987

Wepfer JF, Reed JG, Cullen GM et al: Calcific tendinitis of the gluteus maximus tendon (gluteus maximus tendinitis). Skeletal Radiol 9:198–200, 1983

Weston WJ: Thorn and twig-induced pseudotumours of bone and soft tissues. Br J Radiol 36:323–326, 1963

Whitehouse GH, Bottomley JP, Bradley J: Lymphangiographic appearances in Waldenstrom's macroglobulinemia. Br J Radiol 47:226–229, 1974

Whitfield MF: Chondrodysplasia punctata after warfarin in early pregnancy. Radiology 148:693–698, 1983

Wiesmann VW, Galanski M et al: Radiologische diagnostik der aggressiven fibromatose. Fortschr Geb Roentgenstr 145:555–559, 1986

Winterberger AR: Radiographic diagnosis of lymphangiomatosis of bone. Radiology 102:321–324, 1972

Wong WS, Kaiser LR, Gold RH et al: Radiographic features of osseous metastases of soft-tissue sarcomas. Radiology 143:71–74, 1982

Yousefzadeh DK, Jackson JH: Neonatal and infantile candidal arthritis with or without osteomyelitis: A clinical and radiographical review of 21 cases. Skeletal Radiol 5:77–90, 1980

Yousefzadeh DK, Schumann EM, Mulligan GM et al: The role of imaging modalities in diagnosis and management of pyomyositis. Skeletal Radiol 8:285–289, 1982

Zenny JC, Chevrot A, Sultan Y et al: Lésions hémorragiques intro-osseouses des afibrinémies congénitales. J Radiol 62:263–266, 1981

Zvetina RJ, Demos TC, Rubinstein H: Mycobacterium intracellulare infection of the shoulder and spine in a patient with steroid-treated systemic lupus erythematosus. Skeletal Radiol 8:111–113, 1982

Angiography

Bliznak J, Staple TW: Radiology of angiodysplasias of the limb. Radiology 110:3–44, 1974

Chudacek Z: Angiographic feature of inflammatory fibrous histiocytoma. Br J Radiol 53:1006–1007, 1980

Hudson TM et al: Angiography of malignant fibrous histiocytoma of bone. Radiology 131:9–15, 1979

Hutcheson J, Klatte EC, Kremp R: The angiographic appearance of myositis ossificans circumscripta: A case report. Radiology 102:5–58, 1972

Jaffe N, Knapp J, Chuang VP et al: Osteosarcoma: Intra-arterial treatment of the primary tumor with cis-diamine-dichloroplatinum II (CDP). Angiographic, pathologic, and pharmacologic studies. Cancer 51:402–407, 1983

Karnel VF, Salomonowitz E et al: Digital subtraktionsangiographie: Eine wertvolle methode zum nachweis eines osteoidosteoms. Fortschritte a/d Gebiet Röntgenstrahlen 144:735–736, 1986

Laurin S: Angiography of benign bone tumors. Acta Radiol 22:601–607, 1981

Lindbom A, Lindvall N, Soderberg G, Spjut H: Angiography in osteoid osteoma. Acta Radiol [Diagn] 53:377–384, 1960

Norman A, Ulin R: A comparative study of periosteal new bone response in metastatic bone tumors (solitary) and primary bone sarcomas. Radiology 92:705–708, 1969

Yaghamai I, Abdolmahmoud SZ, Shams S, Afshari R: Value of arteriography in the diagnosis of benign and malignant bone lesions. Cancer 27:1134–1147, 1971

Yaghamai I: Angiographic features of chondromas and chondrosarcomas. Skeletal Radiol 3:91–98, 1978

Yaghamai I: Angiographic features of osteosarcoma. Am J Roentgenol 129:1073–1082, 1977

Yaghmai I: Angiography of Bone and Soft Tissue Lesions. New York, Springer-Verlag, 1979

Ultrasonography

Apple JS, Martinez S, Nelson PA et al: Sonographic correlation in extremity soft-tissue masses. Noninvasive Medical Imaging 1:7–81, 1984

Bernardino ME, Jing BS, Thomas JL et al: The extremity soft-tissue lesion: A comparative study of ultrasound, computed tomography, and xeroradiography. Radiology 139:5–59, 1981

deSantos LA, Goldstein HM: Ultrasonography in tumors arising from the spine and bony pelvis. Am J Roentgenol 129:1061–1064, 1977

Fornage BD: Peripheral nerves of the extremities: Imaging with US. Radiology 167:179–182, 1988

Hermann G, Yeh HC et al: Computed tomography and ultrasonography of the hemophilic pseudotumor and their use in surgical planning. Skeletal Radiol 15:123–128, 1986

Hermann G, Yeh HS, Schwartz I: Computed tomography of soft-tissue lesions of the extremities, pelvic and shoulder girdles: Sonographic and pathological correlations. Clin Radiol 35:193–202, 1984

Macpherson RI, Halvorsen R: Tumors of the pubis: An analysis by probabilities. J Can Assoc Radiol 32:168–170, 1981

Majewski VA, Freyschmidt J, Steinmeyer R et al: Das ossifizierende knochenfibrom (OF). Fortschritte a/d Gebiet Röntgenstrahlen 140:179–187, 1984

Majid MA, Mathias PF, Seth HN, Thirumalachar MJ: Primary mycetoma of the patella. J Bone Joint Surg [Am] 46:1283–1286, 1964

Marchal AL, Hoeffel JC et al: Atteintes pleurales par contiguiete ou metastases dans les tumeurs osseuses malignes primitives de l'enfant. J Radiol 67:303–307, 1986

Computed Tomography

Balck WC, Armstrong P et al: Computed tomography of aggressive fibromatosis in the posterior mediastinum. J Comput Assist Tomogr 11:153–155, 1987

Berger PE, Kuhn JP: Computed tomography of tumors of the musculoskeletal system in children. Radiology 127:171–175, 1978

Bernardino ME, Jing BS, Thomas JL et al: The extremity soft-tissue lesion: A comparative study of ultrasound, computed tomography, and xeroradiography. Radiology 139:5–59, 1981

Bressler EL, Marn CS et al: Evaluation of ectopic bone by CT. AJR Am J Roentgenol 148:931–935, 1987

Coppola J, Mueller NL et al: Computed tomography of musculoskeletal tuberculosis. J Can Assoc Radiol 38:199–203, 1987

deSantos LA et al: Computed tomography in the evaluation of musculoskeletal neoplasms. Radiology 128:89–94, 1978

Engdahl DE, Kaufman RA, Hospson CN: Computed tomography in the diagnosis of rare plantar ganglion cyst in a child. J Bone Joint Surg [Am] 65:1348–1349a, 1983

Farmlett EJ, Fishman EK et al: Computed tomography in the assessment of myonecrosis. J Can Assoc Radiol 38:278–282a, 1987

Fink IJ, Lee MA et al: Case reports: Radiographic and CT appearance of intraosseous xanthoma mimicking a malignant lesion. Br J Radiol 58:262–264, 1985

Haaga JR, Alfidi RJ: Computed Tomography of the Whole Body, Vol 11. St. Louis, CV Mosby, 1983

Heiken JP, Lee JKT, Smathers RL et al: CT of benign soft tissue masses of the extremities. AJR Am J Roentgenol 142:575–580, 1984

Helms CA, Jeffrey RB et al: Computed tomography and plain film appearance of a bony sequestration: Significance and differential diagnosis. Skeletal Radiol 16:117–120, 1987

Hermann G, Leviton M et al: Osteosarcoma: Relation between extent of marrow infiltration on CT and frequency of lung metastases. Am J Roentgenol 149:1203–1206, 1987

Hermann G, Yeh HC et al: Computed tomography and ultrasonography of the hemophilic pseudotumor and their use in surgical planning. Skeletal Radiol 15:123–128, 1986

Hermann G, Yeh HS, Schwartz I: Computed tomography of soft-tissue lesions of the extremities, pelvic and shoulder girdles: Sonographic and pathological correlations. Clin Radiol 35:193–202, 1984

Hudson TM, Springfield DS et al: Computed tomography of parosteal osteosarcoma. Am J Roentgenol 144:961–965, 1985

Jones ET, Kuhns LR: Pitfalls in the use of computed tomography for musculoskeletal tumors in children. J Bone Joint Surg [Am] 63:1297–1304, 1981

Lee KR, Tines SC, Yoon JW: CT findings of suprapatellar synovial cysts. J Comput Assist Tomogr 8:296–299, 1984

Levine E, Neff JR: Dynamic computed tomography scanning of benign bone lesions: Preliminary results. Skeletal Radiol 9:238–245, 1983

Lindell MM Jr, Shirkhoda A et al: Parosteal osteosarcoma: Radiologic–pathologic correlation with emphasis on CT. Am J Roentgenol 148:323–328, 1987

Lukens JA, McLeod RA, Sim FH: Computed tomographic evaluation of primary osseous malignant neoplasma. Am J Roentgenol 139:45–48, 1982

Mendelsohn DB, Hertzanu Y, Glass RBJ: Computed tomographic findings in primary mandibular osteosarcoma. Clin Radiol 34:153–155, 1983

Mink JH, Weitz I et al: Bone scan-positive and radiography-and CT-negative vertebral lesion in a woman with locally advanced breast cancer. AJR Am J Roentgenol 148:341–348, 1987

Mourad K, Katz D, Paradinas FJ: Case reports: Extravisceral diffuse infiltration of adult histiocytosis X demonstrated by CT. Br J Radiol 56:879–881, 1983

Murcia M, Brennan RE, Edeiken J: Computed tomography of stress fracture. Skeletal Radiol 8:193–195, 1982

Nelson OA, Greer RB: Localization osteoid osteoma of the spine using computerized tomography. J Bone Joint Surg [Am] 65:263–265, 1983

Orcutt J, Ragsdale BD, Curtis DJ et al: Misleading CT in parosteal osteosarcoma. Am J Roentgenol 136:1233–1235, 1981

Pakter RL, Fishman EK et al: Calf hematoma-computed tomographic and magnetic resonance findings. Skeletal Radiol 16:393–396, 1987

Pawar S, Kay CJ, Anderson HH et al: Primary amyloidoma of the spine. J Comput Assist Tomogr 6:1175–1177, 1982

Schreiman JS, McLeod RA et al: Multiple myeloma: Evaluation by CT. Radiology 154:483–486, 1985

Solomon A, Rahamni R, Seligsohn U et al: Multiple myeloma: Early vertebral involvement assessed by computerised tomography. Skeletal Radiol 11:258–261, 1984

Soye I, Levine E, Batnitzky S et al: Computed tomography of sacral and presacral lesions. Neuroradiology 24:71–76, 1982

Sundaram M, McGuire MH: Computed tomography or magnetic resonance for evaluating the solitary tumor or tumor-like lesion of bone? Skeletal Radiol 17:393–401, 1988

Sundaram M, McGuire MH: Computed tomography or magnetic resonance for evaluating the solitary tumor or tumor-like lesion of bone? Skeletal Radiol 17:393–401, 1988

Van Lom KJ, Kellerhouse LE et al: Infection versus tumor in the spine: Criteria for distinction with CT Radiology 166:851–855, 1988

Vogelzang RL, Hendrix RW, Neiman HL: Computed tomography of tuberculous osteomyelitis of the pubis. J Comput Assist Tomogr 7:914–915, 1983

Weinberger G, Levinsohn EM: Computed tomography in the evaluation of sarcomatous tumors of the thigh. AJR Am J Roentgenol 130:115–118, 1978

Whelan MA, Gold RP: Computed tomography of the sacrum: 1. Normal anatomy. AJR Am J Roentgenol 139:1183–1190, 1982

Whelan MA, Hilal SK, Gold RP et al: Computed tomography of the sacrum: 2. Pathology. AJR Am J Roentgenol 139:1191–1195, 1982

Yousem D, Magid D et al: Computed tomography of stress fractures. J Comput Assist Tomogr 10:92–95, 1986

Magnetic Resonance

Algra PR, Postma T, Van Groeningen CJ et al: MR imaging of skeletal metastases from medulloblastoma. Skeletal Radiol 21:425–430, 1992

Beltran J, McGhee RB et. al.: Experimental infections of the musculoskeletal system: Evaluation with MR imaging and Tc-99m MDP and Ga-67 scintigraphy. Radiology 167:167–172, 1988

Beltran J, Simon DC et al: Increased MR signal intensity in skeletal muscle adjacent to malignant tunors: Pathologic correlation and clinical relevance. Radiology 162:251–255, 1987

Berquist TH, Ehman RL, Richardson ML: Magnetic Resonance of the Musculoskeletal System. New York, Raven Press, 1987

Bohndrof K, Reiser M et al: Magnetic resonance imaging of primary tumors and tumor-like lesions of bone. Skeletal Radiol 15:511–517, 1986

Cohen EK, Kressel HY et al: Hyaline cartilage-origin bone and soft-tissue neoplasma: MR appearance and histologic correlation. Radiology 167:477–481, 1988

Cohen MD, Klatte EC, Baehner R et al: Magnetic resonance imaging of bone marrow disease in children. Radiology 151:715–718, 1984

Daffner RH, Lupetin AR et al: MRI in the detection of malignant infiltration of bone marrow. AJR Am J Roentgenol 146:353–358, 1986

Fobben ES, Dalinka MK et al: The magnetic resonance imaging appearance at 1.5 Tesla of cartilaginous tumors involving the epiphysis. Skeletal Radiol 16:647–651, 1987

Frouge C, Vanel D et al: The role of magnetic resonance imaging in the evaluation of Ewing's sarcoma. Skeletal Radiol 17:387–392, 1988

Fruehwald FJ, Tscholakoff T et al: Magnetic resonance imaging of the lower vertebral column in patients with multiple myeloma. Invest Radiol 23:193–199, 1988

Hajek PC, Baker LL et al: Focal fat deposition in axial bone marrow: MR characteristics. Radiology 162:245–249, 1987

Herman SD, Mesgarzadeh M et al: The role of magnetic resonance imaging in giant cell tumor of bone. Skeletal Radiol 16:635–643, 1987

Huber DJ, Sumers E et al: Soft tissue pseudotumor following intramuscular injection of "DPT": A pitfall in magnetic resonance imaging. Skeletal Radiol 16:469–473, 1987

Lee JK, Yao L: Stress fractures: MR imaging. Radiology 169:217–220, 1988

Mirowitz SA: Fast scanning and fat-suppression MR imaging of musculoskeletal disorders. Am J Roentgen 161:1147–1157, 1993

Moon KL, Genant HK, Helms CA et al: Musculoskeletal applications of nuclear magnetic resonance. Radiology 147:161–171, 1983

Nidecker AC, Mueller S et al: Extremity bone tumors: Evaluation by P-31 MR spectroscopy. Radiology 157:167–174, 1985

Pakter RL, Fishman EK et al: Calf hematoma-computed tomographic and magnetic resonance findings. Skeletal Radiol 16:393–396, 1987

Pettersson H, Gillespy T III et al: Primary musculoskeletal tumors: Examination with MR imaging compared with conventional modalities. Radiology 164:237–241, 1987

Pettersson H, Slone RM et al: Musculoskeletal tumors: T1 and T2 relaxation times. Radiology 167:783–785, 1988

Richardson ML, Kilcoyne RF et al: Magnetic resonance imaging of musculoskeletal neoplasma. Radiol Clin North Am 24:259–268, 1986

Schweitzer ME, Levine C, Mitchell DG et al: Bull's-eyes and halos: Useful MR discriminators of osseous metastases. Radiology 188:249–252, 1993

Shuman WP, Patten RM, Baron RL et al: Comparison of STIR and spin-echo MR imaging at 1.5 T in 45 suspected extremity tumors: Lesion conspicuity and extent. Radiology 179:247–252, 1991

Sundaram M, Awwad EE: Magnetic resonance imaging of arachnoid cysts destroying the sacrum. Am J Roentgenol 146:359–360, 1986

Sundaram M, McGuire MH: Computed tomography or magnetic resonance for evaluating the solitary tumor or tumor-like lesion of bone? Skeletal Radiol 17:393–401, 1988

Vanel D, Lacombe MJ et al: Musculoskeletal tumors: Follow-up with MR imaging after treatment with surgery and radiation therapy. Radiology 164:243–245, 1987

Yuh WTC, Schreiber AE et al: Magnetic resonance imaging of pyomyositis. Skeletal Radiol 17:190–193, 1988

Nuclear Medicine

Anscombe A, Walkden SB: An interesting bone scan in multiple myeloma: Myeloma superscan? Br J Radiol 56:489–492, 1983

Arrington ER, Eisenberg B, Orrison WW et al: Scintigraphic appearance of uncommon soft-tissue osteogenic sarcoma metastases. J Nucl Med 31:679–681, 1990

Bataille R, Chevalier J, Rossie M et al: Bone scintigraphy in plasma-cell myeloma. Radiology 145:801–804, 1982

Beltran J, McGhee RB et. al.: Experimental infections of the musculoskeletal system: Evaluation with MR imaging and Tc-99m MDP and Ga-67 scintigraphy. Radiology 167:167–172, 1988

Brady AW, Croll MN: The role of bone scanning in the cancer patient. Skeletal Radiol 3:217–222, 1979

Burkhalter JL, Patel BR, Harrison RB: Radionuclide bone scan as an aid in localizing lesions for bone biopsy. Skeletal Radiol 9:246–247, 1983

d'Avigon MB, Baum S: Increased jaw radioactivity on bone imaging. Semin Nucl Med 12:219, 1982

El-Khoury GY, Wehbe MA, Bonfiglio M et al: Stress fractures of the femoral neck: A scintigraphic sign for early diagnosis. Skeletal Radiol 6:271–273, 1981

Farrands PA, Perkins A, Sully L et al: Localisation of human osteosarcoma by antitumour monoclonal antibody. J Bone Joint Surg [Br] 65:638–640, 1983

Fordham EW, Ali A, Turner DA, Charters JR: Atlas of Total Body Radionuclide Imaging, Vol 1. Philadelphia, Harper & Row, 1982

Gilday et al: Radionuclide skeletal survey for pediatric neoplasms. Radiology 123:399–406, 1977

Gold RH, Bassett LW: Radionuclide evaluation of skeletal metastases: Practical considerations. Skeletal Radiol 15:1–9, 1986

Hudson TM, Chew FS, Manaster BJ: Radionuclide bone scanning of medullary chondrosarcoma. AJR Am J Roentgenol 138:1071–1076, 1982

Hudson TM, Chew FS, Manaster BJ: Scintigraphy of benign exostoses and exostotic chondrosarcomas. AJR Am J Roentgenol 140:581–586, 1983

Inoue Y: A new finding in bone scintigram: Three cases of defect findings. Fortschr Geb Rontgenstr 128:258–261, 1978

Kalin B, Jacobsson H: Misleading renal stasis on bone scintigraphy in diffuse symmetrical skeletal metastases of prostatic carcinoma. Fortschr Geb Rontgenstr 147:465–466, 1987

Kaufman RA et al: False negative bone scans in neuroblastoma metastatic to the ends of long bones. AJR Am J Roentgenol 130:131–135, 1978

Kunkler IH, Merrick MV et al: Bone scintigraphy in breast cancer: A nine year follow-up. Clinical Radiol 36:279–282, 1985

Leonard RCF, Owen JP, Proctor SJ et al: Multiple myeloma: Radiology or bone scanning? Clin Radiol 32:291–295, 1981

Ludwig H, Kumpan W, Sinzinger H: Radiography and bone scintigraphy in multiple myeloma: A comparative analysis. Br J Radiol 55:173–181, 1982

Madkour MM, Sarif HS et al: Osteoarticular brucellosis: Results of bone scintigraphy in 140 patients. AJR Am J Roentgenol 150:1101–1105, 1988

Manier SM, Nostrand DV: Super bone scan. Semin Nucl Med 14:46–47, 1984

Miller JH, Hayon I: Bone scintigraphy in hypervitaminosis A. AJR Am J Roentgenol 144:767–768, 1985

Mink JH, Weitz I et al: Bone scan-positive and radiography-and CT-negative vertebral lesion in a woman with locally advanced breast cancer. AJR Am J Roentgenol 148:341–348, 1987

Moon KL, Genant HK, Helms CA et al: Musculoskeletal applications of nuclear magnetic resonance. Radiology 147:161–171, 1983

Moon KL, Genant HK, Helms CA et al: Musculoskeletal applications of nuclear magnetic resonance. Radiology 147:161–171, 1983

Naji AF et al: So-called adamantinoma of long bones: Report of a case with massive pulmonary metastases. J Bone Joint Surg [Am] 46:151–158, 1964

Nidecker AC, Mueller S et al: Extremity bone tumors: Evaluation by P-31 MR spectroscopy. Radiology 157:167–174, 1985

Podrasky AE, Stark DD, Hattner RS et al: Radionuclide bone scanning in neuroblastoma: Skeletal metastases and primary tumor localizaton of 128mTc-MDP. AJR Am J Roentgenol 141:469–472, 1983

Riddel RJ, Louis CJ, Bromberger NA: Pulmonary metastases from chondroblastoma of the tibia: Report of a case. J Bone Joint Surg [Br] 55:848–853, 1973

Terry DW, Isitman AT, Holnes RA: Radionuclide bone images in hypertrophic pulmonary osteoarthropathy. AJR Am J Roentgenol 124:571–576, 1975

Plain Film Radiographs

Agha FP, Lilienfeld RM: Roentgen features of osseous neurilemmoma. Radiology 102:325–326, 1972

Blaquiere RM, Guyer PB, Buchanan RB et al: Sclerotic bone deposits in multiple myeloma. Br J Radiol 55:591–593, 1982

Gardner DJ, Azouz EM: Solitary lucent epiphyseal lesions in children. Skeletal Radiol 17:497–504, 1988

Janecki CJ, Nelson CL, Dohn DF: Intrasacral cyst: Report of a case and review of the literature. J Bone Joint Surg [Am] 54:423–428, 1972

Kirkpatrick DJ: Donovanosis (granuloma inguinale): A rare cause of osteolytic bone lesions. Clin Radiol 21:101–105, 1970

Kolawole TM, Bohrer SP: Ulcer osteoma: Bone response to tropical ulcer. Am J Roentgenol 109:611–618, 1970

Levick RK, Steiner GM: Skeletal survey in Wilms' tumour assessment. Radiology 149:894, 1983

Sebes JI, Niell HB et al: Skeletal surveys in multiple myeloma. Skeletal Radiol 15:354–359, 1986

NEOPLASMS

General Neoplasms

Alho A, Connor JF, Mankin HJ et al: Assessment of malignancy of cartilage tumors using flow cytometry. J Bone Joint Surg [Am] 65:779–785, 1983

Angervall L, Enzinger FM: Extraskeletal neoplasm resembling Ewing's sarcoma. Cancer 36:240–251, 1975

Apple JS, Martinez S, Nelson PA et al: Sonographic correlation in extremity soft-tissue masses. Noninvasive Medical Imaging 1:7–81, 1984

Ayala AG, Zornosa J: Primary bone tumors: Percutaneous needle biopsy. Radiology 149:675–679, 1983

Baltzer G, Jacob H, Esselborn H: Contrast media and renal function in multiple myeloma. Fortschr Geb Rontgenstr 129:208–211, 1978

Baudrillard JC, Lerair JM et al: Compression medullaire dorsale par chondrome sous-perioste vertebral. J Radiol 68:527–531, 1987

Bell RS, Goodman SB, Fornasier VL: Coccygeal glomus tumors: A case of mistaken identity. J Bone Joint Surg [Am] 64:595–597, 1982

Beltran J, Simon DC et al: Increased MR signal intensity in skeletal muscle adjacent to malignant tumors: Pathologic correlation and clinical relevance. Radiology 162:251–255, 1987

Bohlman HH, Sachs BL et al: Primary neoplasms of the cervical spine. J Bone Joint Surg 68:483–493, 1986

Bohndrof K, Reiser M et al: Magnetic resonance imaging of primary tumors and tumor-like lesions of bone. Skeletal Radiol 15:511–517, 1986

Booker RJ: Lipoblastic tumors of the hands and feet: Review of the literature and report of 33 cases. J Bone Joint Surg [Am] 47:727–740, 1965

Brady AW, Croll MN: The role of bone scanning in the cancer patient. Skeletal Radiol 3:217–222, 1979

Bronsky D, Bernstein A: Acute gout secondary to multiple myeloma: A case report. Ann Intern Med 41:820–822, 1954

Buirski G, Ratliff AHC et al: Cartilage cell containing tumours of the pelvis: A radiological review of 40 patients. Br J Radiol 59:197–204, 1986

Burgener FA, Landman S: The radiological manifestations of fibroxanthosarcomas. Fortschr Geb Roentgenstr 125:123–128, 1976

Cavanagh RC: Tumors of the soft tissues of the extremities. Semin Roentgenol 8:7–89, 1973

Charneux F, Bretagne MC, Hoeffel JC et al: Tumeur rare du naso pharynx. J Radiol 62:335–337, 1981

Cheyne C: Histiocytosis X. J Bone Joint Surg [Br] 53:366–382, 1971

Chudacek Z: Angiographic feature of inflammatory fibrous histiocytoma. Br J Radiol 53:1006–1007, 1980

Clarisse PDT, Staple TW: Diffuse bone sclerosis in multiple myeloma. Radiology 99:327–328, 1971

Cohen EK, Kressel HY et al: Hyaline cartilage-origin bone and soft-tissue neoplasma: MR appearance and histologic correlation. Radiology 167:477–481, 1988

Crone M, Watt I: Case of the month: A lump on the thigh. Br J Radiol 60:1035–1036, 1987

Dahlin DC: Bone Tumors: General Aspects and Data on 6,221 Cases. Springfield, IL, Charles C Thomas, 1978

Das Gupta T: Tumors of Soft Tissues. New York, Appleton–Century–Crofts, 1983

deSantos LA et al: Computed tomography in the evaluation of musculoskeletal neoplasms. Radiology 128:89–94, 1978

Enneking WF, Spanier SS, Goodman MA: Current concepts review: The surgical staging of musculoskeletal sarcoma. J Bone Joint Surg [Am] 62:1027–1030, 1980

Enneking WF: Staging of musculoskeletal neoplasma. Skeletal Radiol 13:183–194, 1985

Fobben ES, Dalinka MK et al: The magnetic resonance imaging appearance at 1.5 Tesla of cartilaginous tumors involving the epiphysis. Skeletal Radiol 16:647–651, 1987

Fruehwald FJ, Tscholakoff T et al: Magnetic resonance imaging of the lower vertebral column in patients with multiple myeloma. Invest Radiol 23:193–199, 1988

Gardner DJ, Azouz EM: Solitary lucent epiphyseal lesions in children. Skeletal Radiol 17:497–504, 1988

Giangarra C, Gallo G et al: Endometriosis in the biceps femoris. J Bone Joint Surg 69:290–292, 1987

Gilday et al: Radionuclide skeletal survey for pediatric neoplasms. Radiology 123:399–406, 1977

Gold RH, Bassett LW: Radionuclide evaluation of skeletal metastases: Practical considerations. Skeletal Radiol 15:1–9, 1986

Gompels BM, Vataw ML, Martel W: Correlation of radiological manifestations of multiple myeloma with immunoglobulin abnormalities and prognosis. Radiology 104:509–514, 1972

Gonzales-Crussi F, Enneking WF, Arean VM: Infiltrating angiolipoma. J Bone Joint Surg [Am] 48:1111–1124, 1966

Hall FM, Gore SM: Osteosclerotic myeloma variants. Skeletal Radiol 17:101–105, 1988

Hermann G, Yeh HS, Schwartz I: Computed tomography of soft-tissue lesions of the extremities, pelvic and shoulder girdles: Sonographic and pathological correlations. Clin Radiol 35:193–202, 1984

Herold CJ, Wittich GR et al: Skeletal involvement in hairy cell leukemia. Skeletal Radiol 17:171–175, 1988

Hill JA et al: Myxoma of the toes: A case report. J Bone Joint Surg [Am] 60:128–130, 1978

Himmelfarb E, Sebes J, Rainowitz J: Unusual roentgenographic presentations of multiple myeloma: Report of 3 cases. J Bone Joint Surg [Am] 56:1723–1728, 1974

Humphrey M, Neff J et al: Leiomyosarcoma of the saphenous vein. J Bone Joint Surg 69:282–286, 1987

Jaffe HL: Histogenesis of bone tumors. In Anderson MD: Hospital and Tumor Institute: Tumors of Bone and Soft Tissue, pp 41–44. Chicago, Year Book Medical Publishers, 1965

Jaffe HL: Tumors and Tumorous Conditions of the Bones and Joints. Philadelphia, Lea & Febiger, 1958

Jones ET, Kuhns LR: Pitfalls in the use of computed tomography for musculoskeletal tumors in children. J Bone Joint Surg [Am] 63:1297–1304, 1981

Karasick D, O'Hara EA: Juvenile aponeurotic fibroma. Radiology 123:725–726, 1977

Kim KS, Rogers LF, Lee C: The dural lucent line: Characteristic sign of hyperostosing meningioma en plaque. AJR Am J Roentgenol 141:1217–1221, 1983

Levick RK, Steiner GM: Skeletal survey in Wilms' tumour assessment. Radiology 149:894, 1983

Levine HA, Enrile F: Giant-cell tumor of patellar tendon coincident with Paget's disease. J Bone Joint Surg [Am] 53:335–340, 1971

Macpherson RI, Halvorsen R: Tumors of the pubis: An analysis by probabilities. J Can Assoc Radiol 32:168–170, 1981

McDonald DJ, Capanna R, Gherlinzoni F et al: Influence of chemotherapy on perioperative complications in limb salvage surgery for bone tumors. Cancer 65:1509–1516, 1990

McDonald P: Malignant sacrococcygeal teratoma: A report of 4 cases. AJR Am J Roentgenol 118:444–449, 1973

Nessi R, Gattoni F, Mazzoni R et al: Lipoblastic tumours of somatic soft tissues: A xerographic evaluation of 67 cases. Skeletal Radiol 5:137–143, 1980

Nidecker AC, Mueller S et al: Extremity bone tumors: Evaluation by P-31 MR spectroscopy. Radiology 157:167–174, 1985

Nuss DD, Aeling JL et al: Multiple hamartoma syndrome (Cowden's disease). Arch Dermatol 114:743–746, 1978

O'Connor MI, Sim FH: Salvage of the limb in the treatment of malignant pelvic tumors. J Bone Joint Surg [Am] 71:481–494, 1989

Ogilvie JW: Malignant eccrine acrospiroma. J Bone Joint Surg [Am] 64:780–782, 1982

Pastershank SP, Yip S, Sodhi HS: Cerebrotendinous xanthomatosis. J Can Assoc Radiol 25:282–286, 1974

Pettersson H, Gillespy T III et al: Primary musculoskeletal tumors: Examination with MR imaging compared with conventional modalities. Radiology 164:237–241, 1987

Pettersson H, Slone RM et al: Musculoskeletal tumors: T1 and T2 relaxation times. Radiology 167:783–785, 1988

Pinckney L, Parker BR: Myelosclerosis and myelofibrosis in treated histiocytosis X. AJR Am J Roentgenol 129:521–523, 1977

Podrasky AE, Stark DD, Hattner RS et al: Radionuclide bone scanning in neuroblastoma: Skeletal metastases and primary tumor localizaton of 128mTc-MDP. AJR Am J Roentgenol 141:469–472, 1983

Rao AS, Vigorita VJ: Pigmented villonodular synovitis (giant-cell tumor of the tendon sheath and synovial membrane). J Bone Joint Surg [Am] 66:7–94, 1984

Rich PJ, King W III: Benign cortical hyperostosis underlying soft-tissue tumors of the thigh. AJR Am J Roentgenol 138:419–422, 1982

Richardson ML, Kilcoyne RF et al: Magnetic resonance imaging of musculoskeletal neoplasma. Radiol Clin North Am 24:259–268, 1986

Rodde A, Becker S et al: Chordomes du rachis cervical: Aspects radiologiques caracteristiques: A propos de 2 observations. J Radiol 68:587–591, 1987

Rodriguez AR, Lutcher CL, Coleman FW: Osteosclerotic myeloma. JAMA 236:1872–1874, 1976

Schaffzin EA, Chung SMK, Kay R: Congenital generalized fibromatosis with complete spontaneous regression: A case report. J Bone Joint Surg [Am] 54:657–662, 1972

Schajowicz F: Tumors and Tumorlike Lesions of Bone and Joints. New York, Springer-Verlag, 1981

Schey WL, Shkolnik A, White H: Clinical and radiographic considerations of sacrococcygeal teratomas: An analysis of 26 new cases and review of the literature. Radiology 125:189–195, 1977

Schreiman JS, McLeod RA et al: Multiple myeloma: Evaluation by CT. Radiology 154:483–486, 1985

Schwaighofer VB, Markl-Pohl H et al: Der diagnostische stellenwert des ultraschalls beim malignen melanom. Fortschritte a/d Gebiel Röntgenstrahlen 146:409–411, 1987

Sebes JI, Niell HB et al: Skeletal surveys in multiple myeloma. Skeletal Radiol 15:354–359, 1986

Seth HN, Majid MA, Rao BDP: Giant-cell tumor arising from the periosteum: Report of a case occurring in the femur. J Bone Joint Surg [Am] 46:844–847, 1964

Shuman WP, Patten RM, Baron RL et al: Comparison of STIR and spin-echo MR imaging at 1.5 T in 45 suspected extremity tumors: Lesion conspicuity and extent. Radiology 179:247–252, 1991

Singleton EB, Rosenberg HS, Dodd GD, Dolan PA: Sclerosing osteogenic sarcomatosis. Am J Roentgenol 88:483–490, 1962

Smith J, McLachlan DL, Huvos AG, Higinbotham NL: Primary tumors of the clavicle and scapula. AJR Am J Roentgenol 124:113–123, 1975

Som PM, Lawson W, Cohen BA: Giant-cell lesions of the facial bones. Radiology 147:129–134, 1983

Soye I, Levine E, Batnitzky S et al: Computed tomography of sacral and presacral lesions. Neuroradiology 24:71–76, 1982

Spagnoli I, Gattoni F, Viganotti G: Roentgenographic aspects of

non-Hodgkin's lymphomas presenting with osseous lesions. Skeletal Radiol 8:39–41, 1982

Staple TW, Melson GL, Evens RG: Miscellaneous soft-tissue lesions of the extremities. Semin Roentgenol 8:117–127, 1973

Steel HH: Turtle-egg tumors: A late sequel of parenteral quinine. J Bone Joint Surg [Am] 46:134–136, 1964

Stewart JR, Dahlin DC, Pugh DG: Pathology and radiology of solitary bone tumors. Semin Roentgenol 1:268–292, 1966

Tang TT et al: Angioglomoid tumor of bone. J Bone Joint Surg [Am] 58:873–876, 1976

Tiedjen KU: Ewing's–sarkom bei einem 13 monate alten jungen. Fortschritte a/d Gebiet Röntgenstrahlen 129:798–800, 1978

Vanel D, Lacombe MJ et al: Musculoskeletal tumors: Follow-up with MR imaging after treatment with surgery and radiation therapy. Radiology 164:243–245, 1987

Yaghamai I, Abdolmahmoud SZ, Shams S, Afshari R: Value of arteriography in the diagnosis of benign and malignant bone lesions. Cancer 27:1134–1147, 1971

Yaghamai I: Intra- and extraosseous xanthomata associated with hyperlipidemia. Radiology 128:49–54, 1978

Yasko AW, Lane JM: Current concepts review: Chemotherapy for bone and soft-tissue sarcomas of the extremities. J Bone Joint Surg [Am] 73:1263–1271, 1991

Metastatic Neoplasms

Algra PR, Postma T, Van Groeningen CJ et al: MR imaging of skeletal metastases from medulloblastoma. Skeletal Radiol 21:425–430, 1992

Amin R: Orbital metastasis from prostatic carcinoma. Br J Radiol 56:56–58, 1983

Aoki J, Yamamoto I et al: Sclerotic bone metastasis: Radiologic–pathologic correlation. Radiology 159:127–132, 1986

Arrington ER, Eisenberg B, Orrison WW et al: Scintigraphic appearance of uncommon soft-tissue osteogenic sarcoma metastases. J Nucl Med 31:679–681, 1990

Bloon RA, Libson E et al: The periosteal sunburst reaction to bone metastases: A literature review and report of 20 additional cases. Skeletal Radiol 16:629–634, 1987

Case records of the Massachusetts General Hospital (osteogenic sarcoma of humerus, with ossifying metastases in the regional nodes). N Engl J Med 225:953, 1941

DuBois PJ, Orr DP, Meyersen EN, Barnes LE: Undifferentiated parotid carcinoma with osteoblastic metastases. AJR Am J Roentgenol 129:744–746, 1977

Gatti JM, Morvan GG, Henin D et al: Leiomyomatosis metastasizing to the spine. J Bone Joint Surg [Am] 65:1163–1165, 1983

Gillison EW, Grainger RG, Fernandez D: Osteoblastic metastases in carcinoma of the pancreas. Br J Radiol 43:818–820, 1970

Gyepes MT, D'Angio GJ: Extracranial metastases from CNS tumors in children and adolescents. Radiology 87:55–63, 1966

Hermann G, Leviton M et al: Osteosarcoma: Relation between extent of marrow infiltration on CT and frequency of lung metastases. Am J Roentgenol 149:1203–1206, 1987

Krishnamurthy GT et al: Distribution pattern of metastatic bone disease. JAMA 237:2504–2506, 1977

Lamego CMB, Zerbini MCN: Bone-metastasizing primary renal tumors in children. Radiology 147:449–454, 1983

Lehrer HZ, Maxfield WS, Nice CM: The periosteal "sunburst" pattern in metastatic bone tumors. AJR Am J Roentgenol 108:154–161, 1970

Marchal AL, Hoeffel JC et al: Atteintes pleurales par contiguiete ou metastases dans les tumeurs osseuses malignes primitives de l'enfant. J Radiol 67:303–307, 1986

Mitchell ML, Ackerman LV: Metastatic and pseudomalignant osteoblastoma: A report of two unusual cases. Skeletal Radiol 15:213–218, 1986

Naji AF et al: So-called adamantinoma of long bones: Report of a case with massive pulmonary metastases. J Bone Joint Surg [Am] 46:151–158, 1964

Norman A, Ulin R: A comparative study of periosteal new bone response in metastatic bone tumors (solitary) and primary bone sarcomas. Radiology 92:705–708, 1969

O'Connell DJ, Frank PH, Riddel RH: The metastases of meningioma: Radiologic and pathologic features. Skeletal Radiol 3:30–35, 1978

Raskin P, McClain CJ, Medsger TA: Hypocalcemia associated with metastatic bone disease: A retrospective study. Arch Intern Med 132:539–543, 1973

Reed MH, Shokeir MHK, Macpherson RI: Skeletal metastases from retinoblastoma. J Can Assoc Radiol 26:249–254, 1975

Reese EJ, Baker HL, Scanlon PW: The roentgenologic aspects of metastatic pheochromocytoma. AJR Am J Roentgenol 115: 783–793, 1972

Riddel RJ, Louis CJ, Bromberger NA: Pulmonary metastases from chondroblastoma of the tibia: Report of a case. J Bone Joint Surg [Br] 55:848–853, 1973

Rock MG, Pritchard DJ, Unni KK: Metastases from histologically benign giant-cell tumor of bone. J Bone Joint Surg [Am] 66:269–274, 1984

Rock MG, Sim FH et al: Secondary malignant giant-cell tumor of bone. J Bone Joint Surg 68:1073–1078, 1986

Scalley JR, Collins J: Thymoma metastatic to bone: Report of a case diagnosed by percutaneous biopsy. Radiology 96:423–424, 1970

Schweitzer ME, Levine C, Mitchell DG et al: Bull's-eyes and halos: Useful MR discriminators of osseous metastases. Radiology 188:249–252, 1993

Steinbach LS, Johnston JO: Case report Skeletal Radiol 22:203–205, 1993

Vandevoort PLM, Rosenbusch G: Ossifizierende lymph kontenmetastasen eines osteosarcoms. Fortschritte a/d Gebiet Röntgenstrahlen 126:492–494, 1977

Vilar J, Lezana AH, Pedrosa CS: Spiculated periosteal reaction in metastatic lesions of bone. Skeletal Radiol 3:230–233, 1979

Wong WS, Kaiser LR, Gold RH et al: Radiographic features of osseous metastases of soft-tissue sarcomas. Radiology 143:71–74, 1982

Yaghamai I: Angiographic features of chondromas and chondrosarcomas. Skeletal Radiol 3:91–98, 1978

Yaghamai I: Angiographic features of osteosarcoma. Am J Roentgenol 129:1073–1082, 1977

Zollikofer C, Zuniga WC, Stenlund R et al: Lung metastases from synovial sarcoma simulating granulomas. AJR Am J Roentgenol 135:161–163, 1980

Benign Primary Neoplasms of Bone

Agha FP, Lilienfeld RM: Roentgen features of osseous neurilemmoma. Radiology 102:325–326, 1972

Anderson RL, Popowitz L, Li JKH: An unusual sarcoma rising in a solitary osteochondroma. J Bone Joint Surg [Am] 51:1199–1204, 1969

Arata MA, Peterson HA, Dahlin DC: Pathological fractures through non-ossifying fibromas. J Bone Joint Surg [Am] 63:980–988, 1981

Assor D: Chondroblastoma of the rib: Report of a case. J Bone Joint Surg [Am] 55:208–210, 1973

Bertoni F, Calderoni P et al: Benign fibrous histiocytoma of bone. J Bone Joint Surg [Am] 68:1225–1230, 1986

Bohlman HH, Sachs BL et al: Primary neoplasms of the cervical spine. J Bone Joint Surg 68:483–493, 1986

Braddock GTF, Hadlow VD: Osteosarcoma in enchondromatosis (Ollier's disease): Report of a case. J Bone Joint Surg [Br] 48:145–149, 1966

Buirski G, Ratliff AHC et al: Cartilage-cell containing tumours of the pelvis: A radiological review of 40 patients. Br J Radiol 59:197–204, 1986

Buirski G, Watt I: The radiological features of "solid" aneurysmal bone cysts. Br J Radiol 57:1057–1065, 1984

Capanna R, Springfield DS et al: Juxtaepiphyseal aneurysmal bone cyst. Skeletal Radiol 13:21–25, 1985

Cary GR: Juxtacortical chondroma: A case report. J Bone Joint Surg [Am] 47:1405–1407, 1965

Chudacek Z: Angiographic feature of inflammatory fibrous histiocytoma. Br J Radiol 53:1006–1007, 1980

Dahlin DC, McLeod RA: Aneurysmal bone cyst and other nonneoplastic conditions. Skeletal Radiol 8:243–250, 1982

Dahlin DC: Giant cell tumor of bone: Highlights of 407 cases. AJR Am J Roentgenol 144:955–960, 1985

Dalinka MK, Chunn SP: Osteoblastoma—benign or malignant precursor? Report of a case. J Can Assoc Radiol 23:214–216, 1972

deSantos LA, Goldstein HM: Ultrasonography in tumors arising from the spine and bony pelvis. Am J Roentgenol 129:1061–1064, 1977

Destouet JM, Kyriakos M, Gilula LA: Fibrous histiocytoma (fibroxanthoma) of a cervical vertebra. Skeletal Radiol 5:241–246, 1980

Donner R, Dickland R: Adamantinoma of the tibia: A longstanding case with unusual histological features. J Bone Joint Surg [Br] 48:139–144, 1966

Dorfman HD, Bhagavan BS: Malignant fibrous histiocytoma of soft tissue with metaplastic bone and cartilage formation: A new radiologic sign. Skeletal Radiol 8:145–150, 1982

Dunlop JAY, Morton KS, Elliott GB: Recurrent osteoid osteoma: Report of a case with a review of the literature. J Bone Joint Surg [Br] 52:128–133, 1970

Fink IJ, Lee MA et al: Case reports: Radiographic and CT appearance of intraosseous xanthoma mimicking a malignant lesion. Br J Radiol 58:262–264, 1985

Fobben ES, Dalinka MK et al: The magnetic resonance imaging appearance at 1.5 Tesla of cartilaginous tumors involving the epiphysis. Skeletal Radiol 16:647–651, 1987

Giustra PE, Freiberger RH: Severe growth disturbance with osteoid osteoma: A report of 2 cases involving the femoral neck. Radiology 96:285–288, 1970

Gohel VK, Dalinka MK, Edeiken J: Ischemic necrosis of the femoral head simulating chondroblastoma. Radiology 107:545–546, 1973

Goldenberg RR, Campbell CJ, Bonfiglio M: Giant-cell tumor of bone: An analysis of 218 cases. J Bone Joint Surg [Am] 52:619–664, 1970

Greenspan A, Elguezbel A, Bryk D: Multifocal osteoid osteoma: A case report and review of the literature. AJR Am J Roentgenol 121:103–106, 1974

Greyson-Fleg RT, Reichmister JP et al: Post-traumatic osteochondroma. J Can Assoc Radiol 38:195–198, 1987

Hamilton WC, Ramsey PL, Hanson SM, Schiff DC: Osseous xanthoma and multiple hand tumors as a complication of hyperlipidemia. J Bone Joint Surg [Am] 57:551–553, 1975

Hamlin JA, Adler L, Greenbaum EI: Central enchondroma: A precursor to chondrosarcoma. J Can Assoc Radiol 22:206–209, 1971

Hardy R, Lehrer H: Desmoplastic fibroma vs desmoid tumor of bone. Radiology 88:899–901, 1967

Herman SD, Mesgarzadeh M et al: The role of magnetic resonance imaging in giant cell tumor of bone. Skeletal Radiol 16:635–643, 1987

Hill JA et al: Myxoma of the toes: A case report. J Bone Joint Surg [Am] 60:128–130, 1978

Horner K, Forman GH: Atypical simple bone cysts of the jaws. II: A possible association with benign fibro-osseous (cemental) lesions of the jaws. Clin Radiol 39:59–63, 1988

Howie JL: CT of osteoid osteoma of the femoral neck: The value of oblique reformatting. J Assoc Can Radiol 36:254–257, 1985

Hudson TM, Chew FS, Manaster BJ: Scintigraphy of benign exostoses and exostotic chondrosarcomas. AJR Am J Roentgenol 140:581–586, 1983

Joannides T, Pringle JA, Shaw DG et al: Giant cell tumour of bone in focal dermal hypoplasia. Br J Radiol 56:684–685, 1983

Johnson GF: Osteoid osteoma of the femoral neck. AJR Am J Roentgenol 74:65–69, 1955 236. Johnson LC: A general theory of bone tumors. Bull NY Acad Med 29:164–171, 1953

Kaibara N, Mitsuyasu M, Katsuki I et al: Generalized enchondromatosis with unusual complications of soft tissue calcifications and hemangiomas. Skeletal Radiol 8:43–46, 1982

Kenin A, Levine J, Spinner M: Parosteal lipoma: A report of 2 cases with associated bone changes. J Bone Joint Surg [Am] 41:1122–1126, 1959

Kim KS, Rogers LF, Lee C: The dural lucent line: Characteristic sign of hyperostosing meningioma en plaque. Am J Roentgenol 141:1217–1221, 1983

Kricun ME: Red-yellow marrow conversion: Its effect on the location of some solitary bone lesions. Skeletal Radiol 14:10–19, 1985

Kumar R, Swischuk LE et al: Benign cortical defect: Site for an avulsion fracture. Skeletal Radiol 15:553–555, 1986

Laurin S, Ekelund L, Persson B: Late recurrence of giant-cell tumor of bone: Pharmacoangiographic evaluation. Skeletal Radiol 5:227–231, 1980

Laurin S: Angiography of benign bone tumors. Acta Radiol 22:601–607, 1981

Levine E, Neff JR: Dynamic computed tomography scanning of benign bone lesions: Preliminary results. Skeletal Radiol 9:238–245, 1983

Lindbom A, Lindvall N, Soderberg G, Spjut H: Angiography in osteoid osteoma. Acta Radiol [Diagn] 53:377–384, 1960

McGrath PJ: Giant-cell tumour of bone. J Bone Joint Surg [Br] 54:216–229, 1972

McLaughlin RE, Sweet DE, Webster T, Merritt WM: Chondroblastoma of the pelvis suggestive of malignancy: Report of an unusual case treated by wide pelvic excision. J Bone Joint Surg [Am] 57:549–550, 1975

Milgram JW: Intraosseous lipomas: Radiologic and pathologic manifestations. Radiology 167:155–160, 1988

Mitchell ML, Ackerman LV: Metastatic and pseudomalignant osteoblastoma: A report of two unusual cases. Skeletal Radiol 15:213–218, 1986

Moore TM, Row JB, Harvey JP: Chondroblastoma of the talus. J Bone Joint Surg [Am] 59:830–831, 1977

Moser RP Jr, Sweet DE et al: Multiple skeletal fibroxanthomas: Radiologic–pathologic correlation of 72 cases. Skeletal Radiol 16:353–359, 1987

Murphy FD, Blount WB: Cartilaginous exostosis following irradiation. J Bone Joint Surg [Am] 44:662–668, 1962

Murphy NB, Price CHG: The radiological aspects of chondromyxoid fibroma of bone. Clin Radiol 22:261–269, 1971

Naji AF et al: So-called adamantinoma of long bones: Report of a case with massive pulmonary metastases. J Bone Joint Surg [Am] 46:151–158, 1964

Nelson OA, Greer RB: Localization osteoid osteoma of the spine using computerized tomography. J Bone Joint Surg [Am] 65:263–265, 1983

Omojola MF, Cockshott WP, Beatty EG: Osteoid osteoma: An evaluation of diagnostic modalities. Clin Radiol 32:199–204, 1981

Picci P, Baldini N et al: Giant cell reparative granuloma and other giant cell lesions of the bones of the hands and feet. Skeletal Radiol 15:415–421, 1986

Picci P, Manerini M, Zucchi V et al: Giant-cell tumor of bone in skeletally immature patients. J Bone Joint Surg [Am] 65: 486–490, 1983

Prichard RW, Stoy RP, Barwick JTF: Chondromyxoid fibroma of the scapula: Report of a case. J Bone Joint Surg [Am] 46: 1759–1760, 1964

Rock MG, Pritchard DJ, Unni KK: Metastases from histologically benign giant-cell tumor of bone. J Bone Joint Surg [Am] 66: 269–274, 1984

Rockwell MA, Enneking WF: Osteosarcoma developing in solitary enchondroma of the tibia. J Bone Joint Surg [Am] 53:341–344, 1971

Rosenfeld K, Bora FW, Lane JM: Osteoid osteoma of the hamate: A case report and review of the literature. J Bone Joint Surg [Am] 55:1085–1087, 1973

Ross P: Gardner's syndrome. AJR Am J Roentgenol 96:298–301, 1966

Schwimer SR, Bassett LW, Mancuso AA et al: Giant cell tumor of the cervicothoracic spine. Am J Roentgenol 136:63–67, 1981

Scott I, Connell DG et al: Regression of aneurysmal bone cyst following open biopsy. J Can Assoc Radiol 37:198–200, 1986

Sim FH, Danlin DC, Beabout JW: Multicentric giant-cell tumor of bone. J Bone Joint Surg [Am] 59:1052–1060, 1977

Spence AJ, Lloyd-Roberts GC: Regional osteoporosis in osteoid osteoma. J Bone Joint Surg [Br] 43:501–507, 1961

Sung HW, Kuo DP, Shu WP et al: Giant-cell tumor of bone: Analysis of two hundred and eight cases in Chinese patients. J Bone Joint Surg [Am] 64:755–761, 1982

Sybrandy S, de la Fuente AA: Multiple giant-cell tumour of bone. J Bone Joint Surg [Br] 55:350–356, 1973

Vallance R, Hamblen DL et al: Vascular complications of osteochondroma. Clin Radiol 36:639–642, 1985

Vinstein AL, Franken EA: Hereditary multiple exostoses: Report of a case with spinal cord compression. AJR Am J Roentgenol 112:405–407, 1974

Wright JL, Sherman MS: An unusual chondroblastoma. J Bone Joint Surg [Am] 46:597–600, 1964

Malignant Primary Neoplasms of Bone

Ahuja SC, Villacin AB, Smith J et al: Juxtacortical (parosteal) osteogenic sarcoma. J Bone Joint Surg [Am] 59:532–547, 1977

Alho A, Connor JF, Mankin HJ et al: Assessment of malignancy of cartilage tumors using flow cytometry. J Bone Joint Surg [Am] 65:779–785, 1983

Anderson RL, Popowitz L, Li JKH: An unusual sarcoma rising in a solitary osteochondroma. J Bone Joint Surg [Am] 51:1199–1204, 1969

Anscombe A, Walkden SB: An interesting bone scan in multiple myeloma: Myeloma superscan? Br J Radiol 56:489–492, 1983

Arrington ER, Eisenberg B, Orrison WW et al: Scintigraphic appearance of uncommon soft-tissue osteogenic sarcoma metastases. J Nucl Med 31:679–681, 1990

Bahr AL, Gayler BW: Cranial chondrosarcomas. Radiology 124:151–156, 1977

Blaquiere RM, Guyer PB, Buchanan RB et al: Sclerotic bone deposits in multiple myeloma. Br J Radiol 55:591–593, 1982

Bohlman HH, Sachs BL et al: Primary neoplasms of the cervical spine. J Bone Joint Surg 68:483–493, 1986

Braddock GTF, Hadlow VD: Osteosarcoma in enchondromatosis (Ollier's disease): Report of a case. J Bone Joint Surg [Br] 48:145–149, 1966

Buckwalter JA: The structure of human chondrosarcoma proteoglycans. J Bone Joint Surg [Am] 65:958–974, 1983

Buirski G, Ratliff AHC et al: Cartilage-cell containing tumours of the pelvis: A radiological review of 40 patients. Br J Radiol 59:197–204, 1986

Case records of the Massachusetts General Hospital (osteogenic sarcoma of humerus, with ossifying metastases in the regional nodes). N Engl J Med 225:953, 1941

Cooper RR: Juxtacortical chondrosarcoma: A case report. J Bone Joint Surg [Am] 47:524–528, 1965

Dahlin DC, Unni KK: Osteosarcoma of bone and its important recognizable varieties. Am J Surg Pathol 1:61–72, 1977

Dahlin DC: Giant cell tumor of bone: Highlights of 407 cases. AJR Am J Roentgenol 144:955–960, 1985 deSantos LA, Goldstein HM: Ultrasonography in tumors arising from the spine and bony pelvis. Am J Roentgenol 129:1061–1064, 1977

Dillon E, Parkin GJS: The role of diagnostic radiology in the diagnosis and management of rhabdomyosarcoma in young persons. Clin Radiol 29:5–59, 1978

Dorfman HD, Bhagavan BS: Malignant fibrous histiocytoma of soft tissue with metaplastic bone and cartilage formation: A new radiologic sign. Skeletal Radiol 8:145–150, 1982

Eady JL, McKinney JD et al: Primary leiomyosarcoma of bone: A case report and review of the literature. J Bone Joint Surg 69:287–289, 1987

Edeiken-Monroe B, Edeiken J, Kim EE: Radiologic concepts of lymphoma of bone. Radiol Clin North Am 28:841–864, 1990

Engels EP, Smith RC, Krantz S: Bone sclerosis in multiple myeloma. Radiology 75:242–247, 1960

Farr GH, Huvos AG: Juxtacortical osteogenic sarcoma: An analysis of 14 cases. J Bone Joint Surg [Am] 54:1205–1261, 1972

Feldman F, Norman D: Intra- and extraosseous malignant histocytoma (malignant fibrous xanthoma). Radiology 104:497–508, 1972

Fink IJ, Lee MA et al: Case reports: Radiographic and CT appearance of intraosseous xanthoma mimicking a malignant lesion. Br J Radiol 58:262–264, 1985

Fitzgerald RH, Dahlin DC, Sim FH: Multiple metachonous osteogenic sarcoma: Report of 12 cases with 2 long-term survivors. J Bone Joint Surg [Am] 55:595–605, 1973

Fobben ES, Dalinka MK et al: The magnetic resonance imaging appearance at 1.5 Tesla of cartilaginous tumors involving the epiphysis. Skeletal Radiol 16:647–651, 1987

Frouge C, Vanel D et al: The role of magnetic resonance imaging in the evaluation of Ewing's sarcoma. Skeletal Radiol 17:387–392, 1988

Gitelis S, Bertoni F, Campanacci M: Chondrosarcoma of bone. J Bone Joint Surg [Am] 63:1248–1257, 1981

Glasser DB, Lane JM: Stage IIB osteogenic sarcoma. Clin Orthop 270:29–39, 1991

Goorin AM, Abelson HT, Frei E: Osteosarcoma: Fifteen years later. N Engl J Med 313:1637–1643, 1985

Hamlin JA, Adler L, Greenbaum EI: Central enchondroma: A precursor to chondrosarcoma. J Can Assoc Radiol 22:206–209, 1971

Herman SD, Mesgarzadeh M et al: The role of magnetic resonance imaging in giant cell tumor of bone. Skeletal Radiol 16:635–643, 1987

Hermann G, Leviton M et al: Osteosarcoma: Relation between extent of marrow infiltration on CT and frequency of lung metastases. Am J Roentgenol 149:1203–1206, 1987

Hudson TM et al: Angiography of malignant fibrous histiocytoma of bone. Radiology 131:9–15, 1979

Hudson TM, Chew FS, Manaster BJ: Radionuclide bone scanning of medullary chondrosarcoma. AJR Am J Roentgenol 138:1071–1076, 1982

Hudson TM, Chew FS, Manaster BJ: Scintigraphy of benign exostoses and exostotic chondrosarcomas. AJR Am J Roentgenol 140:581–586, 1983

Hudson TM, Springfield DS et al: Computed tomography of parosteal osteosarcoma. Am J Roentgenol 144:961–965, 1985

Huvos AG, Butler A, Bretsky SS: Osteogenic sarcoma associated with Paget's disease. Cancer 52:1489–1495, 1983

Huvos AG, Woodard HQ, Cahan WG et al: Postradiation osteosarcoma of bone and soft tissues. Cancer 55:1244–1255, 1985

Jaffe N, Knapp J, Chuang VP et al: Osteosarcoma: Intra-arterial treatment of the primary tumor with cis-diamine-dichloroplatinum II (CDP). Angiographic, pathologic, and pharmacologic studies. Cancer 51:402–407, 1983

Jarde O, Desablens B et al: Difficultes diagnostiques du sarcome de Parker et Jackson. J Radiol 68:305–307, 1987

Jokl P, Albright JA, Goodman AH: Juxtacortical chondrosarcoma of the hand. J Bone Joint Surg [Am] 53:1370–1376, 1971

Kenney PJ, Siegel MJ, McAlister WH: Congenital intraspinal neuroblastoma: A treatable simulant of myelodysplasia. Am J Roentgenol 138:166–167, 1982

Larsson SE, Lorentzon R: The incidence of primary malignant bone tumors in relation to age, sex, and site. J Bone Joint Surg [Am] 56:534–540, 1974

Leonard RCF, Owen JP, Proctor SJ et al: Multiple myeloma: Radiology or bone scanning? Clin Radiol 32:291–295, 1981

Lindell MM Jr, Shirkhoda A et al: Parosteal osteosarcoma: Radiologic–pathologic correlation with emphasis on CT. Am J Roentgenol 148:323–328, 1987

Link MP, Goorin AM, Miser AW et al: The effect of adjuvant chemotherapy on relapse-free survival in patients with osteosarcoma of the extremity. N Engl J Med 314:1600–1606, 1986

Lodwick GS: Solitary malignant tumors of bone: The application of predictor variables in diagnosis. Semin Roentgenol 1:293–313, 1966

Ludwig H, Kumpan W, Sinzinger H: Radiography and bone scintigraphy in multiple myeloma: A comparative analysis. Br J Radiol 55:173–181, 1982

Lukens JA, McLeod RA, Sim FH: Computed tomographic evaluation of primary osseous malignant neoplasma. Am J Roentgenol 139:45–48, 1982

Marcove RC et al: Osteogenic sarcoma under the age of 21: A review of 145 operative cases. J Bone Joint Surg [Am] 52:411–423, 1970

Mendelsohn DB, Hertzanu Y, Glass RBJ: Computed tomographic findings in primary mandibular osteosarcoma. Clin Radiol 34:153–155, 1983

Mitchell ML, Ackerman LV: Metastatic and pseudomalignant osteoblastoma: A report of two unusual cases. Skeletal Radiol 15:213–218, 1986

Naji AF et al: So-called adamantinoma of long bones: Report of a case with massive pulmonary metastases. J Bone Joint Surg [Am] 46:151–158, 1964

Ngan H, Preston BJ: Non-Hodgkin's lymphoma presenting with osseous lesions. Clin Radiol 26:351–356, 1975

O'Hara JM et al: An analysis of 30 patients surviving longer than 10 years after treatment for osteogenic sarcoma. J Bone Joint Surg [Am] 50:335–354, 1968

Parker F, Jackson H: Primary reticulum-cell sarcoma of bone. Surg Gynecol Obstet 68:45–51, 1939

Pasquel PM, Levet SN, DeLeon B: Primary rhabdomyosarcoma of bone: A case report. J Bone Joint Surg [Am] 58:1176–1178, 1976

Phillips WC, Kattapuram SV, Doseretz DE et al: Primary lymphoma of bone: Relationship of radiographic appearance and prognosis. Radiology 144:285–290, 1982

Picci P, Baldini N et al: Giant cell reparative granuloma and other giant cell lesions of the bones of the hands and feet. Skeletal Radiol 15:415–421, 1986

Picci P, Campanacci M et al: Medullary involvement in parosteal osteosarcoma. J Bone Joint Surg 69:131–136, 1987

Riddel RJ, Louis CJ, Bromberger NA: Pulmonary metastases from chondroblastoma of the tibia: Report of a case. J Bone Joint Surg [Br] 55:848–853, 1973

Rockwell MA, Enneking WF: Osteosarcoma developing in solitary enchondroma of the tibia. J Bone Joint Surg [Am] 53:341–344, 1971

Ros PR, Viamonte M, Rywlin AM: Malignant fibrous histiocytoma: Mesenchymal tumor of ubiquitous origin. Am J Roentgenol 142:753–759, 1984

Rosen G, Caparros B, Huvos AG et al: Preoperative chemotherapy for osteogenic sarcoma: Selection of postoperative adjuvant chemotherapy based on the response of the primary tumor to preoperative chemotherapy. Cancer 49:1221–1230, 1982

Rossleigh MA, Smith J et al: Case reports: A photopenic lesion in osteosarcoma. Br J Radiol 60:497–499, 1987

Schajowicz F, Araujo ES, Berenstein M: Sarcoma complicating Paget's disease of bone. J Bone Joint Surg [Br] 65:299–307, 1983

Schajowicz F, Lemos C: Malignant osteoblastoma. J Bone Joint Surg [Br] 58:202–211, 1976

Smith J, Ahuja SC, Huvos AG, Bullough P: Parosteal (juxtacortical) osteogenic sarcoma: A roentgenological study of 30 patients. J Can Assoc Radiol 29:167–174, 1978

Solomon A, Rahamni R, Seligsohn U et al: Multiple myeloma: Early vertebral involvement assessed by computerised tomography. Skeletal Radiol 11:258–261, 1984

Spiers FW, King SD, Beddoe AH: Measurements of endosteal surface area in human long bones: Relationship of sites of occurrence of osteosarcoma. Br J Radiol 50:769–776, 1977

Sung HW, Kuo DP, Shu WP et al: Giant-cell tumor of bone: Analysis of two hundred and eight cases in Chinese patients. J Bone Joint Surg [Am] 64:755–761, 1982

Sybrandy S, de la Fuente AA: Multiple giant-cell tumour of bone. J Bone Joint Surg [Br] 55:350–356, 1973

Taber DS, Libshitz HI, Cohen MA: Treated Ewing's sarcoma: Radiographic appearance in response, recurrence, and new primaries. Am J Roentgenol 140:753–758, 1983

Toland J, Phelps PDD: Plasmacytoma of the skull base. Clin Radiol 22:93–96, 1971

Torrance DJ: "Negative" bone density in a case of multiple myeloma. Radiology 70:864–865, 1958

Unni KK, Dahlin DC, Beaubout SW, Ivins JC: Parosteal osteogenic sarcoma. Cancer 37:2466–2475, 1976

Unni KK, Dahlin DC, McLeod RA et al: Interosseous well-differentiated osteosarcoma. Cancer 40:1337–1347, 1977

Vandevoort PLM, Rosenbusch G: Ossifizierende lymph kontenmetastasen eines osteosarcoms. Fortschritte a/d Gebiet Röntgenstrahlen 126:492–494, 1977

Winkler K, Beron G, Kotz R et al: Neoadjuvant chemotherapy for osteogenic sarcoma: Results of a cooperative German/Austrian study. J Clin Oncol 2:617–624, 1984

Benign Soft-Tissue Neoplasms

Balck WC, Armstrong P et al: Computed tomography of aggressive fibromatosis in the posterior mediastinum. J Comput Assist Tomogr 11:153–155, 1987

Coventry MB, Harrison EG, Martin JF: Benign synovial tumors of the knee: A diagnostic problem. J Bone Joint Surg [Am] 48:1350–1358, 1966

Heiken JP, Lee JKT, Smathers RL et al: CT of benign soft tissue masses of the extremities. AJR Am J Roentgenol 142:575–580, 1984

Leffert RD: Lipomas of the upper extremity. J Bone Joint Surg [Am] 54:1262–1266, 1972

Louis DS, Dick HM: Ossifying fibrolipoma of the median nerve. J Bone Joint Surg [Am] 55:1082–1084, 1973

McCook TA, Martinez S, Korobkin M et al: Intramuscular myxoma. Skeletal Radiol 7:1–19, 1981

Schwimer SR, Bassett LW, Mancuso AA et al: Giant cell tumor of the cervicothoracic spine. Am J Roentgenol 136:63–67, 1981

Sim FH, Danlin DC, Beaubout JW: Multicentric giant-cell tumor of bone. J Bone Joint Surg [Am] 59:1052–1060, 1977

Weitzman G: Lipoma arborescens of knee: Report of a case. J Bone Joint Surg [Am] 47:1030–1034, 1965

Malignant Soft-Tissue Neoplasms

Ahmed MJ, Omar YT et al: Soft tissue sarcoma in Kuwait: A review of 114 patients. Clin Radiol 38:2–29, 1987

Brodsky AE, Dennis MD, Sassard WR: Alveolar soft part sarcoma. J Bone Joint Surg [Am] 65:841–842, 1983

Hamilton A, Davis RI et al: Synovial chondrosarcoma complicating synovial chondromatosis. J Bone Joint Surg 69:1084–1088, 1987

Jessurun J, Rojas ME, Saavendra JA: Congenital extraskeletal embryonal chondrosarcoma. J Bone Joint Surg [Am] 64:293–296, 1982

Liefeld PA, Ferguson AB, Fu FH: Focal myositis: A benign lesion that mimics malignant disease. J Bone Joint Surg [Am] 64:1371–1373, 1982

Linscheid RL, Soule EH, Henderson ED: Pleomorphic rhabdomyosarcomata of the extremities and limb girdles: A clinicopathological study. J Bone Joint Surg [Am] 47:715–726, 1965

Reszel PA, Soule EH, Coventry MB: Liposarcoma of the extremities and limb girdles: A study of 222 cases. J Bone Joint Surg [Am] 48:229–244, 1966

Smith J: Radiation-induced sarcoma of bone: Clinical and radiographic findings in 43 patients irradiated for soft tissue neoplasms. Clin Radiol 33:205–221, 1982

Watt AC, Haggar AM, Krasicky GA: Extraosseous osteogenic sarcoma of the breast: Mammographic and pathologic findings. Radiology 150:34, 1984

Weinberger G, Levinsohn EM: Computed tomography in the evaluation of sarcomatous tumors of the thigh. AJR Am J Roentgenol 130:115–118, 1978

Zollikofer C, Zuniga WC, Stenlund R et al: Lung metastases from synovial sarcoma simulating granulomas. AJR Am J Roentgenol 135:161–163, 1980

General References

Castleman B, McNeill MJ: Bone and Joint Clinicopathological Conferences of the Massachusetts General Hospital. Boston, Little, Brown & Co, 1966

Dahlin DC, Unni KK: Bone Tumors, 4th ed. Springfield, IL, Charles C Thomas, 1986

Dodds WJ, Steinbach HL: Gout associated with calcification of cartilage. N Engl J Med 275:745–749, 1966

Doe WF, Henry K, Doyle FH: Radiological and histological findings in 6 patients wiht alpha-chain disease. Br J Radiol 49:3–11, 1976

Draper MW, Chafetz N, Weinberg GL et al: Distinct form of osteosclerosis in identical twins with mental retardation. AJR 1Am J Roentgenol 39:1205–1209, 1982

Edeiken B, de Santos LA: Percutaneous needle biopsy of the irradiated skeleton. Radiology 146:653–655, 1983

El-Khoury GY, Wehbe MA, Bonfiglio M et al: Stress fractures of the femoral neck: A scintigraphic sign for early diagnosis. Skeletal Radiol 6:271–273, 1981

Elson MW: The syndrome of exophthalmos, hypertrophic osteoarthropathy, and pretibial myxedema. AJR Am J Roentgenol 85:114–118, 1961

Evans GA, Park WM: Familial multiple nonosteogenic fibromata. J Bone Joint Surg [Br] 60:416–419, 1978

Ewald FC: Unilateral mixed sclerosing bone dystrophy associated with unilateral lymphangiectasis and capillary hemangioma: A case report. J Bone Joint Surg [Am] 54:878–880, 1972

Fornasier VL: Hemangiomatosis with massive osteolysis. J Bone Joint Surg [Br] 52:444–451, 1970

Frangione B, Franklin EC: Heavy chain diseases: Clinical features and molecular significance of the disordered immunoglobulin structure. Semin Hematol 10:53–64, 1973

Greenspan A, Steiner G et al: Mixed sclerosing bone dysplasia coexisting with dysplasia epiphysealis hemimelica (Trevor-Fairbank disease). Skeletal Radiol 15:452–454, 1986

Harris IE, Leff AR, Gitelis S et al: Function after amputation, arthrodesis, or arthroplasty for tumors about the knee. J Bone Joint Surg [Am] 72:1477–1485, 1990

Harris JR, Brand PW: Patterns of disintegration of the tarsus in the anaesthetic foot. J Bone Joint Surg [Br] 48:4–16, 1966

Haverbush TJ, Wilde AH, Hawk WA, Scherbel AL: Osteolysis of the ribs and cervical spine in progressive systemic sclerosis (scleroderma). J Bone Joint Surg [Am] 56:637–640, 1974

Hemingway SP, Leung A, Lavender JP: Familial vanishing limbs: Four generations of idiopathic multicentric osteolysis. Clin Radiol 34:585–588, 1983

Ho A, Williams DM et al: Unilateral hypertrophic osteoarthropathy in a patient with an infected axillary–axillary bypass graft. Radiology 162:573–574, 1987

Jensen WN, Lasser EC: Urticaria pigmentosa associated with widespread sclerosis of the spongiosa of bone. Radiology 71:826–832, 1958

Kanis JA, Thomson JG: Mixed sclerosing bone dystrophy with regression of melorheostosis. Br J Radiol 48:400–402, 1975

Kittredge RD, Finby N: The many facets of lymphangioma. AJR Am J Roentgenol 95:56–66, 1965

Kozlowski K, Anderson R, Tink A: Multifocal recurrent periostitis. Fortschr Geb Rontgenstr 135:597–602, 1981

Kyle RA, Greipp PR: Amyloidosis (AL): Clinical and laboratory features in 229 cases. Mayo Clin Proc 58:665–683, 1983

Lagier R, Mbakop A, Bigler A: Osteopoikilosis: A radiological and pathological study. Skeletal Radiol 11:161–168, 1984

Macpherson RI, Letts RM: Skeletal diseases associated with angiomatosis. J Can Assoc Radiol 29:90–100, 1978

McNulty JG, Pim P: Hyperphosphatasia: A report of a case with a 30-year follow-up. AJR Am J Roentgenol 115:614–618, 1972

Mirra JM, Arnold WD: Skeletal hemangiomatosis in association with hereditary hemorrhagic telangiectasia: A case report. J Bone Joint Surg [Am] 55:850–854, 1973

Moule B, Grant MC, Boyle IT, May H: Thyroid acropachy. Clin Radiol 21:329–333, 1970

Murphy WA, Seligman PA, Tillack T et al: Osteosclerosis, osteomalacia, and bone marrow aplasia: A combined late complication of Thorotrast administration. Skeletal Radiol 3:234–238, 1979

Parker LN, Wu SY, Lai MK et al: The early diagnosis of atypical thyroid acropachy. Arch Intern Med 142:1749–1751, 1982

Pastakia B, Horvath K et al: Seventeen-year follow-up and autopsy findings in a case of massive osteolysis. Skeletal Radiol 16:291–297, 1987

Patrick JH: Melorheostosis associated with arteriovenous aneurysm of the left arm and trunk. J Bone Joint Surg [Br] 51:126–129, 1969

Resnick D, Vint V, Poteshman NL: Sternocostoclavicular hyperostosis. J Bone Joint Surg [Am] 63:1329–1332, 1981

Rubin P: Dynamic Classification of Bone Dysplasias. Chicago, Year Book Medical Publishers, 1964

Russell WJ, Bizzozero OJ, Omori Y: Idiopathic osteosclerosis. Radiology 90:70–76, 1968

Sartoris DJ, Clopton P et al: Vertebral-body collapse in focal and diffuse disease: Patterns of pathologic processes. Radiology 160:479–483, 1986

Soffa DJ, Sire DJ, Dodson JR: Melorheostosis with linear sclerodermatous skin changes. Radiology 114:577–578, 1975

Solomon A, McLaughlin CL: Immunoglobulin structure determined from products of plasma cell neoplasms. Semin Hematol 10:3–17, 1973

Stringer DA, Hall CM: Juvenile hyaline fibromatosis. Br J Radiol 54:473–478, 1981

Teplick JG et al: Ghost infantile vertebrae and hemipelves within adult skeleton from thorotrast administration in childhood. Radiology 129:657–660, 1978

Van Den Bout AG, Dreyer L: Malacoplakia of bone. J Bone Joint Surg [Br] 63:254–256, 1981

Vichi GF et al: Diagnosis: Idiopathic carpal/tarsal osteolysis (ICTO) associated with nephropathy.

Whitehouse GH, Bottomley JP, Bradley J: Lymphangiographic appearances in Waldenstrom's macroglobulinemia. Br J Radiol 47:226–229, 1974

Wolfson JJ, Kane WJ, Laxdal SD et al: Bone findings in chronic granulomatous disease of childhood: A genetic abnormality of leukocyte function. J Bone Joint Surg [Am] 51:1572–1583, 1969

Infections

Alderson M, Speers D et al: Acute haematogenous osteomyelitis and septic arthritis: A single disease. J Bone Joint Surg 68:268–274, 1986

Behr JR, Daluga DJ et al: Herpetic infections in the fingers of infants. J Bone Joint Surg 69:137–139, 1987

Beltran J, McGhee RB et. al.: Experimental infections of the musculoskeletal system: Evaluation with MR imaging and Tc-99m MDP and Ga-67 scintigraphy. Radiology 167:167–172, 1988

Bergdahl S, Fellander M, Robertson B: BCG osteomyelitis. J Bone Joint Surg [Br] 58:212–216, 1976

Blockey NJ: Chronic osteomyelitis. J Bone Joint Surg [Br] 65:120–123, 1983

Braithwaite PA, Lees RF: Vertebral hydatid disease: Radiological assessment. Radiology 140:763–766, 1981

Chang AC, Destouet JM, Murphy WA: Musculoskeletal sporotrichosis. Skeletal Radiol 12:23–28, 1984

Claudon M, Bracard S et al: Spinal involvement in alveolar echinococcosis: Assessment of two cases. Radiology 162:571–572, 1987

Cockshott WP, Davies AGM: Tumoural gummatous yaws: Two case reports. J Bone Joint Surg [Br] 42:785–787, 1960

Comstock C, Wolson AH: Roentgenology of sporotrichosis. Am J Roentgenol 125:651–655, 1975

Coppola J, Mueller NL et al: Computed tomography of musculoskeletal tuberculosis. J Can Assoc Radiol 38:199–203, 1987

Dalinka MK, Dinnenberg S, Greendyke WH, Hopkins R: Roentgenographic features of osseous coccidioidomycosis and differential diagnosis. J Bone Joint Surg [Am] 53:1157–1164, 1971

Danigelis JA, Long RE: Anonymous mycobacterial osteomyelitis: A case report of a 6-year-old child. Radiology 93:353–354, 1969

Davidson JC, Palmer PES: Osteomyelitis variolosa. J Bone Joint Surg [Br] 45:687–693, 1963 Davidson JW, Chacha PB, James W: Multiple osteosarcomata: Report of a case. J Bone Joint Surg [Br] 47:537–541, 1965

del Busto R, Quinn EL, Fisher EJ et al: Osteomyelitis of the pubis. JAMA 248:1498–1500, 1982

Dismukes WE et al: Destructive bone disease in early syphilis. JAMA 236:2646–2648, 1976

Donovan RM, Shah KJ: Unusual sites of acute osteomyelitis in childhood. Clin Radiol 33:222–230, 1982

Duran H et al: Osseous hydatidosis. J Bone Joint Surg [Am] 60:685–690, 1978

Ellis W: Multiple bone lesions caused by Avian–Battey mycobacteria. J Bone Joint Surg [Br] 56:323–326, 1974

Erikson V, Hjelmstedt A: Roentgenologic aspects of BCG osteomyelitis. Radiology 101:575–578, 1971

Fernandez F, Pueyo I, Jiménez JR et al: Epiphysiometaphyseal changes in children after severe meningococcic sepsis. AJR Am J Roentgenol 136:1236–1238, 1981

Frazier JK, Anzel SH: Osteomyelitis of the greater trochanter in children. J Bone Joint Surg [Am] 63:833–835, 1981

Gantz NM: Gonococcal osteomyelitis: An unusual complication of gonococcal arthritis. JAMA 236:2431–2432, 1976

Gehweiler JA, Capp MP, Chick EW: Observations on the roentgen patterns in blastomycosis of bone: A review of cases from the blastomycosis cooperative study of the Veterans Administration and Duke University Medical Center. Am J Roentgenol 108:497–510, 1970

Green NE, Beauchamp RD, Griffin PP: Primary subacute epiphyseal osteomyelitis. J Bone Joint Surg [Am] 63:107–114, 1981

Grossman M: Aspergillosis of bone. Br J Radiol 48:57–59, 1975

Heitzman ER, Bornhurst RA, Russell JP: Disease due to anonymous mycobacteria. AJR Am J Roentgenol 103:533–539, 1968

Helms CA, Jeffrey RB et al: Computed tomography and plain film appearance of a bony sequestration: Significance and differential diagnosis. Skeletal Radiol 16:117–120, 1987

Highland TR, LaMont RL: Osteomyelitis of the pelvis in children. J Bone Joint Surg [Am] 65:230–234, 1983

Hsieh CK: Echinococcus involvement of bone with x-ray examination. Radiology 14:562–575, 1930

Israel O, Gips S et al: Osteomyelitis and soft-tissue infection: Differential diagnosis with 24 hour/4 hour ration of Tc-99m MDP uptake. Radiology 163:725–726, 1987

Jenkins FH, Raff MJ, Florman LD et al: Pubic osteomyelitis due to anaerobic bacteria. Arch Intern Med 144:842–843, 1984

Johns D: Syphilitic disorders of the spine. J Bone Joint Surg [Br] 52:724–731, 1970

Johnson AC, James AE, Reddy ER, Johnson S: Relation of vascular and osseous changes in leprosy. Skeletal Radiol 3:36–41, 1978

Joyce PF et al: A rare clinical presentation of blastomycosis. Skeletal Radiol 2:239–242, 1977

Jurik AG, Moller SH et al: Chronic sclerosing osteomyelitis of the iliac bone: Etiological possibilities. Skeletal Radiol 17:114–118, 1988

Kirkpatrick DJ: Donovanosis (granuloma inguinale): A rare cause of osteolytic bone lesions. Clin Radiol 21:101–105, 1970

Kolawole TM, Bohrer SP: Ulcer osteoma: Bone response to tropical ulcer. Am J Roentgenol 109:611–618, 1970

Kumar R, Smissen EVD, Jorizzo N: Systemic sporotrichosis with osteomyelitis. J Can Assoc Radiol 35:83–84, 1984

Lagier R: Coexistence of staphylococcic spondylitis and spinal hyperostosis. Fortschr Geb Rontgenstr 147:452–453, 1987

Lee SM, Lee RGL et al: Magnification radiograpy in osteomyelitis. Skeletal Radiol 15:625–627, 1986

Lewall DB, Ofole S et al: Mycetoma. Skeletal Radiol 14:257–262, 1985

Lifeso R: Atlanto-axial tuberculosis in adults. J Bone Joint Surg 69:183–187, 1987

Lord CF, Gebhardt MC, Tomford WW et al: Infection in bone allografts: Incidence, nature, and treatment. J Bone Joint Surg [Am] 70:369–376, 1988

Madkour MM, Sarif HS et al: Osteoarticular brucellosis: Results of bone scintigraphy in 140 patients. AJR Am J Roentgenol 150:1101–1105, 1988

Majid MA, Mathias PF, Seth HN, Thirumalachar MJ: Primary mycetoma of the patella. J Bone Joint Surg [Am] 46:1283–1286, 1964

McCrea ES, Wagner E: Femoral osteomyelitis secondary to diverticulitis. J Can Assoc Radiol 32:181–182, 1981

McGahan JP, Gravers DS, Palmer ES: Coccidioidal spondylitis. Radiology 136:5–9, 1980

Miller EH, Semian DW: Gram-negative osteomyelitis following puncture wounds of the foot. J Bone Joint Surg [Am] 57:535–537, 1975

Mok PM, Reilly BJ, Ash JM: Osteomyelitis in the neonate. Radiology 145:677–682, 1982

Moore RM, Green NE: Blastomycosis of bone. J Bone Joint Surg [Am] 64:1097–1101, 1982

Morris E, Wolinsky E: Localized osseous cryptococcosis: A case report. J Bone Joint Surg [Am] 47:1027–1029, 1965

Mortensson W, Eklof O, Jorulf H: Radiologic aspects of BCG osteomyelitis in infants and children. Acta Radiol [Diagn] 17:845–855, 1976

Musher DM et al: Vertebral osteomyelitis. Arch Intern Med 136:105–110, 1976

Nathan PA, Trung NB: Osteomyelitis variolosa: Report of a case. J Bone Joint Surg [Am] 56:1525–1528, 1974

O'Reilly GV, Clark TM, Crum CP: Skeletal involvement in mycosis fungoides. AJR Am J Roentgenol 129:741–743, 1977

Parker MD, Irwin RS: Mycobacterium kansasii tendinitis and fasciitis. J Bone Joint Surg [Am] 57:557–559, 1975

Pearl KN, Dearlove J, Chin KS: Periostitis in an infant with cytomegalovirus infection acquired after birth. Br J Radiol 57:638–640, 1984

Pintilie DC, Panoza GH, Hatman VD, Fahrer M: Echinococcosis of the humerus: Treatment by resection and bone grafting. J Bone Joint Surg [Am] 48:957–962, 1966

Probst FP: Chronic multifocal cleidometaphyseal osteomyelitis of childhood. Acta Radiol [Diagn] 17:531–537, 1976

Resnick D, Pineda CJ et al: Osteomyelitis and septic arthritis of the hand following human bites. Skeletal Radiol 14:263–266, 1985

Ribner BS, Freimer EH: Osteomyelitis caused by viridans streptococci. Arch Intern Med 142:1739, 1982

Rong SH, Nie ZQ: Hydatid disease of bone. Clin Radiol 36:301–305, 1985

Rosen RS, Jacobson G: Fungus disease of bone. Semin Roentgenol 1:370–391, 1966

Rosenthal RE, Spickard WA, Markham RD et al: Osteomyelitis of the symphysis pubis: A separate disease from osteitis pubis. J Bone Joint Surg [Am] 64:123–128, 1982

Rudwan MA, Sheikh NA: Aspergilloma of paranasal sinuses: A common cause of unilateral proptosis in Sudan. Clin Radiol 27:497–502, 1976

Satin R, Usher MS, Goldenberg M: More causes of button sequestrum. J Can Assoc Radiol 27:288–289, 1976

Silverman FN: Virus diseases of bone: Do they exist? AJR Am J Roentgenol 126:677–703, 1976

Singson RD, Berdon WE et al: "Missing" femoral condyle: An unusual sequela to neonatal osteomyelitis and septic arthritis. Radiology 161:359–361, 1986

Spiegel PG, Kengla KW, Isaacson AS, Wilson JC: Intervertebral disc-space inflammation in children. J Bone Joint Surg [Am] 54:284–296, 1972

Sugarman B, Hawes S, Musher DM et al: Osteomyelitis beneath pressure sores. Arch Intern Med 143:683–688, 1983

Swischuk LE, Jorgenson F, Caden D: Wooden splinter induced "pseudotumors" and "osteomyelitis-like" lesions of bone and soft tissue. Am J Roentgenol 122:176–179, 1974

Taylor CR, Lawson JP: Periostitis and osteomyelitis in chronic drug addicts. Skeletal Radiol 15:209–212, 1986

Torgerson WR, Hammond G: Osteomyelitis of the sesamoid bones of the 1st metatarsophalangeal joint. J Bone Joint Surg [Am] 51:1420–1422, 1969

Tuazon CU: Teichoic acid antibodies in osteomyelitis and septic arthritis caused by staphylococcus aureus. J Bone Joint Surg [Am] 64:762–765, 1982

Tumeh SS, Aliabadi P et al: Disease activity in osteomyelitis: Role of radiography. Radiology 165:781–784, 1987

Van Lom KJ, Kellerhouse LE et al: Infection versus tumor in the spine: Criteria for distinction with CT Radiology 166:851–855, 1988

Versfeld GA, Solomon A: A diagnostic approach to tuberculosis of bone and joints. J Bone Joint Surg [Br] 64:446–449, 1982

Vogelzang RL, Hendrix RW, Neiman HL: Computed tomography of tuberculous osteomyelitis of the pubis. J Comput Assist Tomogr 7:914–915, 1983

Williams CS, Riordan DC: Mycobacterium marinum (atypical acid-fast bacillus): Infections of the hand: A report of 6 cases. J Bone Joint Surg [Am] 55:1042–1050, 1973

Yocum RC, McArthur J, Petty GE et al: Septic arthritis caused by Propionibacterium acnes. JAMA 248:1740–1741, 1982

Yousefzadeh DK, Jackson JH: Neonatal and infantile candidal arthritis with or without osteomyelitis: A clinical and radiographical review of 21 cases. Skeletal Radiol 5:77–90, 1980

Fractures

Arata MA, Peterson HA, Dahlin DC: Pathological fractures through non-ossifying fibromas. J Bone Joint Surg [Am] 63:980–988, 1981

Aymard A, Chevrot A et al: Fracture spontanee du sternum. J Radiol 68:593–595, 1987

Berrey BH Jr, Lord CF, Gebhardt MC et al: Fractures of allografts: Frequency, treatment, and end-results. J Bone Joint Surg [Am] 72:825–833, 1990

Bersani D, Riwer-Mugel B, Watrin MP: Ostéolyse post-traumatique de l'extrémité distale de la clavicule. J Radiol 65:47–49, 1984

Daffner RH, Martinez S, Gehweiler JA et al: Stress fractures of the proximal tibia in runners. Radiology 142:63–65, 1982

Daffner RH: Stress fractures: Current concepts. Skeletal Radiol 2:221–229, 1978

Gaucher A, Regent D et al: Les fractures par insuffisance osseouse du sacrum. J Radiol 68:433–440, 1987

Goergen TG, Resnick D, Riley RR: Posttraumatic abnormalities of the pubic bone simulating malignancy. Radiology 126:85–87, 1978

Greaney RB, Gerber FH, Laughlin RL et al: Distribution and natural history of stress fractures in U.S. Marine recruits. Radiology 146:339–346, 1983

Kaltsas DS: Stress fractures of the femoral neck in young adults. J Bone Joint Surg [Br] 63:33–37, 1981

Kumar R, Swischuk LE et al: Benign cortical defect: Site for an avulsion fracture. Skeletal Radiol 15:553–555, 1986

Lee JK, Yao L: Stress fractures: MR imaging. Radiology 169:217–220, 1988

Levin DC, Blazina ME, Levine E: Fatigue fractures of the shaft of the femur: Simulation of malignant tumor. Radiology 89:883–885, 1967

Miller B, Markheim HR, Towbin MN: Multiple stress fractures in rheumatoid arthritis: A case report. J Bone Joint Surg [Am] 49:1408–1414, 1967

Murcia M, Brennan RE, Edeiken J: Computed tomography of stress fracture. Skeletal Radiol 8:193–195, 1982

Nussbaum AR, Treves ST et al: Bone stress lesions in ballet dancers: Scintigraphic assessment. Am J Roentgenol 150:851–855, 1988

Yousem D, Magid D et al: Computed tomography of stress fractures. J Comput Assist Tomogr 10:92–95, 1986

Tumor-like Lesions

Abdelwahab IF, Present DA et al: Tumorlike tuberculous granulomas of bone. AJR Am J Roentgenol 149:1207–1208, 1987

Abdelwhab IF, Norman A: Osteosclerotic sarcoidosis. AJR 150:161–162, 1988

Abramson MN: Disseminated asymptomatic osteosclerosis with features resembling melorheosis, osteopoikilosis, and osteopathia striata: A case report. J Bone Joint Surg [Am] 50:991–996, 1968

Adler CP: Tumour-like lesions in the femur with cementum-like material: Does a "cementoma" of long bone exist? Skeletal Radiol 14:26–37, 1985

Allen BL, Jinkins WJ: Vertebral osteonecrosis associated with pancreatitis in a child: A case report. J Bone Joint Surg [Am] 60:985–987, 1978

Arlart IP, Maier W, Leupold D et al: Massive periosteal new bone formation in ulcerative colitis. Radiology 144:507–508, 1982

Barnes GR, Gwinn JL: Distal irregularities of the femur simulating malignancy. Am J Roentgenol 122:180–185, 1974

Blane CE, Perkash I: True heterotopic bone in the paralyzed patient. Skeletal Radiol 7:2–25, 1981

Blank N, Lieber A: The significance of growing bone islands. Radiology 85:508–511, 1965

Bohndrof K, Reiser M et al: Magnetic resonance imaging of primary tumors and tumor-like lesions of bone. Skeletal Radiol 15:511–517, 1986

Bressler EL, Marn CS et al: Evaluation of ectopic bone by CT. AJR Am J Roentgenol 148:931–935, 1987

Cannon SR: Massive osteolysis: A review of seven cases. J Bone Joint Surg 68:24–28, 1986

Capanna R, Van Horn J et al: Epiphyseal involvement in unicameral bone cysts. Skeletal Radiol 15:428–432, 1986

Castle WB, Drinker KR, Drinker CK: Necrosis of the jaw in workers employed in applying a luminous paint containing radium. J Industrial Hygiene 7:371, 1925

Chetta SG, Weber MJ, Nelson CL: Non-traumatic clostridial myonecrosis. J Bone Joint Surg [Am] 64:456–457, 1982

Chevrot A, Pallardy G, Ledoux P, Lebard G: Skeletal manifestations of hyperthyroidism. J Radiol 59:167–173, 1978

Chung SMK, Janes JM: Diffuse pigmented villonodular synovitis of the hip joint: Review of the literature and report of 4 cases. J Bone Joint Surg [Am] 47:292–303, 1965

Condon RR, Allen RP: Congenital generalized fibromatosis. Radiology 76:444–448, 1961

Dahlin DC, McLeod RA: Aneurysmal bone cyst and other non-neoplastic conditions. Skeletal Radiol 8:243–250, 1982

Edelstein G, Kyriakos M: Focal hematopoietic hyperplasia of the rib: A form of pseudotumor. Skeletal Radiol 11:108–118, 1984

Engdahl DE, Kaufman RA, Hospson CN: Computed tomography in the diagnosis of rare plantar ganglion cyst in a child. J Bone Joint Surg [Am] 65:1348–1349a, 1983

Farmlett EJ, Fishman EK et al: Computed tomography in the assessment of myonecrosis. J Can Assoc Radiol 38:278–282a, 1987

Ferriter P, Hirschy J, Kesseler H et al: Popliteal pseudoaneurysm. J Bone Joint Surg [Am] 65:695–697, 1983

Gardner DJ, Azouz EM: Solitary lucent epiphyseal lesions in children. Skeletal Radiol 17:497–504, 1988

Glass TA, Mills SE et al: Giant cell reparative granuloma of the hands and feet. Radiology 149:65–68, 1983

Goergen TG, Resnick D, Riley RR: Posttraumatic abnormalities of the pubic bone simulating malignancy. Radiology 126:85–87, 1978

Gohel VK, Dalinka MK, Edeiken J: Ischemic necrosis of the femoral head simulating chondroblastoma. Radiology 107:545–546, 1973

Gunn DR, Young WB: Myositis ossificans as a complication of tetanus. J Bone Joint Surg [Br] 41:535–540, 1959

Healey JH, Buss D: Radiation and pagetic osteogenic sarcomas. Clin Orthop 270:128–134, 1991

Hermann G, Yeh HC et al: Computed tomography and ultrasonography of the hemophilic pseudotumor and their use in surgical planning. Skeletal Radiol 15:123–128, 1986

Hermann G, Yeh HS, Schwartz I: Computed tomography of soft-tissue lesions of the extremities, pelvic and shoulder girdles: Sonographic and pathological correlations. Clin Radiol 35:193–202, 1984

Horner K, Forman GH et al: Atypical simple bone cysts of the jaws. I: Recurrent lesions. Clin Radiol 39:53–57, 1988

Horner K, Forman GH: Atypical simple bone cysts of the jaws. II: A possible association with benign fibro-osseous (cemental) lesions of the jaws. Clin Radiol 39:59–63, 1988

Huber DJ, Sumers E et al: Soft tissue pseudotumor following intramuscular injection of "DPT": A pitfall in magnetic resonance imaging. Skeletal Radiol 16:469–473, 1987

Hutcheson J, Klatte EC, Kremp R: The angiographic appearance of myositis ossificans circumscripta: A case report. Radiology 102:5–58, 1972

Huvos AG, Butler A, Bretsky SS: Osteogenic sarcoma associated with Paget's disease. Cancer 52:1489–1495, 1983

Janecki CJ, Nelson CL, Dohn DF: Intrasacral cyst: Report of a case and review of the literature. J Bone Joint Surg [Am] 54:423–428, 1972

Jernstrom P, Stark HH: Giant-cell reaction of a metacarpal. Am J Clin Pathol 55:77–81, 1971

Jokl P, Federico J: Myositis ossificans traumatica association with hemophilia (factor XI deficiency) in a football player. JAMA 237:2215–2216, 1977

Karlin CA, De Smet AA, Neff J et al: The variable manifestations of extraarticular synovial chondromatosis. AJR Am J Roentgenol 137:731–735, 1981

Kirkpatrick DJ: Donovanosis (granuloma inguinale): A rare cause of osteolytic bone lesions. Clin Radiol 21:101–105, 1970

Lee KR, Tines SC, Yoon JW: CT findings of suprapatellar synovial cysts. J Comput Assist Tomogr 8:296–299, 1984

Lerner MR, Southwick WO: Keratin cysts in phalangeal bones: Report of an unusual case. J Bone Joint Surg [Am] 50:365–372, 1968

Levin DC, Blazina ME, Levine E: Fatigue fractures of the shaft of the femur: Simulation of malignant tumor. Radiology 89:883–885, 1967

Levine HA, Enrile F: Giant-cell tumor of patellar tendon coincident with Paget's disease. J Bone Joint Surg [Am] 53:335–340, 1971

Liefeld PA, Ferguson AB, Fu FH: Focal myositis: A benign lesion that mimics malignant disease. J Bone Joint Surg [Am] 64:1371–1373, 1982

Malghem J, Maldague B: Transient fatty cortical defects following fractures in children. Skeletal Radiol 15:368–371, 1986

Manaster BJ, Anderson TM: Tumoral calcinosis: Serial images to monitor successful dietary therapy. Skeletal Radiol 8:123–125, 1982

McCarthy EF et al: Parosteal (nodular) fasciitis of the hand. J Bone Joint Surg [Am] 58:714–716, 1976

Mitra M, Sen AK, Deb HK: Myositis ossificans traumatica: A complication of tetanus. A report of a case and review of the literature. J Bone Joint Surg [Am] 58:885–886, 1977

Morton KS, Bartlett LH: Benign osteoblastic change resembling osteoid osteoma: A report of 3 cases with unusual radiologic features. J Bone Joint Surg [Br] 48:478–487, 1966

Mourad KA, Grant RW: Unusual post-traumatic ossification within the intertransversarius muscle. Br J Radiol 56:5–57, 1983

Pakter RL, Fishman EK et al: Calf hematoma-computed tomographic and magnetic resonance findings. Skeletal Radiol 16:393–396, 1987

Paling MR, Herdt JR: Radiation osteitis: A problem of recognition. Radiology 137:339–342, 1980

Pawar S, Kay CJ, Anderson HH et al: Primary amyloidoma of the spine. J Comput Assist Tomogr 6:1175–1177, 1982

Pazzaglia UE, Beluffi G et al: Myositis ossificans in the newborn. J Bone Joint Surg 68:456–458, 1986

Proctor SLP, Jones RB, Nagel DA: Iatrogenic soft-tissue calcification in an extremity. J Bone Joint Surg [Am] 64:449–450, 1982

Rao AS, Vigorita VJ: Pigmented villonodular synovitis (giant-cell tumor of the tendon sheath and synovial membrane). J Bone Joint Surg [Am] 66:7–94, 1984

Resnick D, Conne RO: The nature of humeral pseudocysts. Radiology 150:27–28, 1984

Rhea JT, Weber AL: Giant-cell granuloma of the sinuses. Radiology 147:135–137, 1983

Roberts JA: Paget's disease and metastatic carcinoma: A case report. J Bone Joint Surg 68:22–23, 1986

Roth SI: Squamous cysts involving the skull and phalanges. J Bone Joint Surg [Am] 46:1442–1450, 1964

Rubin P: Dynamic Classification of Bone Dysplasias. Chicago, Year Book Medical Publishers, 1964

Sartoris DJ, Pate D et al: Plasma cell sclerosis of bone: A spectrum of disease. J Can Assoc Radiol 37:25–34, 1986

Sazbon L, Najenson T, Tartakovsky M et al: Widespread periarticular new-bone formation in long-term comatose patients. J Bone Joint Surg [Br] 63:120–125, 1981

Schajowicz F, Araujo ES, Berenstein M: Sarcoma complicating Paget's disease of bone. J Bone Joint Surg [Br] 65:299–307, 1983

Schajowicz F: Tumors and Tumor-like Lesions of Bones and Joints. New York, Springer–Verlag, 1981 426. Schajowicz F: Juxtacortical chondrosarcoma. J Bone Joint Surg [Br] 59: 473–480, 1977

Schlenker JD, Clark DD, Weckesser EC: Calcinosis circumscripta of the hand in scleroderma. J Bone Joint Surg [Am] 55:1051–1056, 1973

Soye I, Levine E, Batnitzky S et al: Computed tomography of sacral and presacral lesions. Neuroradiology 24:71–76, 1982

Sundaram M, Awwad EE: Magnetic resonance imaging of arachnoid cysts destroying the sacrum. Am J Roentgenol 146:359–360, 1986

Sundaram M, McGuire MH: Computed tomography or magnetic resonance for evaluating the solitary tumor or tumor-like lesion of bone? Skeletal Radiol 17:393–401, 1988

Swischuk LE, Jorgenson F, Caden D: Wooden splinter induced "pseudotumors" and "osteomyelitis-like" lesions of bone and soft tissue. Am J Roentgenol 122:176–179, 1974

Tucker RE et al: Pyomyositis mimicking malignant tumor: Three case reports. J Bone Joint Surg [Am] 60:701–703a, 1978

Valderrama JAF, Matthews JM: The haemophilic pseudotumour or haemophilic subperiosteal haematoma. J Bone Joint Surg [Br] 47:256–265, 1965

Viau MR, Pedersen HE, Salciccioli GG et al: Ectopic calcification as a late sequela of compartment syndrome. Clin Orthop 176:178–180, 1983

Weston WJ: Thorn and twig-induced pseudotumours of bone and soft tissues. Br J Radiol 36:323–326, 1963

Wolfe MS, North ER: Extravasation of injected calcium solution leading to calcifications in the upper extremity of the neonate. J Bone Joint Surg [Am] 65:558–559, 1983

Zadek I: Ossifying hematoma in the thigh: A case report. J Bone Joint Surg [Am] 51:386–390, 1969

Bone Marrow

Cohen MD, Klatte EC, Baehner R et al: Magnetic resonance imaging of bone marrow disease in children. Radiology 151:715–718, 1984

Daffner RH, Lupetin AR et al: MRI in the detection of malignant infiltration of bone marrow. AJR Am J Roentgenol 146:353–358, 1986

Edelstein G, Kyriakos M: Focal hematopoietic hyperplasia of the rib: A form of pseudotumor. Skeletal Radiol 11:108–118, 1984

Kricun ME: Red-yellow marrow conversion: Its effect on the location of some solitary bone lesions. Skeletal Radiol 14:10–19, 1985

Murphy WA, Seligman PA, Tillack T et al: Osteosclerosis, osteomalacia, and bone marrow aplasia: A combined late complication of Thorotrast administration. Skeletal Radiol 3:234–238, 1979

INDEX

Page numbers followed by *f* indicate figures; those followed by *t* indicate tabular material.